Human Anatomy and Physiology
For NURSING
and Allied Sciences

About author

Mahindra Kumar Anand MBBS, MS, DO, PhD, Associate Professor of Anatomy, Muzaffarnagar Medical College, Muzaffarnagar, Uttar Pradesh, India. He has already written successful books on Human Anatomy for MBBS and Dental students. He has to his credit a number of national and international publications.

About coauthor

Meena Verma, BSc (Hons) Nursing, AIIMS, BSc (App) Optometry. She has an excellent academic record and has received awards for best nurse in 1994 and Aiimsonians of America award for best nurse in 2000. She completed her BSc (App) Optometry with distinction and was ranked first in the University in 2005. She has contributed earlier in an 1000 pages quarterly medical magazine 'Advance Drug Review'. She is at present independently handling the investigative part of Cornea Research Laboratory, Dr Rajendra Prasad Eye Centre, AIIMS, New Delhi. She is actively involved in Eye Banking.

Publisher

Human Anatomy and Physiology
For NURSING
and Allied Sciences

SECOND EDITION

MAHINDRA KUMAR ANAND

MBBS, MS, DO, PhD
Associate Professor
Department of Anatomy
Muzaffarnagar Medical College
Muzaffarnagar, Uttar Pradesh, India

Formerly
Lady Hardinge Medical College, New Delhi
Maulana Azad Medical College, New Delhi
Pramukhswami Medical College, Karamsad, Gujarat
SR College of Dental Sciences and Research, Faridabad, Haryana

MEENA VERMA

BSc (Hons) Nursing, AIIMS, BSc (App) Optometry
Cornea Research Laboratory
Dr Rajendra Prasad Eye Centre
AIIMS, New Delhi, India

JAYPEE BROTHERS MEDICAL PUBLISHERS (P) LTD

St Louis (USA) • Panama City (Panama) • New Delhi • Ahmedabad • Bengaluru
Chennai • Hyderabad • Kochi • Kolkata • Lucknow • Mumbai • Nagpur

Published by
Jitendar P Vij
Jaypee Brothers Medical Publishers (P) Ltd

Corporate Office
4838/24 Ansari Road, Daryaganj, **New Delhi** - 110002, India, Phone: +91-11-43574357
Fax: +91-11-43574314

Registered Office
B-3, EMCA House, 23/23B Ansari Road, Daryaganj, **New Delhi** 110 002, India
Phones: +91-11-23272143, +91-11-23272703, +91-11-23282021, +91-11-23245672
Rel: +91-11-32558559, Fax: +91-11-23276490, +91-11-23245683
e-mail: jaypee@jaypeebrothers.com, Website: www.jaypeebrothers.com

Branches

❑ 2/B, Akruti Society, Jodhpur Gam Road Satellite, **Ahmedabad** 380 015, Phones: +91-79-26926233
Rel: +91-79-32988717, Fax: +91-79 26927094, e-mail: ahmedabad@jaypeebrothers.com
❑ 202 Batavia Chambers, 8 Kumara Krupa Road, Kumara Park East, **Bengaluru** 560 001
Phones: +91-80-22285971, +91-80-22382956, +91-80-22372664, Rel: +91-80-32714073
Fax: +91-80-22281761, e-mail: bangalore@jaypeebrothers.com
❑ 282 IIIrd Floor, Khaleel Shirazi Estate, Fountain Plaza, Pantheon Road, **Chennai** 600 008
Phones: +91-44-28193265, +91-44-28194897, Rel: +91-44-32972089, Fax: +91-44-28193231
e-mail: chennai@jaypeebrothers.com
❑ 4-2-1067/1-3, 1st Floor, Balaji Building, Ramkote Cross Road, **Hyderabad** 500 095
Phones: +91-40-66610020, +91-40 24758498, Rel:+91-40-32940929, Fax:+91-40-24758499
e-mail: hyderabad@jaypeebrothers.com
❑ No. 41/3098, B & B1, Kuruvi Building, St. Vincent Road, **Kochi** 682 018, Kerala
Phone: +91-484-4036109, +91-484-2395739, +91-484-2395740, e-mail: kochi@jaypeebrothers.com
❑ 1-A Indian Mirror Street, Wellington Square, **Kolkata** 700 013, Phones: +91-33-22651926
+91-33-22276404, +91-33-22276415, Fax: +91-33-22656075
e-mail: kolkata@jaypeebrothers.com
❑ Lekhraj Market III, B-2, Sector-4, Faizabad Road, Indira Nagar, **Lucknow** 226 016
Phones: +91-522-3040553, +91-522-3040554, e-mail: lucknow@jaypeebrothers.com
❑ 106 Amit Industrial Estate, 61 Dr SS Rao Road, Near MGM Hospital, Parel, **Mumbai** 400012
Phones: +91-22-24124863, +91-22-24104532, Rel: +91-22-32926896 Fax: +91-22-24160828
e-mail: mumbai@jaypeebrothers.com
❑ "KAMALPUSHPA" 38, Reshimbag, Opp. Mohota Science College, Umred Road, **Nagpur** 440 009 (MS)
Phone: Rel: +91-712-3245220, Fax: +91-712 2704275, e-mail: nagpur@jaypeebrothers.com

North America Office
1745, Pheasant Run Drive, Maryland Heights (Missouri), MO 63043, USA, Ph: 001-636-6279734
e-mail: jaypee@jaypeebrothers.com, anjulav@jaypeebrothers.com

Central America Office
Jaypee-Highlights Medical Publishers Inc., City of Knowledge, Bld. 237, Clayton,
Panama City, Panama, Ph: (507)317-0160

Human Anatomy and Physiology for Nursing and Allied Sciences

This book has been published in good faith that the material provided by authors is original. Every effort is made to ensure accuracy of material, but the publisher, printer and authors will not be held responsible for any inadvertent error(s). In case of any dispute, all legal matters are to be settled under Delhi jurisdiction only.

First Edition: **2007**

Second Edition: **2010**

ISBN 978-81-8448-780-0

Typeset at JPBMP typesetting unit
Printed & Bound in India by Nutech Print Services, New Delhi

*Dedicated
to
Infinity*

Foreword

The subjects of human anatomy and physiology form the foundation of study of medical sciences. They are very important in understanding human body and form the base for a sound clinical practice in future.

Anatomy has always been considered as a difficult subject to learn and understand by the students. It is therefore, a difficult task to write a book on this basic but vast subject in a manner that would appeal to the students. Very few authors have attempted to write a textbook on human anatomy and even fewer have attempted to write an integrated book of human anatomy and physiology. It gives me immense pleasure to introduce this book written by Dr Mahindra Kumar Anand, an eminent teaching faculty at our institution. He is a keen academician with great interest in teaching human anatomy in an integrated manner. Dr Anand already has to his credit successful publications of textbooks of Human Anatomy for MBBS and Human Anatomy for Dental Students. He has now written this book of Human Anatomy and Physiology for Nursing and Allied Sciences.

This book has comprehensive and up-to-date text with excellent illustrations. The chapters have been divided systematically and are well organized. The approach to writing text is very reader friendly. It makes it easy for any beginner to understand the anatomy and physiology with the functional and clinical correlation.

I am sure this book will be appreciated not only by students but also the teaching faculty and I wish Dr Mahindra Kumar Anand all the very best in his endeavor.

DK Sharma
Director
Muzaffarnagar Medical College
Muzaffarnagar, UP, India

Preface

The fundamental subjects of medical sciences are human anatomy and physiology. A sound knowledge of these subjects lays the foundation for understanding body changes in various physiological and pathological conditions, their clinical manifestations and the treatment options that ultimately help to provide appropriate patient care in future.

This book provides a comprehensive and up-to-date overview of human anatomy and physiology. The book is divided into five sections. The first section deals with the general approach to the subjects—cell and tissues. This is followed by a section on organization of body. These two sections provide a complete overview of human body. The third section deals with various systems of the human body. Each chapter has adequate text with extensive illustrations that would we hope enable the students to follow the subjects in a sequential manner. Clinical aspect is given at end of each chapter which makes clinical correlation simple to understand in a logical manner. The fourth section deals with elementary genetics that provides basic knowledge of chromosomes, genes and DNA. The fifth section is devoted to radiological anatomy and anatomical basis for clinical examination with the aim to provide students an integrated knowledge of structure and function of the body with clinical correlation that would help them in subsequent clinical postings.

We hope that our efforts would make these difficult subjects easy to understand and assimilate for all students. Any feedback regarding the book is always welcome.

Mahindra Kumar Anand

Meena Verma

Acknowledgements

We would like to acknowledge Dr DK Sharma, Director, Muzaffarnagar Medical College, Muzaffarnagar, Uttar Pradesh, India for his cooperation and encouragement in the making of this book. We extend our thanks to Mr SC Goel, Chairman and Dr RK Srivastava, Principal of Muzaffarnagar Medical College, Muzaffarnagar Uttar Pradesh, India for providing a conducive environment for our efforts.

We highly appreciate Dr GV Shah, Dean, SBKS Medical College, Piparia, Vadodra and Dr TC Singel, Professor and Head, Department of Anatomy, MP Shah Medical College, Jamnagar, Gujarat, India for their valuable review comments.

Our sincere thanks to Shri Jitendar P Vij (Chairman and Managing Director), Mr Tarun Duneja (Director-Publishing) and Mr Bhupesh Arora (General Manager-Publishing) of M/s Jaypee Brothers Medical Publishers (P) Ltd for their dedicated enthusiasm and help throughout writing of the book. Mr Sudhir Sharma deserves special thanks for his excellent formatting of the book.

Contents

Section-1: General Anatomy and Physiology

1. Introduction to Human Anatomy and Physiology 3–16
2. Cell, Cell Cycle and Cell Division 17–26
3. Tissues 27–42
4. Histological Techniques 43–46

Section-2: Organisation of Body

5. Organisation of Body 49–98

Section-3: Systemic Anatomy and Physiology

6. Skeletal System 101–156
7. Muscular System 157–202
8. Anatomical and Functional Organization of Nervous System 203–244
9. Peripheral Nervous System 245–290
10. Somatosensory, Somatomotor and Autonomic Nervous System 291–320
11. Special Senses 321–350
12. Respiratory System 351–392
13. Cardiovascular System 393–452
14. Blood and its Components 453–462
15. Lymphatic System 463–480
16. Digestive System 481–530
17. Urinary System 531–550
18. Endocrine System 551–570
19. Reproductive System 571–600
20. Skin 601–606

Section-4: Genetics

21. Genetics 609–618

Section-5: Basis of Radiological Anatomy and Clinical Examination

22. Basics of Radiological Anatomy 621–628
23. Anatomical Basis of Clinical Examination 629–640

   Appendix 641–641

   Index 643–655

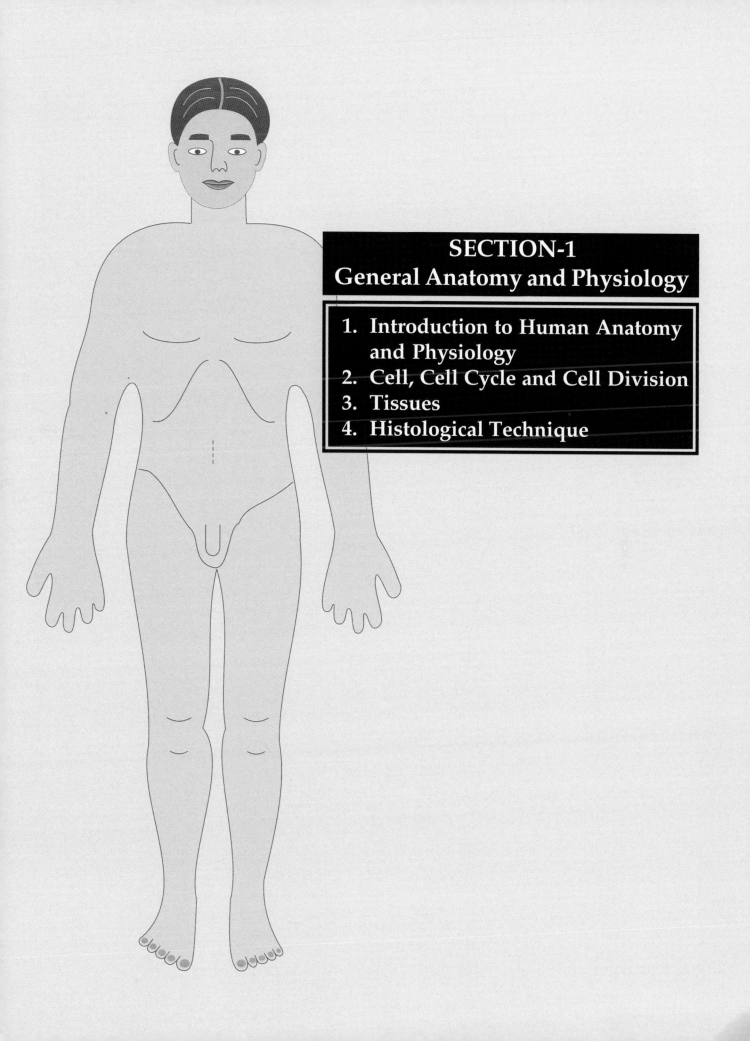

SECTION-1
General Anatomy and Physiology

1. Introduction to Human Anatomy and Physiology
2. Cell, Cell Cycle and Cell Division
3. Tissues
4. Histological Technique

Chapter 1

Introduction to Human Anatomy and Physiology

Anatomy is the oldest medical science. History of anatomy traces its origin to early Greek civilizations around 400 B.C. The word anatomy is derived from Greek word **"anatome"** which means taking apart.

Anatomy is the study of various structures and their relations in the body. Physiology is the science that deals with functioning of various parts and structures of body.

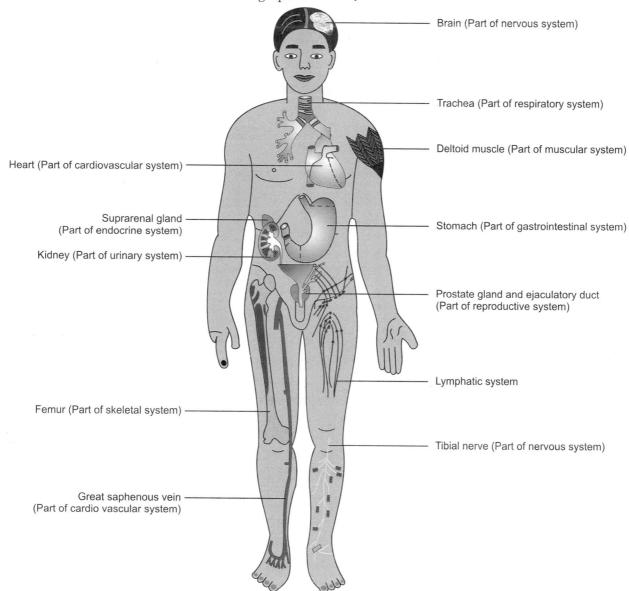

Brain (Part of nervous system)

Trachea (Part of respiratory system)

Deltoid muscle (Part of muscular system)

Heart (Part of cardiovascular system)

Suprarenal gland (Part of endocrine system)

Kidney (Part of urinary system)

Stomach (Part of gastrointestinal system)

Prostate gland and ejaculatory duct (Part of reproductive system)

Lymphatic system

Femur (Part of skeletal system)

Tibial nerve (Part of nervous system)

Great saphenous vein (Part of cardio vascular system)

Fig. 1.1: Different systems of the body

SUBDIVISIONS OF ANATOMY

Gross Anatomy or Macroscopic Anatomy

It is the study of various structures of human body (usually carried out by dissection of cadavers or dead bodies) usually with naked eyes. Gross anatomy can be studied under the subdivisions of systemic anatomy and regional anatomy.

Systemic Anatomy

It is the study of structure of various systems in the body (Fig. 1.1).

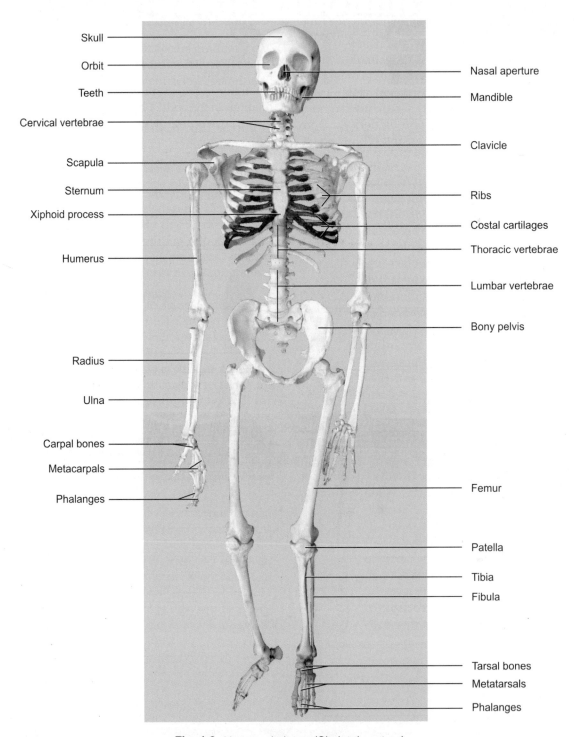

Skull

Orbit

Teeth

Cervical vertebrae

Scapula

Sternum

Xiphoid process

Humerus

Radius

Ulna

Carpal bones

Metacarpals

Phalanges

Nasal aperture

Mandible

Clavicle

Ribs

Costal cartilages

Thoracic vertebrae

Lumbar vertebrae

Bony pelvis

Femur

Patella

Tibia

Fibula

Tarsal bones

Metatarsals

Phalanges

Fig. 1.2: Human skeleton (Skeletal system)

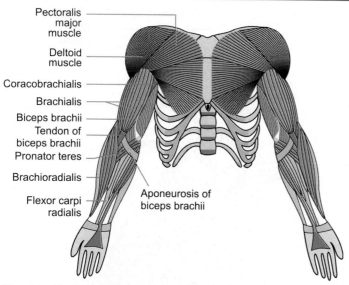

Fig. 1.3: Muscles of pectoral region, arm and forearm (Muscular system)

1. **Skeletal system:** It consists of bones, ligaments, cartilage and joints (Fig. 1.2).
   Functions of skeletal system:
   1. Supports body
   2. Forms framework of body
   3. Protects internal organs
   4. Transmits body weight
2. **Muscular system:** It consists of muscles and tendons (Fig. 1.3).
   Functions of muscular system:
   1. Responsible for movement of skeleton and various hollow viscera of the body.
   2. Is the site of heat production in body.
3. **Nervous system:** It includes brain, spinal cord, spinal nerves, cranial nerves and sympathetic and parasympathetic ganglia (Figs 1.4 and 1.5)

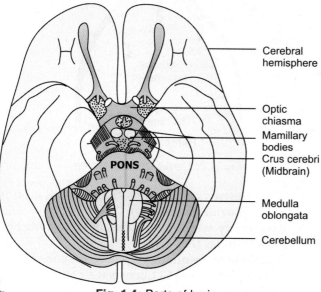
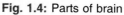

Fig. 1.4: Parts of brain

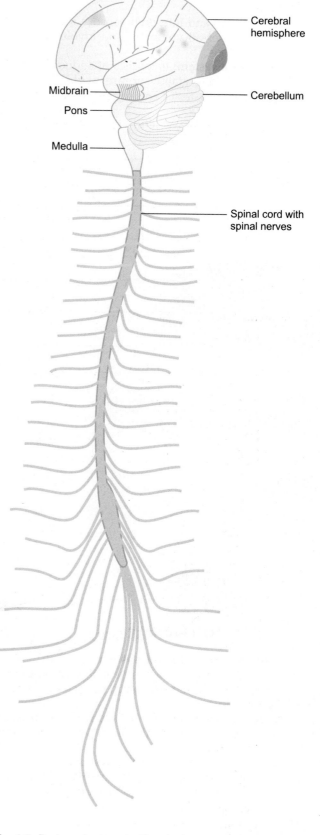

Fig. 1.5: Brain, spinal cord with spinal roots and spinal nerves

Functions of nervous system: It maintains internal homeostasis.
1. Receives and interprets sensory information
2. Regulates all voluntary and involuntary body functions.

4. **Endocrine system:** It consists of endocrine glands namely thyroid gland, suprarenal gland, pituitary gland, ovaries, testes and pancreas, etc. (Fig. 1.6).

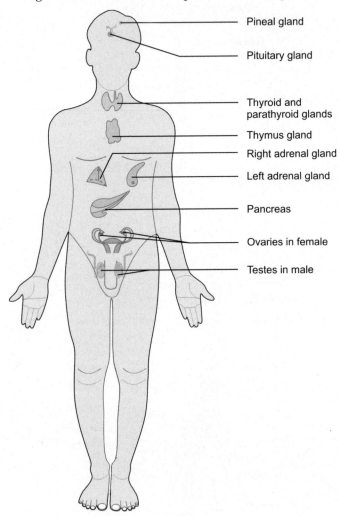

Fig. 1.6: Endocrine system

Functions of endocrine system:
Regulates various body functions, normal growth development and metabolism by secreting various hormones.

5. **Cardiovascular system:** It includes heart, arteries, veins, blood, lymphatics and lymphoid organs (Fig. 1.7).
Functions of cardiovascular system:
1. Transports oxygen and nutrients to tissues and removes waste products from tissues.
2. Lymphatic system
   a. Carries macromolecules
   b. Returns tissue fluids to blood

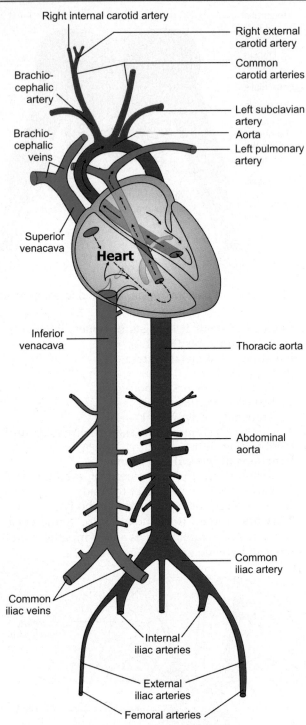

Fig. 1.7: Cardiovascular system

   c. Destroys pathogens that enter the body (provides immunity)
6. **Respiratory system:** It consists of larynx, trachea, bronchi, lungs (Fig. 1.8).
Functions of respiratory system: Responsible for exchange of O_2 and CO_2 between air and blood. O_2 is taken up and CO_2 is excreted out.

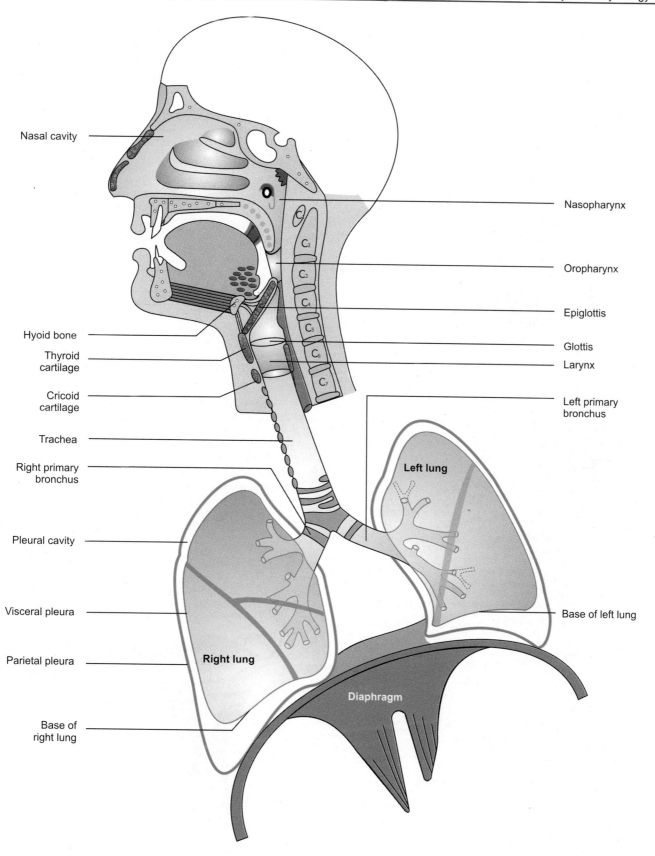

Nasal cavity

Nasopharynx

Oropharynx

Epiglottis

Hyoid bone

Glottis

Thyroid cartilage

Larynx

Cricoid cartilage

Left primary bronchus

Trachea

Right primary bronchus

Left lung

Pleural cavity

Visceral pleura

Base of left lung

Parietal pleura

Right lung

Base of right lung

Diaphragm

Fig. 1.8: Respiratory system

7. **Gastrointestinal or digestive system:** It includes oral cavity, oesophagus, stomach, small intestine, large intestine, anal canal and associated glands (Fig. 1.9).

   Functions of digestive system:
   1. Ingestion of food
   2. Digestion and absorption of food: Changes food to simple chemicals that can be absorbed and assimilated or used by the body.
   3. Detoxification and elimination of waste products (by liver and large intestine).

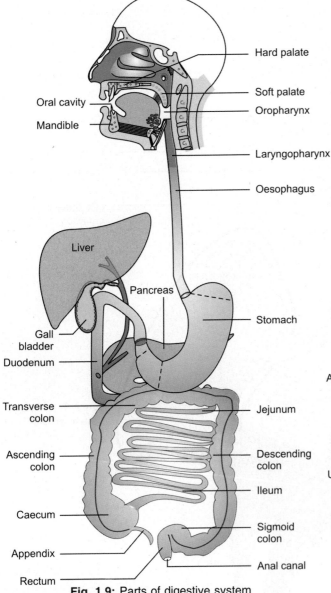

Fig. 1.9: Parts of digestive system

8. **Urinary system:** It includes kidney, urinary bladder, ureters and urethra (Fig. 1.10).

   Functions of urinary system:
   1. Removes waste products from blood in the form of urine.

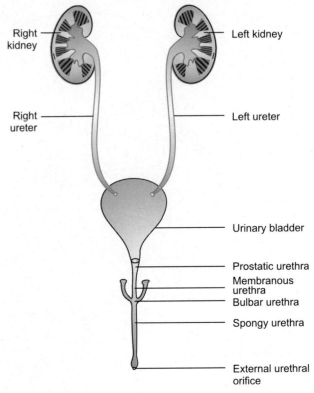

Fig. 1.10: Parts of urinary system in male

   2. Regulates the volume and pH of extra cellular fluid.

9. **Reproductive system:** It is formed by a pair of testis, prostate gland, vas deferens, ejaculatory duct and penis in male; vagina, uterus, uterine tubes and a pair of ovaries in female (Figs 1.11 and 1.12)

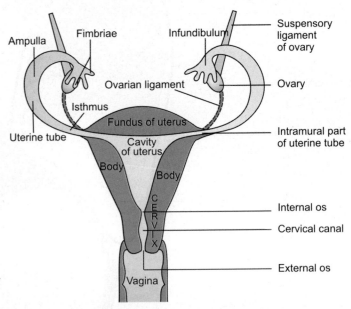

Fig. 1.11: Female reproductive system; diagrammatic representation of internal genital organs

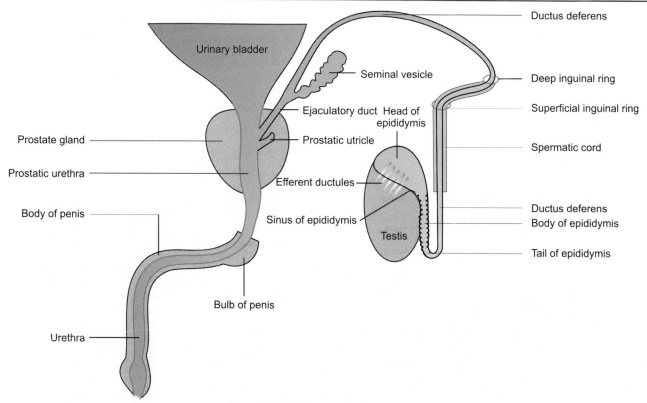

Fig. 1.12: Male reproductive system

Functions of reproductive system:
Propogation of species for survival and existence.

10. **Integumentary system:** It consists of skin, hair, nails and subcutaneous tissue (Fig. 1.13).

    Functions of integumentary system:
    1. Is a barrier to pathogens and chemicals.
    2. Protects internal structures physical and chemical excesses.
    3. Prevents excessive water loss.
    4. Is a major sensory organ.

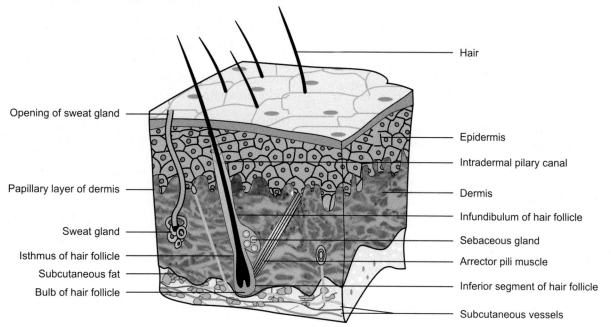

Fig. 1.13: Diagrammatic representation of various layers of skin

CHAPTER-1

Regional Anatomy

It is the study of structure and organisation of a definitive part of the body (Figs 1.14 and 1.15). The various parts or regions of the body studied are:
1. Head and neck
2. Thorax
3. Abdomen
4. Pelvis
5. Back
6. Extremities: Upper and lower limbs

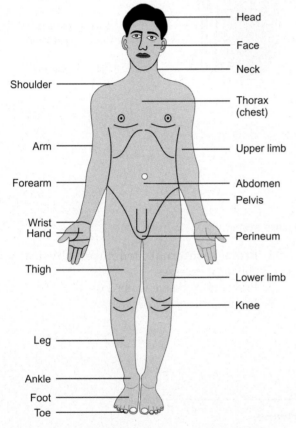

Fig. 1.14: Anterior aspect showing different regions

Functional Anatomy
Study of anatomy which provides correlation between structure and function of various organs.

Developmental Anatomy
Study of prenatal and postnatal developmental changes of the human body.

Histology and Cytology
Study of various body structures organs, tissues and cells, in greater details with the help of microscope.

Surface Anatomy
Study of projection of internal body parts on the corresponding external surface area of the body. This helps in clinical corelation with normal and abnormal anatomy.

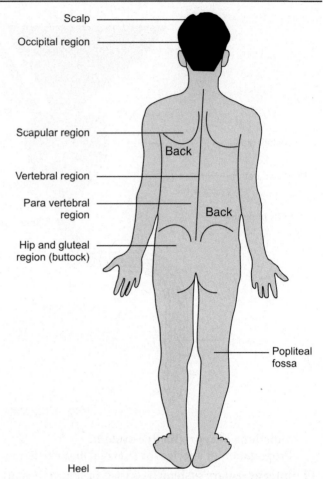

Fig. 1.15: Posterior aspect showing different regions

Radiographic Anatomy
Study of various organs of the body with the help of plain or contrast radiography (X-ray, CT scan, MRI).

Physical Anthropology
Study of external features and variations in their measurements of different races and groups of people and their comparison with the prehistoric remains.

Clinical Anatomy
It emphasizes the structure and function of a part of body or the entire body in relation to the practice of medicine and other health related professions.

Experimental Anatomy
Study of factors, with the help of experiments, which determine the form, structure and function of different parts of the body.

Comparative Anatomy
Study of structural variation between other animals and human beings. This helps to trace the sequence of events in the structural evolution of human beings.

SUBDIVISIONS OF PHYSIOLOGY

The study of functioning of each system of the body can be studied under the following subdivisions of physiology:
- Neuromuscular physiology
- Respiratory physiology
- Cardiovascular physiology
- Physiology of excretory system
- Digestion and metabolism
- Immunology
- Endocrinology

ANATOMICAL TERMINOLOGY
Anatomical Position

This is the conventional position of the body according to which all anatomical descriptions are made.

"Body is erect, the eyes face forward, arms are kept by the side with palms facing forward. The legs are kept together with feet directed forwards" (Fig. 1.16).

Importance of Anatomical Positon

All structures of our body are described in relation to this position, irrespective to any body posture in space.

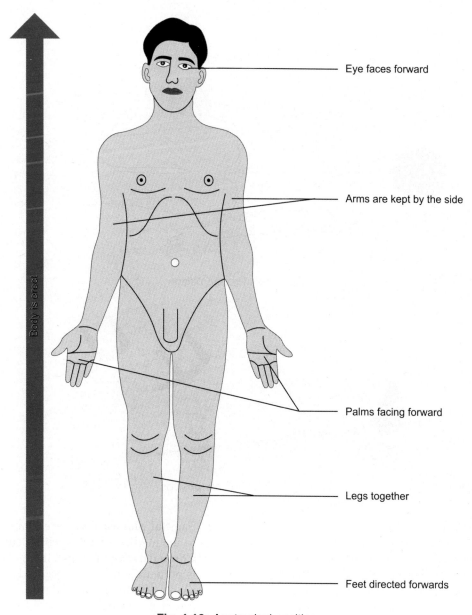

Eye faces forward

Arms are kept by the side

Palms facing forward

Legs together

Feet directed forwards

Body is erect

Fig. 1.16: Anatomical position

Other Positions of the Body

1. **Supine position:** Person lies straight on the back with face directed upwards (Recumbent) (Fig. 1.17).
2. **Prone position:** Person lies straight on the abdomen and face is directed downwards (Fig. 1.18).

3. **Lithotomy position:** Person lies supine with hips and knees semiflexed, thighs abducted and feet strapped in position (Fig. 1.19). This position is useful in the examination of pelvic viscera of female and is commonly practiced for delivery of a baby.

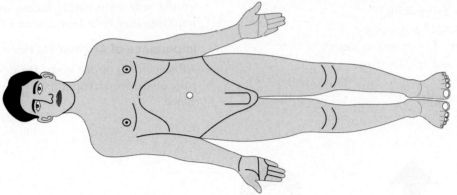

Fig. 1.17: Supine position

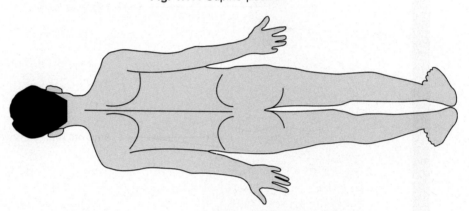

Fig. 1.18: Prone Position

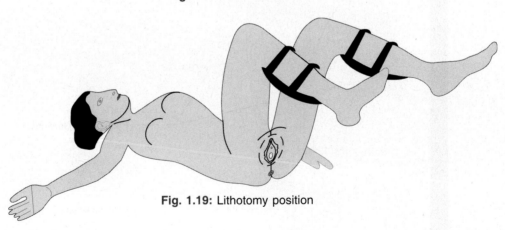

Fig. 1.19: Lithotomy position

Anatomical Planes (Fig. 1.20)

Description of the various parts of the body is based on the following four imaginary planes that divide the body

1. **Midsagittal or median plane:** It is a vertical plane that passes between anterior midline and posterior midline of the body dividing it into left and right halves.

2. **Sagittal planes:** These are planes passing parallel to the median plane on either side.
3. **Coronal or frontal plane:** It is a vertical plane which is perpendicular to midsagittal plane. Mid coronal plane divides the body into equal anterior and posterior halves.

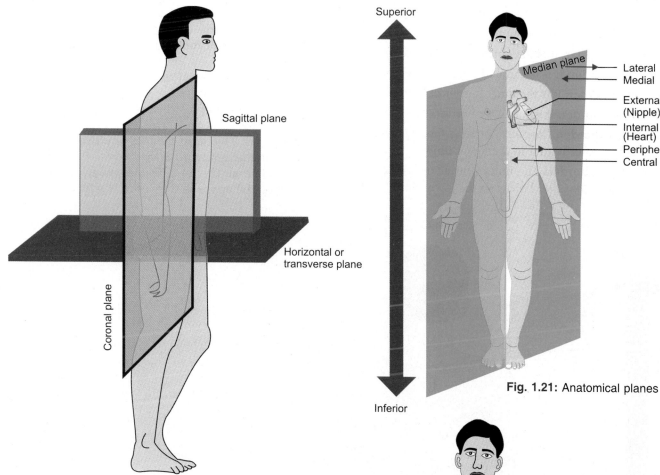

Fig. 1.20: Anatomical planes

Fig. 1.21: Anatomical planes

4. **Transverse planes:** These are planes that pass perpendicular to the midsagittal and coronal planes, dividing the body transversely.

Commonly used anatomical terms to describe the position of a body part and structure (Figs 1.21 to 1.23).

a. **Anterior:** Towards the front aspect of the body.

b. **Posterior:** Towards the back of the body.

c. **Superior:** Towards the head of the body.

d. **Inferior:** Towards the feet of the body.

e. **Central:** Towards the centre of mass of body.

f. **Peripheral:** Away from the centre of mass of body.

g. **Medial:** Towards the median plane.

h. **Lateral:** Away from the median plane.

i. **External:** Close to the surface of the body.

j. **Internal:** Close to the centre or interior of the body.

k. **Ventral:** Towards the anterior aspect of the body (in reference to belly).

l. **Dorsal:** Towards the posterior aspect of the body (in reference to back of the trunk).

m. **Proximal:** This term is used for limbs. Proximal structure is the one which is nearer to the trunk.

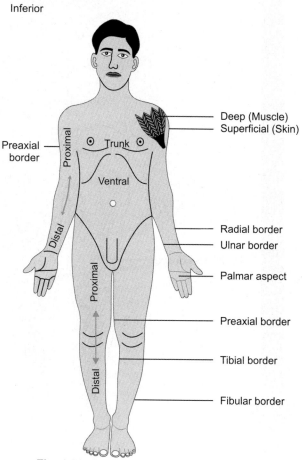

Fig. 1.22: Anterior or ventral aspect of body

n. **Distal:** This term is used for limbs. Distal structure is the one which is away from the trunk.

o. **Radial border:** It is the outer border of forearm.

p. **Ulnar border:** It is the inner border of forearm.

q. **Tibial border:** It is the inner border of leg.

r. **Fibular border:** It is the outer border of leg.

s. **Preaxial border:** The outer border in the upper limb, and the inner border in the lower limb.

t. **Postaxial border:** The inner border in the upper limb, and the outer border in the lower limb.

u. **Palmar or volar aspect of hand:** This pertains to the palm of hand.

v. **Plantar aspect of foot:** This pertains to the sole of foot.

w. **Superficial:** Location of a structure towards the surface of the body.

x. **Deep:** Location of a structure inner to the surface of the body.

y. **Ipsilateral:** This term denotes any two structures lying on the same side of the body.

z. **Contralateral:** This term denotes any two structures lying on the opposite sides of the body.

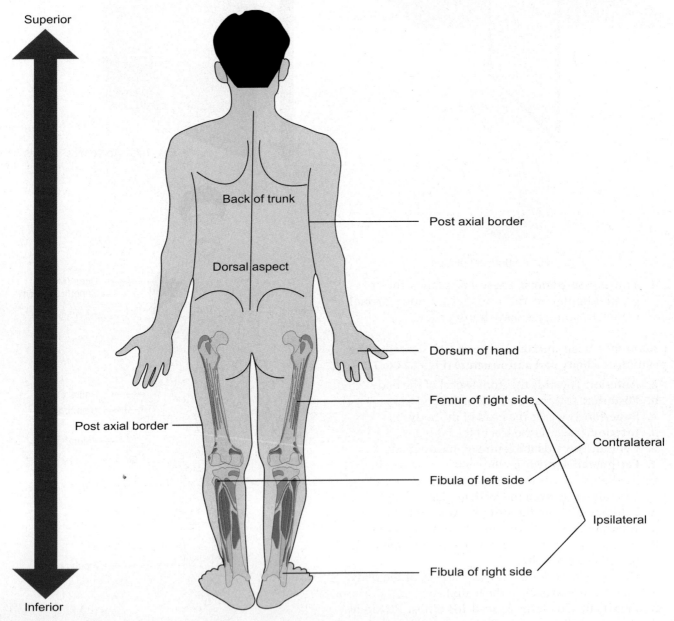

Fig. 1.23: Posterior or dorsal aspect of body

Terms Used for Various Anatomical Movements

1. **Flexion:** In this movement two flexor surfaces come in approximation and angle of the joint is reduced (Fig. 1.24).

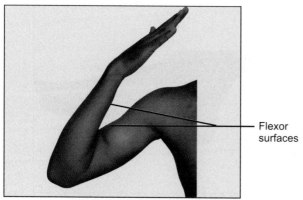

Fig. 1.24: Flexion of forearm

2. **Extension:** In this movement there is approximation of extensor surfaces whereby angle of joint increases (Fig. 1.25).

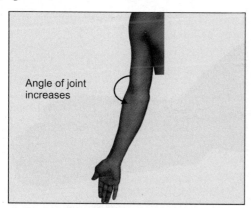

Fig. 1.25: Extension of forearm

3. **Abduction:** It describes the movement away from the median plane, away from the middle finger in hand or away from the 2nd toe in foot (Fig. 1.26).

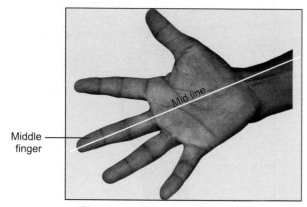

Fig. 1.26: Abduction of digits

4. **Adduction:** This describes the movement towards the median plane or towards the middle finger in hand or towards the 2nd toe of foot (Fig. 1.27).

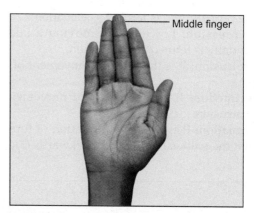

Fig. 1.27: Adduction of digits

5. **Medial rotation:** Medial rotation denotes movement towards median plane or inward rotation (Fig. 1.28).

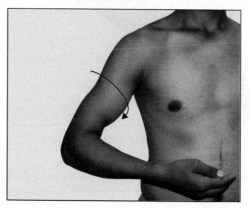

Fig. 1.28: Medial rotation of arm

6. **Lateral rotation:** Lateral rotation denotes rotation away from the median plane or outward rotation (Fig. 1.29).

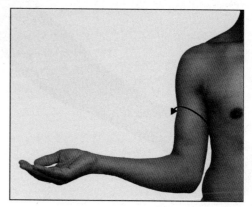

Fig. 1.29: Lateral rotation of arm

7. **Circumduction:** Combined movement of flexion, extension, adduction and abduction in a circular manner is termed as circumduction.
8. **Elevation:** Raising or moving a body part towards the cephalic end is termed as elevation.
9. **Depression:** Lowering or moving a body part caudally is termed as depression.
10. **Protrusion:** It is the forward movement of a body part.
11. **Retraction:** It is the backward movement from protrusion.
12. **Pronation:** It is the medial rotation of forearm so that the palm comes to face backwards (Fig. 1.30).

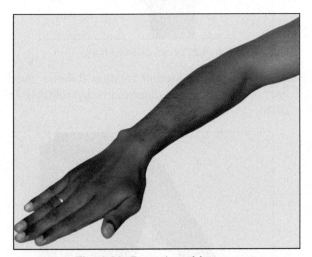

Fig. 1.30: Pronation of forearm

13. **Supination:** It is the lateral rotation of forearm so that the palm comes to face anteriorly (forwards) (Fig. 1.31).

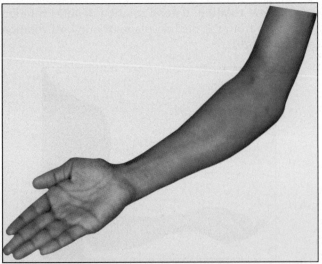

Fig. 1.31: Supination of forearm

14. **Inversion of foot:** It is the movement that causes the plantar surface of foot to face inwards and downwards (Fig. 1.32).

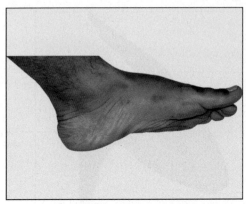

Fig. 1.32: Inversion of foot

15. **Eversion of foot:** It is the movement that causes the plantar surface of foot to face laterally and downwards (Fig. 1.33).

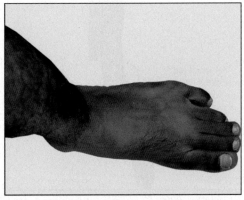

Fig. 1.33: Eversion of foot

16. **Opposition:** It is a combination of abduction, medial rotation and flexion. This movement characteristically occurs in the thumb (Fig. 1.34).

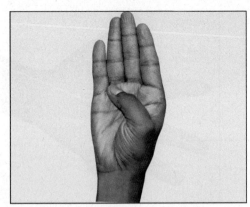

Fig. 1.34: Opposition of thumb

Chapter 2

Cell, Cell Cycle and Cell Division

INTRODUCTION

Cell is the smallest independent unit of life. Cells with similar functions and structures are grouped together to form tissues. The cells that make the body are bathed in extracellular fluid and are enclosed by the integument of the body.

STRUCTURE OF CELL

The study of structure and function of cells is known as cell biology. Human body cells are eukaryotic (Fig. 2.1). Each cell consists of three primary parts. These are:

1. Cell membrane
2. Cytoplasm
3. Nucleus

CELL MEMBRANE

It is also known as plasma membrane and it forms the external envelope of the cell. It separates the intracellular compartment from the extracellular fluid which bathes the cell. Thickness of the membrane is $75\overset{\circ}{A}$. It is semipermeable. Electron microscopy reveals that it consists of three layers:

1. **Outer protein layer:** Consists of protein. It provides elasticity and mechanical resistance. Its thickness is $25\overset{\circ}{A}$.
2. **Intermediate lipid layer:** It is also known as the bimolecular phospholipid layer. It is 25 to $35\overset{\circ}{A}$ thick and consists of two rows of phopholipids. It is permeable to those substances which are soluble in lipid.
3. **Inner protein layer:** It is $25\overset{\circ}{A}$ thick.

The phospholipids are arranged in a double layer. The hydrophobic part (water insoluble) of the phospholipids face each other and the hydrophilic (water soluble) part face extra cellular fluid on one side and cytoplasm of cell on other. Membrane proteins are arranged either in the periphery of membrane (known as peripheral proteins) or may extend throughout its thickness (these are known as integral proteins). Most proteins are glycoproteins.

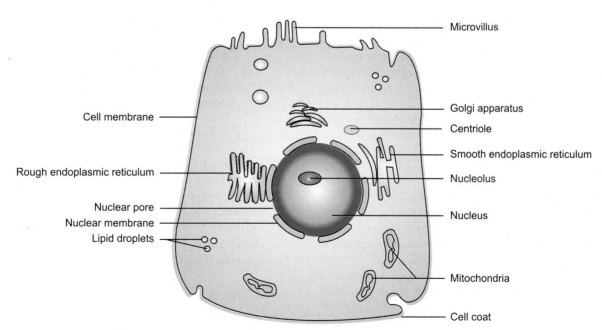

Fig. 2.1: Structure of cell (diagrammatic picture on electron microscopy)

Functions of membrane proteins are as follows
- Anchor cells to one another and to the basement membrane.
- Act as pumps which actively transport ions across membrane.
- Act as carriers: Carry various molecules along their concentration gradient that is, they provide facilitated transport.
- Act as ion channels: Form gateway for passage of ions and water. They may be constantly open (example water channels) or remain closed (example sodium channels). The closed channels open on activation by a chemical or electrical stimulus.
- Function as receptors or recognition sites for various hormones and other chemical messengers that further activate intracellular reactions.
- Function as enzymes: Catalyze various reactions within the cell.
- Provide immunological identity to the cell.

Functions of Plasma Membrane
1. It helps to maintain the shape of a cell.
2. **It is selectively permeable:** Thus, it regulates movements of various ions and molecules in and out of the cell. This is essential to maintain the internal melieu of the cell for its proper functioning.
3. Various receptors are present on the cell membrane.
4. It aids in recognition of identical cells with the help of cell coat which is specific to those cells. It plays an important role in intercellular communication.
5. It helps in the process of endocytosis and exocytosis.

Glycocalyx

The outer protein layer of plasma membrane is covered by a **cell coat** known as **glycocalyx**. It is made up of a carbohydrate rich layer consisting of the carbohydrate components of membrane glycoproteins and glycolipids. This layer has various cell antigens including histocompatibility antigens, blood group antigens and adhesion molecules. It helps to maintain the integrity of the tissues.

TRANSPORT ACROSS CELL MEMBRANE

- The cell membranes are semipermeable, that is they allow only selected substances to pass across them.
- Cell membranes do not allow transport of intracellular proteins and other organic anions to the exterior.
- Transport of various substances across cell membrane depends on their molecular size, lipid solubility, electronic charge, presence of transport proteins and transmembrane channels for the substances.

- Oxygen (O_2) and nitrogen (N_2) have no charge, are non polar and diffuse easily across cell membrane. CO_2 is polar with low molecular weight and it also diffuses easily.
- The lipid bilayer is permeable to water and also has water channels that facilitate diffusion along its concentration gradient.
- Substances like glucose, aminoacids and various ions cannot permeate cell membrane directly. Na^+, K^+, Ca^{++}, Cl^- and HCO_3^- are transported through special channels. Amino acids, proteins, nucleic precursors pass through channels in the membrane, either actively or passively. Lipid soluble substances usually pass easily through the cell membrane.
- The transport across cell membrane is primarily of two types, passive which does not require energy and active, which is energy dependant. Energy is mostly derived from hydrolysis of ATP.

Passive Transport

It is of the following types:
1. **Passive diffusion**
   - The transport of substances occurs down their concentration and electrical gradient. This does not use any energy.
   - Lipid soluble molecules like O_2 and CO_2 diffuse rapidly across cell membrane.
   - Presence of transmembrane protein channels also allows diffusion of various substances and ions.
   - Some channels like water channels are always open and help to equalize water content on both sides.
   - Most of channels for ion transport are gated, that is they open and close in response to various stimuli. These are:
     — **Electrical potential changes:** Voltage gated channels. Examples are Na^+ channels in muscles and nerve cells.
     — **Binding to ligand:** Ligand gated channels. The ligand is usually an hormone or a neurotransmitter which binds to the channel and opens it. Example, acetylcholine binds to and opens Na^+ channels in the post synaptic neuron.
     — **Mechanical stretch:** Example mechanosensitive channels in muscle cell.
2. **Facilitated diffusion:** The transport of substances occurs along their concentration or electrical gradient with the help of carrier proteins present in the cell membrane. Example, transport of glucose is facilitated by presence of glucose transporter protein channel in intestinal cells, RBCs and muscle cells. This does not require any energy input (Fig. 2.2).

Active Transport

- The transport of substances with help of carrier proteins against their concentration gradient is

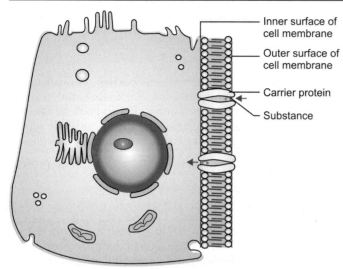

Fig. 2.2: Diagrammatic representation of transport across cell membrane

active transport. This mostly involves hydrolysis of ATP to provide energy for the process.

- The most common and abundant example in our body of active transport is Na^+ K^+ ATPase pump. This transports intracellular Na^+ out of the cell in exchange for K^+. Thus, intracellular concentration of Na^+ is kept low and of K^+ is high.

- In nerve and muscle cells excess intra-cellular K^+ diffuses out of cell along its concentration gradient into ECF via K^+ channels. Thus a positive charge (due to Na^+ and K^+) is maintained on outer surface of cell membrane with respect to inner aspect of the membrane The cell membrane is said to be polarised. This is termed as the resting membrane potential.

- Other examples of active transporters are H^+ K^+ ATPase pump present on basolateral aspect of epithelial cells of stomach and renal tubules.

Secondary Active Transport

- This is mostly carried out as a result of the chemical gradient created by Na^+ K^+ ATPase pump.

- Low intracellular Na^+ levels creates a gradient for this ion and uptake of Na^+ is coupled with transport of other substances. This is brought about by carrier proteins in the cell membrane.

- Example, facilitated diffusion of glucose and aminoacids across cell membrane in intestinal cells and proximal convoluted tubules of kidney is dependant on absorption of Na^+ ions along with them along its electrochemical gradient.

Carrier Proteins

These are proteins with specific affinity to various substances and ions. On binding to the specific substance, they change their configuration and allow the passage of that substance across cell membrane. They take part in both active and passive transport across cell membranes. They are named as follows:

1. **Uniporters:** These transport only one substance. Examples GLUT–Glucose transporter which allows facilitated diffusion of glucose into muscle cells, red blood cells.

2. **Symporters or co-transporters:** These transport more than one substance and both have to bind to the protein transporter. Example is the Na^+ dependant glucose transporter (SGLT) in intestinal epithelium and renal tubules.

3. **Antiporters:** These transport one substance into cell in exchange for another that is extruded out of cell. Example is Na^+ K^+ ATPase pump.

Exocytosis (Fig. 2.3)

- The products of cellular biosynthesis, usually proteins, are enclosed in membrane vesicles and are then secreted by the cell.

- These vesicles fuse with the cell membrane which then breaks down at the site of fusion to release the proteins outside the cell. This is known as exocytosis.

- It usually requires Ca^{2+} and ATP for energy.

- Examples: Hormone secretion by cells, secretion of neurotransmitters at synapses.

Membrane bound vesicle containing product of cellular biosynthesis   Exocytosis

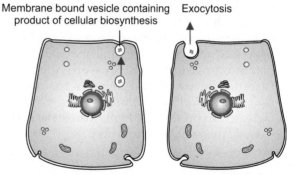

Fig. 2.3: Diagrammatic representation of exocytosis

Endocytosis (Fig. 2.4)

- It is the reverse of exocytosis. In this a substance comes in contact with the cell membrane and at this site the membrane invaginates to enclose the substance. A membrane bound vesicle containing the substance is pinched off from cell membrane and enters the cell.

- Phagocytosis is the process of endocytosis by which bacteria, dead tissue or foreign particles are taken up by cells. The cells responsible for phagocytosis are neutrophils and lymphocytes in blood and tissue macrophages derived from blood. The ingested vesicle or endosome is then delivered to the lysosomes for degradation.

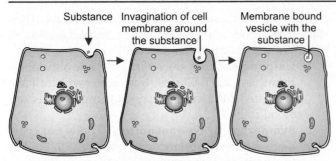

Fig. 2.4: Diagrammatic representation of endocytosis

- Pinocytosis is the process of endocytosis by which substances in solution form are taken up as vesicles.
- Endocytosis may also be receptor mediated in which the substance binds to its receptor and the entire complex is then ingested by the cell. Examples are
  a. Iron and vitamin transport into cells.
  b. Uptake of LDL-cholesterol by liver.
  c. Neurotransmitter uptake by postsynaptic cells.

Filtration

- Filtration is the process by which fluid, mostly water, is forced across the cell membranes due to differences in the hydrostatic pressure across it. It is also dependant on the osmotic pressure difference across the membrane.
- Filtration is characteristically seen in the capillary circulation. Fluid filters out at the arteriolar end due to high pressure. The presence of various colloids, molecules and ions in the capillary blood exert an osmotic pressure. This pressure opposes the filtration of water and helps to maintain the osmolality of plasma solution. Thus, filtration is increased in presence of high hydrostatic and low osmotic pressure and vice versa.

CYTOPLASM

Cytoplasm or cytosol is the intracellular fluid. It intervenes between cell membrane and the nucleus. It is mostly (75 to 90%) made up of water and consists of two parts:

1. **Organelles:** These are as follows:
   a. Ribosomes
   b. Mitochondria
   c. Golgi apparatus
   d. Endoplasmic reticulum
   e. Phagosomes
   f. Lysosomes
   g. Peroxisomes
   h. Cytoskeleton (microtubules)
   i. Filaments and fibrils

2. **Inclusion substances:** Glycoproteins, pigments, fat globules.

Ribosomes

Ribosomes are round to oval bodies, composed of ribosomal RNA and proteins. Each ribosome granule consists of two subunits namely, 40S and 60S. Within the cytoplasm, some of the ribosomes are free while others are attached to the endoplasmic reticulum of the cells.

Functions of ribosomes: They are the site of protein synthesis in the cell.

Mitochondria

Mitochondria are oval shaped vesicles bounded by double membrane. They are seen under microscope with the help of acid fuchsin and supravital stains like Janus green. Mitochondria consist of two membranous walls separated by an intermembranous space. Each membranous wall is made up of an unit membrane. The interior of each mitochondrion is filled with fluid, the mitochondrial matrix. Mitochondrial matrix contains DNA. Thus, they have the power of division.

Functions of mitochondria: Important functions are
- Synthesis of ATP from citric acid (Kreb's cycle).
- Steroid biosynthesis, fatty acid oxidation, nucleic acid synthesis.

Golgi Apparatus

It is made up of vesicles and anastomosing tubules of membranes arranged in discoid lamellae. It contains an outer convex surface or immature face and a concave inner surface known as the mature face.

Function of Golgi apparatus: It helps in the formation of glycoproteins and cell coat.

Endoplasmic Reticulum

It is a system of intercommunicating membranous vesicles or tubules which may extend from the nuclear membrane to cell membrane. There are two types of endoplasmic reticulum:
1. **Smooth endoplasmic reticulum**
   — This is arranged in a plexiform network of tubules, vesicles or lamellae.
   — Its outer surface is devoid of ribosomes.
   — Smooth endoplasmic reticulum is involved in lipid and steroid synthesis.
   Functions: It metabolizes small molecules and contains the cellular detoxification mechanism.
2. **Rough endoplasmic reticulum**
   — Rough endoplasmic reticulum primarily consists of a lamellar form.
   — Ribosome granules are attached to its outer membrane which gives it a rough appearance.

Functions: It helps in the synthesis and storage of proteins.

Phagosomes

When a particle or a living micro-organism enters the cytoplasm of a cell from outside, it gets covered by the infolding of cell membrane. Such a membranous vesicle is known as phagosome. As the phagosome comes in contact with the lysosome, the common wall between them disappears and hydrolytic enzymes of the lysosome cause lysis of the contained material. This process is known as phagocytosis.

Lysosomes

They are thick walled membranous vesicles derived from rough endoplasmic reticulum and golgi apparatus. They are of two types:
1. **Primary lysosomes:** these have not participated in any other metabolic event.
2. **Secondary lysosomes:** engaged in degrading activities.

Functions of lysosomes: Lysosomes contain various enzymes namely esterases, glycosidases, peptidases and hydrolytic enzymes. They help in degrading old cells, ingested foreign particles etc.

Peroxisomes

These are membrane bound spherical or oblique shaped structures. Peroxisomes help in detoxification of various substances. They are predominantly found in thyroid follicles.

Cytoskeleton

It consists of interconnected filamentous proteins present within the cell which provide shape and stability to the cell. It is made up of microfilaments, intermediate filaments and microtubules.

Function of cytoskeleton: It is dispersed within the cell and gives shape to the cell. It helps in transport of various substances and is concerned with cellular movements.

Microfilaments: These are long, solid, fibres, 4 to 6 nm in diameter and are made up of the protein, actin. They bind with various intercellular proteins and provides structure to the cytoplasm and shape to the cell.

Intermediate filaments: These are thicker, 10 to 14 nm diameter fibres of protein which provide intracellular stability and structural strength to the cell. They are characteristic of a particular cell type and hence are of value in histopathology studies. e.g., are keratin in epithelial cells, vimentin in connective tissue, desmin in muscle cells and neurofilaments in neurons, etc.

Microtubules: They are made up of polymers of protein, tubulin which is arranged in the form of long, hollow cylindrical structres. They provide for the dynamic part of the cytoskeleton and are constantly changing in structure. they form centrioles, mitotic spindles, motile hair like projections from cell surface like cilia and flagellum.

Cilia: These are numerous short, hair like projections from surface of cell. Examples are ciliated cells in epithelium of respiratory tract and fallopian tubes.

Flagellum: It is usually a single, long hair like structure. The only example of a cell with flagellum in our body is mature spermatozoa.

Centriole: Each cell possesses two centrioles within the cytoplasm, close to the nuclear membrane. Each centriole presents two cylindrical bodies which are placed at right angles to each other. The wall of the cylinder consists of nine longitudinal bundles and each bundle is composed of three microtubules embedded in fibrillar materials.

Functions of centrioles: Centrioles help in synthesis of microtubules of the achromatic spindle during cell division.

Filaments and fibrils: These are ultra-microscopic network of filamentous structures. They are composed of G-actin subunits. Thicker components are known as fibrils. They act as an internal support frame work of the cells and enter into the central core of microvilli and stereocilia. They form the actin and myosin filaments of contractile muscles.

NUCLEUS

All human cells contain a nucleus, except erythrocytes. It is a round or ellipsoid mass covered by an envelope known as nuclear membrane and is situated with in the cytoplasm. The location of nucleus within the cell depends on the cell type. It may appear in the centre of the cell (e.g., in leucocytes) or near the base (e.g., tall columnar cells) or near the periphery (e.g., in skeletal muscle). Nucleus consists of:
- Nuclear envelope
- Chromatin threads in a resting cell or chromosomes in a dividing cell
- Nucleolus
- Nuclear sap
- Sex chromatin or Barr bodies

Nuclear Envelope

It is 7 to 8 nm thick, double layer of unit membrane. Outer membrane is studded with ribosomes and is actually derived from the rough endoplasmic reticulum of the cytoplasm. The inner membrane is ribosome free. It gives attachment to the ends of chromosomes and has a dense coating of chromatin during interphase. Several hundred nuclear pores, 60 nm diameter, are present in the nuclear envelope. Each pore consists of 8 subunits. Large macromolecules, e.g., mRNA, rRNA pass from the nucleus to cytoplasm through these pores.

Chromatin Threads and Chromosomes

- In the resting phase of interphase of cell, nucleoplasm consists of a large amount of fibrous material called chromatin. The fibres are approximately 20 nm in diameter and consist of straight smooth areas of DNA interspersed with nucleosomes where the DNA is tightly coiled into chromatin fibres. One length of chromatin contains 30 lengths of DNA.
- Uncoiled segments of chromosomes are known as **euchromatin.** These are the genetically active sites. The coiled segments of chromosomes are called **heterochromatin,** which is genetically inert.

CHAPTER-2

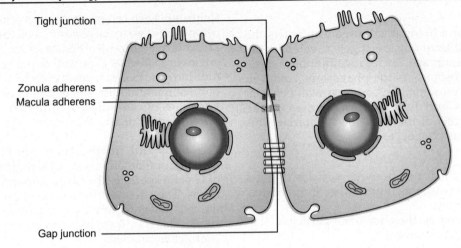

Fig. 2.5: Cell junctions

- During cell division, each chromosome becomes thicker, shorter and tightly coiled along its entire length. In human beings, the total number of chromosomes are 46 (diploid) in all cells except in mature germ cells where they are 23 (haploid) in number.

Nucleolus

Nucleolus is a dense mass in the centre of the nucleus. It is a highly refractile, spherical mass without a membrane. It is made up of a compressed mass of RNA (ribosome), granules and proteins. Nucleoli are most prominent during interphase, disappear during metaphase and reappear during telophase. Ribosomal RNA (rRNA) synthesis occurs in the nucleolus. The nucleolar organiser region contains genes that encode rRNA.

Nuclear Sap

It is the fluid containing proteins which fills up the interspaces between the chromatin threads and the nuclear membrane. It serves as a medium for the transport of ribosomal RNA and messenger RNA to the nuclear pores.

Sex Chromatin or Barr Bodies

This is the characteristic feature of cells of normal females. During interphase, a heterochromatin, plano-convex body is found beneath the nuclear membrane in a cell. This is known as sex chromatin or Barr body.

Intercellular or Extracellular Matrix Junctions

The cell coat helps to maintain an intercellular distance of 20 to 25 nm between two adjacent cells. The plasma membrane of adjacent cells establishes contact by means of cell adhesion molecules (Fig. 2.5). These are of the following types:

1. **Macula adherens (desmosomes):** They are strong intercellular contacts bridged by filaments. They can be circumferential or basal in location. They provide structural integrity to the surface.
2. **Zonula adherens:** These junctions are found in the apical perimeters of epithelial, endothelial and mesothelial cells in a continuous manner. The intercellular gap of 20 nm is filled by adhesive non-stainable material and there are no filaments.
3. **Zonula occludens (tight junction):** This is an occluding junction where the membrane of adjacent cells come in close contact and the intercellular gap is obliterated. These junctions are also found in the apical perimeters of epithelial, endothelial and mesothelial cells in a continuous manner.
4. **Gap junctions:** These are similar to tight junction but have a gap of 3 nm between the cells. This intercellular gap is traversed by numerous trans membrane channels or connexons.
5. **Fascia adherens:** It is similar to zonula adherens but its location is more limited to one side of the cell. Example, it is present between adjacent smooth muscle cells, intercalated discs of cardiac muscle cells.
6. **Hemidesmosomes:** These are anchoring junctions between bases of epithelial cells and basal lamina.

Junctional complex: It is made up of tight junction—macula adherens—desmosome—intercellular gap.

Microvilli

Microvilli are finger like extensions of cell surfaces, usually 0.1 micron in diameter and 5 microns in length. Regularly arranged microvilli are known as stereocilia. Example, microvilli are present on epithelial cells of small intestine and they increase the surface area of absorption.

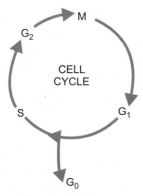

Fig. 2.6: Cell cycle

CELL CYCLE

It is the period extending from the formation of a cell from its parent cell to its own division that further gives rise to daughter cells (Fig. 2.6). The cell cycle is divided into four phases namely:

1. G_1 phase
2. S phase
3. G_2 phase
4. M phase

G_1, S and G_2 phases together form the interphase. This period lies between successive mitosis (M phase) in dividing cells. Complete cell cycle is seen in dividing cells while in non-dividing cells, e.g., neurons, the cells arrest in G_1 phase and enter the G_0 or non-cyclic stage.

Characteristic features of different phases of cell cycle

G_1 phase

- It starts at the end of M phase
- Metabolites required to complete cell division are formed in this phase
- This phase regulates the division of cells
- G_1 phase cyclin is accumulated
- Enzyme P34 kinase is present

S phase
- This phase is present between G_1 and G_2 phases
- DNA replication occurs and by the end of this phase DNA content of the cell is doubled
- Each chromosome consists of a pair of chromatids
- M phase cyclin is accumulated
- Enzyme P34 kinase is present

G_2 phase
- It is a short phase that precedes the M phase
- Cell prepares for division and nuclear membrane breakdown occurs
- Onset of chromosome condensation is seen
- M phase cyclin is accumulated
- Enzyme P34 kinase is present

M phase
- In this phase the cell divides and gives rise to two daughter cells
- Enzyme P34 kinase is present

Cell cycle is regulated by the protein cyclin and the enzyme P34 kinase. Decision for division of a cell is taken during the G_1 phase.

CELL DIVISION

Cell division involves both division of nucleus called karyokinesis and division of cytoplasm known as cytokinesis. There are two types of cell division namely:
- Mitosis
- Meiosis or maturation division

MITOSIS

It is also known as homotypical or equating division because the two daughter cells obtained after mitotic division of a cell contain the same number of chromosomes and the identical distribution of genes as the parent cell. It occurs in most somatic cells and in immature germ cells (Fig. 2.7) .

Characteristic Features of Mitosis

- Mitosis results in 2 daughter cells.
- Chromosome number remains the same in daughter cells as in the parent cell.
- Mitosis is preceded by DNA synthesis in S-phase and the dividing cell becomes tetraploid with each chromosome consisting of two identical strands known as chromatids.
- It is responsible for the growth of an individual and helps in the repair and replacement of old cells.
- The duration of mitosis is generally 1 to 2 hours.
- Mitosis can be further divided into the following four successive phases primarily based on the nuclear changes seen in each.

Stages of Mitosis
1. Prophase
2. Metaphase
3. Anaphase
4. Telophase

Nuclear Changes

- Individual chromosomes are visualized due to condensation.
- Each chromosome is made up of two chromatids joined at the centromere.
- Nucleoli disappear and nucleolar RNA disappears from cytoplasm.
- Nuclear envelope disintegrates into small vesicles and releases the chromosomes into the cytoplasm.

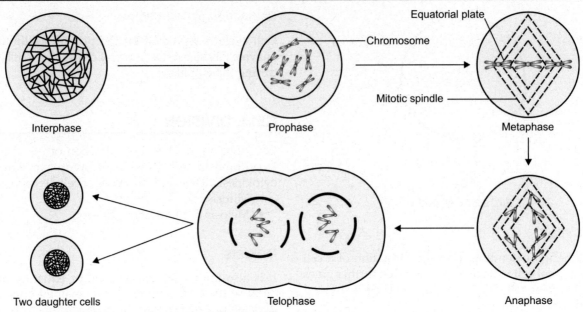

Fig. 2.7: Stages of mitosis

Cytoplasmic Changes

- A pair of centrioles separate and move to opposite poles of the cell. Duplication of each centriole occurs.
- Microtubules are synthesized which radiate from the migrating centrioles and form a meshwork known as aster.

Metaphase (Fig 2.7)

Nuclear Changes

- Chromosomes move towards the equator of the spindle or the equatorial plate of the cell.
- They get attached to the microtubules with the help of their centromeres forming the mitotic spindle.
- A star shaped ring is seen at the equator due to the attachment of chromosomes via centromeres to the microtubules at the equator.
- The chromosomes are maximally contracted in this phase and hence easily visible under microscope.

Cytoplasmic Changes

- Part of spindle that lies at the equator is known as the equatorial plate or the metaphase plate.
- There is equal distribution of mitochondria and other organelles on each side of the cell.

Anaphase (Fig 2.7)

Nuclear Changes

- The centromere of each chromosome splits longitudinally and the two chromatids separate to form two new chromosomes.

- One chromosome from each pair of the newly formed chromosomes separates and migrates to opposite poles due to the contraction of spindle fibres.

Cytoplasmic Changes

- There is infolding at the cell equator and a cleavage furrow appears which progresses further.

Telophase (Fig 2.7)

Nuclear Changes

- The newly formed chromosomes are grouped at each end of the cell.
- Nuclear envelope reappears.
- Nucleoli reappear.
- Spindle remnants disappear.

Cytoplasmic Changes

- The cleavage furrow divides the cell into two.
- The remains of the spindle and the dense cytoplasm at the level of cleavage furrow forms the midbody.
- This midbody disappears later.

MEIOSIS

It is also called reduction or heterotypical division. It occurs during the maturation division of sex cells i.e., the primary oocytes and spermatocytes (Fig. 2.8).

Characteristic features of meiosis

- Meiosis results in four daughter cells.

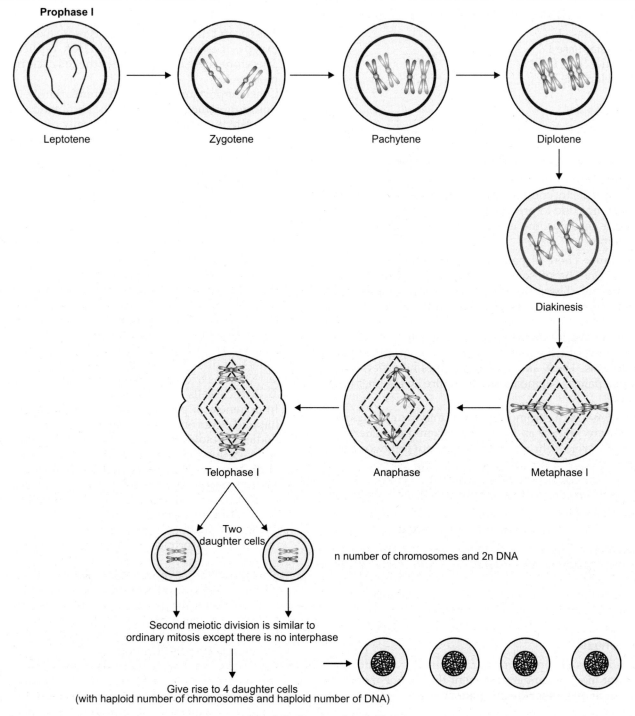

Fig. 2.8: Stages of meiosis

- Meiosis consists of two consecutive cell divisions, meiosis I and meiosis II. There is a very short interphase or no interphase between meiosis I and meiosis II.
- During meiosis I the chromosome number is reduced to haploid but DNA content is diploid in each of the two resultant cells.
- After meiosis II, the daughter cells have haploid (n)

number of chromosomes and haploid DNA. This helps to restore the diploid (2n) number of chromosomes after fertilization.

- There is exchange of genetic material between the homologous chromosomes in meiosis I.
- The duration of meiosis is 24 days in males and it lasts for many years in females.

Meiosis I is divided into the following four phases

1. Prophase I
2. Metaphase I
3. Anaphase I
4. Telophase I

Prophase I

The prophase of meiosis I is a complex and prolonged process. It is divided into 5 stages namely leptotene, zygotene, pachytene, diplotene and diakinesis.

Leptotene: Long thin thread like chromosomes are visible due to condensation. They have a beaded appearance due to presence of chromomeres. One end of each chromosome is seen attached to the nuclear envelope.

Zygotene: There is pairing of homologous chromosomes. One chromosome is of maternal origin and other is paternal. These homologous chromosomes come together lengthwise, side by side, with a point to point relationship. This process is known as **synapsis.** The homologous chromosomes are held together at various points by fibrillar bands known as **synaptonemal complexes.** The X and Y chromosomes however, have limited pairing segments and therefore lie together end to end.

Pachytene: Each chromosome splits into two chromatids which are known as the sister chromatids. There is crossing over of chromatin material between two sister chromatids of a homologous pair. This occurs in the forms of breaks in the DNA which then cross over to the opposite chromatid and reunite at a similar site.

Diplotene: Homologus chromosomes start separating except at the site of crossing over (chiasmata).

Diakinesis: Chiasmata disappear and the two homologus chromosomes separate from each other completely.

At the end of the prophase I the nuclear membrane disappears and spindle formation take place.

Metaphase I

Homologus chromosomes are arranged around the equator in a bivalent arrangement that is, one member is present on either side of equator.

Anaphase I

There is no division of centromere. The homologous pair separate from each other and migrate two opposite poles of the spindle.

Telophase I

Two cells are formed at the end of telophase each having half the number of chromosomes (haploid number) with a pair of chromatid each (thus diploid DNA).

Meiosis II

- The second division of meiosis is more like mitosis except, it is not preceded by DNA replication. Therefore, there is no S phase of the cell cycle before meiosis II.
- Other important point of differentiation between mitosis and meiosis II is that, the chromatids which separate in metaphase are genetically dissimilar.
- Meiosis II also consists of four phases, prophase, metaphase, anaphase and telophase. Ultimately meiosis gives rise to 4 daughter cells with haploid number of chromosomes and haploid DNA.

CLINICAL AND APPLIED ASPECT

- The largest round cell in the human body is Ovum. It measures about 120 to 140 m.
- Crossing over during meiosis varies according to the type of chromosomes. Small, medium and large size chromosomes usually show 1, 2 and 3 crossing over sites respectively during meiosis. 50 recombinations is the average number of crossing over per meiosis per gamete.
- Cells that do not divide after birth are:
  a. Neurons except olfactory neurons.
  b. Muscle cells
- In oogenesis a primary oocyte gives rise to one haploid ovum and three polar bodies. These polar bodies are biologically inert. In spermatogenesis a primary spermatocyte give rise to 4 spermatids and ultimately four functional spermatozoa.
- Meiosis results in the following:
  a. Reduction of number of chromosome to haploid (n) in daughter cells.
  b. Recombination of genetic material.
  c. Random assortment of chromosomes (Mendel's 3rd law).
  This ultimately gives rise to haploid cells with a variant composition from the parents which is responsible for the genetic diversity in the human species. This also enables in reproduction and maintenance of the species. The diploid number is restored after fertilization.
- Colchicine is a drug that arrests mitosis of cells in the metaphase by affecting the formation of microtubules. It is added to cell cultures during preparations for study of chromosomes as they are maximally visible during metaphase.
- **Apoptosis:** Apoptosis is the programmed death of a cell. It is decided by the genetic programming of each cell. There is activation of intracellular enzymes and degranulation of lysosomes leading to degeneration of cell components and its death. The examples of these are cyclical breakdown of endometrium of uterus causing menstruation, removal of old cells of intestinal epithelium etc.

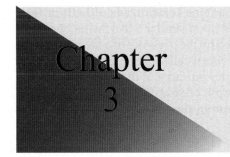

Chapter 3

Tissues

INTRODUCTION

Tissues are made up of groups of cells with similar functions. There are primarily four types of tissues classified on the basis of structure:

1. Epithelial tissue
2. Connective tissue
3. Muscular tissue
4. Nervous tissue

EPITHELIAL TISSUE

It is also known as epithelium. It lines the body cavities and tubes and covers the outer surface of the body (Figs 3.1 to 3.7). Classification of epithelium is based on the number of layers of cells, shape of cells and the cell surface modifications. Epithelium is classified into

1. Simple epithelium
2. Pseudostratified epithelium
3. Stratified epithelium

Simple Epithelium

It is made up of a single layer of cells which lie on a basal lamina. It is present on the absorptive and secretory surfaces of the body and at sites of exchange of substances which are not subjected to stress. It is further divided into squamous, cuboidal and columnar epithelium on the basis of variation in shape of cells:

1. **Simple squamous epithelium (Fig. 3.1):** It consists of a single layer of flat cells lying on the basement membrane. They lie adjacent to each other. This epithelium is meant for exchange of substances which occurs across the cells or intercellular spaces.

   It is present at the following sites
   a. Blood vessels
   b. Alveoli

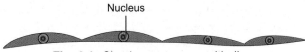

Fig. 3.1: Simple squamous epithelium

c. Bowman's capsule
d. Peritoneum
e. Pleura

2. **Simple cuboidal epithelium (Fig. 3.2):** It is made up of a single layer of cells. The cells are cubical in shape. It is found in the ducts of various glands.

   It is found at the following sites
   a. Thyroid
   b. Small ducts of digestive glands
   c. Germinal epithelium of ovary
   d. Retinal pigment epithelium
   e. Respiratory bronchiole

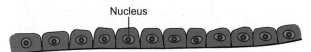

Fig. 3.2: Simple cuboidal epithelium

3. **Columnar epithelium (Fig. 3.3):** It is made up of a single layer of cells which are shaped like column, height being more than the width. This epithelium is present on secretory and absorptive surfaces.

   It is present at the following sites
   a. Uterine tube and uterus
   b. Small bronchi and bronchioles
   c. Tympanic cavities
   d. Eustasian tube
   e. Epididymis
   f. Ependyma of spinal cord
   g. Gall bladder
   h. Gastro-intestinal tract

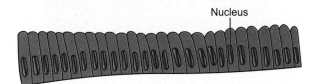

Fig. 3.3: Simple columnar epithelium

Pseudostratified Epithelium

It consists of a single layer of cells which are of different heights, mostly they are tall columnar. The location of nucleus is at different levels in the adjacent cells. This gives a false appearance of multilayering or stratification (Fig. 3.4).

It is present at the following sites
1. In respiratory tract, trachea and bronchi.
2. Male genital system, ductus deferens and male urethra.

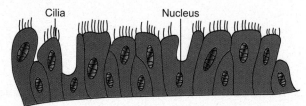

Fig. 3.4: Pseudostratified ciliated columnar epithelium

Stratified Epithelium

Stratified epithelium is made up of more than one layer of cells. It is present at sites subjected to mechanical or other stress. It is further classified into the following types:

1. **Stratified squamous non-keratinized epithelium (Fig. 3.5):** It is made up of 5-6 layers of cells. Basal layer consists of a single layer of columnar cells. 2-3 layers of polygonal cells lie over it. Superficial cells are flat, squamous. It is protective in nature.

   It is present at the following sites:
   a. Oral cavity
   b. Tongue
   c. Tonsils
   d. Pharynx
   e. Esophagus
   f. Vagina
   g. External urethral orifice
   h. Cornea
   i. Conjunctiva

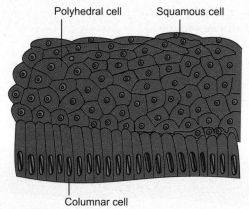

Fig. 3.5: Stratified squamous epithelium

2. **Stratified squamous keratinized epithelium (Fig. 3.6):** It is made up of similar 5 to 6 layers of cells. It is characterized by the presence of a layer of keratin over the superficial cells. This epithelium protects the exposed, dry surfaces of the body. **Skin is the primary example of stratified squamous keratinized epithelium in the body.**

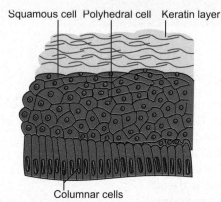

Fig. 3.6: Keratinized stratified squamous epithelium

3. **Stratified cuboidal epithelium:** It consists of two layers of cuboidal cells (Fig. 3.7). **This epithelium is present in large ducts at the following sites**
   a. Ducts of sweat glands and mammary gland
   b. Seminiferous tubules
   c. Ovarian follicles

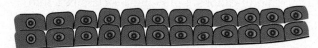

Fig. 3.7: Stratified cuboidal epithelium

4. **Stratified columnar epithelium (Fig. 3.8):** It consists of two layers of columnar cells. It is found at the following sites
   a. Fornix of conjunctiva
   b. Anal mucous membrane
   c. Urethra

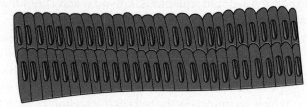

Fig. 3.8: Stratified columnar epithelium

5. **Transitional epithelium (Fig. 3.9):** It is made up of 5 to 6 layers of cells. In this epithelium there is a characteristic transition in shape of cells from basal to superficial layers. Basal layer consists of a single layer of columnar cells. 2 to 3 layers of polygonal cells are present above it. Superficial most cells are umbrella shape.

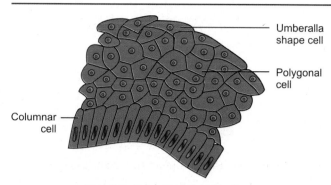

Fig. 3.9: Transitional epithelium

It is present in the urinary tract at the following sites:
a. Pelvis of kidney
b. Ureter
c. Urinary bladder
d. Urethra

GLANDS

Glands are tissues specialized for synthesis and secretion of macromolecules. Glands are formed by the invagination of epithelial cells into the surrounding connective tissue.

Classification of Glands

Glands can be classified in the following ways:

According to Mode of Secretion

1. **Exocrine glands:** The secretions of exocrine glands are carried through ducts to the target surface, e.g., parotid gland.
2. **Endocrine glands:** The secretions of endocrine glands are directly poured into the circulatory system. These are ductless glands. Secretion is carried to the distant target cells by circulation, e.g., Pituitary gland.
3. **Paracrine glands:** These glands are similar to endocrine glands but their secretions diffuse locally to cellular targets in the immediate surrounding.

According to Mechanism of Secretion

1. **Merocrine glands (Fig. 3.10):** The cells of merocrine glands produce secretions that are packaged into vesicles. The vesicle membranes fuse with the

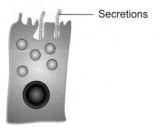

Fig. 3.10: Merocrine gland

plasma membrane to release their contents to the exterior, e.g., simple sweat glands.

2. **Apocrine glands (Fig. 3.11):** In these glands the secretions are present as free droplets within the cytoplasm of the cells and some of the apical cytoplasm along with cell membrane is also extruded along with the secretions, e.g., mammary gland.

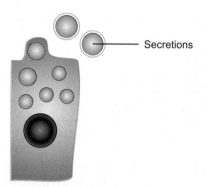

Fig. 3.11: Apocrine gland

3. **Holocrine glands (Fig. 3.12):** Cells are filled with secretory products and the entire cell disintegrates to release its secretions, e.g., sebaceous glands.

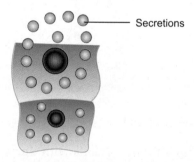

Fig. 3.12: Holocrine gland

Structural and Functional Classification

Exocrine glands are classified further as given below:
1. **Unicellular glands (Fig. 3.13):** These are made of single cells, which are usually interspersed between a non secretory epithelial lining, e.g., goblet cells seen in intestinal and respiratory epithelium.

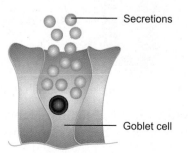

Fig. 3.13: Unicellular gland

2. **Multicellular glands (Fig. 3.14):** These glands consist of cells arranged either in sheets with a common secretory function, e.g., Mucus lining of stomach or as clusters of cells which form invaginated structures into the surrounding submucosa, e.g., Salivary glands. The invaginated glands are the following types:

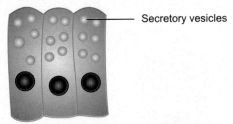

Fig. 3.14: Multicellular gland

a. **Simple tubular glands without ducts (Fig. 3.15):** Cells are arranged in a tubular fashion and open on the epithelial surface without a duct.

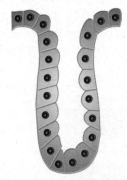

Fig. 3.15: Simple tubular without duct

b. **Simple tubular glands with ducts (Fig. 3.16):** Secreting cells are arranged in tubular shaped structures with upper non-secretory parts, which act as the ducts.

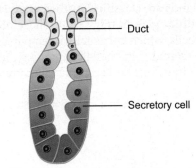

Fig. 3.16: Simple tubular with duct

c. **Simple branched tubular glands (Fig. 3.17):** These glands have a single duct and the secretory cells are arranged in a tubular fashion with branches.

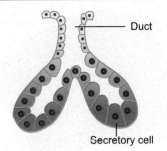

Fig. 3.17: Simple branched tubular gland

d. **Simple coiled tubular glands (Fig. 3.18):** Secretory part is coiled and they have a single duct.

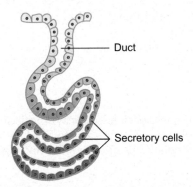

Fig. 3.18: Simple coiled tubular gland

e. **Simple acinar or alveolar glands (Fig. 3.19):** Secretory part is flask shaped with a single connecting duct.

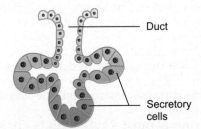

Fig. 3.19: Simple alveolar gland

f. **Compound glands (Figs 3.20 and 3.21):** In these glands the ducts are branched. The secretory part of such glands may be branched tubulo-alveolar or branched tubular or branched alveolar type.

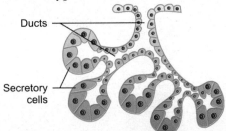

Fig. 3.20: Compound alveolar gland

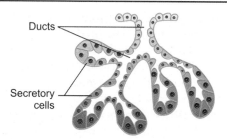

Fig. 3.21: Compound tubular gland

According to Type of Secretion

Exocrine glands may produce mucus or serous secretions or can be of mixed variety.

1. **Mucus secreting or mucus glands:** The cells of mucus glands are filled with mucus which gives the cytoplasm a hazy appearance. The nucleus is flat and located at the base, e.g., sublingual salivary glands.
2. **Serous glands:** These glands secrete thin serum like secretions. The cells have a central nucleus with a granular eosinophilic cytoplasm, e.g., Parotid salivary gland.

CONNECTIVE TISSUE

Connective tissue is characterised by the presence of abundant intercellular material known as extracellular matrix present between the connective tissue cells.

Functions of Connective Tissue

- It connects different tissues and facilitates passage of the neurovascular bundles in different tissues.
- It also helps to give shape to an organ and protects and supports the various organs of the body.
- Special connective tissue cells are involved in defence mechanism of the body, e.g., macrophages.

Connective tissue is classified into general connective tissue which is present all over the body and specialised connective tissue consisting of bones, cartilages and blood and lymph.

Components of Connective Tissue

Connective tissue is made up the following:

1. Cellular components
2. Matrix
3. Fibres

Cellular Components

There are of two types of cells in a connective tissue.

1. **Resident cells:** These consist primarily of fibroblasts, adipocytes and mesenchymal stem cells. Cartilage has special cells named chondroblasts and chondrocytes while bone has osteoblasts, osteocytes and osteoclasts.

2. **Migrant cells:** These consist of cells derived from bonemarrow. They reach the connective tissue via blood and lymphatic circulation. These are macrophages or histocytes, plasma cells, mast cells, pigment cells, lymphocytes and monocytes.

Fibroblasts: Fibroblasts are the most numerous resident cells of connective tissue. They are large, spindle shaped cells with irregular processes and a central oval nucleus. They produce collagen and elastic fibres. Fibrocyte is the mature form of fibroblast (Figs 3.22, 3.23 and 3.29).

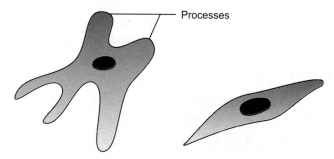

Fig. 3.22: Fibroblast   **Fig. 3.23:** Fibrocyte

Adipocytes: These cells are oval to spherical in shape and are filled with large lipid droplets. The cytoplasm and nucleus are present as a small rim at the periphery. Thus, the cells look empty on routine haematoxylin and eosin (H and E) staining. The total number of fat cells in the body are determined at birth. In obese state, fat cells get enlarged (Figs 3.24 and 3.30).

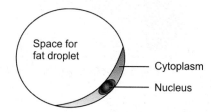

Fig. 3.24: Adipocytes

Mesenchymal stem cells: These cells are derived from the embryonic mesenchyme. They are pluripotent cells and have the capacity to differentiate into various mature cells of connective tissue during growth and development (Fig. 3.25).

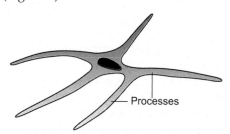

Fig. 3.25: Mesenchymal stem cell

Macrophages: They are relatively large, irregular cells with a large nucleus. The cytoplasm contains numerous granules. They are responsible for the phagocytosis of foreign bodies (Fig. 3.26).

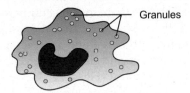

Fig. 3.26: Macrophage

Plasma cells: They are large, round to oval cells with an eccentric nucleus that has a characteristic cart-wheel appearance. They are responsible for production of antibodies in the body. (Fig. 3.27).

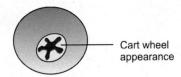

Fig. 3.27: Plasma cell

Mast cells: They are large round to oval shaped cells with a central large nucleus. They contain numerous membrane bound vesicles or granules containing heparin and histamine. They are mostly located around blood vessels (Fig. 3.28).

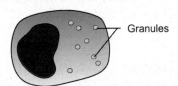

Fig. 3.28: Mast cell

Matrix (Ground Substance)

It is made up of ground substance which consists of soluble complexes of carbohydrate and proteins along with the systematically arranged insoluble protein fibres. The ground substance is made up of amorphous substances of proteoglycans and glycosaminoglycans namely keratan sulphate and mucopolysaccharides.

Fibres

There are three types of fibres present in the matrix of connective tissue (Fig. 3.29).
1. **Collagen fibres:** Collagen fibres are made up of collagen protein. They are secreted by fibroblasts, chondroblasts, osteocytes and chondrocytes. They are present as thick branched bundles of colourless fibres.

2. **Elastic fibres:** They are produced by fibroblasts and mainly contain elastin protein. These fibres are thinner than collagen fibres. They are seen as single, yellow fibres which show extensive branching and cross linking with each other. The broken ends of these fibres are seen to recoil.
3. **Reticular fibres:** They are fine collagen fibres which form a supporting framework for various tissues and organs. They are characteristically present in lymph nodes.

The elastic and reticular fibres are not clearly seen on routine H and E staining and require special stains like orcein and silver stain respectively.

Classification of Connective Tissue

General connective tissue is further classified into the following types based on relative proportion of cells, fibres and ground substance in the connective tissue.
1. **Irregular connective tissue:** It is further classified as
   a. **Loose areolar connective tissue:** It is the most generalized form of connective tissue and is widely distributed in the body. It consists of a meshwork of thin collagen and elastin fibres. Loose areolar connective tissue is present around and within the blood vessels and the submucosa of various organs.
   b. **Dense irregular connective tissue:** It is found in those regions which are subjected to considerable mechanical stress. Matrix is relatively acellular and consists of thick collagen bundles. Dense irregular connective tissue is present as sheaths around blood vessels and nerves, dermis of skin, periosteum and perichondrium and in the capsules of organs like liver.
   c. **Adipose tissue (Fig. 3.30):** It contains abundant fat cells in a vascular loose connective tissue network. Adipose tissue is present in certain regions like subcutaneous tissue, bone marrow, mammary gland, omenta and mesenteries, surrounding kidneys and behind the eye balls.
2. **Regular connective tissue (Fig. 3.31):** This type of connective tissue is characterised by presence of abundant fibrous tissue, mostly made up of collagen fibres with few elastin fibres. The fibres are regularly oriented forming sheets and bundles and they run in one direction. This is also known as white fibrous tissue and it is seen in tendons, ligaments and aponeurosis.

Mucoid tissue: It is fetal or embryonic type of connective tissue which consists of mesenchymal fibroblasts and loose areolar connective tissue with mucoid matrix. It is present in Wharton's jelly, vitreous body of the eye, nucleus pulposus of intervertebral disc and pulp of developing tooth.

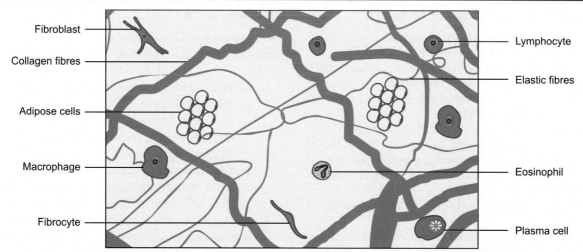

Fibroblast

Collagen fibres

Adipose cells

Macrophage

Fibrocyte

Lymphocyte

Elastic fibres

Eosinophil

Plasma cell

Fig. 3.29: Loose areolar connective tissue (Stain-hematoxylin-eosin under low magnification)

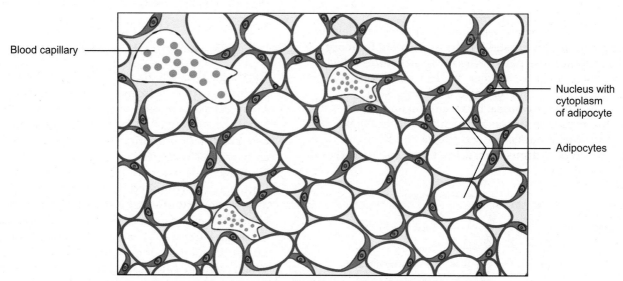

Blood capillary

Nucleus with cytoplasm of adipocyte

Adipocytes

Fig. 3.30: Adipose tissue (Stain-hematoxylin-eosin under low magnification)

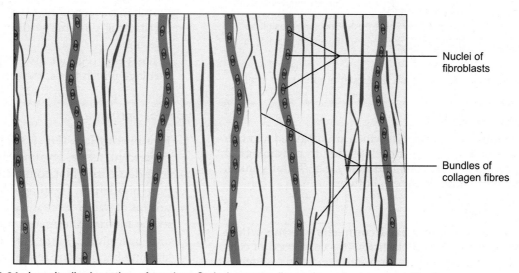

Nuclei of fibroblasts

Bundles of collagen fibres

Fig. 3.31: Longitudinal section of tendon: Stain-hematoxylin-eosin under low magnification

CHAPTER-3

Functions of General Connective Tissue

1. Binds together various structures.
2. Facilitates passage of neurovascular bundle.
3. In the form of deep fascia, connective tissue keeps the muscles and tendons in position, gives origin to muscles and forms different functional compartment of muscles.
4. In the form of ligaments, binds the bones.
5. Attaches muscle to the bone with the help of tendons and facilitates a concentrated pull.
6. Facilitates venous return in lower limb with the help of deep fascia.
7. Helps in wound repair due to the presence of fibroblasts.
8. Aponeurosis is a regular dense connective tissue associated with the attachment of muscles. It is made up of densely arranged collagen fibres.

Bursa

It is a sac of synovial membrane supported by dense irregular connective tissue. It reduces the friction. Hence, it is found at those places where two structures which move relative to each other are in tight apposition. Bursae present at different places are (Fig. 3.32):

a. **Subcutaneous bursa:** between skin and bone.
b. **Submuscular bursa:** between muscle and bone.
c. **Subfascial bursa:** between fascia and bone.
d. **Interligamentous bursa:** the bursa between two ligaments.

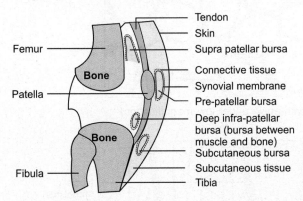

Fig. 3.32: Different type of bursae around knee joint

Adventitious Bursa

It develops over bony parts which are subjected to much friction or pressure. It develops due to physiological reasons and is not present normally. e.g., Tailor's ankle, Porter's shoulder, Weaver's bottom.

CARTILAGE

Cartilage is a specialized connective tissue which provides strength and elasticity. It is composed of cells and fibres embedded in firm gel like matrix which is rich in mucopolysaccharides.

Structure of Cartilage

The cartilage is covered by a fibrous covering named perichondrium and it consists of the following components.

1. **Cells:** Cartilage has two types of specialised cells:
   a. **Chondroblasts:** These are young cells which have the ability to divide. On microscopy, the cells are seen to be arranged singly or in groups of 2 to 3 surrounded by a lacuna in the matrix.
   b. **Chondrocytes:** These are mature cells derived from chondroblasts. They cannot divide but are very active in producing and secreting proteins.
2. **Intercellular substance:** Matrix is predominant and is primarily made up of chondroitin sulphate and hyaluronic acid.
3. **Fibres:** Cartilage is made up of collagen type II fibres and elastic fibres in the matrix.

Characteristic Features of Cartilage

1. **Cartilage is avascular:** It receives its nutrition through diffusion from the nearest capillaries. Many cartilage masses are traversed by cartilage canals which convey blood vessels. These cartilage canals provide nutrition to the deepest core of cartilaginous mass.
2. Cartilage has no nerves. Hence it is insensitive.
3. Cartilage is surrounded by a fibrous layer known as perichondrium except at its junction with the bone. Fibrocartilage does not have perichondrium.
4. Cartilage grows by appositional as well as interstitial method of growth.
5. When cartilage calcifies, chondrocytes die because they are deprived of nutrition as diffusion caeses.
6. Cartilage has low antigenicity because it lacks lymphatics. Hence, homologus transplantation of cartilage is possible without much risk of graft rejection.
7. It has poor regenerative capacity except fibrocartilage which has some capacity to regenerate.

Types of Cartilage

1. **Hyaline cartilage (Fig. 3.33):** It appears as a bluish, opalescent, tissue. Hyaline cartilage is surrounded by a dense irregular connective tissue layer called perichondrium. Cartilage cells are arranged in groups of two or more which occupy small lacunae in the matrix. The matrix appears homogeneous and basophilic. Fibres are not seen on routine staining because the refractive index of fibres and ground substance is similar.

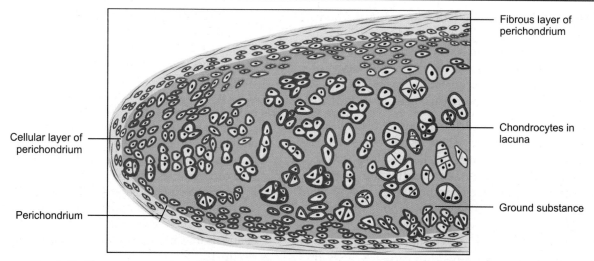

Fig. 3.33: Transverse section of hyaline cartilage (Stain-hematoxylin-eosin under high magnification)

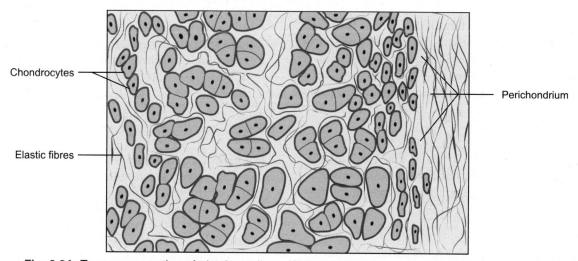

Fig. 3.34: Transverse section of elastic cartilage (Stain-hematoxylin-eosin under high magnification)

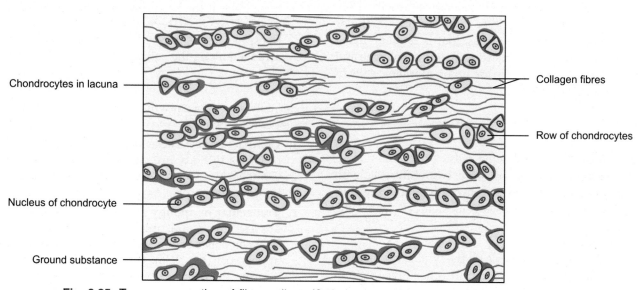

Fig. 3.35: Transverse section of fibrocartilage (Stain-hematoxylin-eosin under high magnification)

Distribution: It is widely distributed in the body and is present at the epiphyseal ends of the bone in children. It is also present in articular cartilage, thyroid cartilage, cricoid cartilage, lower part of arytenoid cartilage, tracheal rings, costal cartilages, bronchial cartilages, nasal cartilage.

2. **Elastic cartilage (Fig. 3.34):** In elastic cartilage the matrix is traversed by yellow elastic fibres which anastomose and branch in all directions. Extra-cellular matrix is metachromatic due to high concentration of glycosaminoglycans. Cells are present in ground substance in groups of 2 to 3. Outer most covering is the perichondrium.
   Distribution: Pinna of external ear, epiglottis, corniculate cartilage, cuneiform cartilage, apex of arytenoid cartilage, auditory tube, external auditory meatus.

3. **White fibro-cartilage (Fig. 3.35):** Fibrocartilage is a dense opaque fibrous tissue. It consists of regularly arranged collagen fibres, in the form of fascicles. It is less cellular than hyaline cartilage and chondrocytes are scattered in the matrix. It also consists of fibroblasts. It does not have any perichondrium.
   Distribution: Intervertebral disc, interpubic disc, menisci of knee joint, articular discs of tempora-omandibular, sternoclavicular and inferior radio-ulnar joints, labra of glenoid and acetabular cavities.

BONES

Bones are specialized, highly vascular, constantly changing, mineralized connective tissue. They are hard, resilient and have enormous regenerative capacity. They are made up of cells and inter cellular matrix. Cellular component is 2% of bone mass. Matrix is made up of 40% organic substance consisting mainly of collagen and 60% inorganic substance made up of, inorganic salts of calcium and phosphate.

Cellular Components

These consist of the following cells:
1. **Osteoblasts:** These are large, basophilic cells with a round, and slightly eccentrically placed nucleus. They originate from osteogenic stem cells from bone marrow.
   Functions:
   a. They are responsible for the synthesis of organic matrix, i.e., collagen and other glycoprotein molecules, which is called osteoid.

   b. Osteoblasts also play a significant role in mineralization of the osteoid.
   c. They have a role in bone remodeling.
2. **Osteocytes:** They form the majority of the cellular component. They are mature bone cells derived from osteoblats which do not produce matrix and have lost their ability to divide. They form the cellular architecture of bone. The cells lie singly, embedded in the matrix and are surrounded by a lacuna. They are large cells with numerous dendritic processes that branch and are interconnected to the processes of adjacent cells. The dendrites are surrounded by extensions of lacunae forming canaculi which serve the function of providing channels for diffusion of nutrients, gases and waste products.
   Functions: Osteocytes play significant role in maintainance of bone.
3. **Osteoclasts:** These are large multinucleated cells with eosinophilic cytoplasm. They arise from monocytes in bone marrow.
   Functions: They help in resorption and remodeling of bones.

Matrix

It is the extracellular component of bone which is made up of
1. **Organic component:** This is mostly made up of collagen with small amount of proteoglycans and glycoproteins. Collagen fibres are arranged in bundles. In woven, immature bones they form an interwoven meshwork. In mature bones they have lamellar arrangement which is in the form of regular parallel laminae.
2. **Inorganic component:** The mineral component of bone gives it the hardness and rigidity. It consists of hydroxyapatite crystals of calcium and phosphate. These crystals are closely packed and arranged along the collagen fibers.

Gross Anatomy of Bone

Externally bones appear white to off-white in colour and are of two types:
1. **Compact bones:** These are dense bones. 70 to 75% of bones in body are compact bones (Fig. 3.36). Compact bone form the external cylinder of all the bones in the body.
2. **Trabecular or spongy or cancellous bones:** They are less dense and present with large cavities in between plates of bones giving them a honey-comb appearance (Fig. 3.36). This type of bone is present inner to the compact bone and supports the bone marrow.

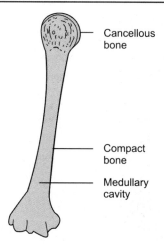

Fig. 3.36: Compact and cancellous bones

Classification of Bones

Bones can be classified into the following according to shape (Figs 3.37 to 3.42).
1. Long bone
2. Short bone
3. Flat bone
4. Irregular bone
5. Pneumatic bone

Long Bones

- Long bones are those bones in which the length exceeds the breadth (Fig. 3.37).
- Each long bone presents a tubular shaft and two ends. Shaft is made up of compact bone which encloses a large cavity in centre known as medullary cavity. It is filled with bone marrow. The ends are expanded and modified according to the type of articular surface. The ends are composed of cancellous bone.
- Long bones ossify in cartilage.

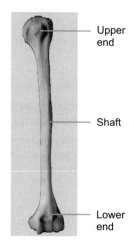

Fig. 3.37: Humerus-long bone

Functions:
- They act as levers for muscles.
- All long bones are weight bearing.

Example: Humerus, femur, radius, ulna, tibia, fibula.

Short Bones (Fig. 3.38)

- Short bones are cubical in shape and present with six surfaces, out of which four surfaces are articular and the remaining two surfaces give attachment to various muscles, ligaments and are pierced by blood vessels.
- Short bones have a central marrow cavity which is surrounded by trabecular bone with a plate of compact bone externally.
- All short bones ossify after birth in cartilage, except talus, calcaneus and cuboid bones which start ossification in intrauterine life.

Example: Carpal bones, Tarsal bones.

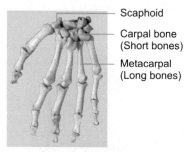

Fig. 3.38: Short and long bones

Flat Bones

Flat bones consist of two plates of compact bone with intervening spongy bone and marrow. The intervening spongy tissue in the bones of the vault of skull is known as the diploe which contain numerous veins. Flat bones form boundaries of some bony cavities and appear in those areas where protection of essential organs is of paramount importance (Fig. 3.39).

Example: Parietal bones , Frontal bone, Ribs, Sternum, Scapula.

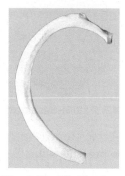

Fig. 3.39: Rib-Flat bone

Irregular Bones

These bones are irregular in shape. They consist mostly of spongy bone and marrow and have an outer thin covering of compact bone (Fig. 3.40).
Example: Vertebra, Hip bone, Sphenoid, Maxilla.

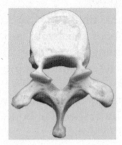

Fig. 3.40: Vertebra-Irregular bone

Pneumatic Bones

These are similar to irregular bones and have air filled cavities in them (Fig. 3.41).
Example: Maxilla, Sphenoid, Ethmoid.

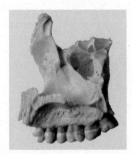

Fig. 3.41: Maxilla-Pneumatic bone

Sesamoid Bones

These bones develop in the tendon of a muscle. They help share the load of the tendon and they may also be responsible in changing the direction of pull of the tendon. Periosteum is absent in these bones (Fig. 3.42).
Example: Patella, Pisiform, Fabella.

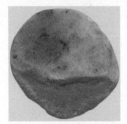

Fig. 3.42: Patella-Sesamoid bone

Parts of a Young Long Bone (Fig. 3.43)

A young long bone presents with
1. Diaphysis
2. Epiphysis

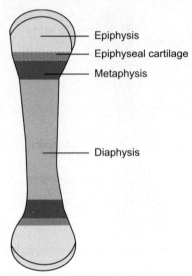

Fig. 3.43: Parts of young long bone

3. Epiphyseal cartilage
4. Metaphysis.

Diaphysis

It is the part of bone which ossifies from the primary centre and forms the shaft of bone. It is composed of a thick collar of dense compact bone, beneath which is a thin layer of spongy trabecular bone enclosing the marrow cavity.

Epiphysis

It is the part of bone which ossifies from the secondary centres. Epiphyses are functionally of three basic types:
a. **Pressure epiphysis:** It helps to transmit the weight of body and protects the epiphyseal cartilage, e.g., Head of femur, head of humerus.
b. **Traction epiphysis:** It is produced due to the pull of muscles., e.g., Trochanters of femur, tubercles of humerus.
c. **Atavistic epiphysis:** It is phylogenetically an independent bone which gets attached to the host bone secondarily, to receive nutrition, e.g., coracoid process of scapula, posterior tubercle of talus or trigonum.

Epiphyseal Cartilage

It is a plate of cartilage which intervenes between the epiphysis and diaphysis of a growing bone. Epiphyseal cartilage persists till the bone is growing. When the full length is achieved, epiphyseal cartilage is replaced by bone and further growth stops.

Metaphysis

The end of diaphysis facing towards the epiphyseal cartilage is known as metaphysis. Characteristics of metaphysis

a. It is the most actively growing area of long bone
b. Metaphysis has a rich blood supply derived from nutrient, periosteal and juxtra-epiphyseal arteries. Nutrient arteries form pin head like capillary loops in the metaphysis. Hence, any circulating micro-organisms can settle in these loops. Thus, infections of long bones primarily affect the metaphysis.

Blood Supply of A Typical Long Bone (Fig. 3.44)

A long bone is supplied by four sets of blood vessels.

1. **Nutrient artery:** Nutrient artery supplies the bone marrow and inner 2/3rd of cortex.

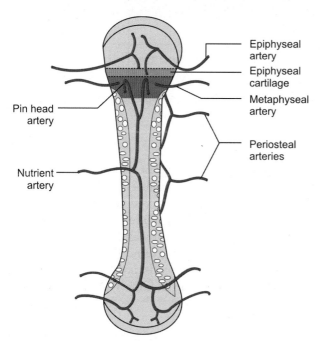

Fig. 3.44: Blood supply of a long bone

2. **Metaphyseal arteries:** They are also known as juxta-epiphyseal arteries.
3. **Epiphyseal arteries**
4. **Periosteal arteries:** They ramify beneath the periosteum and supply the Haversian system in outer 1/3rd of the cortex.

Arterial Supply of Short Long Bone

1. **Nutrient artery**
2. **Epiphyseal and Juxta epiphyseal arteries**
3. **Periosteal arteries:** Periosteal arteries supply the major part of the bone and replace the nutrient artery in these bones.

Arterial Supply of Flat Bones

1. **Periosteal arteries:** Supply major part of the bone.
2. **Nutrient arteries**

Nerve Supply of Bones

Nerves accompany the blood vessels. Most of them are sympathetic and vasomotor in function. Sensory supply is distributed to the periosteum and articular ends of the bones, vertebra and large flat bones.

Microscopic Structure of Bone

Histologically bones are of two types namely:

1. Compact bone
2. Trabecular or spongy bone

Compact Bone

- It is characterized by presence of Haversian systems or osteons (Fig. 3.45).
- Each Haversian system consists of concentrically arranged lamellae around a central Haversian canal.

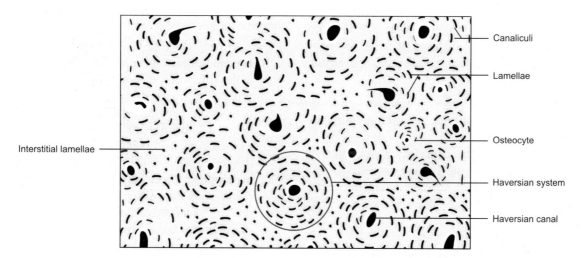

Fig. 3.45: Transverse section of compact bone (Dried section—under high magnification)

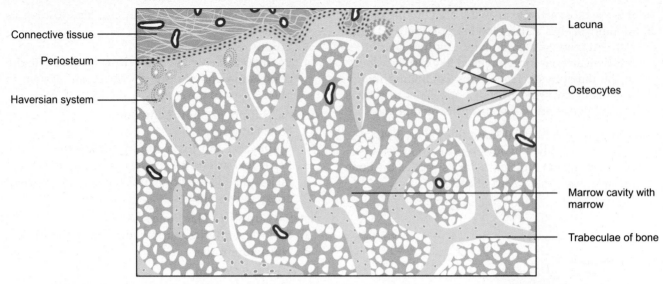

Fig. 3.46: Transverse section of cancellous bone (Stain—hematoxylin-eosin under high magnification)

- Haversian canal contains capillaries and axons of nerves (Neurovascular channel).
- Lamellae are made up of bundles of collagen within a sheet of mineralized matrix.
- In between lamellae are present osteocytes with their canaliculi.
- The Haversian system are arranged adjacent and parallel to each other. Vascular channels known as Volkmann's channels are present obliquely or horizontally, perpendicular to the Haversian systems that connect adjacent Haversian systems to each other and connect the Haversian system to marrow cavity.
- The outer most covering of bone is fibrous layer of dense collagen tissue called periosteum. It has an inner cellular layer of osteoblasts, osteoprogenitor cells and osteoclasts. Inner layer covering the marrow cavity is known as endosteum. Periosteum is absent on articular surfaces of bone where is replaced by hyaline cartilage and at sites of insertion of muscles or tendons.

Functions of Periosteum
1. Receives attachment of muscles and maintains the shape of the bone.
2. Provides nutrition to outer 1/3rd of cortex of compact bone by periosteal blood vessels.
3. Helps in formation of subperiosteal deposits, increasing the width of the bone.
4. Protects the bone.
5. Periosteum is sensitive to pain.
6. It is important in the healing of bone injuries or fractures.

Trabecular Bone

- These consists of plates of bones of varying width and length known as trabeculae (Fig. 3.46).
- These trabeculae are curved and branched enclose a number of marrow cavities in between.
- Each trabecula is lined by endosteum.
- The arrangement of ground substance of matrix, collagen fibres are cells is lamellar, in regular parallel fashion. No definite Haversian system is seen.

Ossification of Bone

Ossification literally means deposition of the proteo-osseous substance or the process of bone formation. It involves the differentiation of osteoblasts which secrete organic intercellular substance or matrix and deposition of Ca^{2+} crystals and salts. Ossification is of two types:

1. **Intramembranous or membranous ossification:** It is the formation of bone from primitive mesenchyme. The mesenchymal cells differentiate to osteogenic progenitor cells and then osteoblasts around a branch of the capillary network of mesenchyme. The osteoblasts proliferate and lay down lamellae of collagen and ground substance molecules. Calcification of matrix occurs and continuous deposition of matrix and calcification with proliferation of osteoblasts results in formation of trabecular bone. This gradually thickens to form compact bone.

   Example: Bones of the vault of skull.

Zone of proliferation   Zone of maturation   Zone of hypertrophy   Calcification of matrix   New bone formation

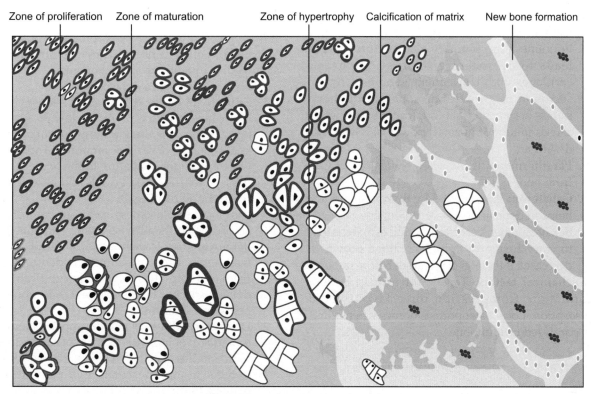

Fig. 3.47: Endochondral ossification

2. **Endochondral or cartilaginous ossification (Fig. 3.47):** The basic principle of endochondral ossification is that bone formation occurs over templates of hyaline cartilage. It means that cartilage dies and bone forms. Most bones ossify in cartilage. At the site of future bone formation mesenchymal cells get collected. These mesenchymal cells becomes chondroblasts and form hyaline cartilage. Mesenchymal cells on the surface of cartilage forms perichondrium. Cells mature and secrete matrix. Hypertrophic cells secrete alkaline phosphatase. Alkaline phosphatase helps in deposition of calcium salts. Due to calcium salt deposition there is no diffusion of nutrition in cartilage, leading to death of cells. This leaves spaces around them known as primary areola. Inner layer of perichondrium (now periosteum) give rise to osteoprogenitor cells. These cells enter along with nutrient artery inside the cartilaginous matrix and proliferate to form the **periosteal bud.** These osteoprogenitor cells eat away the wall of primary areola and these cavities become larger and now called as secondary areola. Osteoprogenitor cells get converted into osteoblasts and lines the walls of these cavities. Osteoblasts lay down the ground substance and collagen fibres to form osteoids. These osteoids become calcified and called as lamellae of new bone.

Growth of Bones

The long bones increase in length by interstitial growth of cells of the epiphyseal cartilage. Width of the long bone increases by subperiosteal deposition of bone formation. Short bones increase in size by the interstitial growth of the articular cartilage.

Factors Affecting Bone Growth

1. **Vitamin A:** Vitamin A controls the activity, distribution and co-ordination of osteoblasts and osteoclasts. High vitamin A concentration leads to resorption of bone. Deficiency of vitamin A causes slow destruction of bone. This reduces the size of spinal and cranial foramina that leads to compression of nerve roots and cranial nerves.

2. **Vitamin C:** Vitamin C helps in formation of intercellular matrix. Deficiency of vitamin C leads to decrease production of trabeculae on the diaphyseal side of epiphyseal cartilage. This, can cause separation of epiphyseal plate.

3. **Vitamin D:** It is essential for the absorption of calcium and phosphorus from intestine. In deficiency of vitamin D, calcification of osteoid matrix is interfered. This leads to osteomalacia and rickets.

4. **Hormonal factors**
   a. **Growth hormone:** Hypersecretion of growth hormone from pituitary gland before puberty leads to persistent growth at epiphyseal cartilages with consequent gigantism hypersecretion of growth hormone after puberty causes acromegaly. Hypopituitarism of infant causes failure of normal growth of bones with dwarfism.
   b. **Parathormone:** It increases resorption of Ca^{2+} from bones.
   c. **Calcitonin:** It is secreted by thyroid gland and helps in deposition of Ca^{2+} in bones.
   d. **Sex hormones:** Testosterone and estrogens lead to early fusion of epiphysis. Bone growth is decreased if their level increases before puberty.
5. **Mechanical factors:** Tensile forces help in bone formation. Compression force favours bone resorption. Local osteoporosis occurs when a limb is paralysed or immobile.

SUPPORTING TISSUES

Mucosa

It is also known as the mucous membrane and consists of:
- Epithelium lying on basement membrane
- Epithelial invaginations that form glands
- Lamina propria: It is a loose connective tissue layer present below the epithelium
- Smooth muscle layer: A thin layer of smooth muscle fibers lies outer to the lamina propria.

Mucosa is the innermost lining of various hollow organs of the body like, stomach and intestines, parts of respiratory, urinary and genital tracts.

A layer of loose connective tissue with fine terminal branches of vessels and nerves is present below the mucosa. It is known as submucosa. It also contains glandular tissue, lymphoid follicles at places and few smooth muscle fibers.

Serosa

It is also known as serosal membrane and is made up of a single layer of flattened, squamous type cells present over a loose connective tissue layer containing a fine network of blood vessels and lymphatic vessels. Serosa lines the pleural, pericardial and peritoneal cavities and forms the external covering of the various viscera present in these cavities.

Fascia

It is a type of connective tissue consisting of interwoven bundles of collagen fibers. They are not as regularly arranged as in tendons and ligaments..

There are two types of fascia:
1. **Superficial fascia:** It consists of a loose connective tissue layer which is present below the skin all over body. Hence, it is also known as subcutaneous tissue and it consists of variable amounts of adipose tissue which provides insulation to the body. It provides passage for the blood vessels and nerve endings to reach the skin.
   It is of variable thickness in various parts of the body according to its adipose tissue content. It is well demarcated in lower part of anterior abdominal wall, limbs and perineum. It is dense over scalp, palm and soles. It is thin and insignificant over the dorsal aspect of hands and feet, side of neck, face, penis and scrotum.
2. **Deep fascia:** It lies below the superficial fascia and is made up of more dense form of connective tissue with bundles of collagen fibers. It provides support to the skin and musculature of body. It provides passage to the neurovascular supply to the underlying muscles. It is well developed functionally in the region of neck and limbs. It is condensed to form specialized binding structures at certain area especially in limbs, forming intermuscular sheaths and retinaculae. The various modifications of deep fascia are described in the respective chapters.

BLOOD AND LYMPH

This is a form of specialised connective tissue. Blood is described in chapter no. 14 (see page no. 453) Lymph is described in lymphatic system (see page no. 463).

MUSCULAR TISSUE

The muscular tissue is organised to form the musculature of the body. It helps in the movements of various parts of the body. It is described in muscular system (see page no. 157).

NERVOUS TISSUE

It is responsible for the maintenance of internal homeostasis by controling the responsiveness of various organs and tissues of the body. It is described in nervous system (see page no. 203).

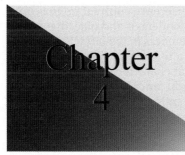

Chapter 4

Histological Techniques

HISTOLOGY

Histology is study of microscopic structure of various tissues of the body with their function.

HISTOLOGICAL TECHNIQUES

The specimens of tissues are first prepared and then stained with appropriate staining dyes after which they are examined under microscopes.

Specimen Preparation

The specimen to be studied under microscope is prepared in the following steps:

1. **Fixation:** It is the first step in specimen preparation. Fixation preserves cell structures while introducing a minimal number of artifacts. The most common fixative used is 10% formaldehyde and glutaraldehyde.

   For electron microscopy specimens typically are immersed in a buffer solution of Osmuim Tetra-oxide (OSO_4) after fixation with glutaraldehyde.

2. **Dehydration:** After fixation, specimens are dehydrated by immersion in a series of solutions containing increasing concentrations of ethanol or acetone. Dehydration is necessary because most embedding media (e.g., Paraffin, Plastic monomers) are immiscible in water.

3. **Embedding:** Next step is embedding of specimen in liquid medium that infiltrates and hardens the specimen so that it can be sliced into thin sections suitable for staining and microscopic examination.

   a. **Paraffin** is often used as the embedding medium in light microscopy.

      Advantage: It is easy to work with paraffin. It allows for a speedy specimen preparation and stains reliably

      Disadvantage: It has a low tensile strength and hence cannot be cut into very thin sections.

   b. **Plastic monomers** are used as the embedding medium in electron microscopy.

4. **Sectioning:** Sections are made from the embedded tissues with the help of microtome.

For light microscope sections are usually 5 to 10 mm thick.

For electron micorscope the sections obtained are 0.02 to 1.0 mm thick.

5. **Staining:** Sections are stained with dyes and fluorescent tags before examination under microscope. The most common stain used in routine microscopy is haemotoxylin and eosin (H and E stain) stain. For electron microscopy specimens are stained with heavy metal salts.

Staining of Specimens

The specimens are stained usually with a combination of acidic and basic dyes which stain specific structures of the tissues and cells and improves their visualization under microscope. The various cell components stain differently according to their chemical composition. These are described below.

Acidophilic Structures

Tissue components that bind to acidic dyes are known as acidophilic. The acidophilic structures include

   a. Cytoplasm of erythrocyte
   b. Collagen fibres
   c. Mitochondria
   d. Lysosomes

Acidic dyes are: Eosin, Orange G.

Basophilic Structures

Tissue components that bind to basic dyes are known as basophilic. The basophilic structures include

1. Nuclei of cells
2. Rough endoplasmic reticulum
3. Extra cellular matrix

Basic dyes are

1. Hematoxylin
2. Methylene blue
3. Toludine blue

Metachromatic Structures

Literal meaning of metachromasia is 'change in colour'. Structures that stain with these dyes are known as metachromatic, e.g., cartilage.
Metachromatic dyes: Toludine blue.

Periodic acid–Schiff (PAS) Reaction

This reaction is used to identify tissue and cells which contain carbohydrates by exposing tissue sections to periodic acid oxidation and then reacting them with Schiff's reagent. PAS positive cell structures include
a. Glycocalyx
b. Basement membrane

Miscellaneous Stains

1. **Special stains**
   a. Orcein—for elastic fibres
   b. Weighert's—for elastic fibres
   c. Silver nitrate—for reticular fibres
2. **Fluorescent tags:** Fluorescent molecules are tagged with antibodies to specific tissue antigens so they can be localized and examined under a fluorescent microscope, e.g., fluorescein isothiocynate
3. **Staining for transmission electron microscope:** Sections are stained with heavy metal salts, e.g., uranyl acetate.

EXAMINATION UNDER MICROSCOPE

Microscopes are primarily of two types, light microscope and electron microscope.

Light Microscope

Modern day light microscopes have a resolution limit of 0.2 to 0.4 mm. This is approximately 1/10th of the diameter of the human erythrocyte. These microscopes utilise day light for illumination or have an inbuilt electrical illumination system.

Types of Light Microscope

They are of two types:
1. **Simple microscope:** This is primarily a magnifying glass with magnification power of 2 to 200X.
2. **Compound microscope:** It consists of two or more lenses set in a specific optical fashion. Compound microscopes are of the following types depending on the different modifications of light system in them.
   i. **Bright-field microscope:** This uses standard lenses and condensers. The limit of resolution of bright field microscope is approximately 0.3 mm (Fig. 4.1).
   ii. **Phase contrast microscope:** It permits direct examination of living cells without fixation or staining.

iii. **Differential interference contrast microscope:** It uses a special condensor and objective lenses to transform differences in the refractive indices between cells of a tissue to give an image with three dimensional characters.
iv. **Fluorescence light microscope:** It is used to localize the inherently fluorescent substances or substances labeled with fluorescent tags.

MONOCULAR COMPOUND LIGHT MICROSCOPE

This is the most common microscope used in laboratories (Fig. 4.1). It consists of the following parts:
1. **Stand:** It is the base of microscope. It is usually horse shoe shaped.
2. **Body:** It is attached to the stand below at a joint and carries the following parts on it:
   a. Limb
   b. Body tubes
   c. Stage
   d. Sub stage
   e. Knobs for focus and fine adjustment
   Limb: It is attached to the base by means of a swivel which allows forward and backward inclination of the microscope. It carries the body tube, stage, sub stage and mirror. The microscope can be held from the limb and shifted to a comfortable position.
   Body tubes: These consist of an external tube which has a revolving nose piece attached to a set of three objective lenses inferiorly and an inner tube designed to hold a single eye piece superiorly. It is attached to the limb.
   Stage: It is a plate like platform attached to the limb below the level of lower end of objective lenses. It bears clips on its superior surface to hold the slide to be viewed. The slide can be moved from side to side or anteroposteriorly by knobs attached to slide holder. The platform has an aperture in the centre for transmission of light to the slide.
   Substage: It is attached to lower end of the limb below the stage. It consists of a condenser through which light is focused on the aperture of stage over which lies the object to be studied.
   Knobs for adjustment: Two sets of knobs are provided on either side of the limb which moves the external body tube up and down with its lenses. This helps to achieve coarse and fine adjustments in focusing the specimen.

Optical System of the Microscope

It consists of the following lenses:
1. **Eye piece:** It has two planoconvex lenses with magnification of 10 X usually. Monocular microscope has a single eye piece mounted on the body to while binocular microscope has two eyepieces mounted on body tubes (Fig. 4.2).

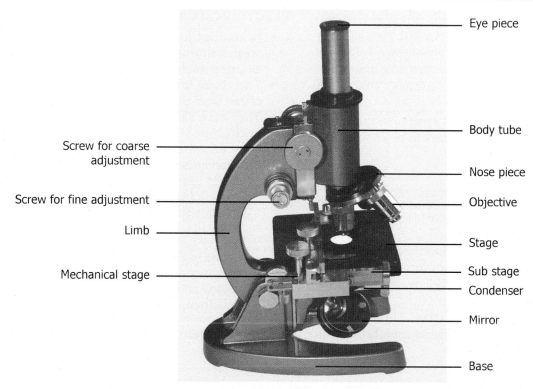

Fig. 4.1: Monocular compound light microscope (Bright-field microscope)

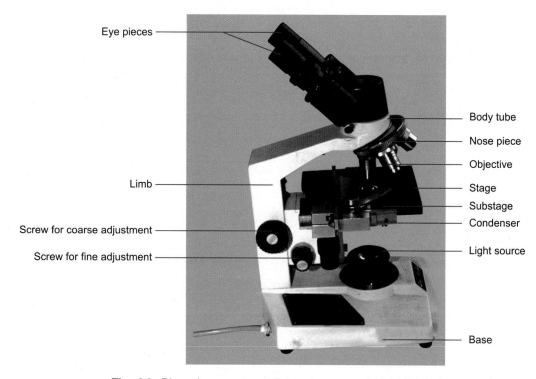

Fig. 4.2: Binocular compound light microscope (Bright-field microscope)

2. **Objective lenses:** They usually consist of three sets of lenses fitted0 into the nosepiece of outer body tube. Each objective lens consists of a battery of lenses with prism incorporated into them and provide a magnification of 10X, 40X, 100X respectively.

3. **Condenser:** It is made up of a pair of simple lenses that focus light onto the object to be viewed. It is mounted on the sub stage.

Illumination System of Microscope

Microscopes can have two types of systems to provide illumination to see the slide.

1. **Mirror:** A mirror is fitted below the condenser. One side of the mirror has a plane mirror and other side has a concave mirror which is used to direct the daylight on to the condenser.

2. **Built in illumination system:** This system is attached to the stand of the microscope, below with an electrical attachment.

ELECTRON MICROSCOPE

- In contrast to light microscopes, electron microscopes illuminate specimens with a stream of electrons, of short wave lengths, instead of photons.
- They form images with help of magnetic lenses rather than glass lenses.
- They have 1000 times the resolving power of light microscope.
- There are two types of electron microscopes namely:
  — **Transmission electron microscope:** Thinly sliced plastic embedded sections are stained with heavy metals and examined under transmission electron microscope. It is used to study fine details of the cell structure and it can resolve features as small as 0.5 nm
  — **Scanning electron microscope:** The entire specimen is subjected to critical point drying, coated with a thin layer of gold and palladium and then examined under scanning electron microscope. It is used to study the three dimensional features of cell surfaces. It can resolve up to 5 nm.

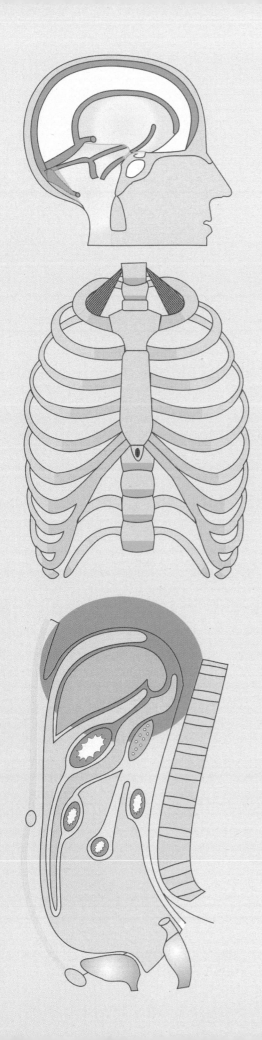

5. Organisation of Body

Chapter 5

Organisation of Body

INTRODUCTION

Anatomy and physiology are integrated. As already described in chapter 1, anatomy deals with study of structure of body while physiology deals with study of functions of various parts and structures of body.

The primary aim of any living organism is survival and existence and it includes basic life processes like

1. **Metabolism:** This includes all chemical processes occurring in the body which facilitate survival and existence.
2. **Homeostasis:** This is the ability of an organism to respond to the external environment and regulate its own internal environment.
3. **Movement:** It includes movement of cells inside the body and of the organism as a whole.
4. **Growth:** It involves increase in size and number of cells, replacement of cells and removal of older cells.
5. **Differentiation:** This is the basic fundamental of formation of various organs of an organism. An unspecialized cell gets converted into a specialized cell during growth and development.
6. **Reproduction:** It includes new cell formation for growth, repair or production of a new individual.

The structural and functional unit of a human body is the cell. A number of cells with similar embryonic origin and function form a tissue (see chapter 3). A number of tissues are organised to form an organ that performs a specific function, e.g., stomach, heart etc.

The various organs and tissues of body are arranged in a systematic manner in order to perform different functions of the body, e.g., gastrointestinal tract, nervous system, etc. These systems perform specific function for survival and maintanance of human body. Each system has an independent function but is interdependent on other systems for its proper functioning.

Composition of Body

In average adults, 60% of total body weight is water, 18% is protein and related substances, 15% is fat and 7% is minerals.

The body water is divided into two parts:

1. **Intracellular fluid (ICF):** It is the fluid contained within the cells. It forms 2/3rd of total body water and 40% total body weight.
2. **Extracellular fluid (ECF):** It forms 1/3rd of total body water and 20% of total body weight. It is further divided into two components:
   a. **Circulating plasma:** It is 25% of ECF and forms 5% of total body weight. Plasma along with various cellular elements forms blood which circulates in the vascular system.
   b. **Interstitial fluid:** It is 75% of ECF and forms 15% of total body weight. This fluid lies outside the blood vessels and bathes the cells.

The normal cell function depends on the composition of interstitial fluid. Thus the internal environment of the body is kept constant by multiple regulatory factors. This is called **homeostasis.** This is a dynamic process that regulates volume, composition, pH, temperature and contents of fluid within physiological limits.

The human body is a well organised unit and it can be studied systematically by dividing it into study of various regions of the body. The various regions are:

1. Head and neck
2. Thorax
3. Abdomen and pelvis
4. Upper limb
5. Lower limb

This chapter describes the general organisation of various regions of the body. The specific skeleto-muscular framework, nerve supply and vascular supply of various regions and the anatomical and functional organisation of various systems of the body are described in subsequent chapters.

HEAD AND NECK

- Head consists of skull and face. Upper part of skull known as calvaria.
- The cavity present inside the skull is known as cranial cavity. Cranial cavity lodges the brain, its coverings known as meninges, cerebrospinal fluid and the vascular supply of brain.

- The anterior part of skull provides the skeletal framework for the face. Face has openings of proximal ends of respiratory tract (nostrils) and digestive tract (oral cavity) that communicate with exterior for intake of air (oxygen) and food. The face and skull also have sockets for eyeballs and organ of hearing (ears) which facilitates the communication with external environment.
- Neck connects head to the upper part of trunk. It gives passage to trachea, esophagus, and spinal cord, spinal nerves with sympathetic nerve trunk and carries the vascular supply (carotid and vertebral vessels with their branches, internal jugular veins) to and from the various structures of head and neck and brain.
- The skeletomuscular framework of neck helps in movement of head over trunk. This helps in search of food, facilitates function of sight and hearing and aids in defense.

SCALP

The soft tissue covering the vault of skull is termed as scalp.
Extent
Anterior : Supraciliary arches
Posterior : External occipital protuberance and superior nuchal lines
Lateral : Superior temporal line on each side

Layers of Scalp

The soft tissues of the scalp are arranged in five layers namely (Fig. 5.1).
S—Skin
C—Connective tissue
A—Aponeurosis
L—Loose areolar tissue
P—Periosteum

Skin
- Skin of the scalp is richly supplied with hairs, sweat glands and sebaceous glands.
- It is thick and has about 1,20,000 hairs.

Subcutaneous Tissue
- It consists of lobules of fat bounded in tough fibrous septae which form a very dense network.
- The blood vessels of the scalp lie in this layer. Any injury here results in failure of the lumen of blood vessels to retract because their walls are adherant to the connective tissue. As a result, lacerations of the scalp bleed profusely. This area, in fact has the richest cutaneous blood supply of the body.

Aponeurotic Layer
- This is formed by the aponeurosis of occipito-frontalis muscle over the dome of the skull.
- **The occipitofrontalis** originates from 2 parts.
  a. **Occipital bellies:** Muscular fibres arise from the lateral 2/3rd of superior nuchal lines on either side. They pass upwards and forewards
  b. **Frontal bellies:** The fibres are attached to the skin of the eye brows and root of nose and pass backwards.
The fibres from both the bellies are inserted into a central fibrous layer known as the galea aponeurotica or epicranial aponeurosis.

Extent of Galea Aponeurotica
Anteriorly : It extends upto the coronal suture.
Posteriorly : It blends with the occipital bellies and extends further to attach over the external occipital protuberance and highest nuchal lines on either side.
Laterally : It extends over the temporal fascia and thins out to attach to the zygomatic arch.

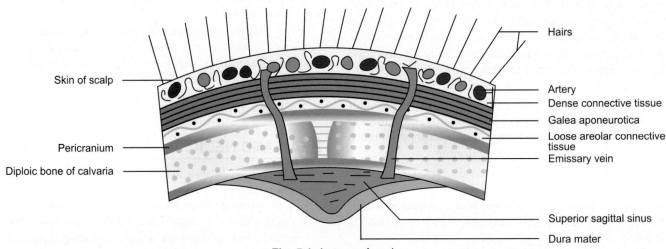

Fig. 5.1: Layers of scalp

Layer of Loose Areolar Tissue

- It lies beneath the aponeurotic layer and accounts for the mobility of scalp on the underlying bone.
- It is in this plane that the surgeons mobilize scalp flaps for reconstructive surgery.
- **Dangerous layer of the scalp:** The layer of loose areolar tissue is often called as dangerous layer of the scalp because it lodges the emissary veins which do not have valves. Hence, if there is any infection of scalp it can travel along the emissary veins into the intracranial dural venous sinuses leading to their thrombosis.

Periosteum

It is the pericranium covering the skull bones and is adherent at the suture-lines of the skull.

FACE

Face is the anterior aspect of head (Fig. 5.2).

Extent

Superior : Hair line of scalp (frontal prominences if person is bald)
Inferior : Chin and base of mandible
Lateral : Tragus of ear on either side

Face consists of two layers of soft tissue namely skin and superficial fascia with facial muscles over the facial skeleton (norma frontalis). There is **no deep fascia in the face.** Face presents with forehead, eyebrows, eyeballs with eyelids, nose (external nose), cheeks, oral cavity (mouth and lips) and chin.

Skin

- Facial skin is thick and elastic and lies loosely over the skeleton except in the area of nose and auricle where it is adherent to the underlying cartilage.
- It is richly supplied by blood vessels. Hence, bleeding is profuse in facial injuries.
- There are numerous sweat glands and sebaceous glands in the skin.
- The facial skin gives attachment to facial muscles.

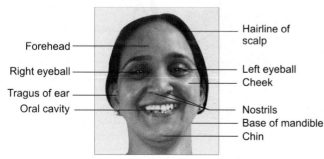

Forehead —
Right eyeball —
Tragus of ear —
Oral cavity —
Hairline of scalp
Left eyeball
Cheek
Nostrils
Base of mandible
Chin

Fig. 5.2: Face

Superficial Fascia

It consists of the following:
1. **Fat:** This is most abundant over the cheeks. It forms the buccal pad of fat especially seen in children. It is absent over the eyelids.
2. Muscles of the face (see page nos 167 to 169)
3. Vessels (see page no. 417)
4. Nerves (see page no. 299)
5. Lymphatics

NECK

Neck is that part of the body which connects the head to the upper part of trunk.

Extent

Superior boundary of neck
- Lower border of body of mandible
- Line joining angle of mandible to mastoid process
- Superior nuchal lines
- External occipital protuberance

Inferior boundary of neck

- Suprasternal notch of manubrium sterni.
- Upper surface of clavicle, on each side.
- Acromian process of scapula on each side.
- Line extending from the acromian process to spine of C_7 vertebra on each side.

It is cylindrical in shape and is covered by skin, superficial fascia and deep fascia. The skeleton of neck consists of cervical vertebrae. The musculature of neck is described on (page nos 170 to 176).

Superficial Fascia of Neck

It is thin and is primarily made up of loose connective tissue. A thin sheet of muscle fibres known as **platysma** is present in this fascia.

Deep Fascia of Neck (Deep Cervical Fascia)

It is well developed and is organied into three layers. From exterior to interior these are:
1. Investing layer
2. Pretracheal layer
3. Prevertebral layer

Investing Layer of Deep Cervical Fascia

The investing layer of cervical fascia lies deep to the subcutaneous tissue and platysma and surrounds the neck completely like a collar (Figs 5.3 and 5.4).

Attachments
Superiorly (on each side): External occipital protuberance, superior nuchal line, mastoid process, lower border of zygomatic arch, lower border of body of mandible upto symphysis menti.

Inferiorly (on each side): Upper border of spine of scapula, acromian process of scapula, upper surface of clavicle, suprasternal notch of manubrium sterni

Posteriorly (from above downwards): Ligamentum nuchae, spine of C_7 vertebra.

Anteriorly (from above downwards): Symphysis menti, hyoid bone, manubrium sterni

Horizontal Extent of Investing Layer (Fig. 5.3)

- The fascia passes anteriorly from the ligamentum nuchae and splits to enclose the trapezius muscle.
- It reunites at the anterior border of trapezius and runs anteriorly. It splits again to enclose the sternocleidomastoid muscle.
- At the anterior border of the muscle it reunites and can be traced to the midline of neck where it proceeds to the opposite side in same manner.

Vertical Extent of Investing Layer (Fig. 5.4)

- The investing layer of deep fascia encloses the neck like a collar.
- Infront of neck, at its inferior end, the deep fascia splits at two sites and encloses the following two spaces:

1. **Suprasternal space or space of Burn's:** The investing fascia splits over the manubrium sterni into two layers. The superficial layer is attached to anterior margin of suprasternal notch and the deep layer gets attached to the posterior margin to enclose the space.

   Contents
   a. Sternal heads of sternocleidomastoid of both sides
   b. Jugular venous arch
   c. Interclavicular ligament
   d. Occasionally, a lymph node

2. **Supraclavicular space:** This is formed over the middle third of clavicle where the investing layer splits into two and is attached to anterior and posterior margins of upper surface of clavicle.

   Contents
   a. Terminal part of external jugular vein
   b. Supraclavicular nerves before they pierce the deep fascia.

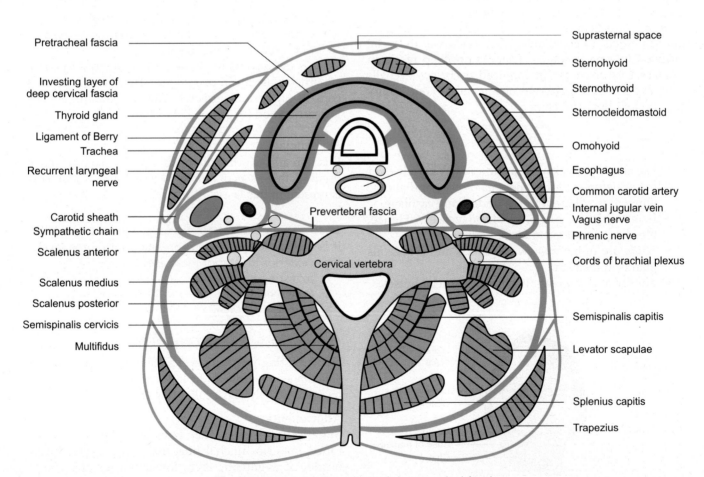

Pretracheal fascia

Investing layer of deep cervical fascia

Thyroid gland

Ligament of Berry

Trachea

Recurrent laryngeal nerve

Carotid sheath

Sympathetic chain

Scalenus anterior

Scalenus medius

Scalenus posterior

Semispinalis cervicis

Multifidus

Suprasternal space

Sternohyoid

Sternothyroid

Sternocleidomastoid

Omohyoid

Esophagus

Common carotid artery

Internal jugular vein

Vagus nerve

Phrenic nerve

Cords of brachial plexus

Semispinalis capitis

Levator scapulae

Splenius capitis

Trapezius

Prevertebral fascia

Cervical vertebra

Fig. 5.3: Horizontal disposition of deep cervical fascia

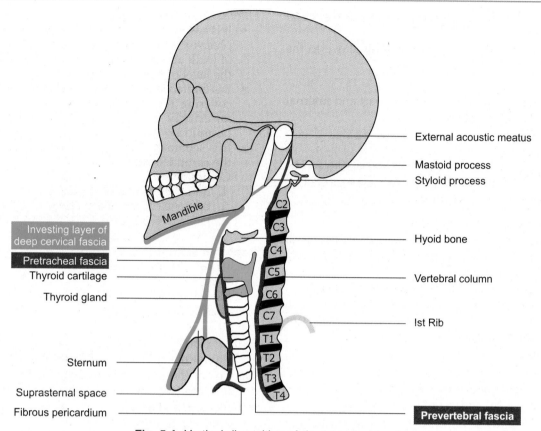

Fig. 5.4: Vertical disposition of deep cervical fascia

- At the upper part the fascia splits to enclose the submandibular glands on either side.
- At the lower pole of parotid gland it splits again to enclose the gland. The superficial layer is thick and merges with the fascia on masseter while the deep layer is thin.
- From the tip of the styloid process to angle of mandible the fascia is thickened to form the stylomandibular ligament.

Pretracheal Fascia

The pretracheal layer of deep cervical fascia lies over the trachea and is also known as pretracheal fascia (Fig. 5.4)

Extent
From above downwards

- It is attached above to the middle of the lower border of body of hyoid bone extending to the oblique line of thyroid cartilage.
- When traced below it encloses the thyroid gland.
- Then it passes in front of trachea.
- Finally, it enters the thorax and blends with the fibrous pericardium.

From medial to lateral

- The layer covers the anterior surface of trachea and passes laterally on each side and merges with the fascia deep to sternocleido-mastoid.

Prevertebral Fascia

This layer of deep fascia lies anterior to the prevertebral muscles (Fig. 5.4). The nerve roots of cervical and brachial plexus along with subclavian vessels lie under it and carry with them a tubular extension from the fascia into the axilla. This forms the axillary sheath which may extend upto the elbow.

Extent
From above downwards

- It is attached to base of skull above.
- It covers the pre and para-vertebral muscles.
- It extends below to the superior mediastinum and is attached to the anterior longitudinal ligament till T_4 vertebra.

From medial to lateral side

- The fascia passes anterior to prevertebral muscles and runs laterally and backwards over the para-vertebral muscles.
- Further posteriorly it blends with the fascia underneath the trapezius, on each side.

Carotid Sheath

The deep cervical fascia forms a tubular sheath around the major vessels of the neck, named the carotid sheath (Fig. 5.3). It is formed by the condensation of fibro-aerolar tissue and is attached to the pretracheal and prevertebral fascia.

Extent: It extends from the base of skull above to the arch of aorta below:

Contents
1. Common carotid artery in lower part and internal carotid artery in upper part
2. Internal jugular vein
3. Vagus nerve

Ansa cervicalis is embedded in its anterior layer. The cervical sympathetic chain lies close to the posterior layer in front of the prevertebral fascia.

Retropharyngeal Space
- It is the potential space present between the fascia covering the muscles of pharynx (buccopharyngeal fascia) and the prevertebral fascia.
- On each side it is limited by the carotid sheath.
- Superiorly, the space is closed by the base of skull while inferiorly it is continuous with superior mediastium of thorax.

Contents
1. Loose aerolar tissue
2. Retropharyngeal lymph nodes
3. Pharyngeal plexus of nerves and vessels

Functions: It allows the pharynx to expand during deglutition.

Lateral Pharyngeal Space
- It is a wedge shaped space present on either side of pharynx with a broad base above formed by base of skull and a narrow apex below extending upto the level of hyoid bone in the neck.
- It is limited laterally by the medial pterygoid muscle covering the inner aspect of ramus of mandible anteriorly and parotid gland with its fascia posteriorly.
- It is separated from the retropharyngeal space by the carotid sheath.

Contents
1. Branches of maxillary nerve
2. Branches of maxillary artery
3. Fibro-fatty tissue

Anatomical Features of Neck
The various features of neck and its contents are studied in two parts:
1. Side of neck
2. Back of neck

Side of Neck
The side of neck encompasses the anterior and lateral surfaces of the neck. It is rectangular in shape and is divided into two triangles by the sternocleidomastoid muscle namely (Fig. 5.5)
1. Anterior triangle
2. Posterior triangle

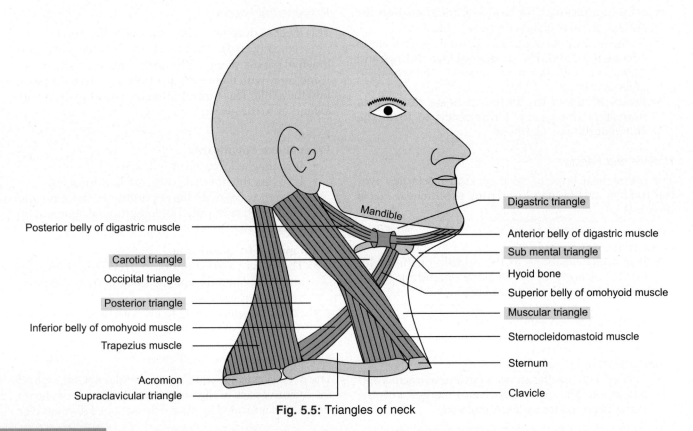

Fig. 5.5: Triangles of neck

Anterior Triangle of Neck (Figs 5.5 and 5.6)

Boundaries of Anterior Triangle of Neck

1. **Anterior:** Anterior midline of the neck extending from symphysis menti above to the middle of suprasternal notch below.
2. **Posterior:** Anterior border of sternocleidomastoid.
3. **Base:** Lower border of the body of mandible and line joining the angle of mandible with the mastoid process
`4. **Apex:** It is formed at the meeting point between anterior border of sternocleidomastoid and anterior midline (vide supra).

The anterior triangle in subdivided by the digastric muscle and superior belly of omohyoid into following four parts (Figs 5.5 and 5.6).

Submental Triangle

Boundaries: Anterior belly of digastric muscles of both sides and upper border of hyoid bone.

Contents
a. Submental lymph nodes.
b. Submental veins, anterior jugular veins.

Digastric Triangle

Boundaries (on each side): Anterior and posterior belly of digastric muscle and inferior border of mandible.

Contents
a. Submandibular salivary gland—Superficial part.
b. Submandibular lymph nodes.
c. Hypoglossal nerve.
d. Submental artery and vein, branches from facial vessels.
e. Mylohyoid nerve and vessels.
f. External carotid artery.
g. Carotid sheath with its contents.

Carotid Triangle

Boundaries (on each side): Superior belly of omohyoid, upper part of sternocleidomastoid and posterior belly of digastric muscles.

Contents
a. Common carotid artery with its terminal branches
    i. Internal carotid artery
    ii. External carotid artery
b. Internal jugular vein
c. Occipital vessels
d. Facial vessels
e. Lingual vessels
f. Superior thyroid vessels.
g. Pharyngeal vessels
h. Last three cranial nerves
    i. Vagus nerve
    ii. Spinal accessory nerve
    iii. Hypoglossal nerve

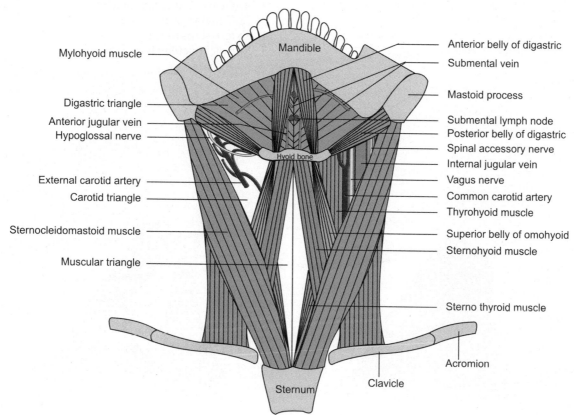

Fig. 5.6: Submental, digastric, carotid, muscular triangles

    i. Sympathetic chain
    j. Cervical part of deep cervical lymph nodes

Muscular Triangle

Boundaries: Superior belly of omohyoid muscle on each side and lower part of sternocleidomastoid muscle below:

Contents

  a. Infrahyoid muscles: They form the floor of muscular triangle and are the contents also. They consist of sternohyoid, omohyoid, sternohyoid and thyrohyoid muscles.

Posterior Triangle of Neck (Figs 5.5, 5.7 to 5.9)

Boundaries of Posterior Triangle of Neck

1. **Anterior:** Posterior border of sternocleidomastoid.
2. **Posterior:** Anterior border of trapezius.
3. **Base:** Middle third of the clavicle.
4. **Apex:** Meeting point of sternocleidomastoid and trapezius on the superior nuchal line.
5. **Roof:** Is formed by investing layer of deep cervical fascia stretching between sternocleidomastoid and trapezius muscles.
6. **Floor:** Is muscular and is formed by following muscles.
    From above downwards.
    a. Semispinalis capitis
    b. Splenius capitis
    c. Levator scapulae
    d. Scalenus posterior
    e. Scalenus medius
    f. Outer border of 1st rib

The prevertebral layer of deep cervical fascia covers all the muscles of the floor thus forming a fascial carpet of the posterior triangle.

The triangle is divided into two parts by the inferior belly of omohyoid over the scalenus medius.

  a. Occipital triangle–Larger, upper part.
  b. Subclavian/supraclavicular triangle—Smaller, lower part.

Occipital Triangle

Contents (From above downwards)

1. Occipital artery at apex
2. Spinal part of accessory nerve
3. Four cutaneous branches of cervical plexus of nerves namely:
    a. Lesser occipital
    b. Great auricular
    c. Transverse cervical
    d. Supra clavicular
4. Muscular branches of C_3 and C_4 nerves
5. Dorsal scapular nerve

Supraclavicular Triangle

Contents

1. Trunks of brachial plexus of nerves with their branches namely:
    a. Dorsal scapular
    b. Long thoracic
    c. Nerve to subclavius
2. 3rd part of subclavian artery
3. Subclavian vein
4. External jugular vein
5. Supraclavicular lymph nodes

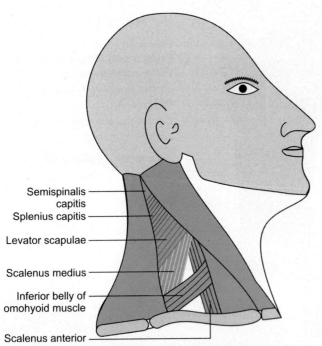

Fig. 5.7: Muscles forming floor of posterior triangle

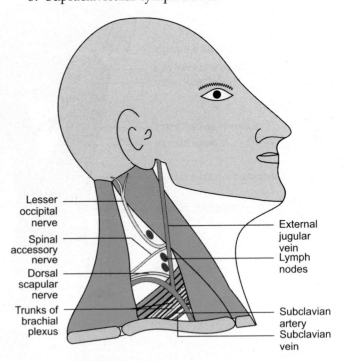

Fig. 5.8: Contents of posterior triangle

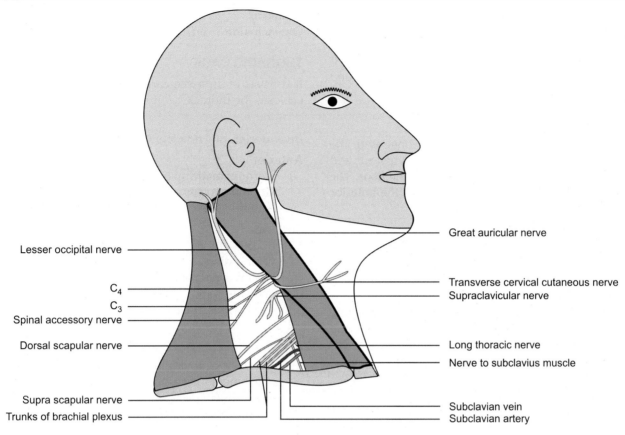

Fig. 5.9: Contents of posterior triangle

Back of Neck

The posterior aspect of neck is primarily muscular.

Ligamentum nuchae: In the median plane beneath the deep fascia lies a fibrous sheath attached to the spines of the cervical vertebrae. This is the ligamentum nuchae. It is attached above to the external occipital protuberance and crest and divides the back of neck into two halves.

Each half of neck is covered by muscles which lie between the deep cervical fascia and posterior aspect of cervical vertebrae. These are (from superficial to deep on each side), trapezius, splenus capitis and cervicis, semispinalis capitis and cervicis, longissimus capitis and cervicis, levator scapula and suboccipital muscles.

Suboccipital Triangles

These are a pair of muscular triangles situated deep in the suboccipital region one on either site of midline and are bounded by four suboccipital muscles (Fig. 7.26).

Boundaries
1. **Superomedial:** Rectus capitis posterior major, supplemented by rectus capitis posterior minor.
2. **Superolateral:** Obliquus capitis superior.
3. **Inferior:** Obliquus capitis inferior.

4. **Roof:** Formed by dense fibrous tissue which is covered by semispinalis capitis medially and longissimus capitis laterally.
5. **Floor:** Is formed by posterior arch of atlas and posterior atlanto-occipital membrane.

Contents
1. Third part of vertebral artery.
2. Dorsal ramus of C_1 (suboccipital nerve).
3. Suboccipital plexus of veins.

Deep Structures and Viscera of Neck

The skin, fascia and external musculature of neck enclosed the following structures. From before backwards these are
1. Thyroid and parathyroid glands.
2. Larynx and trachea.
3. Pharynx and esophagus.

On each side
4. Neurovascular bundle consisting of common carotid (internal carotid) artery, internal jugular vein and vagus nerve. These are present on each side.
5. Cervical sympathetic chain.
6. Origin of cervical and brachial plexuses.
7. Pre and para-vertebral muscles.

THORAX

Thorax is the part of trunk which extends from the thoracic inlet or root of neck upto the abdomen. It presents with the thoracic cavity that contains heart and lungs bounded by the thoracic cage.

Thoracic Inlet

It is reniform in shape and continues above with the neck. The plane of thoracic inlet slopes downwards and forwards and forms an angle of 45° with the floor. The posterior end is about 4 cm. higher than the anterior end.

Boundaries of Thoracic Inlet:
Anterior : Upper border of manubrium.
Posterior : T_1 vertebra.
On each side : 1st rib.

Suprapleural membrane or Sibson's fascia: The thoracic inlet is separated from the root of neck by a supra-pleural membrane. It is a triangular shaped membrane present on either side of inlet with a gap in the centre.

Thoracic Outlet

It is wider than the inlet and continues below with the abdomen. It is separated from the abdomen by a diaphragm which forms the floor of thoracic cavity.

Boundaries of thoracic outlet
Anterior : 7th, 8th, 9th and 10th costal cartilages.

Posterior : T_{12} vertebra.
On each side : 11th and 12th ribs.

THORACIC CAGE

It consists of an osseo-cartilaginous framework which encloses the thoracic cavity.

Boundaries of Thoracic Cage

Anterior
1. Sternum made up of manubrium, body of sternum, xiphoid process.
2. Anterior part of ribs and their costal cartilages.

Posterior
1. Bodies of 12 thoracic vertebrae and their intervening discs.
2. Posterior part of ribs.

On each side
1. Twelve ribs, their cartilages
2. Intercostal spaces.

Functions of Thoracic Cage
1. This osseocartilaginous cage with its muscular attachments is responsible for the movements of respiration.
2. It protects the vital organs namely, lungs and heart.

Thoracic Cavity

Thoracic cavity is the cavity enclosed by the thoracic cage. It communicates above with the neck at the thoracic

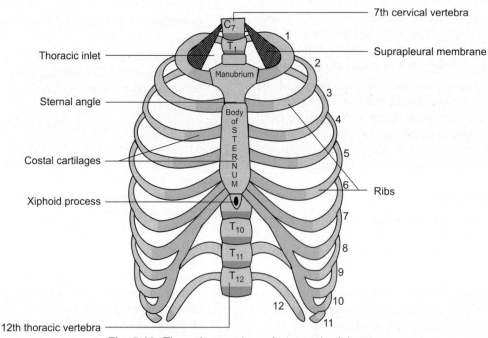

Fig. 5.10: Thoracic cage-bony framework of thorax

inlet and is separated from the abdominal cavity by the diaphragm. It contains right and left pleural sacs (see page nos 374 and 375) which enclose right and left lungs respectively (see page nos 370 to 372). The space between the two sacs is occupied by mediastinum.

MEDIASTINUM

Major part of thoracic cavity is occupied by a pair of lungs covered by its serous covering, the pleura. Mediastinum is the median septum which lies between the two pleural sacs (Figs 5.11 and 5.12).

Boundaries of Mediastinum

Superior : Thoracic inlet
Inferior : Diaphragm
Each side : Mediastinal pleura
Anterior : Sternum
Posterior : Twelve thoracic vertebrae

For the purpose of description mediastinum is divided into superior and inferior mediastinum with the help of an imaginary line extending from the sternal angle to lower border of T_4 vertebra.

Superior Mediastinum

Boundaries of Superior Mediastinum
Anterior : Manubrium sterni.
Posterior : Upper four thoracic vertebrae with their inter-vertebral discs and anterior longitudinal ligament.

Superior : Thoracic inlet.
Inferior : A line passing from the sternal angle to lower border of T_4 vertebra.
Each side : Mediastinal pleura.
Contents: Antero-posteriorly.
1. Origin of sternohyoid muscle and sternothyroid muscle.
2. Thymus gland
3. Right and left brachiocephalic veins
4. Upper part of superior vena cava
5. Left superior intercostal vein
6. Arch of aorta with its three large branches
7. Phrenic nerve
8. Vagus nerve
9. Cardiac nerves
10. Trachea with lymph nodes
11. Esophagus
12. Left recurrent laryngeal nerve
13. Thoracic duct, left to esophagus

Inferior Mediastinum

It is divided into anterior, middle and posterior parts by the pericardium and heart.

Anterior Mediastinum

Boundaries of Anterior Mediastinum
Anterior : Posterior surface of sternum.
Posterior : Anterior surface of pericardium.

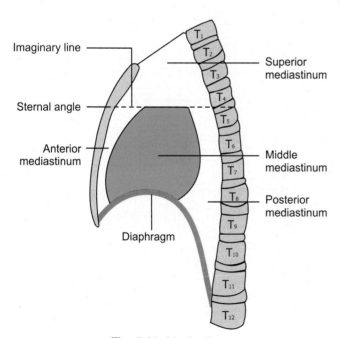

Fig. 5.11: Mediastinum

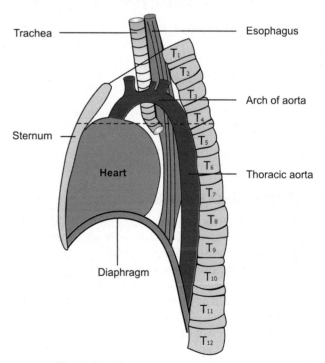

Fig. 5.12: Visceral contents of medastinum

Superior   : Line passing from sternal angle to T₄ vertebra

Inferior   : Diaphragm

On each side : Mediastinal pleura

Contents
1. Superior and inferior sternopericardial ligaments
2. Retro-sternal lymph nodes
3. A few mediastinal branches of internal thoracic artery

Middle Mediastinum

It lies between anterior and posterior mediastinum.

Contents

1. Pericardium enclosing the heart
2. Ascending aorta
3. Pulmonary trunk
4. Four pulmonary veins
5. Lower part of superior vena cava
6. Arch of azygos vein
7. Bifurcation of trachea, with deep cardiac plexus, inferior tracheo-bronchial lymph nodes
8. Phrenic nerve and pericardiophrenic vessels

Posterior Mediastinum

Boundaries of Posterior Mediastinum

Anterior   : Pericardium, bifurcation of trachea.

Anteroinferior : Posterior part of superior surface of diaphragm.

Posterior   : Lower thoracic vertebrae with their intervertebral discs.

On each side   : Mediastinal pleura.

Contents

1. Esophagus
2. Descending aorta
3. Azygos and hemiazygos veins
4. Thoracic duct
5. Vagus nerves
6. Splanchnic nerves
7. Posterior mediastinal lymph nodes
8. Posterior intercostal arteries
9. Some of posterior intercostal veins

ABDOMEN AND PELVIS

Abdomen and pelvis contain the organs of digestive system with its associated glands, urinary system and reproductive system. It gives passage to the neuro-vascular bundle supplying the various organs. Abdomen and pelvis are lined by a serous sac made up of mesothelium known as peritoneum. Various abdominal organs invaginate this peritoneal sac during intrauterine development and result in formation of peritoneal cavity with its folds and ligaments. This facilitates movements of the organs.

ABDOMEN

Abdomen is the part of trunk which lies below the thoraco-abdominal diaphragm.

Boundaries (Fig. 5.13)

Anterior wall : It is musculoaponeurotic and is formed by three flat muscles namely external and internal oblique and transversus abdominis with their aponeurosis. In the mid line it is strengthened by rectus abdominis and pyramidalis muscles.

Posterior wall : It is osseomusculofascial. It is formed by lumbar vertebrae in mid line and the pre and para vertebral muscles on both sides. Principal nerves and vessels of abdomen lie in relation to the posterior wall.

Roof   : It is formed by the undersurface of thoraco-abdominal diaphragm.

Floor   : It is formed by the pelvic diaphragm posteriorly and the urogenital diaphragm in anterior part.

Anterior Abdominal Wall

Extent

Superiorly: Xiphi-sternum, right and left costal margin.
Inferiorly: Iliac crest, fold of groin, pubic tubercle, pubic crest, symphysis pubis
Each side: Mid axillary line

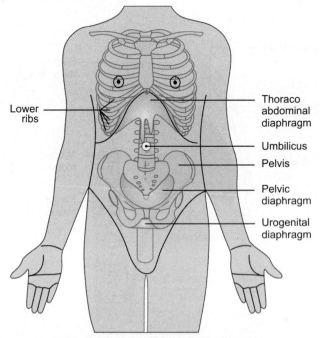

Fig. 5.13: Skeletal boundary of abdomen

Anterior abdominal wall is made up of the following eight layers

1. **Skin:** It is thin and elastic. There is a surface depression present at the level of L_3 and L_4 vertebrae, known as umbilicus. In females, skin in the lower part of abdominal wall may show white lines called as **striae gravidarum.** These are seen in pregnant and parous females due to degenerative fibrosis of subcutaneous fat as a result of stretching by the gravid uterus.
2. **Superficial fascia (Fig. 5.14):** It is a single layer above umbilicus while it splits into two layers in the lower half and forms the:
   a. **Superficial fatty layer:** Camper's fascia
   b. **Deep membranous layer:** Scarpa's fascia
   Extension and modification of fascia Scarpa
   a. Fundiform ligament of penis
   b. Colle's fascia of perineum
3. External oblique muscle and its aponeurosis (see page no. 177).
4. Internal oblique muscle and its aponeurosis (see page no. 177).
5. Transversus abdominis muscle and its aponeurosis (see page no. 177).
6. **Fascia transversalis:** It forms the endo-abdominal fascia and is made up of areolar tissue which lines the inner surface of the transversus abdominis muscle.
   Thomson's ligament: Thickened lower part of fascia transversalis forms the Thomson's ligament. It forms the posterior wall of rectus sheath.
   Deep inguinal ring: It is a deficiency in the fascia transversalis which is situated 1.25 cm above the mid inguinal point. Mid inguinal point is the midpoint of a line joining anterior superior iliac spine and pubic symphysis.
7. **Extra peritoneal tissue:** It is made up of fibro-alveolar fatty tissue
8. **Parietal peritoneum:** It lines the inner surface of anterior abdominal wall beneath extra peritoneal fat.

Other muscles related to anterior abdominal wall (see page no. 177)
1. Cremaster muscle
2. Rectus abdominis
3. Pyramidalis

Inguinal Ligament

It is also known as **Poupart's** ligament. It is the uprolled thickend part of lower part of external oblique aponeurosis (Fig. 5.15).

Extent

It extends from anterior superior iliac spine medially and attaches to pubic tubercle. It is 12 to 14 cm in length. It is slightly convex, towards the thigh, due to traction of fascia lata.

Extensions of Inguinal Ligament
1. Lacunar ligament or Gimbernat's ligament.
2. Reflected part of inguinal ligament.
3. Pectineal ligament of Cooper.

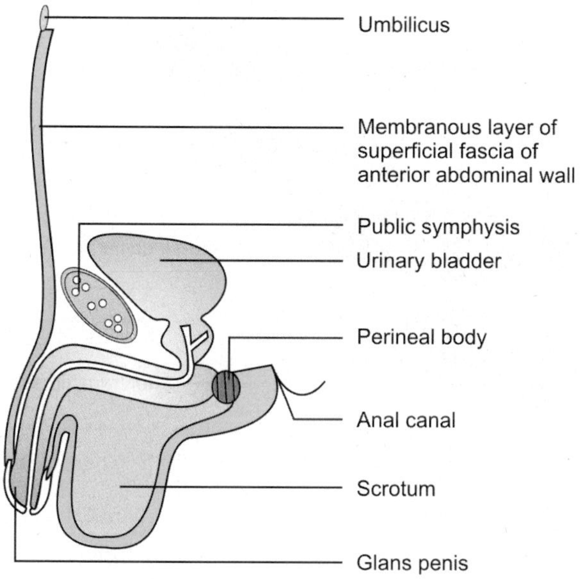

Umbilicus
Membranous layer of superficial fascia of anterior abdominal wall
Public symphysis
Urinary bladder
Perineal body
Anal canal
Scrotum
Glans penis

Fig. 5.14: Extension of membranous layer of superficial fascia of anterior abdominal wall

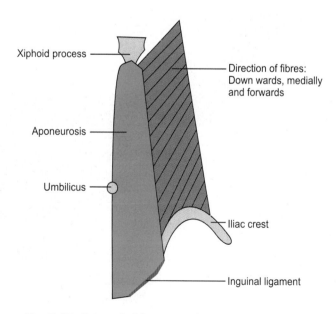

Xiphoid process
Direction of fibres: Down wards, medially and forwards
Aponeurosis
Umbilicus
Iliac crest
Inguinal ligament

Fig. 5.15: External oblique muscle and inguinal ligament

Structures passing behind the inguinal ligament-Lateral to medial side

1. Lateral femoral cutaneous nerve
2. Iliacus muscle
3. Trunk of femoral nerve
4. Tendon of psoas major
5. Femoral artery
6. Femoral branch of genitofemoral nerve
7. Femoral vein
8. Lymphatic
9. Origin of pectineus muscle
10. Accessary obturator nerve, if present

Conjoint Tendon

It is also known as **Falx inguinalis.** It is formed by the fusion of internal oblique and transversus abdominis muscle. 1/3rd of this tendon is formed by internal oblique and 2/3rd is formed by transversus abdominis. It is attached to the pubic crest and medial part of the pecten pubis.

Actions of muscles of anterior abdominal wall

- The muscles retain the viscera in position by providing firm and elastic support. This is chiefly achieved by the tone of external and internal oblique muscles.
- Abdominal muscles increase intra abdominal pressure and compress the viscera during micturition, defecation, parturition, vomiting.

- When rectus abdominis act bilaterally, they cause flexion of the lumbar vertebrae.
- Lateral flexion of spine is caused by unilateral contraction of the oblique muscles.
- Rotation of spine is brought about by unilateral contraction of external oblique with simultaneous contraction of contralateral internal oblique.
- Cremaster muscle pulls the testis towards the superficial inguinal ring, on stimulation. This is known as **cremasteric reflex.**

Inguinal Canal

It is a musculo-aponeurotic passage which lies in the lower part of anterior abdominal wall and extends from the deep inguinal ring to the superficial inguinal ring. It is 4 cm in length in the cadaver. In living state it measures about 3.75 cm (Fig. 5.16).

Superficial inguinal ring: It is the deficiency in aponeurosis of external oblique present superolateral to pubic tubercle. It is bounded by the superior and inferior crura of external oblique aponeurosis which attach to the pubic tubercle and pubic symphysis respectively. Base is formed by the pubic crest.

Boundaries

Anterior Wall

- Skin, superficial fascia.

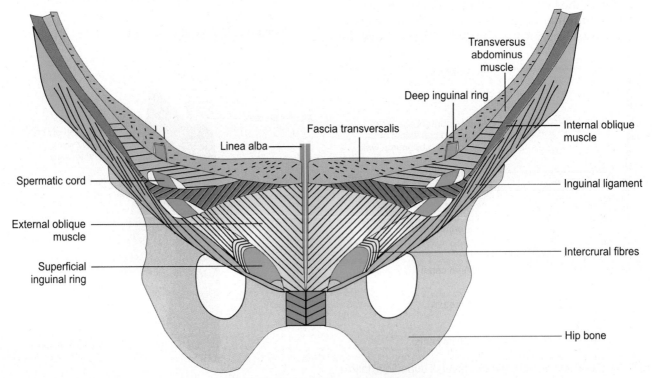

Fig. 5.16: Boundaries of inguinal canal

- External oblique muscle.
- Internal oblique muscle (fleshy fibres), in lateral 1/3rd.

Posterior Wall
- Fascia transversalis, in full length.
- Conjoint tendon, in medial half.
- Reflected part of inguinal ligament, in the medial end.

Floor
- Inguinal ligament

Roof
It is formed by the arched fibres of
- Internal oblique muscle
- Transversus abdominis muscle

Direction of inguinal canal is downwards, forwards and medially

Contents of Inguinal Canal
1. **Spermatic cord** in male or **round ligament** in female with genital branch of genito- femoral nerve.
2. **Ilioinguinal nerve:** It enters the canal through the posterior wall, about 2.5 cm below and medial to the anterior superior iliac spine. It lies superficial to the spermatic cord.

Structures Passing Through the Superficial Inguinal Ring
1. Ilioinguinal nerve.
2. Spermatic cord or round ligament of uterus.

Structures Passing Through Deep Inguinal Ring
1. Spermatic cord or round ligament of uterus.
2. Genital branch of genitofemoral nerve.

Inguinal canal is meant for the descent of gonads, but due to physiological reasons ovaries remain in the pelvis while the testes pass through the canal and descend into the scrotum.

Rectus Sheath

- It is a fibrous sheath formed by the interdigitating aponeurosis of muscles of the anterior abdominal wall. It encloses the rectus abdominis muscles which lie on both sides of the linea alba.
- **The main muscle which forms the rectus sheath is internal oblique.** It splits and encloses the rectus abdominis extending from costal margin above to midway between umbilicus and pubic symphysis below.
- Rectus sheath has an anterior wall and a posterior wall with a medial margin and a lateral margin.

Formation of Rectus Sheath at Different Levels (Fig. 5.17)

1. **Above costal margin**

    Anterior wall : Aponeurosis of external oblique muscle.

    Posterior wall : 5, 6, 7th costal cartilages.

2. **Costal margin to midway between the umbilicus and symphysis pubis.**

    Anterior wall : Aponeurosis of external oblique and anterior lamella of internal oblique muscle.

    Posterior wall : Posterior lamella of internal oblique and transversus abdominus muscle.

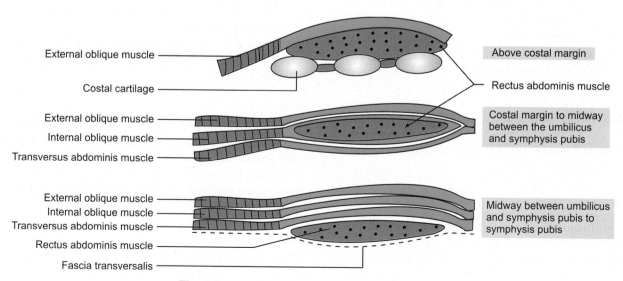

Fig. 5.17: Rectus sheath formation at different level

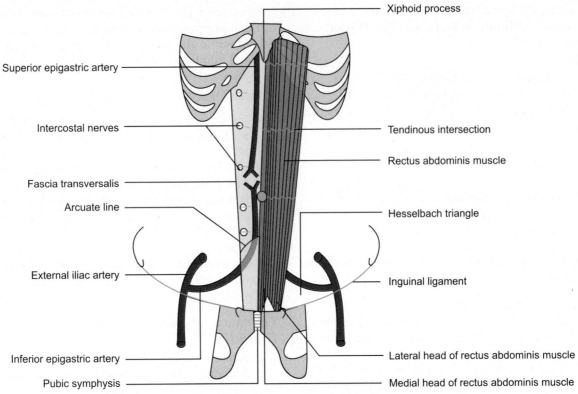

Fig. 5.18: Contents of rectus sheath

3. **Midway between umbilicus and symphysis pubis to symphysis pubis.**
   Anterior wall   :   Aponeurosis of external oblique, internal oblique and transversus abdominis muscles.
   Posterior wall   :   Fascia transversalis (Thompson's ligament)
   Medial Margin   :   It is formed by linea alba

Contents of Rectus Sheath (Fig. 5.18)

1. Rectus abdominis muscle
2. Pyramidalis muscle
3. Superior epigastric vessels
4. Inferior epigastric vessels
5. Lower 5 intercostal nerves
6. Subcostal nerve

Neurovascular bundle of the rectus sheath lies below the rectus abdominus muscle and anastomosis between superior epigastric and inferior epigastric arteries lies in the rectus muscle substance.

Linea Alba

It is a fibrous band which extends in the midline of anterior abdominal wall from xiphoid process above to pubic symphysis below. It is formed by interdigitation of fibres of aponeurosis of external oblique, internal oblique and transversus abdominis muscles.

Expansions of Linea Alba

1. **Suspensory ligament of penis:** Linea alba fibres are attached to the dorsal surface of penis to form the suspensory ligament of penis
2. **Adminiculum linea alba:** Deep fibres which are attached to pubic crest are known as adminiculum linea alba.

Lateral margin of rectus sheath

* Formed by a curved fibrous line extends from tip of 9th costal cartilage to pubic tubercle is known as **linea semilunaris.**
* Ventral rami of lower 6 thoracic nerves (intercostal nerves) enter rectus sheath after passing through linea semilunaris

Umbilicus

Umbilicus represents the attachment of fetal end of umbilical cord. In early part of intrauterine life this acts as a connecting stalk. In embryonic and early fetal life umbilicus transmits umbilical vessels vitello intestinal duct and allantois. In adult these structures either disappear completely or leave their remnants.

Posterior Abdominal Wall

The posterior wall of the abdomen is made up of three components namely bony, muscular and fascial parts (Fig. 5.19).

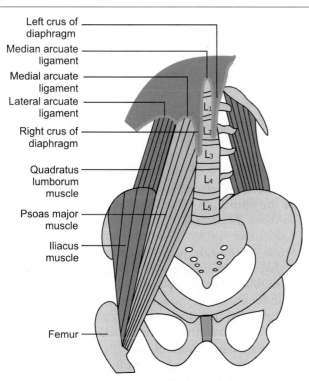

Left crus of diaphragm
Median arcuate ligament
Medial arcuate ligament
Lateral arcuate ligament
Right crus of diaphragm
Quadratus lumborum muscle
Psoas major muscle
Iliacus muscle
Femur

L1
L2
L3
L4
L5

Fig. 5.19: Posterior wall of the abdomen

1. **Bony part:** It lies in the midline and made up of
   a. Inner surface of lower ribs
   b. 5 lumbar vertebrae
   c. Iliac fossa and alae of sacrum
2. **Muscular part:** Medial to lateral side muscles are
   a. Psoas major.
   b. Psoas minor (sometimes)
   c. Quadratus lumborum
   d. Aponeurotic origin of transversus abdominis
   e. Iliacus—(below the iliac crest)
3. **Fascia**
   a. **Thoraco lumbar fascia:** This is also known as lumbar fascia. It is made up of three layers namely: anterior, middle and posterior.
      Muscles enclosed by thoraco-lumbar fascia
      — **Quadratus lumborum:** Between anterior and middle layer.
      — **Errector spinae:** Between middle and posterior layer.
   b. **Fascia iliacus:** This sheet of fascia encloses the iliacus and psoas major muscles.
      It is divided into two parts
      — Iliac part
      — Psoas part

Structures Related to Posterior Abdominal Wall

1. **Blood Vessels**
   a. Abdominal aorta and its branches.
   b. Inferior vena cava and its tributaries.

   c. Ascending lumbar vein.
   d. Lumbar azygos vein.
2. **Lymphatics**
   a. Cisterna chyli.
   b. Para-aortic group of lymph nodes.
   c. Pre-aortic group of lymph nodes.
   d. External iliac group of lymph node.
3. **Nerves**
   a. Lumbar plexus.
   b. Lumbosacral trunk.
   c. Subcostal nerve.
   d. Sympathetic trunk.
4. **Viscera**
   a. Kidney and ureter.
   b. Suprarenal glands.
   c. Duodenum.
   d. Pancreas.

ABDOMINAL CAVITY

It is the cavity enclosed within the abdominal wall. It is lined by peritoneum which consists of a single layer of epithelial cells known as mesothelium with a thin connective tissue layer.

PERITONEUM

Peritoneum is a large serous sac which lines the inner surface of the abdomino-pelvic wall and is invaginated by viscera from different sides. These invaginations throw the peritoneal sac into folds and forms parietal and visceral layers of peritoneum.

Parietal Peritoneum

* Parietal peritoneum lines the inner surfaces of abdominal and pelvic walls and the undersurface of diaphragm.
* It is seperated from the abdominal wall musculature by extra peritoneal tissue which consists of variable amount of fat, areolar tissue and neurovascular bundle. It is loosely attached except under the diaphragm and linea alba.
* Embryologically, it is derived from somatopleuric mesoderm.
* It derives its blood supply and innervation from the body wall. Due to its somatic innervation it is sensitive to pain.

Visceral Peritoneum

* This lines the outer surfaces of the viscera.
* It is firmly adherent to the viscera and cannot be stripped off.
* It develops from the **splanchnopleuric mesoderm** in the embryo.

CHAPTER-5

- It derives its blood supply and nerve supply from the underlying viscera itself. It is insensitive to painful stimuli due to its autonomic innervation. However, pain does occur when it gets stretched over a distended or enlarged viscera.

Functions of the Peritoneum

- The neurovascular bundle is carried along the peritoneal folds to the organs.
- It facilitates movement of viscera by reducing friction.
- It prevents spread of infection. The greater omentum wraps around an inflamed organ to contain the infection. **Greater omentum is known as the policeman of abdomen.**
- Phagocytes and lymphocytes that are present in the tissue provide local cellular and humoral immunity against infection.
- Aids the transfer of oocyte shed from ovary into the uterine tubes
- It has great absorbtive power and can be used to treat local cancers by injecting drugs.
- Peritoneal dialysis is helpful in patients with kidney failure to remove urea.

Peritoneal Cavity

- It is the potential space between the parietal and visceral peritoneum.
- Peritoneal cavity is a closed sac in males. In females however, the cavity communicates to the exterior via the ostia of uterine tubes.
- It contains minimal serous fluid made up of water electrolytes, proteins, few epithelial cells and phagocytes. Normally there is no gas in the cavity.
- Peritoneal cavity is primarily made up of two intercommunicating sacs
  1. **Greater sac (Figs 5.20, 5.22 and 5.23):** It is the larger sac and extends from the diaphragm to the pelvic floor.
  2. **Lesser sac (omental bursa):** It is the smaller sac present behind stomach and liver and opens into the greater sac via the omental foramen.

Peritoneal Folds

- These are folds of the peritoneum which suspend the viscera in the peritoneal cavity.
- The ventral mesentery of alimentary tract mostly disappears during intra-uterine development and the organs are suspended from posterior abdominal wall by remnants of dorsal mesentery.
- They maintain the mobility of the viscera and provide passage for the neurovascular supply to the organ.

Types of Peritoneal Folds

1. **Omenta:** These connect stomach to other organs.
2. **Mesenteries:** These suspend the intestine from the abdominal parieties.
3. **Ligaments:** e.g. gastrosplenic ligament, lienorenal ligament.
4. **Other folds:** e.g. right and left gastro-pancreatic fold, paraduodenal fold, ileo-caecal fold etc.

Vertical Disposition of Peritoneum

For the convenience of study, the peritoneum is traced from the umbilicus (Figs 5.20 and 5.21).

1. Above the umbilicus, the parietal peritoneum lining the inner surface of anterior abdominal wall gives rise to the **falciform ligament.** This is a sickle shaped fold of peritoneum which extends from the midline of inner or posterior surface of anterior abdominal wall and attaches to the antero-superior surface of liver between the anatomical right and left lobes. It continues on the right and left with the visceral peritoneum of liver.
2. The inferior free margin of the falciform ligament contains the ligamentum teres. This is the obliterated left umbilical vein that extends from umbilicus to a notch on inferior border of liver.
3. At the posterior end, falciform ligament diverges into a right and left layer. The right layer is continuous with superior layer of coronary ligament and the left layer is continuous with the anterior layer of left triangular ligament.
4. Parietal peritoneum is reflected from the diaphragm on to the upper part of posterior surface of right lobe of liver in the form of **superior layer of coronary ligament** and **inferior layer of coronary ligament** enclosing a non peritoneal bare area. The peritoneum from superior layer of coronary ligament is then reflected on the superior, right and anterior surface of the right lobe of liver. The peritoneum from inferior layer of coronary ligament is reflected to the inferior surface of liver and also passes on to the right kidney and suprarenal on posterior abdominal wall. **This part is named hepatorenal ligament.**
5. A triangular area present on the posterior surface of right lobe of liver, between the two layers of coronary ligament, is not covered by the peritoneum. This is called the **bare area of liver** and is bounded by
   a. Superior layer of coronary ligament
   b. Inferior layer of coronary ligament
   c. Right triangular ligament
   d. Groove for inferior vena cava.
6. The two layers of coronary ligament fuse on the extreme right to form a small V-shaped fold, the

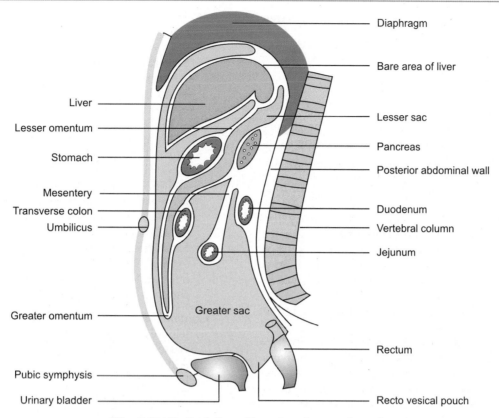

Fig. 5.20: Vertical disposition of peritoneum in male

right triangular ligament. This extends till the diaphragm and right postero-lateral abdominal wall.

7. On the left side, the inferior layer of coronary ligament from the upper part of hepatic groove for inferior vena cava continues over the caudate lobe till the right margin of fissure for ligamentum venosum. It is here that it forms the **posterior layer of lesser omentum**. Potential space between inferior layer of coronary ligament, visceral over caudate lobe and posterior layer of lesser omentum is known as **superior omental recess.**

8. **Hepatorenal pouch or Morrison's pouch:** The inferior layer of coronary ligament, when traced below, is reflected onto the right kidney, second part of duodenum and right colic flexure. This encloses the Morrison's pouch or hepatorenal pouch.

Boundaries

Anteriorly : Inferior surface of right lobe of liver, inferior surface of gall bladder.

Posteriorly : Right suprarenal gland, upper part of right kidney, 2nd part of duodenum, hepatic flexure of colon, transverse mesocolon, part of head of pancreas.

Superiorly : Inferior layer of coronary ligament.
Inferiorly : It opens into the general peritoneal cavity.

• Peritoneum from the hepatorenal pouch continues downwards over the front and sides of the ascending colon and caecum. A right paracolic gutter is formed as the peritoneum reflex to the right antero-lateral abdominal wall.

• **Left triangular ligament:** Peritoneum is reflected from under surface of diaphragm to the superior border of left lobe of liver forming anterior and posterior leaves of left triangular ligament. Medially, it continues with left layer of falciform ligament and laterally it is continues with left layer of lesser omentum at the upper end of fissure for ligamentum venosum.

9. **Lesser Omentum (Fig. 5.20)**
• The peritoneum covering the liver is reflected from inferior surface of liver to the lesser curvature of stomach and the adjoining 1.25cm of first part of duodenum below. This forms the lesser omentum.

• It is attached above in a L-shaped manner, vertical limb arises from margins of fissure for ligamentum venosum and horizontal limb arises from margins of porta-hepatis.

- It has an **anterior and posterior layer with a free margin on the right side.**
- Contents of the free margin from anterior to posterior
  1. Hepatic artery
  2. Bile duct
  3. Portal vein
- Inferiorly, at the lesser curvature, the two layers split to enclosed the stomach continuing as its visceral covering.

10. **Greater Omentum (Figs 5.20 and 5.23)**
    - It is the large peritoneal fold made up of four layers.
    - The 1st and 2nd layer are formed by the peritoneum which descends from the greater curvature of stomach and adjoining 1st part of duodenum. These layer decend down to a variable distance and fold upon themselves to form the 3rd and 4th layer.
    - **The space between 2nd and 3rd layer is the continuation of lesser sac.** It is mostly obliterated due to fusion of the two layers.
    - The greater omentum thus hangs down like a thick curtain of variable length from the stomach. The 4th layer in its uppermost part is fused to transverse colon and mesocolon.

    Contents of Greater Omentum
    1. Right and left gastroepiploic vessels
    2. Fat

    Functions of Greater Omentum
    - It limits the spread of infection from an organ by embracing it and sealing it off from the surrounding areas.
    - It acts as a storehouse of fat.

11. **Transverse mesocolon**
    - It is a fold of peritoneum that suspends the transverse colon from the posterior abdominal wall.
    - Its attachment extends in front of second part of duodenum, head and neck of pancreas, duodeno-jejunal junction and upper pole of left kidney.
    - It continues over the anterior and inferior surfaces of the transverse colon. Superior layer is fused with 4th layer of greater omentum and inferior layer continues back to the abdominal wall.
    - It contains the vessels (middle colic) and lymphatics supplying the transverse colon.

12. **Mesentery (Fig. 5.20)**
    - It is a broad, fan shaped fold of peritoneum that suspends the jejunum and ileum from the posterior abdominal wall.
    - It consists right and left layer which is attached to the posterior abdominal wall and form the **root of mesentery.**

- The root of mesentery is 6 inches long and extends from the duodenojejunal flexure (level of L_2 vertebra) to the right sacroiliac joint.
  Structures crossed by the root of mesentery
  — 3rd part of duodenum
  — Abdominal aorta
  — Inferior vena cava
  — Right ureter
  — Right psoas major muscle
- Right layer continues superiorly towards ascending colon and is continuous with the inferior layer of transverse mesocolon. Inferiorly it invests the coils of jejunum and ileum and folds back to the posterior abdominal wall as the left layer.
- From the root of mesentery the peritoneum extends vertically downwards on to the posterior abdominal wall over the descending and sigmoid colon.

Contents of root of mesentery
1. Jejunal and ileal branches of superior mesenteric vessels
2. Autonomic nerve plexus
3. Lymphatics
4. Fat: It is most abundant near the root of mesentery and in upper part.

13. **Sigmoid mesocolon**
    — It is an inverted V-shaped fold of peritoneum that connects sigmoid colon to lower abdominal wall.
    — Apex of the V lies at the point of division of left common iliac artery into its terminal branches. Right limb extends along left psoas major muscle while left limb extends into pelvis upto S_3 vertebral level.
    — It contains sigmoid and superior rectal vessels, nerves and lymphatics.
    — It then passes down over the rectum and covers the anterior 2/3rd of rectum.

14. **In males** the peritoneum gets reflected from the rectum to the superior surface of the bladder forming a potential space known as recto-vescical space. Further, it passes forwards to line the anterior parietes back to the umbilicus.
    In females, the peritoneum from the anterior surface of rectum is reflected over the upper part of posterior surface of vagina and encloses a potential space called rectouterine pouch. It further extends upwards to cover successively, the posterior surface, fundus and anterior surface of the uterus. Anteriorly at the junction of uterus and cervix, the peritoneum passes forwards over the superior surface of bladder to enclosed vesico-uterine pouch. It then reflected to posterior surface of anterior abdominal wall.

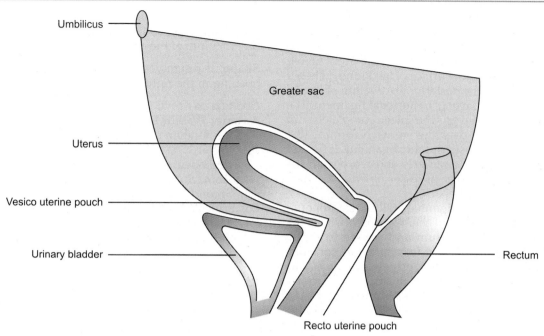

Fig. 5.21: Vertical disposition of peritoneum in pelvis in female

Pouch of Douglas or Rectouterine Pouch

It is the most dependant part of the pelvic peritoneal cavity in females in standing position (Fig. 5.21).

Boundaries

Anteriorly	:	Cervix (supravaginal part), Posterior fornix of vagina.
Posteriorly	:	Middle 1/3rd of rectum.
Floor	:	Formed by the fold of peritoneum passing from rectum to the uterus anteriorly. It lies 5.5 cm above the anus or 7.5 cm above the vaginal introitus.

15. The visceral peritoneum over the urinary bladder is reflected back under the lower part of anterior abdominal wall it raises 5 elevations as follows: From medial to lateral side they are (Fig. 5.23)
    a. **One median umbilical fold:** It extends from umbilicus to apex of urinary bladder. It is formed due to presence of urachus.
    b. **Two medial umbilical folds:** These elevation extend from umbilicus to internal iliac arteries on each side. They are formed due to presence of obliterated umbilical arteries.
    c. **Two lateral umbilical folds:** These folds extend from umbilicus to external iliac arteries. They are formed due to presence of inferior epigastric vessels.

Between median and medial umbilical fold lies supra vesical fossa, between medial and lateral umbilical fold lies medial inguinal fossa. Lateral to lateral umbilical fold lies lateral inguinal fossa.

Horizontal Disposition of Peritoneum

It is divided into two parts and is described below (Figs 5.22 and 5.23).

Right Side

1. **Above the transverse colon:** When traced from the parietal attachment of falciform ligament the peritoneum lines the anterolateral surface of the abdominal wall and is reflected over the superior surface of the liver as the superior layer of coronary ligament. This continues over the anterior and inferior surfaces of the liver and is traced down as the inferior layer of coronary ligament. From here it is reflected over anterior surface of right kidney and part of suprarenal gland. It then continues over the inferior vena cava **forming the posterior boundary of epiploic foramen.**

2. **Below the transverse colon:** The parietal peritoneum of the infra umbilical part of the anterior abdominal wall can be traced laterally and then posteriorly over the quadratus lumborum and is reflected over the front and sides of ascending colon and caecum. It forms the right paracolic gutter which communicates with the hepatorenal pouch above. It then passes over the right psoas major muscle, right ureter and 2nd and 3rd parts of duodenum. As it reaches the inferior vena cava and abdominal aorta, it continues with the right layer of mesentery.

Left Side

1. From the left layer of falciform ligament the peritoneum covers the anterolateral surface of abdominal wall and continues over the left lobe of

liver as the anterior layer of triangular ligament. This continues over the anterior and inferior surface of liver and extends posteriorly and forms the posterior layer of triangular ligament. From here it extends over anterior surface of left kidney. Then it is reflected onto the posterior lip of hilum of spleen to form posterior layer of **lieno-renal ligament.** The peritoneum then invests the spleen completely and passes anteriorly over the stomach forming the anterior layer of **gastrosplenic ligament.** It further covers the stomach anteriorly and reaches on the right as anterior layer of lesser omentum which passes to the porta hepatis.

2. From the anterior abdominal wall the peritoneum is reflected laterally and then posteriorly over the left quadratus lumborum and passes over the descending colon. Here it forms the left paracolic further that communicates with pelvic cavity below. It passes over the left psoas major muscle, ureter and continues as the left layer of mesentery over the abdominal aorta.

Lesser Sac

It is also known as the **omental bursa.** It presents as a diverticulum of the greater sac (Figs 5.20, 5.22 and 5.23).

Shape: It resembles an empty hot water bag with an opening in the right margin.

Boundaries

Anterior Wall of Lesser Sac
1. Peritoneum covering caudate lobe of liver.
2. Posterior layer of lesser omentum.
3. Peritoneum covering the postero-inferior surface of stomach.
4. Second layer of greater omentum.

Posterior Wall of Lesser Sac
1. Third layer of greater omentum.
2. Peritoneum covering the anterosuperior surface of transverse mesocolon.
3. Superior layer of transverse mesocolon

Right Margin of Lesser Sac
1. Below transverse colon, right free margin of greater omentum.

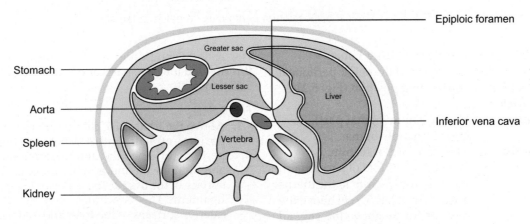

Fig. 5.22: Horizontal disposition of peritoneum at the level of epiploic formen

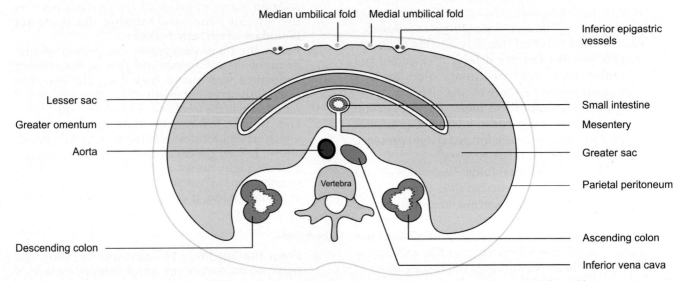

Fig. 5.23: Horizontal section at the level of infracolic compartment to show horizontal disposition

2. **Epiploic foramen:** This lies above the level of transverse colon. This connects the greater sac to the lesser sac.

Boundaries of Epiploic Foramen (Fig. 5.22)

Anterior	:	Right free margin of lesser omentum
Posterior	:	Inferior vena cava, right suprarenal, T_{12} vertebra.
Superior	:	Caudate process of liver with its peritoneal covering.
Inferior	:	Peritoneum over the first part of duodenum.

Left Margin of Lesser Sac
1. Left free margin of greater omentum
2. Gastrosplenic and lieno-renal ligament
3. Gastrophrenic ligament

Upper Margin of Lesser Sac

It is formed by the peritoneum which is reflected from the diaphragm to the upper end of caudate lobe of liver.

Lower Margin of Lesser Sac

It is formed by the lower margin of greater omentum. In adults due to fusion of 2nd and 3rd layers of greater omentum the lower part of lesser sac extends only upto the transverse colon.

Organs covered by peritoneum of lesser sac
1. Caudate lobe of liver
2. Posteroinferior surface of stomach
3. Proximal part of 1st part of duodenum
4. Antero superior surface of transverse colon
5. Anterior surface of neck, body and tail of pancreas
6. Upper part of anterior surface of left suprarenal gland
7. Gastric area of left kidney

Rest of the organs are covered by peritoneum of greater sac.

PELVIS

- Pelvis is the region which lies below the abdomen and consists of structures enclosed within the two hip bones and sacrum.
- **Pelvic cavity** is a bowl shaped cavity enclosed within the hip bones and sacrum. It continues above with the abdominal cavity at the pelvic inlet. Pelvic inlet is formed by sacral promontory, ala of sacrum ileopectineal line and pubic symphysis on each side. It is separated from the perineum below by the pelvic diaphragm.
- It contains the bladder, rectum and anal canal and reproductive tracts of male or female.
- **Pelvic diaphragm:** It is a gutter shaped thin sheet of muscular partition that separates the pelvic cavity from perineum. This forms floor of pelvic cavity. It is formed by two muscles namely levator ani and coccygeus and the fasciae covering them (Fig. 4.9)

PERINEUM

It is a diamond shaped space between the upper part of two thighs lying below the pelvic diaphragm. It fills the pelvic outlet (Fig. 5.24).

Boundaries

Anteriorly: Lower border of symphysis pubis, arcuate pubic ligament.
Posteriorly: Tip of coccyx.

On Each Side
Anterolaterally: Ischiopubic rami, Ischial tuberosities
Postero-laterally: Sacrotuberous ligament

Perineum is divided into anal triangle posteriorly and urogenital triangle anteriorly by an imaginary line passing through the ischial tuberosities.

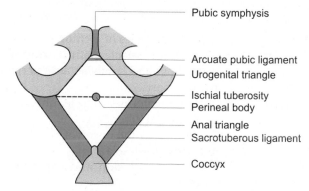

Fig. 5.24: Perineum

ANAL TRIANGLE (FIG. 5.24)

Boundaries

Anteriorly: Line joining the ischial tuberosities
Posteriorly: Tip of coccyx.
On each side: Sacrotuberous ligament
Structures present in anal triangle-(below upward)
1. Skin
2. Superficial fascia
3. Deep fascia
4. Perineal body
5. Terminal part of anal canal
6. Sphincter ani externus
7. Ano coccxygeal ligament
8. Ischiorectal fossa

Perineal Body
- It lies at the centre point of the perineum.
- It is a fibromuscular pyramidal shaped node, located in the median plane, 1.25 cm anterior to the anal orifice.
- It receives the insertion of the following nine perineal muscles.
    1. Levator ani muscle—from both sides.
    2. Sphincter urethrae.
    3. Transverse perinei profundus muscle—from both sides.
    4. Deep part of external sphinter ani.
    5. Bulbospongiosus.
    6. Superficial transverse perinei muscle—from both sides.

ISCHIORECTAL FOSSA

It is a wedge shaped space on each side of the anal canal below the pelvic diaphragm. The apex of the fossa is upwards. The base is present downwards and superficially (Fig. 5.25).

Function: It is filled with fat which acts as an elastic cushion to allow expansion of the rectum and anal canal during defaecation.

Boundaries

The medial boundary is directed upwards and laterally. The lateral boundary is vertical.

Structures forming the boundaries of ischiorectal fossa

Medially	:	Levator ani muscle with its inferior fascia above and sphincter ani externus in lower part.
Laterally	:	Obturator internus muscle, obturator fascia, ischial tuberosity.
Apex	:	It is formed by the fusion of anal fascia and obturator fascia.
Base	:	It is formed by skin and superficial fascia.
Anteriorly	:	It is limited by the superficial and deep perinei muscles with intervening perineal membrane.
Posteriorly	:	Sacrotuberous ligament covered by lower fibres of gluteus maximus.

Spaces and Canals of the Fossa

1. **Pudendal canal:** It is also known as **Alcock's canal:** It lies in relation to lateral wall of the ischiorectal fossa and may be formed by splitting of obturator fascia or separation of lunate and obturator fascia. It extends from lesser sciatic foramen to the posterior limit of deep perineal pouch.

   Contents of the canal
   a. Pudendal nerve
   b. Internal pudendal vessels Pudendal nerve divides within the canal to give rise to the dorsal nerve of penis and perineal nerve

2. **Supra tentorial space:** Lies between apex of the fossa and tegmentum of lunate fascia. It contains loose fat.

3. **Ischio rectal space:** Superiorly bounded by fascia lunata and below by perianal fascia. It contains fat with delicate intervening septae. Hence, there is minimal pain in case of an abscess.

4. **Perianal space:** Superiorly bounded by perianal fascia and below by perianal skin. It is subdivided into compartments by fibroelastic septae. The compartments contain fat. Perianal space of both the sides communicate with each other.

Contents of Ischiorectal Fossa

1. Pudendal nerve
2. Internal pudendal vessels
3. Inferior rectal nerve and vessels
4. Posterior scrotal (or labial in female) nerves and vessels
5. Perineal branch of 4th sacral nerve
6. Perforating branches of S_2, S_3 nerves
7. Pad of fat

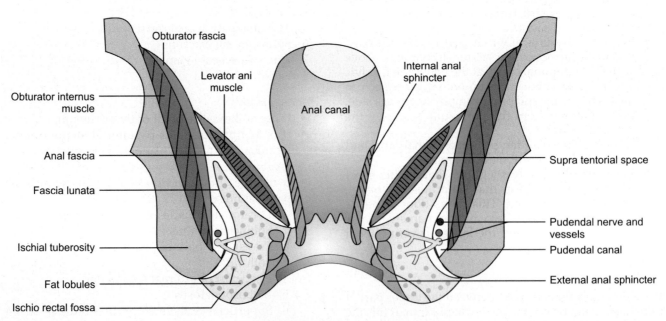

Fig. 5.25: Ischio rectal fossa

UROGENITAL TRIANGLE (FIG. 5.24)

Boundaries

Anteriorly	:	Pubic symphysis with arcuate pubic ligament
Posteriorly	:	An imaginary horizontal line joining two ischial tuberosities
On each side	:	Ischio-pubic rami

Structures present in urogenital triangle—Anterior to posterior

1. **Skin**
   — In males, a median raphae is present which is continuous with the median raphae of scrotum.
   — In females, a median cleft is present known as vestibule.
2. **Fatty layer of superficial fascia**
3. **Membranous layer of superficial fascia or colles fascia:** It is the continuation of membranous layer of superficial fascia of anterior abdominal wall.

   Extent

In front	:	Continuous with dartos muscle of scrotum, fascia of penis and fascia of anterior abdominal wall.
Behind	:	Continuous with posterior margin of perineal membrane
On each side	:	Attached to ischio-pubic ramus at the lower margin

   Structures piercing the Colles fascia
   a. Perineal branch of posterior femoral cutaneous nerve.
   b. In female, urethra and vagina and in male urethra only.

4. **Contents of superficial perineal pouch**
5. **Perineal membrane:** It is the inferior fascia of urogenital diaphragm extends across the pubic arch

   Extent

In front	:	Thickened to form transverse perineal ligament it is continuous with superior fascia of urogenital diaphragm around sphincter urethrae.
Behind	:	Attached to perineal body and split into two layers, get attached to deep transverse perinei and superficial transverse perinei muscles.
On each side	:	Inner surface of ischio pubic ramus above the attachment of crus perinei

   Structures pierce the perineal membrane (Fig. 5.26)
   a. Dorsal artery of the penis or clitoris
   b. Deep artery of penis or clitoris
   c. Artery to the bulb of penis or clitoris
   d. Duct of bulbo urethral gland in male
   e. Membranous urethra in male, urethra and vagina in female
   f. 2 posterior scrotal or labial nerves and vessels on each side
   g. The oval gap between arcuate pubic ligament and transverse perineal ligament transmits the deep dorsal vein of penis and dorsal nerve of penis.

6. **Contents of deep perineal pouch.**
7. **Superior fascia of urogenital diaphragm**

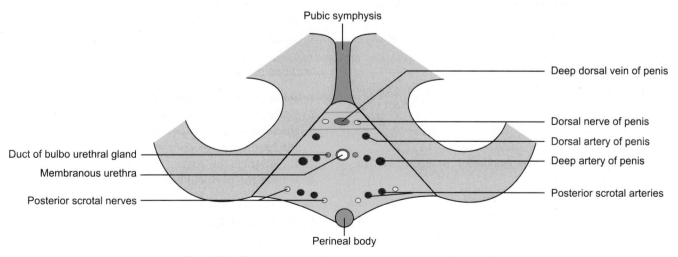

Fig. 5.26: Structures piercing perineal membrane (in male)

Superficial Perineal Space

It is an interfascial space which lies in the urogenital triangle of perineum (Figs, 5.27 and 5.28).

Boundaries

Superiorly	: Perineal membrane
Inferiorly	: Colles fascia
On each side	: Inner surface of ischio-pubic ramus
Anteriorly	: Continuous with superficial inguinal space in anterior abdominal wall, fascia of penis and scrotum
Posteriorly	: Pouch is closed by fusion of Colles fascia with perineal membrane around superficial transverse perinei muscle

Contents of Superficial Perineal Space

1. **Muscles:** Total six in number, three on each side.
   a. Ischiocavernosus
   b. Superficial transverse perinei
   c. Bulbospongiosus
2. **Arteries and veins:** Six in number, three on each side.
   a. Two posterior scrotal or labial vessels, branch of internal pudendal vessel.
   b. Transverse perineal vessels, branches of scrotal or internal pudendal.
3. **Nerves:** Six in number, three on each side.
   a. Two posterior scrotal or labial nerves branches of perineal nerve.
   b. Perineal branch of posterior femoral cutaneous nerve.
4. Crus penis or clitoridis, attached on each side of the ischio-pubic ramus.
5. Bulb of penis with urethra in male.
6. Urethra and vagina in female, with bulb of vestibule and greater vestibular glands present on each side of the vagina.

Deep Perineal Space

It is an interfascial space that lies superior to the perineal membrane in the urogenital triangle of perineum (Figs 5.27 and 5.28).

Boundaries

Superiorly	: Superior fascia of urogenital diaphragm.
Inferiorly	: Perineal membrane.
Posteriorly	: Fusion of perineal membrane with superior fascia of urogenital diaphragm.
Anteriorly	: Transverse perineal ligament.
On each side	: Inner surface of ischiopubic ramus.

Contents of Deep Perineal Space

1. **Muscles:** Two in number
   a. Sphincter urethrae
   b. Deep transverse perinei
2. **Vessels:** Internal pudendal artery and its branches
   a. Deep artery of penis or clitoris
   b. Dorsal artery of penis or clitoris
   c. Artery to bulb of penis or vestibule
3. **Nerves:** Dorsal nerve of penis or clitoris
4. Membranous urethra
5. Bulbo-urethral glands and ducts in male
6. Urethra and vagina in female

UROGENITAL DIAPHRAGM

It is a musculo fascial partition which separates the pelvic cavity from anterior part of outlet. It is made up of a sheet of muscles namely, sphincter urethrae and a pair of deep transverse perinei. This sheet is covered by condensations of pelvic connective tissue which forms fascia covering the muscles and are named as
1. Superior fascia of urogenital diaphragm
2. Inferior fascia of urogenital diaphragm (perineal membrane)

Structures Piercing the Diaphragm

1. Urethra in male
2. Urethra and vagina in female

Superior Relations of Urogenital Diaphragm

1. Apex of prostate in male or neck of urinary bladder in female
2. Anterior fibres of both levator ani muscles
3. Anterior recesses of ischiorectal fossae

Functions of Urogenital Diaphragm

1. It supports the prostate or bladder
2. Sphincter urethrae exerts voluntary control of micturation, and expels the last drop of urine after the bladder stops contraction
3. It constricts the vagina in female
4. It fixes the perineal body

PELVIC DIAPHRAGM

Described in muscular system (see page no. 179).

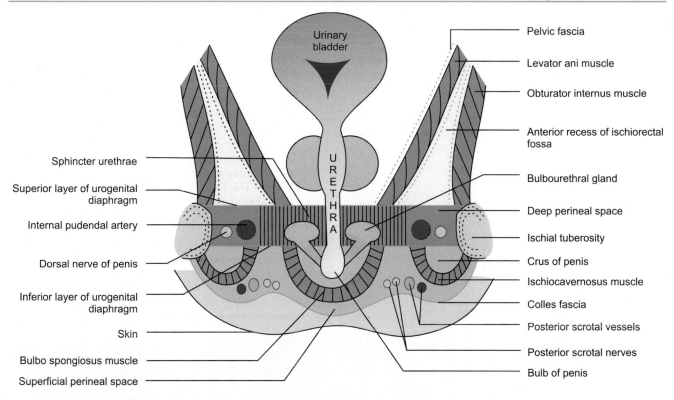

Urinary bladder

Pelvic fascia

Levator ani muscle

Obturator internus muscle

Anterior recess of ischiorectal fossa

Sphincter urethrae

URETHRA

Bulbourethral gland

Superior layer of urogenital diaphragm

Deep perineal space

Internal pudendal artery

Ischial tuberosity

Dorsal nerve of penis

Crus of penis

Ischiocavernosus muscle

Inferior layer of urogenital diaphragm

Colles fascia

Posterior scrotal vessels

Skin

Posterior scrotal nerves

Bulbo spongiosus muscle

Bulb of penis

Superficial perineal space

Fig. 5.27: Coronal section of urogenital triangle of male showing deep and superficial perineal spaces

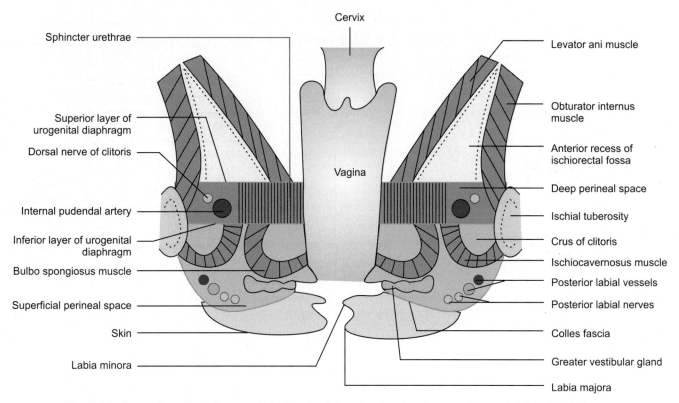

Cervix

Sphincter urethrae

Levator ani muscle

Obturator internus muscle

Anterior recess of ischiorectal fossa

Superior layer of urogenital diaphragm

Dorsal nerve of clitoris

Vagina

Deep perineal space

Internal pudendal artery

Ischial tuberosity

Crus of clitoris

Inferior layer of urogenital diaphragm

Ischiocavernosus muscle

Bulbo spongiosus muscle

Posterior labial vessels

Superficial perineal space

Posterior labial nerves

Skin

Colles fascia

Labia minora

Greater vestibular gland

Labia majora

Fig. 5.28: Coronal section of urogenital triangle of female showing deep and superficial perineal spaces

UPPER LIMB

Upper limb is also known as upper extremity. Adaptating to the upright posture in human being, upper limb is the prehensile organ that helps to manipulate the environment for survival and existence. The characteristic feature is the grasping mechanism of the hand. Arm and forearm are meant to increase the range of movement of hand to manipulate the external environment.

Functions of Upper Limb
1. Defence
2. Grasping
3. Tactile apparatus

Parts of Upper Limb

Upper limb can be studied as follows:
1. **Shoulder region:** It is the region in relation to shoulder girdle with the help of which upper limb proper is attached to the trunk. It consists of the following parts:
   a. **Shoulder region:** Region in relation to shoulder girdle with the help of which upper limb proper is attached to the trunk.
   b. **Pectoral region:** It lies on the front of the chest.
   c. **Scapular region:** Part around shoulder joint and over the scapula on the back of the body is the scapular region.

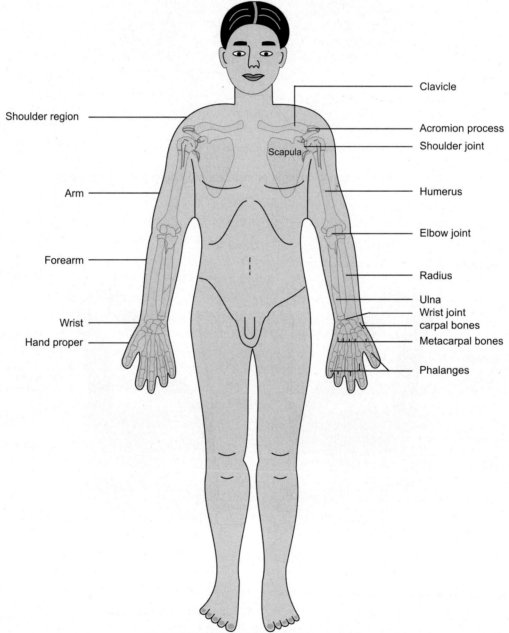

Fig. 5.29: Parts and bones of upper limb

d. **Axilla or arm pit:** Pyramidal space between pectoral region and scapular region is known as axilla or arm pit.

2. **Upper limb proper:** This part of the limb is free and is attached to the trunk with the help of shoulder region. It consists of the following parts:
   a. **Arm:** It extends from shoulder joint to elbow joint.
   b. **Forearm:** It extends from elbow joint to wrist joint.
   c. **Hand:** It is further divided into two parts:
      i. **Wrist:** It is the region in relation to carpal bones.
      ii. **Hand proper:** It is the region in relation to metacarpals, and phalanges.

Skin: Skin of upper limb is hairy except in region of palm.

Superficial Fascia: It consists of fibro-areolar tissue. In the pectoral region it splits to enclose mammary gland. Superficial fascia contains veins, lymphatic and cutaneous nerves

Shoulder region: Region in relation to shoulder girdle with the help of which upper limb proper is attached to the trunk.

Pectoral region or breast region: It lies on the front of the chest

Scapular region: Part around shoulder joint and over the scapula on the back of the body is the scapular region.

Axilla or arm pit: Pyramidal space between pectoral region and scapular region.

Deep fascia: It is modified in the different regions of the upper limb.

Bones Forming Upper Limb

They are thirty-two in number (Fig. 5.29).

Bones and Joints Present in Upper Limb

Region	Bones	Joints
Shoulder region	Clavicle, Scapula	a. Sterno-clavicular joint b. Acromio-clavicular joint
Arm	Humerus	a. Gleno-humeral joint or shoulder joint
Forearm	Radius, Ulna	a. Elbow joint b. Superior radio-ulnar joint c. Middle radio-ulnar joint d. Inferior radio-ulnar joint
Hand	Eight carpals Five metacarpals Fourteen phalanges	a. Wrist joint b. Inter carpal joints c. Carpo metacarpal joints d. Inter metacarpal joints e. Metacarpo-phalangeal joints f. Proximal interpha-langeal joints g. Distal interphalangeal joints

PECTORAL REGION

It lies on the front of the chest.

Skin

Skin of the pectoral region is supplied by medial, intermediate and lateral supraclavicular nerves. The intercosto brachial nerve and anterior and lateral cutaneous branches of second to sixth intercostal nerves also supply skin of pectoral region.

Superficial Fascia

It contains following structures:
   a. Cutaneous nerves as described above.
   b. Cutaneous vessels: They are, perforated branches of internal thoracic artery and lateral cutaneous branches of posterior intercostal artery.
   c. Platysma muscle.
   d. Mammary gland (see page no. 581).

Deep Fascia of Pectoral Region

The deep fascia of pectoral region is given the following names at special sites.
   1. Fascia over deltoid muscle
   2. Subscapular fascia
   3. Supraspinous fascia
   4. Infraspinous fascia
   5. Pectoral fascia
   6. **Clavipectoral fascia:** It is a strong fibrous sheet behind clavicular part of pectoralis major. It covers the axillary vessels and nerves.

Muscles of Pectoral Region

   1. Pectoralis major
   2. Pectoralis minor
   3. Subclavius
   4. Serratus anterior

AXILLA (ARMPIT)

It is a pyramidal shaped space present between the upper part of arm and the lateral thoracic wall. It acts as a passage for the neurovascular bundle from neck to upper limb.

Boundaries (Figs 5.30 and 5.31)

Apex	:	It is triangular in shape and is also called as cervico-axillary canal. It continues upwards into the root of the neck. It is bounded by the following
In front	:	Clavicle.
Behind	:	Superior border of scapula.
Medially	:	Outer border of first rib.

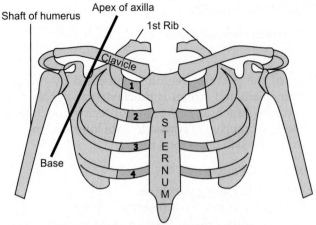

Fig. 5.30: Skeletal boundaries of axilla

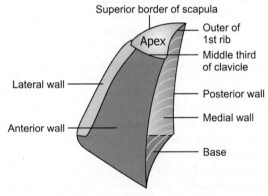

Fig. 5.31: Boundaries of axilla

Base: It is convex upwards and faces downwards. It forms the armpit and is lying by
- Skin and superficial fascia,
- Axillary fascia and suspensory ligament of axilla

Anterior Wall: It is formed by
- Pectoralis major muscle
- Pectoralis minor muscle
- Subclavius muscle

Posterior Wall: It is formed by
- Subscapularis muscle
- Latissimus dorsi muscle
- Teres major muscle

Medial Wall: It is made up of
- Upper 4 or 5 ribs and corresponding intercostal muscles
- Upper part of serratus anterior muscle

Lateral Wall: It is made up of
- Upper 1/3rd of humerus.
- Biceps brachii muscle.
- Coracobrachialis muscle

Contents of Axilla

1. Axillary artery and its branches (see page no. 417).
2. Axillary vein and its tributaries (see page no. 433).
3. Cords of brachial plexus and their branches (see page no. 246).

4. Axillary lymph nodes and their afferent and efferent connections (see page no. 473).
5. Axillary fat and occasionally axillary tail of the breast.

SHOULDER REGION

Region in relation to shoulder girdle with the help of which upper limb proper is attached to the trunk.

SCAPULAR REGION

Part around shoulder joint and over the scapula on the back of the body is the scapular region.

Skin of shoulder region is supplied by

a. **Lateral supraclavicular nerve:** It supplies skin over the upper half of deltoid muscle.
b. **Upper lateral cutaneous nerve of the arm:** It supplies skins over the lower half of deltoid muscle.
c. **Dorsal rami of the upper thoracic nerves:** They supply skin over the back of scapula.

Muscles of Scapular Region (see page no. 185)

1. Deltoid
2. Supraspinatus
3. Infraspinatus
4. Teres minor
5. Teres major
6. Subscapularis

UPPER BACK

Skin and Fascia

- Skin of upper back is relatively thick as compare to rest of body.
- Superficial fascia in this region is thick and strong with adipose tissue. It is attached to the skin in the region of the neck.
- Cutoneous nerve supply of this region comes from dorsal rami of thoracic spinal nerves. Each dorsal ramus divides into medial and lateral branches. Medial branches of dorsal rami of upper six thoracic spinal nerves supply the skin in upper part while the lateral branches of dorsal rami of lower six thoracic spinal nerves supply the skin in lower part.
- Deep fascia in this region is thin and fibrous.

Superficial Group of Muscles of Upper Back

This group consists of muscles which connect upper limb to the axial skeleton, i.e., skull, ribs and verterbral column (see page no. 185).

1. Trapezius
2. Latissimus dorsi
3. Levator scapulae
4. Rhomboideus major
5. Rhomboideus minor

ARM

Arm extends from shoulder joint to elbow joint.

Deep Fascia of Arm

The deep fascia of arm is known as brachial fascia and it continues above with the fascia over deltoid and pectoralis major muscle and below with fascia of fore arm. It gives rise to medial and lateral intermuscular septa which divides the arm into anterior and posterior compartments. The lateral intermuscular septum is attached distally to lateral lip of intertubercular sulcus, lateral supra condylar ridge and lateral epicondyle. It is perforated by radial nerve and radial collateral branch of arteria profunda brachii near the junction of upper 2/3rd and lower 1/3rd. The medial intermuscular septum is attached to medial lip of intertubercular sulcus, medialsupracondylar ridge and medial epicondyle. It is perforated by ulnar nerve and superior ulnar collateral artery (Fig. 5.32).

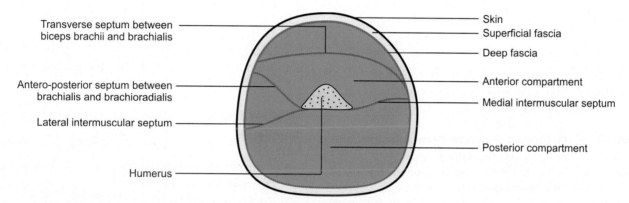

Fig. 5.32: Transverse section through lower 1/3rd of arm showing intermuscular septa and compartments

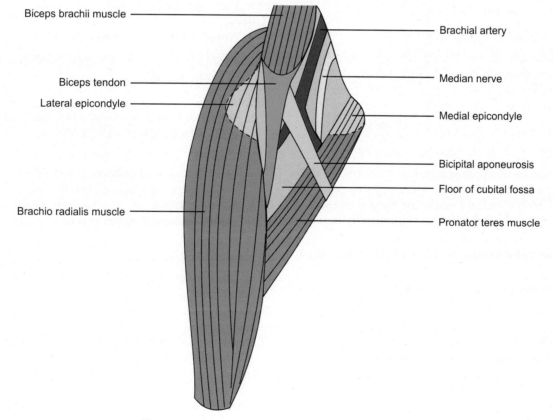

Fig. 5.33: Boundaries and contents of cubital fossa

Contents of Anterior Compartment of Arm (Fig. 5.32)
1. Muscles: Coracobrachialis, biceps brachii, brachialis (see page no. 187)
2. Brachial artery
3. Nerves: Musculorcutaneous, Ulnar, Median

Contents of Posterior Compartment of Arm (Fig. 5.32)
1. Triceps brachii muscle (See page no. 187).
2. Profunda brachii artery.
3. Radial nerve.

CUBITAL FOSSA

It is a triangular space in front of the elbow (Fig. 5.33).

Boundaries

Medially : Lateral border of pronator teres.
Laterally : Medial border of brachioradialis.
Base : An imaginary line joining both epicondyles of humerus.
Apex : Is formed by convergence of brachioradialis and pronator teres.
Floor : Is formed by brachialis, supinator in lower and lateral part.
Roof : Is made up of deep fascia of forearm, bicipital aponeurosis, median cubital vein, medial and lateral cutaneous nerve of forearm.

Contents (Medial to Lateral Side)
1. Median nerve
2. Brachial artery, ulnar and radial artery
3. Biceps tendon
4. Radial nerve

FOREARM

Forearm extends from elbow joint to wrist joint. The deep fascia of forearm is attached to the apex of posterior surface of olecranon and posterior border of ulna. A number of septae extend forward between the muscles and divide the forearm into an anterior or flexor compartment and a posterior or extensor compartment.

Flexor Compartment of Forearm

Boundaries
Posterior
- Anterior surface of radius
- Anterior and medial surfaces of ulna
- Interrosseous membrane
Medial
- Olecranon process
- Posterior border of ulna

Lateral
- Anterior border of radius
Anterior
- Skin and fascia

Contents
1. **Muscles:** They are arranged in superficial, intermediate and deep groups (see page nos 188, 189)
2. **Vessels**
- Radial artery
- Ulnar artery
- Anterior interosseous artery
3. **Nerves**
- Median nerve
- Ulnar nerve
- Superficial division of radial nerve (only sensory)
- Anterior interosseous nerve

Extensor Compartment of Forearm

Boundaries
Anterior
- Posterior surface of radius
- Posterior surface of ulna
- Intervening interosseous membrane
Medial
- Posterior surface of olecranon
- Posterior border of ulna
Lateral
- Anterior border of radius

Posterior
- Skin and fascia

Contents
1. **Muscles:** They are arranged in superficial and deep groups (see page nos 189, 190).
2. **Vessels**
- Posterior interosseous artery
- Anterior interosseous artery, only in lower part
3. **Nerves:** Trunk of radial nerve. Posterior interosseous branch of radial nerve.

Extensor Retinaculum

It is the condensation of deep fascia in the form of a fibrous band.

Attachments
Lateral : Anterior border of radius, just above styloid process.
Medial : Pisiform bone, triquetal bone.

It gives rise to septae from the deep aspect which extend to the radius and medial carpal bones. This forms six osseo-fascial compartments.

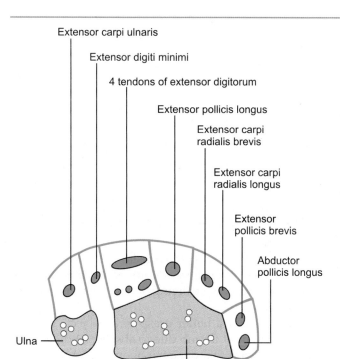

Fig. 5.34: Structures passing deep to extensor retinaculum, seen in transverse section at wrist

Structures passing deep to the extensor retinaculum (Fig. 5.34): From lateral to medial side in each compartment
1. Abductor pollicis longus
   Extensor pollicis brevis
2. Extensor carpi radialis longus
   Extensor carpi radialis brevis
3. Extensor pollicis longus
4. Four tendons of extensor digitorum
   Tendon of extensor indices
5. Tendon of extensor digiti minimi
6. Tendon of extensor carpi ulnaris

Anatomical Snuff Box
Boundaries (Fig. 23.3)
Lateral (Anterior) : Tendon of abductor pollicis longus, tendon of extensor pollicis brevis.
Medial (Posterior) : Tendon of extensor pollicis longus.
Floor : Styloid process of radius, scaphoid, trapezium, base of 1st metacarpal.
Roof : Skin, fascia, cephalic vein, superficial branch of radial nerve.
Content: Radial artery.

HAND
It is divided into two parts
1. Wrist: Region in relation to carpal bones.

2. Hand proper: Region in relation to metacarpals and phalanges.
The hand presents with a palmar and a dorsal surface

Palm of Hand

Skin: It is thick and glabrous. Palmar skin is devoid of hair and sebaceous glands. Has numerous sweat glands. It is immobile because a number of fibrous bands attach it firmly to underlying deep fascia or palmar aponeurosis. Allows for proper grasp and to withstand considerable pressure

Superficial fascia: It contains the following
1. Fat, in numerous small tight compartments.
2. Palmaris brevis, a subcutaneous muscle.
3. Superficial transverse ligament.

Deep fascia: It is thickened and forms three specialized structures namely
1. Flexor retinaculum
2. Palmar aponeurosis
3. Fibrous flexor sheath of digits

Dorsum of Hand

Skin: The skin is thin. It is hairy with sebaceous and sweat glands. It is freely mobile over the deep fascia.

Superficial fascia: It presents a dorsal subcutaneous space which contains the following:
1. Dorsal venous arch–collects blood from dorsal and palmar surfaces of hand.
2. Dorsal digital nerves.

Deep fascia: It is thin and covers extensor tendons of hand. It continues above with extensor retinaculum and on sides with palmar fascia.

Flexor Retinaculum

It is the modification of deep fascia and forms a strong fibrous band attached to the following carpal bones (Figs 5.35 and 5.36).

Laterally : Tubercle of scaphoid, crest of trapezium.
Medially : Pisiform bone, hook of hamate.

It forms a tunnel over the concave surfaces of carpal bones known as carpal tunnel. It continues above with deep fascia of forearm and below with palmar aponeurosis.

Structures passing superficial to flexor retinaculum (Fig. 5.35): From medial to lateral side.
1. Ulnar nerve
2. Ulnar artery
3. Palmar cutaneous branch of ulnar nerve
4. Palmaris longus tendon

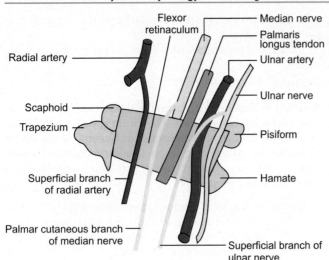

Fig. 5.35: Structures superficial to flexor retinaculum

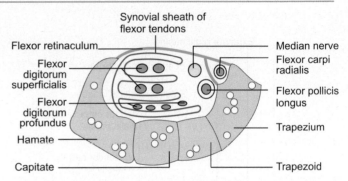

Fig. 5.36: Transverse section of wrist demonstrating carpal tunnel and structures passing deep to flexor retinaculum

5. Palmar cutaneous branch of median nerve
6. Superficial palmar branch of radial artery

Structures passing deep to flexor retinaculum (Fig. 5.36): .
1. Median nerve, lies just below it.
2. Tendons of flexor digitorum superficialis.
3. Tendons of flexor digitorum profundus.
4. Tendon of flexor pollicis longus.
5. Flexor carpi radialis tendon lies between superficial and deep slips of the retinaculum on lateral side.

Palmar Aponeurosis

It is the condensation of deep fascia of palm (Fig. 5.38). It is made up of three parts, namely central, medial and lateral.

Central part: This is the palmar aponeurosis proper. It is thick and triangular in shape. Apex is directed proximally and fuses with flexor retinaculum. Distally, it divides into four digital slips for medial four fingers. Superficial fibres are attached to the dermis and superficial transverse ligament of palm. Deep fibres blend with the fibrous flexor sheaths. Medial and lateral palmar septae extend deep from the respective margins of the central part of palmar aponeurosis.

Medial part: It is thin and covers the hypothenar muscles of palm.

Lateral part: It is thin and covers the thenar muscles of palm. On each side the aponeurosis continues with deep fascia of dorsum of hand.

Functions of Palmar Aponeurosis
1. It protects the palmar neurovascular bundle.
2. It prevents bow-stringing of long tendons of flexor muscles.
3. It allows for a better grasp of an object. The free movement of thumb due to absence of digital slip from it leads to movement of opposition and helps in better grip.

Fibrous Flexor Sheath of Digits (Fig. 5.37A)

Fibrous flexor sheath of digits are formed by condensations of deep fascia which extend over the flexor tendons of forearm. Each sheath extends from the

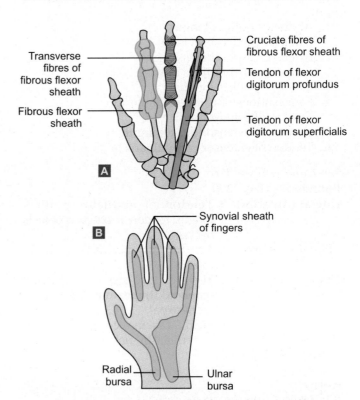

Figs 5.37A and B: (A) Fibrous flexor sheath of digits and (B) Synovial sheath of fingers, radial and ulnar bursae

head of metacarpal bone to base of distal phalanx of each digit. In the thumb it covers the tendon of flexor pollicis longus. In medial four fingers the sheath covers a pair of tendons, flexor digitorum superficialis and flexor digitorum profundus. The fibrous sheath helps to retain the tendons in their position.

Synovial Sheath of Flexor Tendons (Fig. 5.37B)

The flexor tendons in their lower ends are provided with an envelope of synovial sheaths. This helps to prevent friction of the tendons against the osseofibrous canals of lower end of forearm and hand while allowing free movement. In the carpal tunnel two synovial sheaths are present. These are

1. **Radial bursa**: It covers the tendon of flexor pollicis longus.
2. **Ulnar bursa**: It is a common synovial sheath covering the four tendons of flexor digitorum superficialis and four tendons of flexor digitorum profundus.

Digital Synovial Sheaths (Fig. 5.37B)

- Each digit is provided with a tubular synovial sheath covering the flexor tendons. They are present inner to the fibrous flexor sheath.
- In thumb, the synovial sheath encloses tendon of flexor pollicis longus. It continues proximally with radial bursa and distally extends upto attachment of the corresponding tendons.
- In medial four fingers, the tubular sheath covers a each pair of tendons of flexor digitorum superficialis and profundus. The synovial sheath of little finger continues proximally with ulnar bursa. The sheath over 2nd, 3rd and 4th fingers end blindly over head of metacarpal bone.

Vincula Longa and Brevia

These are synovial folds which connect tendons to phalanges. They transmit vessels to the tendons.

Intrinsic Muscles of Hand

See page no. 191.

Fascial Spaces of Hand

Space of parona: It is a potential space present deep to the long flexor tendons of forearm and lined by the fascia of forearm.

Mid palmar space: It is present in the middle of palm betwen medial and intermediate palmar septum and is triangular in shape (Fig. 5.38).

Thenar space: It is also triangular in shape and is present laterally below muscles of thenar eminence. (Fig. 5.38).

Pulp spaces: These spaces intervene between the palmar skin and distal phalanges, lying distal to the fibrous flexor sheath of long flexor tendons. The pulp space of each digit is divided into a number of small compartments by septae which extend from under the skin to the periosteum of the distal phalanx. Each compartment is filled tightly with fat and contains blood vessels and nerves.

Dorsal subcutaneous space: This space lies deep to loose skin of dorsum of hand.

Dorsal subaponeurotic space: This space lies between the metacarpal bones and aponeurosis which connects extensor tendons.

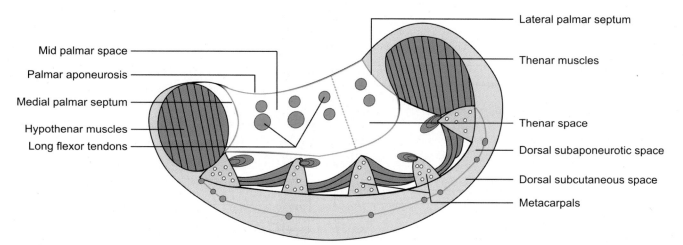

Fig. 5.38: Palmar spaces of hand

LOWER LIMB

Lower limb is also known as inferior extremity. Lower limb is that part of the body which extends from hip and buttock region to toes. It is meant for **locomotion, support and transmitting body weight.** Lower limb is attached to the trunk by the sacro-iliac joint.

Functions of Lower Limb
1. Locomotion
2. Support
3. Transmitting body weight.

The line of centre of gravity passes behind the hip joint but in front of knee and ankle joints.

Parts of Lower Limb (Fig. 5.39)
1. Hip and bottock
2. Thigh
3. Leg
4. Foot and toes

Bones of the Lower Limb—31+2 in Number (Fig. 5.39)
1. Hip bone
2. Femur: bone of thigh

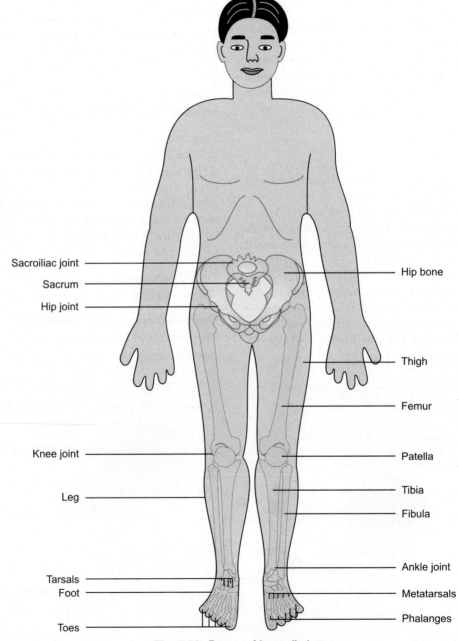

Fig. 5.39: Bones of lower limb

3. Patella
4. Tibia: bone of leg
5. Fibula: bone of leg
6. Tarsal bones—bones of foot
   a. Calcaneus
   b. Talus
   c. Navicular
   d. Cuboid
   e. Cuneiform—three in number
7. 5 Metatarsals—bones of foot
8. 14 Phalanges—bones of foot
9. 2 Seasmoid bones in relation to 1st metatarsal

Main Joints of the Lower Limb

1. Hip joint
2. Knee joint
3. Ankle joint
4. Subtalar joint
5. Joints of the foot

Fascia of Lower Limb

Lower limb has superficial and deep fascia. There are different modifications of deep fascia in different regions of the lower limb.

1. **Superficial fascia:** It is fatty and lobulated. It contains the neurovascular bundle of skin.
2. **Deep fascia:** It is membranous and is modified in various regions.

THIGH

Thigh extends from the hip to knee.

Proximally : It extends anteriorly to groove of groin, posteriorly to gluteal fold, medially upto perineum and laterally upto the hollow on the side of the hip.

Distally : It extends upto knee joint anteriorly and popliteal fossa posteriorly

Superficial Fascia of Thigh

It is made up of loose areolar tissue. It contains
1. Fat
2. Cutaneous nerves
3. Great saphenous vein and its tributaries
4. Cutaneous branches of femoral artery
5. Inguinal lymph nodes with lymph vessels

Deep Fascia of Thigh

It is also known as **fascia lata** because of its wide extent. It is thickened along the lateral surface of the thigh to form the ilio tibial tract. It is modified to form the following:

1. Lateral intermuscular septum
2. Medial intermuscular septum
3. Posterior intermuscular septum (incomplete)
4. Saphenous opening
5. Iliotibial tract

Front of Thigh–Anterior Compartment

It is the region which lies between the medial and lateral intermuscular septum.

Cribriform fascia: It is the deep layer of superficial fascia. It has a sieve like appearance, hence the name cribriform fascia. It covers the saphenous opening.

Saphenous Opening (Fossa Ovalis)

It lies in the deep fascia, fascia lata of thigh (Fig. 5.40). It lies 3 cm below, lateral and inferior to pubic tubercle. It is oval in shape and is a twisted gap. It measures about 3-4 cm vertically. It is covered by cribriform fascia.

Structures passing through saphenous opening
1. Great saphenous vein.
2. Superficial epigastric and external pudendal artery.
3. Lymph vessels.
4. Few branches of medial femoral cutaneous nerves.

Important relation: It lies in relation to the anterior wall of femoral sheath.

Ilio Tibial Tract

It is a modification of deep fascia of thigh. It is in the form of a band about 2.5 cm. wide. Iliotibial tract receives attachment of tensor fascia lata and 3/4th of gluteus maximus muscle.

Actions:
1. When knee is straight, it maintains the knee in extended position.

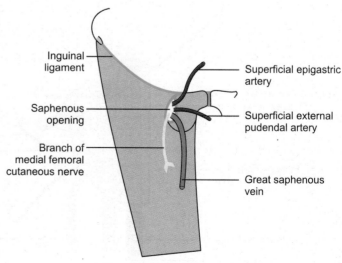

Fig. 5.40: Saphenous opening

2. In semiflexed knee, it exerts an antigravity force to support the knee joint in walking and running.
3. The antigravity pull elongates gluteus maximus which contracts more strongly as the movement proceeds. Therefore iliotibial tract helps in forceful contraction of gluteus maximus in running and walking.

Femoral Sheath

It is a funnel shaped fascial prolongation around proximal part of femoral blood vessels situated in femoral traingle below the inguinal ligament. It is 3 to 4 cm in length (Figs 5.41 and 5.42) and is formed by

Anteriorly : Fascia transversalis.

Posteriorly : Fascia iliacus.

Inferiorly : It merges with perivascular sheath of femoral vessels.

The fascia iliacus and transversalis meet each other at the lateral and medial margins. Lateral margin passes vertical downwards and is perforated by femoral branch of genito femoral nerve. Medial margin slopes downward and laterally, perforated by great saphenous vein.

Contents: Femoral sheath is divided into following three compartments by two septa.
1. **Lateral compartment:** It contains
   a. Femoral artery
   b. Femoral branch of genigofemoral nerve
2. **Middle compartment:** It contains femoral vein
3. **Medial compartment or femoral canal:** It contains

a. Deep inguinal lymph node known as Cloquet's lymph node and lymphatics
b. Fat and aerolar tissue

Functions of Femoral Sheath

It allows femoral vessels to glide freely in and out beneath the inguinal ligament during the movement of hip joint. It is rudimentary in newborn—due to fetal position of flexion.

Femoral Canal

It is the medial compartment of the femoral sheath. It is conical, wider above and narrow below. The wider upper end is known as femoral ring which opens into abdominal cavity (Fig. 5.41).

Dimensions: Length is 1.25 cm, wdth is 1.25 cm

Contents
1. Lymphatics
2. Lymph node
3. Areolar tissue

Boundaries of Femoral Ring
Medially : Lacunar ligament
Anteriorly : Inguinal ligament
Posteriorly : Pectin pubis
Laterally : Septum separating from the femoral vein

Functions of Femoral Canal
• It allows expansion of femoral vein in case of increased venous return.

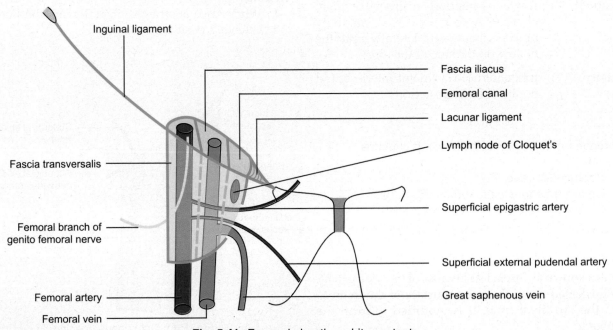

Inguinal ligament

Fascia iliacus

Femoral canal

Lacunar ligament

Lymph node of Cloquet's

Fascia transversalis

Superficial epigastric artery

Femoral branch of genito femoral nerve

Superficial external pudendal artery

Femoral artery

Great saphenous vein

Femoral vein

Fig. 5.41: Femoral sheath and its contents

- There is a communication of lymphatics of lower limb to abdomen through femoral canal via femoral ring.

Femoral Triangle (Fig. 5.42)

It is a triangular depression below the inguinal ligament with the apex directed below, and is present in the upper one-third of the front of thigh.

Boundaries

Base	:	Inguinal ligament.
Apex	:	Meeting point of sartorius and adductor longus muscles.
Medially	:	Medial border of adductor longus.
Laterally	:	Medial border of sartorius
Floor	:	From lateral to medial side it is formed by iliacus, tendon of psoas major, pectineus and adductor longus muscles.

Roof: Fascia lata, superficial fascia, skin.

Contents (Fig. 5.42)

1. Femoral sheath.
2. Femoral artery and its branches.
3. Femoral vein and its tributaries.
4. Deep inguinal lymph nodes.
5. Femoral nerve and its branches.
6. A part of lateral femoral cutaneous nerve.
7. Femoral branch of genito femoral nerve.
8. Some fibro-fatty tissue.

Adductor Canal (Hunter's Canal, Subsartorial Canal)

It is a musculo-aponeurotic tunnel which lies in middle 1/3rd of medial side of thigh. It extends from apex of femoral triangle to 5th osseo-aponeurotic opening of adductor magnus.It is triangular in shape on cross section.

Boundaries

Antero-laterally	:	Vastus medialis muscle.
Posteriorly	:	Adductor longus muscle above. Adductor magnus muscle below.
Apex	:	It is formed by medial lip of linea aspera where vastus medialis and adductor muscles meet.
Roof	:	Fascia of thigh. Saphenous nerve and saphenous branch of descending genicular artery pierce the roof.

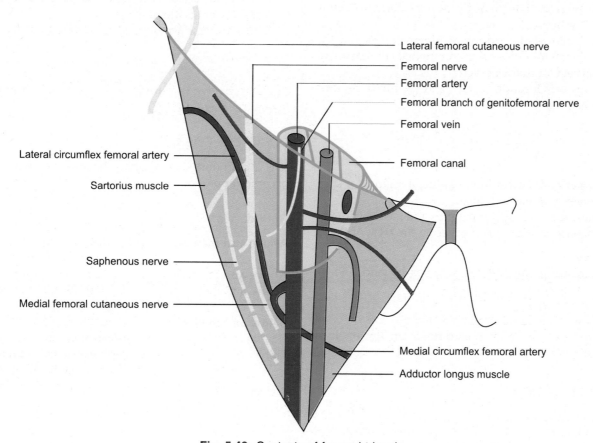

Lateral femoral cutaneous nerve
Femoral nerve
Femoral artery
Femoral branch of genitofemoral nerve
Femoral vein
Femoral canal

Lateral circumflex femoral artery
Sartorius muscle
Saphenous nerve
Medial femoral cutaneous nerve
Medial circumflex femoral artery
Adductor longus muscle

Fig. 5.42: Contents of femoral triangle

Contents

1. Femoral artery: It is deeply situated
2. Femoral vein: It lies posterior to femoral artery in upper part and lateral in lower part.
3. Nerve to vastus medialis
4. Occasionally posterior division of obturator nerve
5. Terminal part of profunda femoris vessels.
6. Descending genicular artery: It is a branch of femoral artery and divides into superficial saphenous branch and deep muscular branch.

Muscles of Front of Thigh

See page no. 196.

Medial Compartment of Thigh

This is also known as the adductor compartment of thigh. It lies between the medial intermuscular septum and the incomplete posterior intermuscular septum.

Contents

1. **Muscles:** Lie in three planes and are innervated by anterior division of obturator nerve (see page no. 197).
   a. **Superficial plane:** Adductor longus, gracilis.
   b. **Intermediate plane** Obturator externus, Adductor brevis.
   c. **Deep plane:** Adductor magnus, it lies at the junction of posterior and medial compartment
2. **Nerve:** Obturator nerve.
3. **Arteries:** Obturator artery and profunda femoris artery.

Back of Thigh (Posterior compartment)
Extent

1. **Upper end:** Lower limit of gluteal region.
2. **Lower end:** Back of knee.
3. **Anteriorly:** Adductor magnus and vastus lateralis.
4. **Posteriorly:** Fascia lata covering the back of thigh.

Contents

1. Hamstring muscles (see page nos 198 and 199).
2. Short head of biceps femoris.
3. Sciatic nerve.
4. Posterior femoral cutaneous nerve.
5. Chain of vascular anastomosis on the back of adductor magnus.

GLUTEAL REGION

Hip and buttock is also called as gluteal region. It extends from small of the back of waist superiorly to the gluteal fold inferiorly and the hollow on lateral side of thigh.

Hip is the upper part and buttock is the rounded bulge behind and below.

Extent

Above: Entire length of iliac crest
Below: Gluteal fold
Behind: Sacral spines in mid-dorsal line
In front: An imaginary vertical line extending downwards from the anterior superior iliac spine to anterior edge of greater trochanter.

Superficial Fascia

It is thick and fatty. Cutaneous nerves and vessels lie in the superficial fascia.

Deep Fascia

It splits to enclose tensor fascia lata and gluteus maximus. It also forms the gluteal aponeurosis.

Skeletal Frame Work of Gluteal Region

1. Dorsal surface of sacrum and coccyx
2. Gluteal surface of ilium
3. Dorsal surface of ischium, ischial tuberosity, greater and lesser sciatic notches.
4. Posterior surface of upper part of femur.

Muscles of Gluteal Region

They are twelve in number and are arranged in three layers (see page no. 197).

POPLITEAL FOSSA

It is a diamond shaped space behind the knee which becomes apparent as a depression in the flexed knee.

Boundaries (Fig. 5.43)

Above and medially	:	Semitendinosus and semimembranosus
Above and laterally	:	Tendon of biceps femoris
Below and laterally	:	Plantaris and lateral head of gastrocnemius
Below and medially	:	Medial head of gastrocnemius
Floor	:	Popliteal surface of femur
	:	Oblique popliteal ligament
	:	Posterior part of upper end of tibia
	:	Fascia covering the popliteal muscle
Roof	:	Popliteal fascia

Roof is pierced by the short saphenous vein and posterior femoral cutaneous nerve.

Contents of Popliteal Fossa (Fig. 5.44)

1. Popliteal artery and its branches
2. Popliteal vein and its tributaries
3. Tibial nerve
4. Common peroneal nerve
5. Termination of short saphenous vein
6. Posterior femoral cutaneous nerve
7. Genicular branch of posterior division of obturator nerve

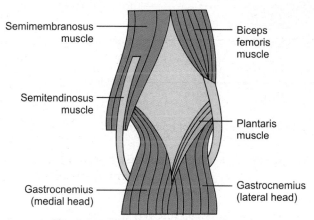

Fig. 5.43: Boundaries of popliteal fossa

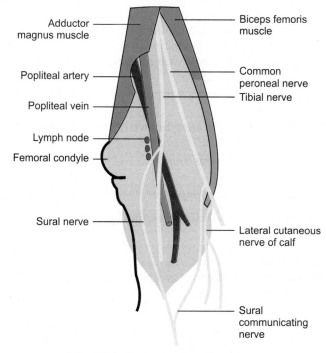

Fig. 5.44: Contents of popliteal fossa

8. Popliteal lymph nodes
9. Pad of fat

LEG

Leg extends from knee joint to ankle joint. The fleshy part of back of leg is known as calf. Deep fascia is attached to anterior and medial border of tibia and is modified into

1. Anterior intermuscular septum
2. Posterior intermuscular septum
3. Transverse intermuscular septum

Leg is divided into three compartments with the help of anterior and posterior intermuscular septae and an interosseous membrane. Anterior and posterior septa are attached to anterior and posterior border of fibula.

Compartments of Leg

1. Anterior or extensor compartment.
2. Lateral or peroneal compartment.
3. Posterior or flexor compartment.

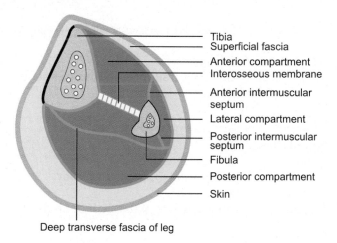

Fig. 5.45: Compartments of right leg

Anterior Crural Compartment (Fig. 5.46)

Boundaries

Anteriorly : Deep fascia.
Posteriorly : Interosseous membrane. Anterior surface of shaft of fibula.
Laterally : Anterior intermuscular septum.
Medially : Lateral surface of the shaft of tibia.

Contents

1. Muscles (see page no. 199)
   a. Tibialis anterior muscle
   b. Extensor digitorum longus muscle
   c. Extensor hallucis longus muscle
   d. Peroneus tertius muscle

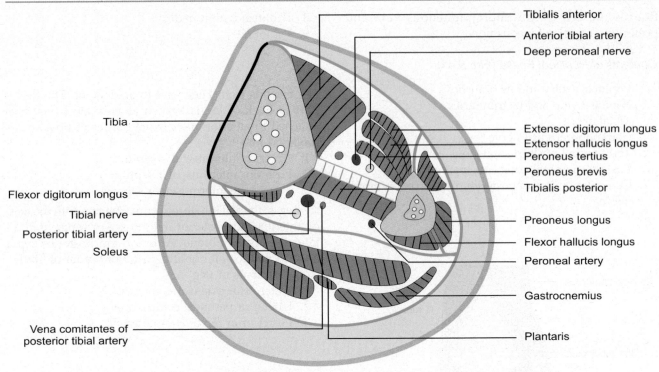

Fig. 5.46: Transverse section of right leg showing muscles of different compartments

2. Anterior tibial vessels.
3. Deep peroneal nerve: It supplies the muscles of this compartment.

Lateral Crural Compartment (Fig. 5.46)
Boundaries

Anterior	:	Anterior intermuscular septum
Posterior	:	Posterior intermuscular septum
Laterally	:	Deep fascia
Medially	:	Lateral surface of the shaft of fibula

Contents
1. Muscles (see page no. 200)
   a. Peroneus longus muscle
   b. Peroneus brevis muscle
2. Superficial peroneal nerve
3. Peroneal branch of posterior tibial artery and veins

Posterior Crural Compartment (Fig. 5.46)

It is further subdivided into three subcompartments by two fasciae namely, deep transverse fascia and fascia covering tibialis posterior muscle

Superficial Compartment

It contains superficial muscles of the calf.

Boundaries

Posteriorly	:	Deep fascia

Anteriorly	:	Deep transverse fascia of leg
	:	Posterior intermuscular septum

Contents
1. Muscles (see page nos 200 and 201).
   a. Gastrocnemius muscle
   b. Soleus muscle
   c. Popliteus muscle.
   d. Tibialis posterior muscle
   e. Flexor hallucis longus muscle
   f. Flexor digitorum longus muscle
   g. Plantaris muscle
2. Sural nerve: It lies between two heads of gastrocnemius.
3. Sural communicating branch of common peroneal nerve.
4. Short saphaneous vein.

Intermediate Compartment

Long flexors of toe lie in this compartment.

Boundaries

Posteriorly	:	Deep transverse fascia of leg.
Anteriorly	:	Medial part of posterior surface of tibial shaft.
		Fascia covering the tibialis posterior.
		Lateral part of the posterior surface of the shaft of the fibula.

Contents
1. Flexor digitorum longus muscle on which lie the posterior tibial vessels and tibial nerve with their branches (see page no. 201).
2. Flexor hallucis longus muscle.
3. Peroneal artery.

Deep Compartment

It contains tibialis posterior muscle.

Boundaries

Posteriorly	:	Fascia covering tibialis posterior.
Anteriorly	:	Lateral part of posterior surface of shaft of tibia.
	:	Interosseous membrane. Medial part of the posterior surface of the shaft of the fibula.

Contents: Tibialis posterior muscle (see page no. 201).

FOOT

Foot extends from the point of heel to the roots of the toes. Superior surface is called dorsum of the foot. Inferior surface is sole or plantar surface.

Dorsum of Foot

Skin: It is thin and mobile over the fascia. It lacks hair.
Superficial fascia: It is thin over dorsum of foot.
Deep fascia: In the region of ankle and dorsum of foot, deep fascia is modified to form the following:
1. Superior extensor retinaculum
2. Inferior extensor retinaculum
3. Flexor retinaculum
4. Superior peroneal retinaculum
5. Inferior peroneal retinaculum
6. Plantar aponeurosis

Superior Extensor Retinaculum

It is the condensation of deep fascia in front of the lower part of the leg (Fig. 5.47).

Attachments

Laterally	:	Lower part of subcutaneous anterior border of fibula.
Medially	:	Anterior border of tibia above the medial malleolus

Structures passing deep to superior extensor retinaculum from medial to lateral side
1. Tibialis anterior muscle
2. Extensor hallucis longus muscle
3. Anterior tibial artery
4. Deep peroneal nerve
5. Extensor digitorum longus muscle
6. Peroneus tertius muscle

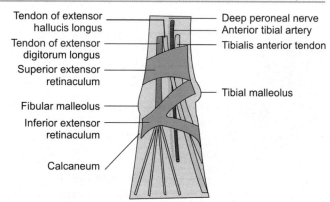

Fig. 5.47: Superior and inferior extensor retinacula

These structures can be memorised with the help of pnemonic.

THE	:	Tibialis anterior
HOSPITALS	:	Extensor hallucis longus
ARE	:	Anterior tibial artery
NEVER	:	Deep peronial nerve
DIRTY	:	Extensor digitorum longus
PLACES	:	Peronius tertius

Inferior Extensor Retinaculum (Fig. 5.47)

It is Y shaped. The stem of the Y is directed laterally, while the two limbs of the retinaculum are directed medially.

Attachments

Stem of the Y: It is attached to the lower surface of calcaneum

Upper limb of Y: It is attached to the medial malleolus

Lower limb of Y: It is attached to the plantar aponeurosis

Structures passing deep to inferior extensor retinaculum: from medial to lateral side
1. Tendon of tibialis anterior muscle
2. Tendon of extensor hallucis longus muscle
3. Anterior tibial artery
4. Extensor digitorum longus muscle
5. Peroneus tertius tendon muscle

Functions of extensor retinaculae: They keep the tendons in position and prevent bow stringing of these tendons forward.

Superior Peroneal Retinaculum (Fig. 5.48)

It is a fibrous band arising from deep fascia, extending from lateral malleolus to calcaneus.

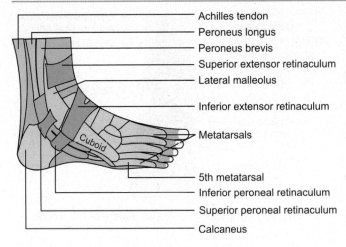

Fig. 5.48: Peroneal retinaculae

Inferior Peroneal Retinaculum

It is the fibrous condensation of deep fascia and extends from peroneal trochlea on calcaneus below to the inferior extensor retinaculum above.

The two peroneal retinaculae bind the tendons of peroneus longus and peroneus brevis to the lateral malleolus.

Flexor Retinaculum (Figs 5.48 and 5.49)

It is the condensation of deep fascia extending from the medial malleolus to the back of calcaneus. It bridges over the deep flexor tendons and neurovascular bundle.

Structures passing under flexor retinaculum: From medial to lateral side (Fig. 5.49).
1. Tendon of tibialis posterior
2. Tendon of flexor digitorum longus
3. Posterior tibial artery with accompanying veins
4. Tibial nerve
5. Tendon of flexor hallucis longus

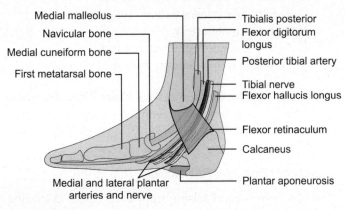

Fig. 5.49: Flexor retinaculum and structures passing under it

To remember these structures the pnumonic is

THE	:	Tibialis posterior
DOCTORS	:	Flexor digitorum longus
ARE	:	Posterior tibial artery
NEVER	:	Tibial nerve
HEALTHY	:	Flexor hallucis longus

Sole of Foot

Skin: Skin of the sole is thick and it is devoid of hairs and sebaceous glands. Numerous sweat glands are present.

Superficial fascia: It contains superficial fat enclosed in lobules of fibrous septa. This helps in proper grip of the sole on to the ground.

Deep fascia: It is modified to form the **plantar aponeurosis** (Fig. 5.50) which lies just below the superficial fascia. It has three parts, namely medial, central and lateral aponeurosis. Medial and lateral part are also called as plantar fascia.

Functions of plantar aponeurosis
1. It maintains the longitudinal arches.
2. It provides origin to superficial group of plantar muscles.
3. It protects plantar nerves and vessels from compression.

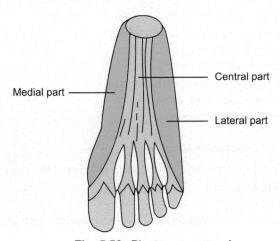

Fig. 5.50: Plantar aponeurosis

Layers of the Sole

Sole is divided into six layers. They are as follows (Fig. 5.51)
1. **1st layer:** It lies beneath the plantar aponeurosis. It is made up of three short intrinsic muscles of foot (see page no. 202).
   a. Abductor hallucis

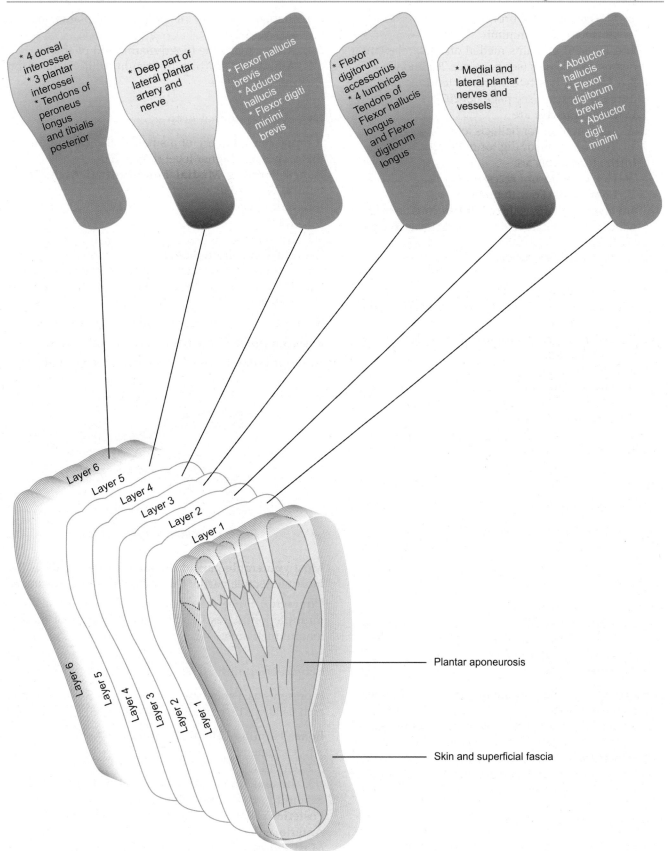

Fig. 5.51 : Layers of the sole

b. Flexor digitorum brevis

c. Abductor digit minimi

2. **2nd layer:** It contains medial and lateral plantar nerves and vessels (see page nos 262 and 426)

3. **3rd layer:** It has two extrinsic tendons and two intrinsic muscles (see page no. 202).

   Extrinsic muscles are
   a. Tendon of flexor hallucis longus
   b. Tendon of flexor digitorum longus

   Intrinsic muscles are
   a. Flexor digitorum accessorius
   b. Lumbricals: Four in number

4. **4th layer:** It contains three intrinsic muscles of foot which are limited to region of metatarsals (see page no. 202).

   a. Flexor hallucis brevis
   b. Adductor hallucis
   c. Flexor digiti minimi brevis

5. **5th layer:** It contains deep part of lateral plantar artery and nerve.

6. **6th layer:** It has seven intrinsic muscles and two extrinsic tendons.

   Intrinsic muscles are
   a. 4 dorsal interossei
   b. 3 plantar interossei

   Extrinsic muscles are
   a. Peroneus longus
   b. Tibialis posterior

ARCHES OF FOOT

Basic Functions of Foot

1. Transmission of body weight and
2. It serves as a lever to propel the body forwards.

Classification of Arches

Arches of foot are classified into the following:

1. **Longitudinal arches**
   a. Medial longitudinal arch
   b. Lateral longitudinal arch
2. **Transverse arch**

Following factors help in the maintenance of arches:
1. Shape of bones
2. Various ligaments and intrinsic muscles of foot act as binding agents between the bones forming **intersegmental tiers** and **tie beams.**
3. Suspension of arches from above by tendons of various extrinsic muscles of foot.

Functions of Arches of Foot

1. Proportional distribution of body weight.
2. Acts as a segmented lever for propulsion of foot.

3. Plantar concavity of foot protects plantar nerves and vessels.
4. Arches make the foot dynamic and pliable.
5. Allows for shifting of weight while moving on uneven surface.

Medial Longitudinal Arch

It represents a big arc of a small circle. The summit of this arch is at a higher level (Fig. 5.52).

Bones Forming Medial Longitudinal Arch (From behind forwards):
1. Calcaneus
2. Talus
3. Navicular
4. Three cuneiform bones
5. Medial three metatarsals upto their heads
6. Two sesamoid bones beneath the head 1st metatarsal

Summit   : Upper trochlear surface of talus.

Posterior pillar : Medial tubercle of calcaneus.

Anterior pillar : Head of medial three metatarsals.

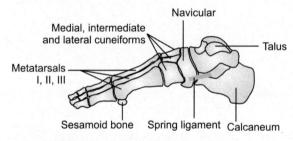

Fig. 5.52: Medial longitudinal arch

Most vulnerable part of the arch: Head of talus is the most vulnerable part of this arch. It acts as a **keystone.**

Character: Since it is made up of more bones and multiple joints, **resiliency** is the character of medial longitudinal arch.

Lateral Longitudinal Arch

It presents as a small arc of a big circle. Summit of this arch is lower than medial arch (Fig. 5.53).

Bones Forming Lateral Longitudinal Arch
1. Calcaneus
2. Cuboid
3. 4th and 5th metatarsals upto their heads.

Summit   : Subtalar joint

Posterior pillar : Medial tubercle of calcaneums

Anterior pillar : Head of 4th and 5th metatarsals

Most vulnerable part of the arch is calcaneo–cuboid joint.

Character: It is formed by less number of bones and joints. Transmits body weight before medial longitudinal arch comes into play. Rigidity is the characteristic of this arch.

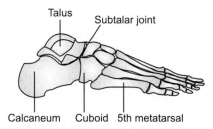

Fig. 5.53: Lateral longitudinal arch

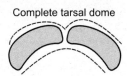

Fig. 5.54: Transverse arch

Transverse Arch

When medial borders of both feet are approximated a complete transverse arch is formed. It basically consists of series of arches (Fig. 5.54).

Bones Forming Transverse Arch

1. Bases of metatarsals.
2. Cuboid
3. 3 Cuneiform bones.

Each foot represents half dome of the arch

CLINICAL AND APPLIED ASPECT

SCALP AND FACE

- The neurovascular bundle of scalp lies in the subcutaneous layer which is made up of tough connective tissue. In case of injury to the scalp, this tough connective tissue prevents the retraction of blood vessels. Therefore, scalp wound bleed profusely.
- Head injury resulting in soft tissue damage can lead to collection of blood in the loose subaponeurotic layer of scalp and results in **black eye.** This is because the loose subaponeurotic layer is continuous over the upper eye lid. The blood easily tracks down anteriorly over the eyelids leading to discoloration of the eye known as black eye.
- **Cephalhaematoma:** It is the collection of blood below the periosteal layer of scalp. It mostly occurs due to an injury. The swelling due to the haematoma is localized over the particular bone involved as the periosteum is adherent to the underlying bone at the sutures which limits its spread. In a new born cephalhaematoma has to be differentiated from caput formation.
- **Caput:** It is the collection of fluid in the loose aerolar tissue of scalp due to forces of labour. The swelling on scalp due to caput is generally diffuse and more on the dependant areas. It is not limited over a particular bone. This collection can cross the midline as the loose aleolar layer is not limited by sutures. Caput usually disappear by 24 hours of birth.
- The loose areolar tissue layer is the dangerous layer of scalp because emissary veins are lodged in this layer which directly communicate with the intra-cranial sinuses.
- Boils in the region of nose and external ear are extremely painful as compared to any other part because the skin in these areas is adherent to the cartilage below:

MEDIASTINUM

- The compression of various contents of the mediastinum due to a tumor or collection of fluid, as seen in infections, leads to mediastinal syndrome. The clinical presentation would vary according to the structure compressed. A few examples are given below.
  - Compression of trachea leads to dyspnea and cough.
  - Compression of esophagus leads to dysphagia.
  - Hoarseness of voice occurs due to compression of left recurrent laryngeal nerve.
  - Superior vena caval obstruction results in engorged neck veins.
  - The diaphragm is paralysed if phrenic nerve is compressed.
- The mediastinum is displaced to the opposite side when there is a large collection of air or fluid in a pleural cavity. It may be shifted to the same side due to collapse of lung of that side. Clinically, the presence of mediastinal shift may be indicated by
  - Displacement of trachea away from midline.
  - Displacement of apex beat of heart.

HAND

- Pus from infected synovial sheaths of flexor tendons can extend into and accumulate in the space of Parona. Incision to drain pus from space of Parona should be given along the medial or lateral borders of forearm. These borders are not crossed by motor nerves and thus allows safe and complete access for surgical explorations.

- The pus from infections of fibrous flexor sheath or digital synovial sheaths of index, middle and ring fingers can burst into midpalmar and thenar spaces. Direct injury may also cause infection of these spaces. The pus in thenar space is drained by giving an incision on the interdigital web between 1st and 2nd fingers whereas, for midpalmar space infections, incision is given at the interdigital cleft of 3rd and 4th fingers.

- Infection of pulp space is called whitlow. The patient comes with complaint of severe throbbing pain in the distal phalanx. This is due to the increase in pressure by accumulation of inflammatory substances in the tight compartments of pulp of fingers. In neglected cases the pressure can lead to avascular necrosis of distal 4/5th of terminal phalanx. Since the proximal 1/5th of this bone is supplied by a separate branch of digital vessels before it enters the pulp space, it is spared. Pus is drained from the pulp space by giving an incision on the lateral aspect of the distal part of finger is given to enable access to interseptal compartments. This allows for drainage of collected pus without damage to skin.

- **Dupuytren's contracture:** Inflammation of palmar aponeurosis results in fibrosis and thickening of the aponeurosis when healing occurs. This results in contracture of aponeurosis which leads to flexion of proximal and middle phalanges of the digits. The most common site of involvement is the ulnar part of apponeurosis and hence it affects the ring finger.

ANTERIOR ABDOMINAL WALL—INGUINAL CANAL

- Internal oblique is the key muscle of the inguinal canal as it forms the anterior wall, roof and posterior wall of the inguinal canal.
- **Inguinal hernia:** It is the protusion of a viscus or part of a viscus through the inguinal canal. It is of two types:
  a. **Direct inguinal hernia:** Whenever the hernia enters through the posterior wall of the inguinal canal directly it is known as direct inguinal hernia
  b. **Indirect inguinal hernia:** When hernia enters through the deep inguinal ring into the inguinal canal it is known as indirect inguinal hernia.
- Clinically direct and indirect inguinal hernia aredifferentiated with the help of ring occlusion test (occlusion of deep inguinal ring by finger).

- During surgery the differentiation between direct and indirect inguinal hernia is done by tracing the **Hesselbach triangle.** It is a triangle formed by the lateral border of rectus abdominis muscle medially, inferior epigastric artery laterally and inguinal ligament inferiorly. If the hernia passes through the triangle, it is direct inguinal hernia and if it passes lateral to the triangle then it is indirect inguinal hernia (Fig. 5.18).
- **Littre's hernial:** When Meckel's diverticulum enters the hernial sac is known as Littre's hernia.
- Differences between indirect and direct inguinal hernia are tabulated below

Indirect hernia	Direct hernia
1. Hernia enters through deep inguinal ring	1. It enters through the posterior wall of the inguinal canal
2. Neck of the sac is lateral to the inferior epigastric artery	2. Neck of the sac is medial to the inferior epigastric artery
3. Directed-downward, forward, medially	3. Directed-straight for ward
4. Occurs in young age	4. Occurs in old age
5. **Cause is**-congenital, due to persistence of processus vaginalis of peritoneum	5. **Cause is**-acquired, due to weakness of the posterior wall of inguinal canal

- Inferior epigastric artery is an important surgical landmark to differentiate direct and indirect inguinal hernia
- Common incisions given for laparotomy are
  a. Longitudinal incisions: These can be midline or paramedian in location.
  b. Transverse incisions: These can be Kocher's of Pfannensteil's incisions.
- Structures cut in a mid line incision are
  — Skin
  — Subcutaneous tissue
  — Linea alba
  — Fascia transversalis
  — Extra peritoneal fat
  — Peritoneum
- Structures cut in a Kocher's incision are
  — Skin
  — Anterior rectus sheath
  — Rectus muscle
  — Posterior rectus sheath
  — Fascia transversalis
  — Extra peritoneal fat
  — Peritoneum

UMBILICUS

- **Watershed line:** Umbilicus acts as a watershed line because subcutaneous lymphatics above the umbilicus drain into axillary group of lymph nodes while below the umbilicus they drain into superficial inguinal group of lymph nodes. Hence umbilicus acts as a demarcation line.
- Referred pain at umbilicus or around umbilicus originates from appendix or gonads.

PERITONEUM

- **Ascites:** It is the accumulation of fluid in the perotineal cavity.
- Hepatorenal pouch is the most dependant part of the peritoneal cavity in supine position. It is the commonest site of location of a subphrenic abscess.
- Pouch of Douglas is the most dependant part of peritoneal cavity in females. Hence, whenever there is any collection of fluid in the abdominal cavity, e.g., pus or blood (in ruptured ectopic pregnancy), it collects in this pouch. The floor of the pouch can be approached pervaginally through the posterior fornix. Incision in the posterior fornix over the bulge of fluid helps in drainage of pus without laparotomy. Aspiration of blood from the posterior fornix helps in diagnosis of suspected case of ectopic pregnancy.

PERINEUM

- Damage to perineal body during parturition can lead to prolapse of uterus, rectum and urinary bladder.
- Perianal and ischiorectal spaces are the common sites for abscess formation.
- Abscess from one ischio rectal fossa can spread to the other side behind anal canal. The pus collects in a horse shoe shape mannure.
- Fat in the perianal space is tightly arranged in small loculi. The infection of this region, therefore very painful due to tension caused by the swelling.
- Injury to membranous part of urethra in males can lead to extravasation of urine into the anterior abdominal wall and can reach upto umbilicus as the membranous layer of superficial fascia of abdomen forms the inferior boundary of superficial perineal pouch.
- If urethra ruptures inferior to the perineal membrane then urine can extravasate into the anterior abdominal wall, penis and scrotum. It can ascend up to the axilla along the fascial planes but cannot extend into thigh.

AXILLA

- Axillary abscess should always be drained by giving incision at the base of axilla midway between the anterior and posterior axillary folds, towards the thoracic side to avoid injury to lateral thoracic, subscapular and axillary vessels.
- Cervicoaxillary canal is a triangular interval bounded by:
  Arteriorly: Posterior surface of clavicle
  Posteriorly: Superior border of scapula
  Medially: Outer border of first rib
  It corresponds to apex of axilla through which axillary vessels and brachial plexus enter the axilla from the neck.

ARM

- **Clinical importance of contents of cubital fossa**
  — Brachial artery pulsations are felt in cubital fossa.
  — Median cubital vein, a superficial vein of upperlimb, is commonly cannulated for admin-istration of intravenous medication and fluids.
- **Carrying angle:** It is the angle between long axis of arm with long axis of forearm, when forearm is extended and supinated. It disappears in full flexion of elbow and in pronation. It is about 12° in males and 15 to 18° in females. The angle appears because medial flange of trochlea of radius is larger than lateral flange and projects downwards to a lower level. Also the superior articular surface of coronoid process of ulna is oblique.

  Importance
  — It allows the arm to swing, clearly away from the body.
  — The forearm in midprone position comes in line with long axis of arm. This is the most comfor-table position used for various functions of the hand.
  Sex difference: Carrying angle is greater in females because of wider pelvis.

THIGH

- **Femoral hernia (Fig. 5.41):** It is defined as protrusion of a viscus or   part of a viscus into the femoral canal through femoral ring. Femoral hernia is more common in females due to a wider pelvis.
  Direction of femoral hernia: It passes through the femoral ring first downwards then forwards through the saphenous opening and ultimately

turns upwards around the upper falciform margin of saphenous opening towards the inguinal ligament. Hernia is reduced in the opposite direction to which it occurs.

- Coverings of complete femoral hernia are from without inward:
  a. Skin
  b. Superficial fascia
  c. Cribriform fascia
  d. Anterior wall of femoral sheath
  e. Femoral septum
  f. Peritoneum of hernial sac
  g. Loose areolar tissue and fat

- **Aberrant obturator artery:** A pubic branch of inferior epigastric artery may replace obturator artery in 30% of cases. It is known as aberrant obturator artery. It forms an important relation with the lacunar ligament. In case of obstructed femoral hernia the lacunar ligament is cut to release the neck of the sac. Hence, care should be taken during surgery to avoid damage to this artery as it can lead to unexpected severe bleeding.

- Muscles of the floor of femoral triangle are attached to the posterior aspect of femur and hence the floor appears like a gutter. The apex continues below with the adductor canal.

- Clinical Importance of adductor canal
  a. Saphenous nerve pierces the roof of adductor canal.
  b. Femoral artery is ligated in the adductor canal in the treatment of popliteal artery aneurysm.

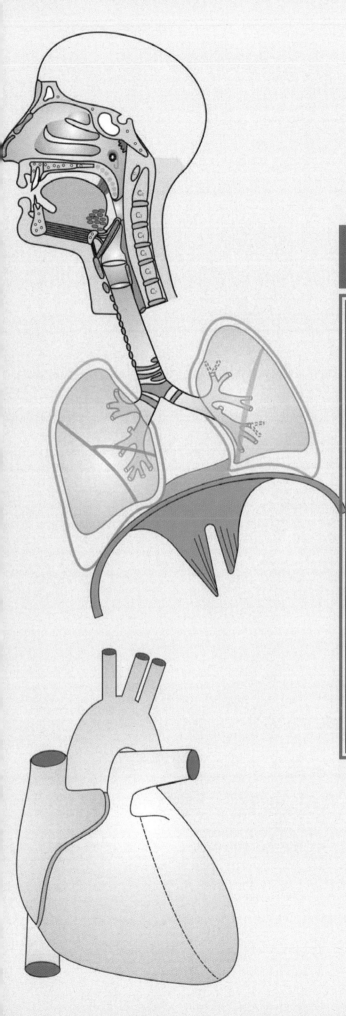

SECTION-3
Systemic Anatomy and Physiology

6. Skeletal System
7. Muscular System
8. Anatomical and Functional Organization of Nervous System
9. Peripheral Nervous System
10. Somatosensory, Somatomotor and Autonomic Nervous System
11. Special Senses
12. Respiratory System
13. Cardiovascular System
14. Blood and its Components
15. Lymphatic System
16. Digestive System
17. Urinary System
18. Endocrine System
19. Reproductive System
20. Skin

Skeletal System

Skeletal system is composed of skeleton.

SKELETON (FIG. 6.1)

Human skeleton is endoskeleton. It forms the structural frame work of the body. Skeleton includes bones, cartilage and joints. It is bilaterally symmetrical. It can be studied in two parts:

a. **Axial skeleton:** This includes bones of head (skull), vertebral column, ribs and sternum. Hyoid bone is also the part of axial skeleton.

b. **Appendicular skeleton:** It consists of bones of extremities, i.e., upper limb and lower limb.

Axial Skeleton (Fig. 6.1)

It consists of skull, vertebral column, thoracic cage and hyoid bone.

Skull

It is made up of 22 bones + 6 ear ossicles.

Paired bones	Unpaired bones
Temporal	Frontal
Parietal	Occipital
Maxilla	Sphenoid
Lacrimal	Ethmoid
Palatine	Vomer
Zygomatic	Mandible
Nasal	
Inferior concha	
Bones of middle ear cavity	
Incus	
Malleus	
Stapes	

Vertebral Column

It is made up of 33 vertebrae, namely, 7 cervical, 12 thoracic, 5 lumbar, 5 sacral and 4 coccygeal vertebrae.

Thoracic Cage

It consists of 12 thoracic vertebrae, 12 pairs of ribs with their costal cartilages, sternum and xiphoid process.

Hyoid Bone

It lies in the mid line.

Appendicular Skeleton (Fig. 6.1)

Bones Forming Upper Limb Skeleton

Clavicle
Scapula
Humerus
Radius
Ulna
8 Carpal bones: Scaphoid, lunate, triquetral, pisiform, trapezium, trapezoid, capitate, hamate
5 Metacarpals
14 Phalanges

Bones Forming Lower Limb Skeleton

Ilium
Ischium
Pubis
Femur
Patella
Tibia
Fibula
8 Tarsal bones: Talus, calcaneum, navicular, cuboid and three cuneiform bones
5 Metatarsals
14 Phalanges

Functions of the Skeleton (Fig. 6.1)

1. Skeleton forms the structural framework of the body.
2. It supports the body.
3. It transmits the weight of the body.
4. Bones and joints act as a biochemical lever on which muscles act to produce motion.
5. Skeleton of head and vertebral column protect the vital organs namely brain and spinal cord.
6. Skeletal frame work of thoracic cage (ribs and sternum) provides for the respiratory movements and protects the heart and lungs. It provides structural support in ear, larynx and trachea where rigidity not required.
7. Bones serve as a reservoir of ions (Ca^{++}, PO_4, CO_3^-) in the mineral homeostasis of the body.
8. Bone marrow in adults is the source of red blood cells, granular white blood cells and platelets.
9. Cartilage is a precursor for formation of bones.

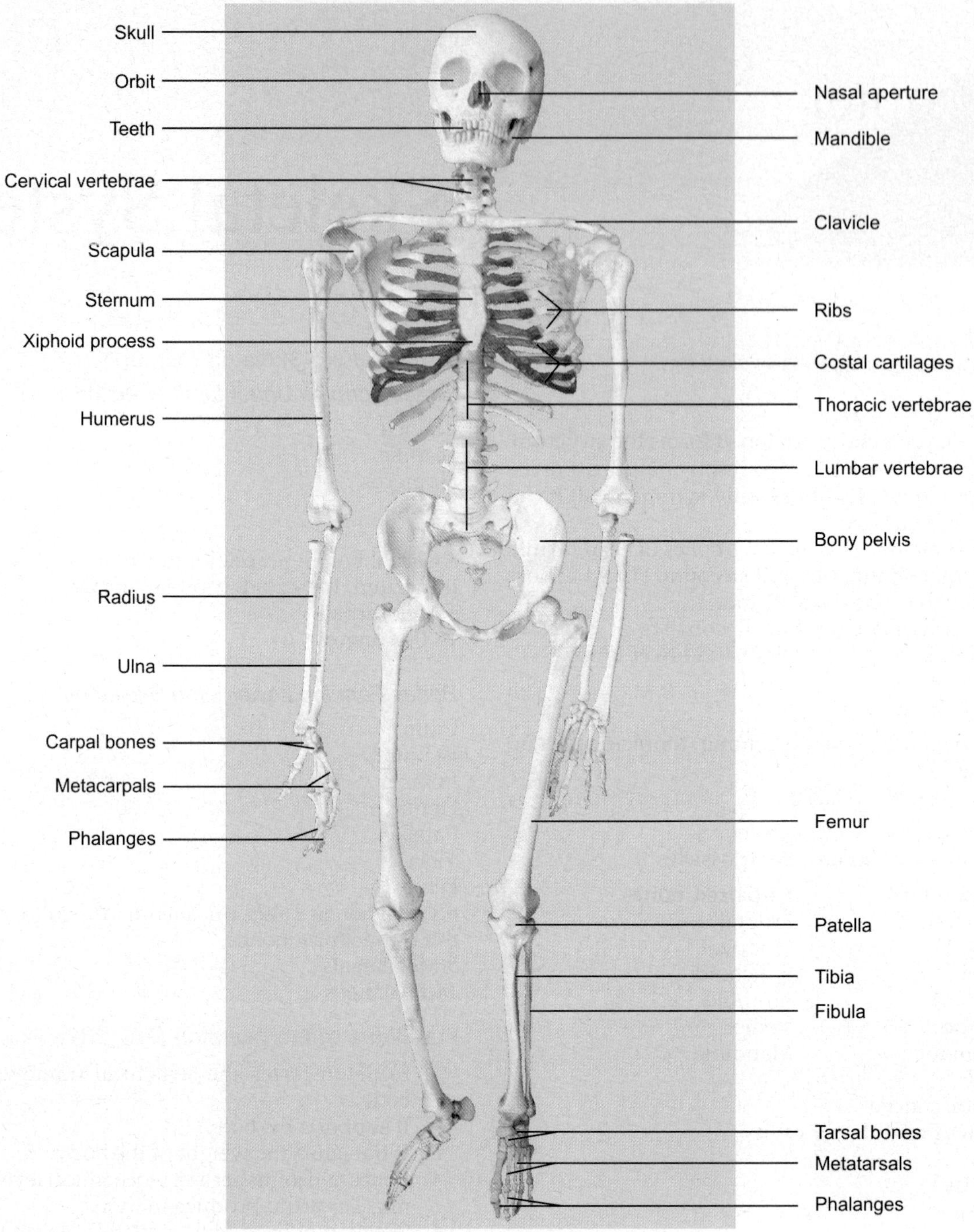

Skull
Orbit
Teeth
Cervical vertebrae
Scapula
Sternum
Xiphoid process
Humerus
Radius
Ulna
Carpal bones
Metacarpals
Phalanges

Nasal aperture
Mandible
Clavicle
Ribs
Costal cartilages
Thoracic vertebrae
Lumbar vertebrae
Bony pelvis
Femur
Patella
Tibia
Fibula
Tarsal bones
Metatarsals
Phalanges

Fig. 6.1: Human skeleton

SKULL

Skull forms the skeleton of head and provides:

1. A case for the brain.
2. Cavities for organs of special sensation (sight, hearing, equilibration, smell and taste).
3. Openings for the passage of air and food.
4. Jaws with sockets for teeth used during mastication.

The term cranium is used for skull without mandible. Skull is made up of 22 bones plus 6 ear ossicles and is divided into the following two parts:

a. Neurocranium: It is also known as calvaria or brain-box.

b. Facial skeleton.

Neurocranium (calvaria) consists of eight bones
  a. **Paired:** Parietal and temporal.
  b. **Unpaired:** Frontal, occipital, sphenoid and ethmoid.
Facial skeleton consists of fourteen bones
  a. **Paired:** Maxilla, zygomatic, nasal, lacrimal, palatine and inferior nasal concha.
  b. **Unpaired:** Mandible and vomer.

EXTERNAL FEATURES OF SKULL

The exterior of the skull is studied in five different views:
  1. Superior view or norma verticalis.
  2. Posterior view or norma occipitalis.
  3. Anterior view or norma frontalis.
  4. Lateral view or norma lateralis.
  5. Inferior view or norma basalis.

Norma Verticalis (Superior Aspect of Skull)

When the skull is viewed from above, it appears oval being wider posteriorly than anteriorly (Fig. 6.2). Four bones can be identified on this aspect namely:

  1. **One frontal bone,** anteriorly.
  2. **Two parietal bones,** one on each side.
  3. **One occipital bone,** posteriorly.

These bones are united by the following sutures:
  1. **Coronal suture:** Present between frontal bone and anterior margins of parietal bones.
  2. **Sagittal suture:** Present between the two parietal bones.
  3. **Lambdoid suture:** Present between occipital bone and posterior margins of parietal bones.
  4. **Metopic suture:** Present between the two halves of frontal bones, is seen in 3 to 8% cases.

Features of Importance
  1. **Bregma:** It is the point at which the coronal and sagittal sutures meet.
  2. **Parietal eminence:** It is the area of maximum convexity of parietal bone.
  3. **Vertex:** Highest point of the skull is known as vertex. It lies on the sagittal suture near its middle and is situated a few centimeters behind the bregma.
  4. **Parietal foramen:** A small foramen is seen in each parietal bone, near the sagittal suture, 2.8 to 4 cm in front of lambda.

Norma Occipitalis (Posterior Aspect of the Skull)

The back of skull is composed of posterior part of parietal bones, occipital bone and mastoid part of temporal bones (Figs 6.3 and 6.6). They are located as follows:
  1. **Parietal bones:** The two lie superiorly, one on each side of midline.
  2. **Occipital bone:** It lies inferiorly.
  3. **Mastoid part of temporal bones:** These are present infero-laterally, one on each side.

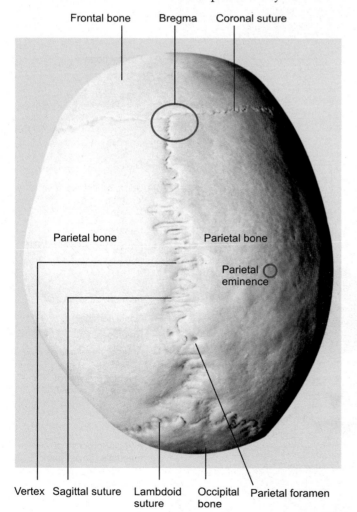

Frontal bone   Bregma   Coronal suture

Parietal bone   Parietal bone

Parietal eminence

Vertex Sagittal suture Lambdoid suture Occipital bone Parietal foramen

Fig. 6.2: Norma verticalis

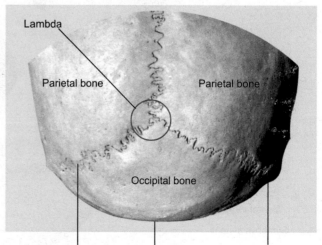

Lambda

Parietal bone   Parietal bone

Occipital bone

Lambdoid suture   External occipital protuberance   Mastoid process

Fig. 6.3: Norma occipitalis

Sutures which unite these bones are:
1. **Lambdoid suture:** It lies between the occipital bone and the two parietal bones.
2. **Occipitomastoid suture:** It is present, between the occipital bone and the mastoid part of temporal bone (Fig. 6.6).
3. **Parietomastoid suture:** It lies on each side between the parietal bone and the mastoid part of temporal bone (Fig. 6.6).

Other features to be noted on the posterior aspect of the skull are (Figs 6.8 and 6.9):
1. **Lambda:** It is the point at which the sagittal and the lambdoid sutures meet.
2. External occipital protuberance
3. Superior nuchal lines
4. External occipital crest
5. Inferior nuchal lines

Norma Frontalis (Anterior Aspect of Skull)

In frontal view, the skull appears oval in shape, being wider above and narrow below (Fig 6.4) The anterior aspect of skull presents with the following bones:
1. **Frontal bone,** forms the forehead.
2. **Right and left nasal bones,** form the bridge of nose.
3. **Right and left maxillae,** form the upper jaw.
4. **Right and left zygomatic bones,** form the malar prominences.
5. **Mandible,** forms the lower jaw.

Features of Importance
1. **Forehead:** It is formed by the frontal bones. On each side of median plane, the frontal bones articulate with the nasal bone at the root of nose. Supraciliary arches arch are arched bony prominences seen above the superior orbital margins.
   Orbits: These are two bony cavities in which the eyes are located.

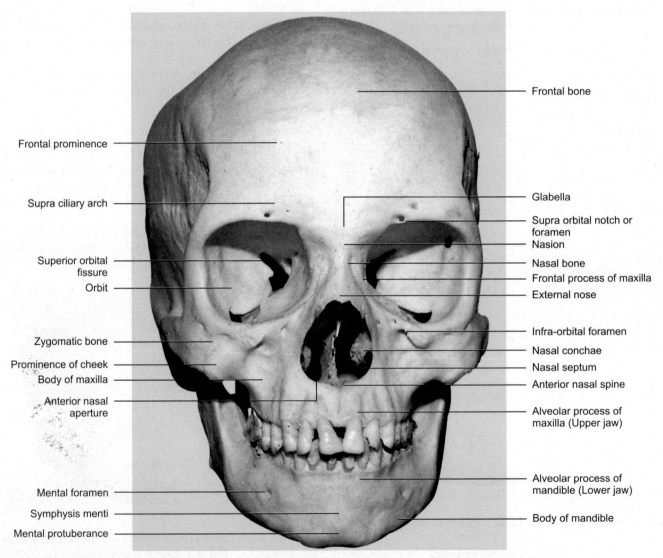

Fig. 6.4: Norma frontalis

2. **Prominence of the Cheek:** It is formed by zygomatic (malar) bone. It is situated on the lower and lateral side of the orbit and rests on the maxilla.

3. **Bony External Nose:** It is formed by the nasal bones above and the maxillae laterally. It terminates as a piriform shaped aperture below called anterior nasal aperture. The aperture is seen to be divided into twp parts by the nasal septum.

4. **Upper and Lower Jaws:** Upper jaw is formed by alveolar process of the two maxillae. It carries the sockets for root of upper teeth. The lower jaw is formed the upper border or alveolar arch of mandible. It carries the lower teeth.

5. **Glabella:** It is a median elevation above the nasion and between the supraciliary arches.

6. **Nasion:** It is the median point at the root of nose where the internasal and frontonasal sutures meet.

7. **Anterior nasal spine:** It is a sharp bony projection, seen in the lower boundary of the piriform aperture in the median plane.

8. **Symphysis menti:** It is the median ridge joining the two halves of the mandible.

9. **Mental protuberance:** It is a triangular elevation at the lower end of symphysis menti.

10. **Mental point (gnathion):** It is the middle point of the base of mandible.

11. **Frontal prominence:** It is a low rounded elevation above the supraciliary arch on each side.

Norma Lateralis (Lateral Aspect of Skull)

The lateral aspect of skull presents with the following bones (Figs 6.5 and 6.6):

1. **Above:** Nasal, frontal, parietal, occipital.
2. **In middle:** Maxilla, zygomatic, sphenoid, temporal.
3. **Below:** Body and ramus of mandible.

The bones are united by the following sutures:

1. **Coronal suture**
2. **Parieto-squamosal suture,** between parietal bone and squamous part of temporal bone.
3. **Parietomastoid suture,** between parietal bone and mastoid part of temporal bone.
4. **Occipitomastoid suture,** between occipital bone and mastoid part of temporal bone.
5. **Lambdoid suture**

Features of Importance

1. **Superior and inferior temporal lines.**
2. **Zygomatic arch:** A horizontal bar of bone formed by the union of temporal process of zygomatic bone and zygomatic process of temporal bone.
3. **External acoustic meatus:** Seen just below the posterior root of the zygoma.
4. **Suprameatal triangle (triangle of McEven):** It is a small triangular depression above the external auditory meatus. The triangle is formed by posterior margin of external auditory meatus, supra nastoid crest and a vertical tangent drawn to the posterior margin of external auditory meatus.
5. **Mastoid process:** A conical process extending down from the mastoid part of temporal bone behind the meatus.

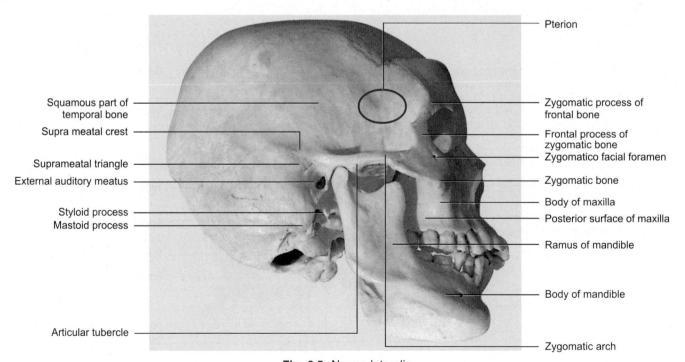

Fig. 6.5: Norma lateralis

CHAPTER-6

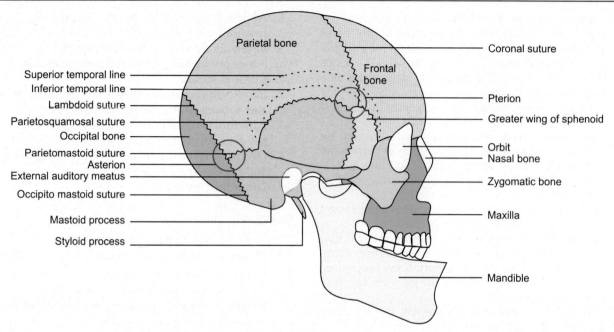

Fig. 6.6: Norma lateralis (diagrammatic representation)

6. **Asterion:** It is the meeting point of parietomastoid, occipitomastoid and lambdoid sutures. In an infant it is the site of posterolateral (mastoid) fontanelle.
7. **Styloid process:** It is a thin long bony process of temporal bone lying anterolateral to the mastoid process. It is directed downwards forwards and slightly medially.
8. **Pterion:** It is the region in the anterior part of temporal fossa where four bones namely, frontal, parietal, squamo-temporal and greater wing of

sphenoid meet to form an H-shaped suture. It is situated 4 cm above the midpoint of the zygomatic arch.

Temporal Fossa

The lateral aspect of skull above the zygomatic arch upto the superior temporal line constitutes the temporal region. The temporal fossa forms the floor of this region (Fig. 6.7).

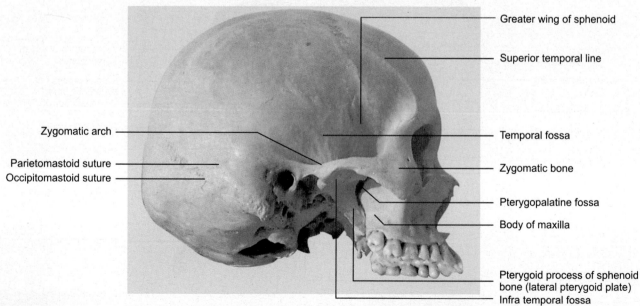

Fig. 6.7: Temporal, infratemporal and pterygopalatine fossae

Boundaries

Anterior	:	Temporal surface of zygomatic bone, Frontal process of zygomatic bone, Adjoining part of greater wing of sphenoid.
Superior	:	Superior temporal line.
Posterior	:	Posterior part of superior temporal line leading to supramastoid crest.
Inferior	:	It communicates with infratemporal fossa, in front.
Floor	:	It is formed by temporal part of frontal bone, antero-inferior part of parietal bone, squamous part of temporal bone, and lateral surface of greater wing of sphenoid.

The four bones meet at an H-shaped suture line termed pterion.

Contents of Temporal Fossa

1. Temporalis muscle
2. Temporal fascia
3. **Vessels:**
    a. Deep temporal vessels.
    b. Superficial temporal vessels.
4. **Nerves:**
    a. Deep temporal nerves, branches of anterior division of mandibular nerve
    b. Auriculotemporal nerve, branch of posterior division of mandibular nerve.

Infratemporal Fossa

When the mandible is disarticulated from the skull infratemporal region is revealed on either side of skull below the level of middle cranial fossa. The space behind maxilla forms the infratemporal fossa (Fig. 6.7).

Boundaries

Anterior	:	Posterior surface of body of maxilla.
Posterior	:	It is open and limited posteriorly by the styloid process of temporal bone and carotid sheath.
Medial	:	Lateral pterygoid plate
Lateral	:	Inner aspect of the ramus and coronoid process of mandible.
Superior	:	Infratemporal or lateral surface of greater wing of sphenoid
Inferior	:	It opens along the sides of the pharynx and esophagus

Contents of Infratemporal Fossa

1. **Muscles**
    - Lower part of temporalis
    - Lateral and medial pterygoids
2. **Nerves**
    - Mandibular nerve and its branches
    - Chorda tympani, branch of facial nerve
    - Otic ganglion

3. **Vessels**
    - Maxillary artery
    - Pterygoid venous plexus

Pterygopalatine Fossa

The pterygopalatine fossa is a pyramidal shaped space situated deep to the infratemporal fossa, below the apex of orbit.

Boundaries

Anterior	:	Posterior surface of body of maxilla.
Posterior	:	Anterior surface of root of pterygoid process and adjoining part of sphenoid bone.
Superior	:	Inferior surface of body of sphenoid bone, inferior orbital fissure.
Inferior	:	This is the apex of the fossa and is formed by meeting of the anterior and posterior boundaries, inferiorly.
Medial	:	Posterosuperior part of lateral surface of perpendicular plate of palatine bone.
Lateral	:	Fissure between anterior border of lateral pterygoid plate and posterior surface of maxilla.

Communications: The pterygopalatine fossa communicates with the following:
- Infratemporal fossa, via the pterygomaxillary fissure.
- Orbit, through the inferior orbital fissure.
- Middle cranial fossa, through foramen rotundum.
- Foramen lacerum via pterygoid canal.
- Pharynx through palato-vaginal canal.
- Nasal cavity via sphenopalatine foramen present in upper part of palatine bone.

Contents of Pterygopalatine Fossa

1. Maxillary nerve
2. Pterygopalatine ganglion
3. 3rd part of maxillary artery

Norma Basalis (Inferior Aspect of Skull)

Norma basalis or inferior surface of cranium is divided into three parts: anterior, middle and posterior (Figs 6.8 and 6.9).

Anterior part is formed by the alveolar arch and hard palate while the middle and posterior parts are separated by a transverse line passing through the anterior margin of the foramen magnum.

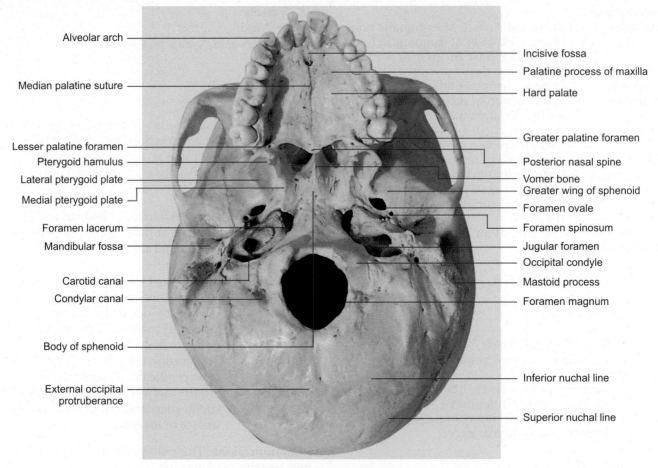

Fig. 6.8: Norma basalis

Features in the Anterior Part

1. **Alveolar arch of maxilla:** It bears sockets for the roots of upper teeth.
2. **Hard palate:** It is formed by the palatine processes of maxillae (3/4th) in front and by horizontal plates of palatine bones behind (1/4th).

Features in the Middle Part

1. Posterior border of vomer is seen separating two posterior nasal apertures
2. A broad bar of bone, formed by the fusion of the body of sphenoid and basilar part of the occipital bone.
3. **Pterygoid process of sphenoid bone:** This projects downwards from the sphenoid bone behind last molar tooth. It divides into medial and lateral pterygoid plates which are separated from each other by pterygoid fossa.
4. **Infra temporal or lateral surface of the greater wing of sphenoid.** It lies lateral to pterygoid process. Four foramina located along the posteromedial margin.

These are
   a. Foramen spinosum
   b. Foramen ovale
   c. Emissary sphenoidal foramen
   d. Canaliculus innominatus
5. **Sulcus tubae:** It is a groove seen between the posterolateral margin of the greater wing of sphenoid and petrous temporal bone. It lodges the cartilaginous part of the auditory tube.
6. **Inferior surface of the petrous temporal bone**
7. **Tympanic part of temporal bone**
8. **Squamous part of temporal bone**
9. **Tegmen tympani:** Thin plate of bone which arises from anterior surface of petrous temporal part.

Features in the Posterior Part

1. **The median area** presents following structures from before backwards
   a. Foramen magnum
   b. External occipital crest
   c. External occipital protuberance

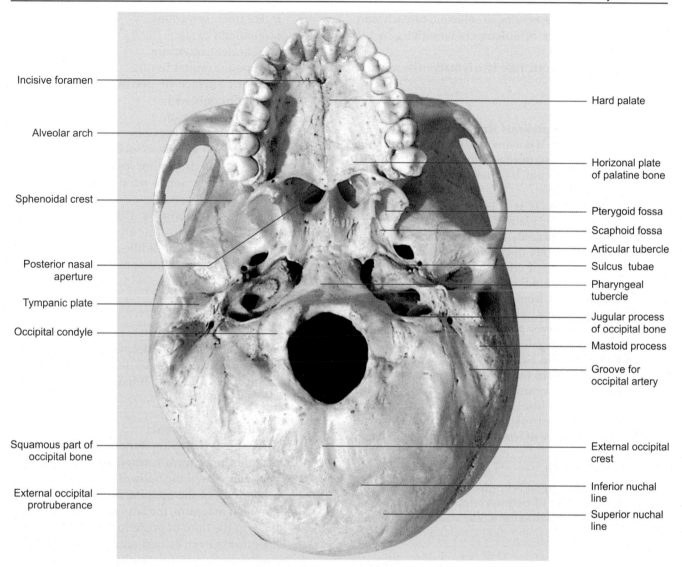

Incisive foramen

Alveolar arch

Sphenoidal crest

Posterior nasal aperture

Tympanic plate

Occipital condyle

Squamous part of occipital bone

External occipital protruberance

Hard palate

Horizonal plate of palatine bone

Pterygoid fossa

Scaphoid fossa

Articular tubercle

Sulcus tubae

Pharyngeal tubercle

Jugular process of occipital bone

Mastoid process

Groove for occipital artery

External occipital crest

Inferior nuchal line

Superior nuchal line

Fig. 6.9: Norma basalis

2. **The lateral area presents on each side:**
   a. **Occipital condyle:** It is an oval condylar process present on the side of foramen magnum.
   b. **Hypoglossal canal:** It is located antero-superior to the occipital condyle.
   c. **Condylar fossa:** It is small fossa located behind the occipital condyle.
   d. **Jugular process of occipital bone:** It lies lateral to the occipital condyle and forms the posterior boundary of jugular foramen.
   e. **Squamous part of occipital bone.**
   f. **Jugular foramen:** It is a large elongated foramen at the posterior end of the petro-occipital suture. Its anterior wall is hollowed out to form the jugular fossa.
   g. **Petrous temporal bone**

   h. **Styloid process:** It is seen projecting externally between the petrous and tympanic part of temporal bone, in the posterior aspect.
   i. **Stylomastoid foramen:** It is situated posterior to root of the process.
   j. **Mastoid process**

Internal Surface of the Base of Skull

The internal surface of the base of the skull is divided into **anterior, middle and posterior cranial fossae** (Figs 6.10 and 6.11).

Anterior Cranial Fossa

Anterior cranial fossa is bounded by the squamous part of frontal bone anteriorly and is limited posteriorly by:

CHAPTER-6

a. Free border of lesser wing of sphenoid on each side.
b. Anterior border of sulcus chiasmaticus in the median region.

The junction between these two is marked by anterior clinoid processes.

Features

1. **Median region presents from before backwards**
   a. Frontal crest: It is a median, vertical crest on the inner aspect of frontal bone.
   b. Foramen caecum: It is present at the inferior end of frontal crest.
   c. Crista galli: It is a bony crest formed by perpendicular plate of ethmoid bone.
   d. Jugum sphenoidale, superior surface of anterior part of the body of sphenoid.
   e. On each side of crista galli lies the cribriform plate of ethmoid which separates the anterior cranial fossa from nasal cavity. It possesses a number of foramina that provide passage for olfactory nerves and a nasal slit, one on either side of crista galli.
2. **Lateral region on each side presents with**
   a. Orbital plate of the frontal bone. This separates the anterior cranial fossa from the orbit and supports the frontal lobe of the brain. It shows impressions of sulci and gyri of brain.
   b. Upper surface of lesser wing of sphenoid bone.

Middle Cranial Fossa

The middle cranial fossa is limited posteriorly by
   a. Superior border of petrous temporal bone
   b. Upper border of dorsum sellae

Features

1. **The median region from before backwards presents with**
   a. **Sulcus chiasmaticus:** This sulcus leads into the optic canal on each side which further leads into the orbit.
   b. **Sella turcica:** It consists of the hypophyseal fossa which lodges the pituitary gland and is bounded in front by an anterior slope, the tuberculum sellae and behind by an upward projection, the dorsum sellae. The lateral ends of tuberculum sellae bear middle clinoid processes and the lateral ends of dorsum sellae bear posterior clinoid processes.
   c. **Carotid groove:** It is present on either side of sella turcica.
2. **The lateral area lodges the temporal lobes of the brain and presents on either side:**
   a. Cranial surface of greater wing of sphenoid. It shows four foramina arranged in a roughly semicircular array.

   i. Foramen spinosum
   ii. Foramen ovale
   iii. Foramen rotundum
   iv. Superior orbital fissure
   b. Anterior surface of petrous temporal bone which presents with:
   i. Foramen lacerum
   ii. Trigeminal impression
   iii. Hiatus and groove for greater petrosal nerve
   iv. Hiatus and groove for lesser petrosal nerve
   v. Arcuate eminence produced by superior semicircular canal.
   vi. Tegmen tympani is a thin plate of bone anteriolateral to the arcuate eminence. It forms the roof of middle ear.
   c. Inner surface of squamous part of temporal bone.

Posterior Cranial Fossa

The posterior cranial fossa is deepest and lies behind the superior border of petrous temporal bone and dorsum sellae of the sphenoid. It lodges the hind brain.

Features

1. **The median area presents**
   a. **Clivus:** It is a sloping surface seen in front of foramen magnum, formed by the fusion of posterior part of the body of sphenoid with the basilar part of the occipital bone.
   b. **Foramen magnum,** the largest foramen of skull. It lies in the floor of posterior cranial fossa. It is bounded in front by basi-occiput, posteriorly by squamous part of the occipital bone and on each side by condylar part of the occipital bone.
   c. **Hypoglossal canal:** It is present on each side of the foramen magnum.
   d. **Squamous part of occipital bone presents with:**
   i. Internal occipital crest: A vertical bony ridge.
   ii. Internal occipital protuberance: It is located opposite the external occipital protuberance.
2. **Lateral area on each side consists of**
   a. Posterior surface of petrous temporal bone. This presents the following features:
   i. A groove made by the sigmoid sinus posteriorly which opens into jugular foramen.
   ii. **Internal acoustic meatus:** It is present above the jugular foramen.
   iii. **Aqueduct of vestibule:** It is a slit like opening behind the meatus for the saccule and the ductus endolymphaticus.
   iv. **Pyramidal notch**

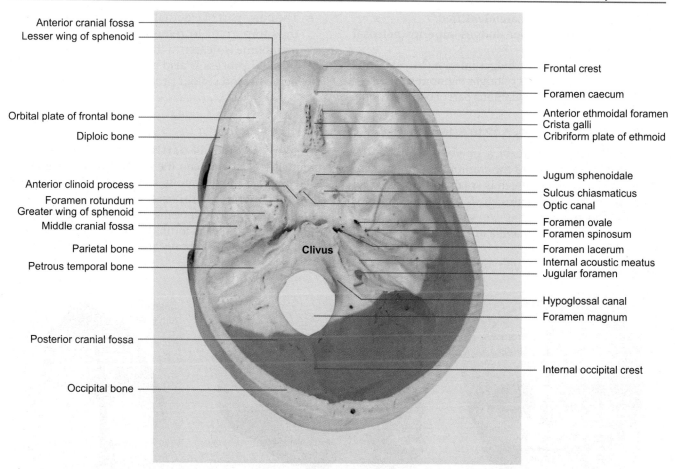

Anterior cranial fossa
Lesser wing of sphenoid

Orbital plate of frontal bone

Diploic bone

Anterior clinoid process
Foramen rotundum
Greater wing of sphenoid
Middle cranial fossa

Parietal bone
Petrous temporal bone

Posterior cranial fossa

Occipital bone

Frontal crest
Foramen caecum
Anterior ethmoidal foramen
Crista galli
Cribriform plate of ethmoid

Jugum sphenoidale
Sulcus chiasmaticus
Optic canal
Foramen ovale
Foramen spinosum
Foramen lacerum
Internal acoustic meatus
Jugular foramen

Hypoglossal canal
Foramen magnum

Internal occipital crest

Clivus

Fig. 6.10: Internal surface of base of skull

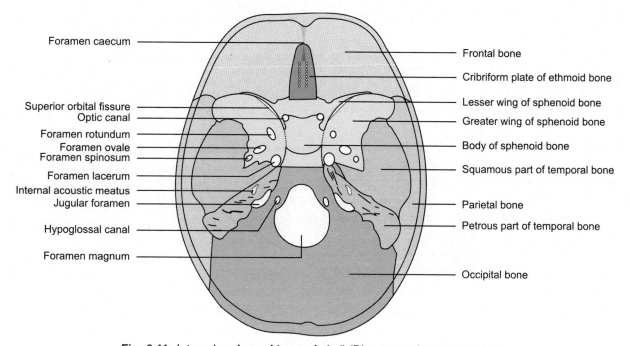

Foramen caecum

Superior orbital fissure
Optic canal
Foramen rotundum
Foramen ovale
Foramen spinosum
Foramen lacerum
Internal acoustic meatus
Jugular foramen
Hypoglossal canal
Foramen magnum

Frontal bone
Cribriform plate of ethmoid bone
Lesser wing of sphenoid bone
Greater wing of sphenoid bone
Body of sphenoid bone
Squamous part of temporal bone
Parietal bone
Petrous part of temporal bone
Occipital bone

Fig. 6.11: Internal surface of base of skull (Diagrammatic representation)

CHAPTER-6

v. **Three borders are identified**
Superior border, lodges superior petrosal sinus
Inferior border, lodges inferior petrosal sinus
Posterior border, lodges sigmoid sinus.
b. Inner surface of squamous part of occipital bone.

NEWBORN SKULL (FIGs 6.12 to 6.16)

- The striking feature of a newborn skull is the relatively large size of the cranium as compared to the facial skeleton which is small and consists of a collection of tiny bones clustered on the anterior end of the cranium.
- The mandible and maxilla are not fully developed as there are no teeth.
- The sinuses are also underdeveloped.

- The bony part of external ear is not developed. It is thus important to remember that the tympanic membrane is nearer to the surface.
- Mastoid process is also absent and thus the facial nerve behind styloid process is also superficial.

Fontanelles

The skull at birth is partly ossified and gaps or fontanelles exist between the various bones. These are filled in by a membranous structure. The fontanelles serve two important purposes:
1. Permit some overlapping of the skull bones during child birth. This is termed as moulding.
2. Permit growth of brain after birth specially in the first year of life.

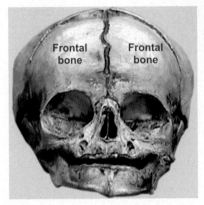

Fig. 6.12: New born skull (anterior aspect)

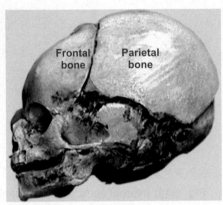

Fig. 6.13: New born skull (lateral aspect)

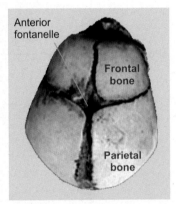

Fig. 6.14: New born skull (superior aspect)

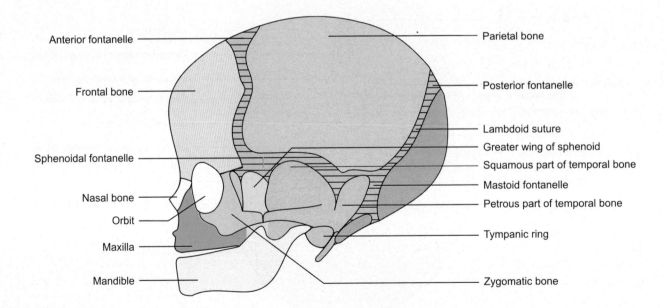

Fig. 6.15: New born skull (lateral aspect, diagrammatic representation)

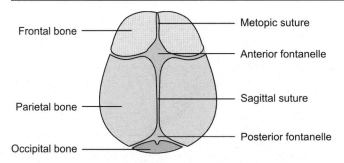

Frontal bone — Metopic suture

— Anterior fontanelle

— Sagittal suture

Parietal bone —

— Posterior fontanelle

Occipital bone —

Fig. 6.16: New born skull (superior aspect)

Number of fontanelles: There are six fontanelles, one situated at each angle of the parietal bone.

1. **Median fontanelles:** These are two in number namely,
   a. **Anterior fontanelle:** It is rhomboid in shape and is present at the meeting point of sagittal, coronal and metopic sutures. It closes by 18 to 24 months of age.
   b. **Posterior fontanelle:** It is triangular in shape and lies at junction of sagittal and lambdoid sutures. It closes by 4 months of age.
2. **Lateral fontanelles:** These are four in number
   a. Two anterolateral fontanelles or **sphenoidal fontanelles.**
   b. Two posterolateral fontanelles or **mastoid fontanelles.**

INDIVIDUAL SKULL BONES

MANDIBLE

Mandible or lower jaw is the largest and the strongest bone of the face (Fig. 6.17). It consists of three parts

1. **Body:** It is horse shoe shaped. External surface presents a faint vertical ridge in the mid-line known as symphysis menti. Upper border is also known as alveolar border and bears sockets for teeth of lower jaw. Lower border is known as base of mandible.
2. **Pair of rami:** One ramus is attached on either side of the body. It is more or less a quadrilateral plate of bone. Lateral surface is overlapped by parotid gland. Superior border presents two processes:
   a. **Coronoid process:** It is a triangular projection from anterior end of superior border.
   b. **Condylar process:** It is an expanded projection from posterosuperior aspect of the ramus. The upper end is the head which articulates with the mandibular fossa of temporal bone to form temporomandibular joint.

MAXILLA

Maxilla is an irregular, pyramidal shaped bone. One maxilla is present on either side of the midline (Figs 6.18A and B). Each maxilla consists of a body and four processes.

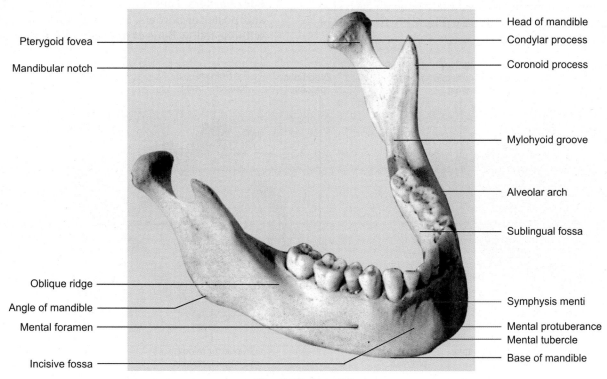

Pterygoid fovea — — Head of mandible

— Condylar process

Mandibular notch — — Coronoid process

— Mylohyoid groove

— Alveolar arch

— Sublingual fossa

Oblique ridge —

Angle of mandible — — Symphysis menti

Mental foramen — — Mental protuberance
— Mental tubercle

Incisive fossa — — Base of mandible

Fig. 6.17: Mandible

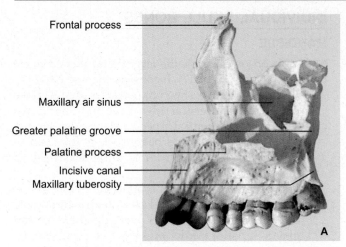
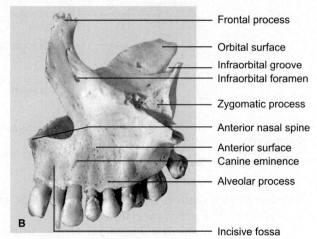

Figs 6.18A and B: (A) Right maxilla (medial view) (B) Left maxilla (lateral view)

1. **Body:** It is pyramidal in shape and contains a cavity called the maxillary air sinus within its substance (see page no. 357). It has an anterior and a posterior surface, a nasal surface which forms the lateral wall of nasal cavity and a orbital surface which forms the floor of orbit.
2. **Four processes:** Frontal process, zygomatic process, alveolar process, palatine process. The alveolar processes of each side join and form the upper alveolar arch or upper jaw. The palatine processes of both sides join to form anterior part of the hard palate.

TEMPORAL BONES

A pair of temporal bones are situated one on each side of the skull extending to its base (Fig. 6.19). It consists of following four basic parts:

1. Squamous part
2. Petro-mastoid part
3. Tympanic part
4. Styloid process

PARIETAL BONES

These are a pair of curved plate of bones which form the major portion of the vault of the skull. Each parietal bone is quadrilateral in shape and presents with two surfaces and four borders (Fig. 6.20):

1. **Two surfaces:** External surface is smooth and convex. Internal surface is concave and covers the parietal lobe of brain.
2. **Four borders:** These are superior, inferior, anterior and posterior borders. Superior border articulates with the fellow bone of opposite side at the sagittal

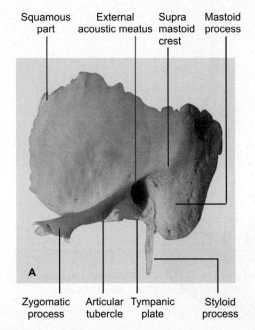
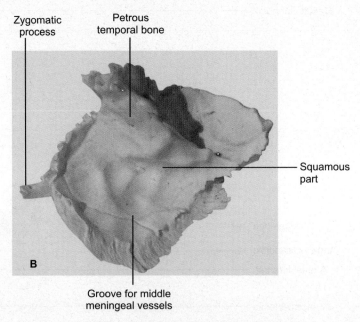

Figs 6.19A and B: (A) Left temporal bone (external view) (B) Left temporal bone (internal view)

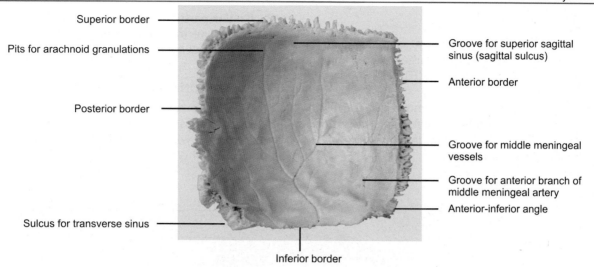

Fig. 6.20: Left parietal bone (internal view)

Superior border

Pits for arachnoid granulations

Posterior border

Sulcus for transverse sinus

Groove for superior sagittal sinus (sagittal sulcus)

Anterior border

Groove for middle meningeal vessels

Groove for anterior branch of middle meningeal artery

Anterior-inferior angle

Inferior border

suture. Inner aspect forms a groove that lodges the superior sagittal sinus.

ZYGOMATIC BONES

The zygomatic bones form the prominence of the cheeks. Each bone has a body and two processes namely: frontal process and temporal process (Fig. 6.21).

FRONTAL BONE

It is located in the region of forehead. It is shaped like a shell and presents with the following parts (Fig. 6.22):

1. Squamous part, forms the region of forehead.
2. Nasal part, articulates with the nasal bones.
3. Two orbital plates: These form the roof of orbit on each side.
4. Two zygomatic processes.
5. Frontal air sinuses (see page no. 357).

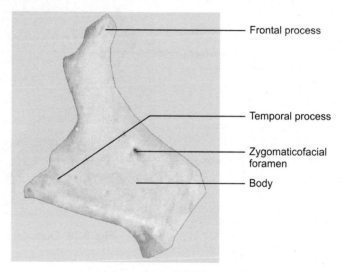

Frontal process

Temporal process

Zygomaticofacial foramen

Body

Fig. 6.21: Right Zygomatic bone (external view)

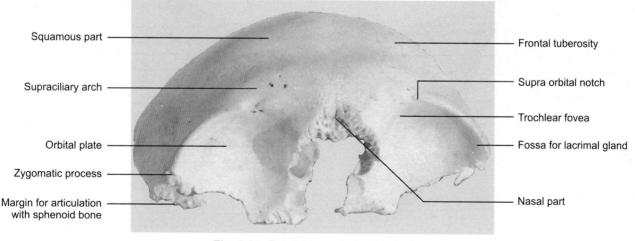

Squamous part

Supraciliary arch

Orbital plate

Zygomatic process

Margin for articulation with sphenoid bone

Frontal tuberosity

Supra orbital notch

Trochlear fovea

Fossa for lacrimal gland

Nasal part

Fig. 6.22: Frontal bone (external view)

OCCIPITAL BONE

Occipital bone occupies the posterior part of skull. It is characterized by the presence of a large foramen known as foramen magnum, in the midline (Fig. 6.23). It consists of following four parts:

1. **Squamous part:** It is an expanded plate of bone present above and behind the foramen magnum.
2. **Two condylar parts** situated externally, one on each side of foramen magnum.

3. **Basilar part:** This projects forwards and upwards in front of the foramen magnum and fuses with the body of sphenoid.

SPHENOID BONE

The sphenoid is an unpaired irregularly shaped bone situated at the base of skull. Its structure resembles a bat with spreadout wings. It consists of the following seven parts (Fig. 6.24)

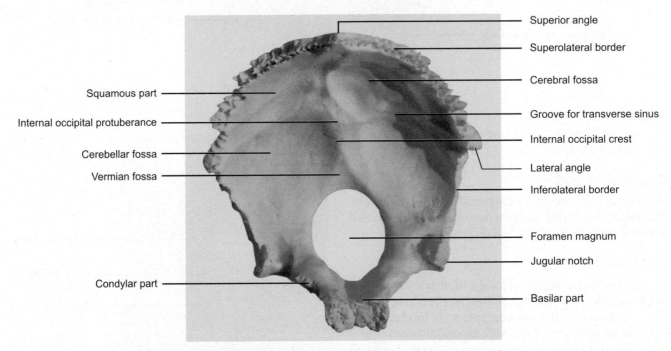

Fig. 6.23: Occipital bone (internal surface)

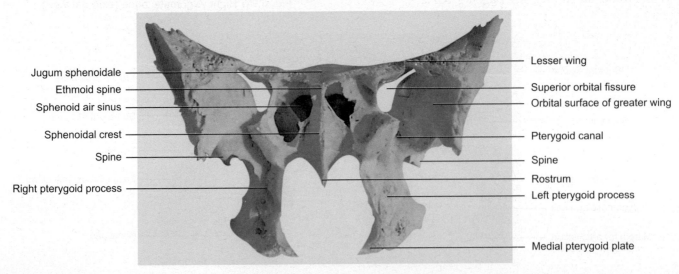

Fig. 6.24: Sphenoid bone (anterior view)

1. Body: It has the sphenoidal air sinuses (see page no. 357)
2. Two lesser wings
3. Two greater wings
4. Two pterygoid processes

ETHMOID BONE (FIG. 6.25)

Ethmoid bone is a single irregular bone located between the two orbital cavities superiorly. It consists of two parts:

1. **Cribiform plate:** It is a central horizontal plate which has numerous pores that transmit olfactory nerve filaments.

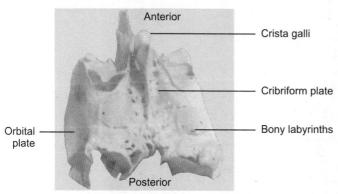

Fig. 6.25: Ethmoid bone (superior view)

2. **Bony labyrinths:** These are cuboidal shaped boxes filled with air cells which extend downwards, one on each side, from the lateral border of the cribiform plate.

PALATINE BONES

Each palatine bone is lodged between the maxilla in front and pterygoid process of sphenoid behind. It is an L-shaped bone with a perpendicular and a horizontal plate. The horizontal plate is quadrilateral in shape and extends medially to join the opposite side plate. The two together form posterior part of the hard palate.

VOMER

It is a thin quadrilateral plate of bone which forms the postero-inferior part of nasal septum.

NASAL BONES

These are a pair of triangular bones which form the bridge of the nose.

LACRIMAL BONES

These are thin plates of bones situated on the medial aspect of the orbit.

INFERIOR NASAL CONCHAE

These are a pair of curved bones, lying in an antero-posterior direction, on the lateral wall of nasal cavity.

HYOID BONE

This U-shaped bone is located in the front portion of the neck between the mandible and the larynx at the level of third cervical vertebra. It does not articulate with any other bone but, is suspended from the styloid processes of temporal bones on each side by stylohyoid ligaments (Fig. 6.26). Hyoid bone consists of the following five parts

1. A body
2. A pair of greater cornu (also called horns).
3. A pair of lesser cornu.

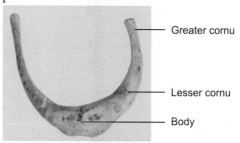

Fig. 6.26: Hyoid bone (anterio-superior view)

VERTEBRAL COLUMN

- Vertebral column is made up of 33 vertebrae articularted with each other in a vertical line (Figs 5.2 to 5.4). These are:
  1. 7 cervical vertebrae
  2. 12 thoracic vertebrae
  3. 5 lumbar vertebrae
  4. 5 sacral vertebrae
  5. 4 coccygeal vertebrae
- The column encloses a vertebral canal formed by joining of the vertebral foramen of the 33 vertebrae. The vertebral canal contains spinal cord with its meninges, nerve roots and blood vessels.
- Length of vertebral column in adult male is 70 cm and in adult female is 60 cm.
- The adjacent vertebrae are join together by intervertebral disc between the vertebral bodies and by synovial joints between the facets on the pedicle of vertebrae (except in sacral vertebrae which are fused to form a single sacrum).
- On each side a gap is present between two adjacent vertebrae known as the intervertebral foramen which transmits spinal nerves and vessels.
- Vertebral column is not linear. It presents with two primary and two secondary curvatures, in the sagittal plane.
- **Primary curvatures:** The vertebral column is curved with concavity facing anteriorly in the thoracic and pelvic (sacral) regions. These are primary curvatures of the column whcih correspond to the flexed attitude of the fetus.
- **Secondary curvatures:** The vertebral column presents with convex curvature anteriorly at the cervical and lumbar regions. These are the secondary curvatures of the vertebral column

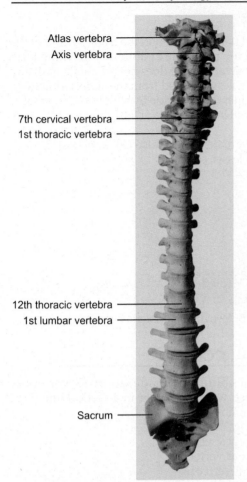

Atlas vertebra
Axis vertebra
7th cervical vertebra
1st thoracic vertebra
12th thoracic vertebra
1st lumbar vertebra
Sacrum

Fig. 6.27: Vertebral column (ventral aspect)

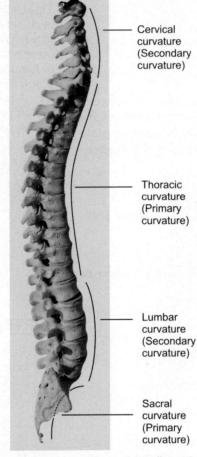

Cervical curvature (Secondary curvature)
Thoracic curvature (Primary curvature)
Lumbar curvature (Secondary curvature)
Sacral curvature (Primary curvature)

Fig. 6.28: Vertebral column (lateral aspect)

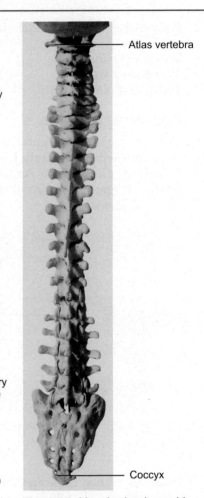

Atlas vertebra
Coccyx

Fig. 6.29: Vertebral column (dorsal aspect)

which help adapt to the upright posture and walking on two legs (bipedal gait).

- There may be a slight lateral curvature seen in the thoracic region which is convex to right side, in right-handed person and left in left-handed person.
- **The line of centre of gravity of vertebral column,** in erect posture, extends through the process of dens to just anterior to body of T_2 vertebra. It then passes down through the center of T_{12} vertebra to the posterior part of body of L_5 vertebra. Further it lies anterior to sacrum.
- A diurnal variation seen in the height of vertebral column from recumbencey to the upright posture. The overall height loss with in 3 hours after rising up in the morning has been found to be upto 16 mm.

Movements of Vertebral Column

Following movements occur at the vertebral column
  a. Flexion
  b. Extension
  c. Lateral flexion
  d. Rotation
  e. Circumduction

These movements are restricted by limited deformation of the intervertebral discs and shape of articular facets in different regions of vertebral column.

Anatomical Features of A Vertebra

- Vertebra is made up of a ventral body and a dorsal vertebral or neural arch that encloses the vertebral foramen.
- The body of vertebra is like a small cylinder which varies in size and shape in the various regions. The size of body increases from cervical to lumbar regions. This is associated with an increase in load of weight on lower vertebra.
- Vertebral arch is made up of a pedicle and a lamina on each side.
- Each pedicle is a short and thick projection from superior part of body projecting dorsally. The superior and inferior borders of the pedicle are notched and when two adjacent vertebrae are joined they are converted to intervertebral foramen.
- Lamina is a broad, vertically flattened part which is dorsal to pedicle and continues medially to meet the lamina of other side.

- A spinous process or vertebral spine projects from dorsal surface of junction of laminae posteriorly.
- The junction of pedicle and lamina bears superior and inferior articular facets on each side.
- Two small bony processes known transverse processes extend laterally on each side from junction of pedicle and lamina.

CERVICAL VERTEBRAE

There are seven cervical vertebrae. They are small in size as compared to thoracic vertebrae as they have to carry less weight. **They are identified by the presence of foramen transversarium—the cardinal feature of cervical vertebrae.** The foramen transmits vertebral artery on each side.

General Features of Typical Cervical Vertebrae (Fig. 6.30)

1. The body is small.
2. Vertebral foramen is roughly triangular in shape.
3. The pedicles project posterolaterally. The lamina are thin and long and project posteromedially.
4. The superior and inferior articular facets are flat.

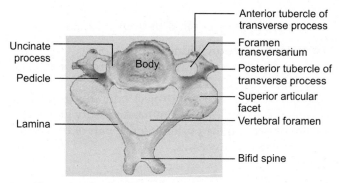

Fig. 6.30: Typical cervical vertebra (superior view)

5. Transverse processes are short and present with a foramen known as foramen transversarium.
6. The spine is short and bifid.

First Cervical Vertebra

The first cervical vertebra is called **atlas** because it supports the globe of the head. It is in the shape of a ring and has neither a body nor a spine. It consists of right and left lateral masses, right and left transverse processes with the foramen transversaria and two arches, anterior and posterior arches (Fig. 6.31).

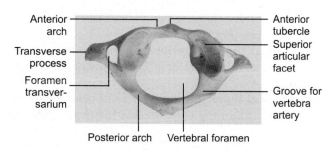

Fig. 6.31: Atlas vertebra (superior view)

Second Cervical Vertebra

The second cervical vertebra is called **axis** because the atlas rotates like a wheel around the axis provided by its odontoid process or dens (Fig. 6.32). It has a strong tooth like process projecting upwards from the body called the **odontoid process**. The dens articulates anteriorly with the anterior arch of the atlas and posteriorly with the transverse ligament of the atlas. The spine is massive, i.e., it is large, thick and very strong. It is deeply grooved inferiorly. The transverse processes are very small and lack the anterior tubercles. The foramen transversarium is directed upwards and laterally. The laminae are thick and strong.

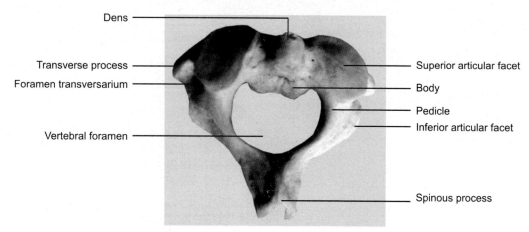

Fig. 6.32: Axis vertebra (superior view)

Seventh Cervical Vertebra

The seventh cervical vertebra is called as vertebra prominens because it's spine is very long and prominent. It is visible through the skin in the lower part of the nuchal furrow. The spine is thick, long and nearly horizontal. It is not bifid and ends in a tubercle. The transverse processes are comparatively larger in size and lacks the anterior tubercles. The foramen transversarium is relatively small and does not transmit the vertebral artery. It transmits only accessory vertebral vein.

THORACIC VERTEBRAE

There are twelve thoracic vertebrae. They are divided into two types (Fig. 6.33).

1. **Typical thoracic vertebrae:** These have similar characteristics. Vertebrae T_2 to T_8 are of the typical type.
2. **Atypical thoracic vertebrae:** Their basic structure is that of thoracic vertebrae but they have peculiar

characteristics of their own. T_1 and T_9 to T_{12} vertebrae belong to this group.

Identification of thoracic vertebrae: Thoracic vertebrae are identified with the help of following features
1. Heart shaped bodies.
2. Presence of costal facets on the sides of the bodies.
3. Presence of costal facets on the transverse processes, except in the 11 and 12th thoracic vertebrae.

Features of Thoracic Vertebra

1. Body is heart shaped.
2. Vertebral foramen is small and circular.
3. Pedicles are short and present with two notches.
4. Transverse processes are large and project laterally and backwards from the junction of the pedicles and the laminae.
5. Laminae are short, thick and broad.
6. Spinous processes are long and slope downwards.

LUMBAR VERTEBRAE

There are five lumbar vertebrae. The size of bodies of lumbar vertebrae increases from above downward. Upper four lumbar vertebrae are typical (Fig. 6.34).

Features of Typical Lumbar Vertebra

1. Massive reniform (kidney shaped) body.
2. Conspicuous vertebral notches are present on pedicles.
3. Transverse processes project laterally from the junction of pedicle and lamina. Accessory tubercles are present on the posteroinferior part of the roots of transverse processes.

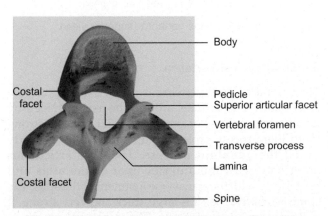

Fig. 6.33: Typical thoracic vertebra (superior view)

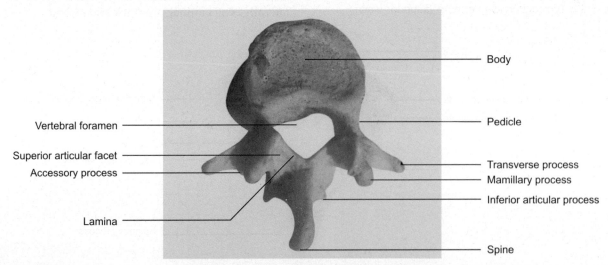

Fig. 6.34: Lumbar vertebra (superior aspect)

4. Superior articular facets are concave facing backward and medially. They lie further apart from inferior articular facet.
5. A mamillary tubercle is present at the posterior margin of each superior articular facet.
6. Spine is quadrangular and horizontal.

5th lumbar vertebra is atypical and presents the following features
1. Body of L$_5$ is the largest
2. Anterior surface of 5th lumbar vertebra is more extensive than posterior surface.
3. Distance between superior and inferior articular facets is identical.
4. Transverse processes encroach on the sides of the body. They are short and large.
5. Vertebral canal is triangular.

SACRUM

It is a large, flattened, triangular bone formed by fusion of 5 sacral vertebrae. The upper part of sacrum is broad and stout as it supports the body weight. The lower part is narrow and tapers downwards. The sacrum articulates with the two hip bones on either side in its upper part. Weight transmission of the body occurs from sacrum through each of the sacro-iliac joints to the hip and thence to the lower limb (Figs 6.35 and 6.36).

Anatomical Features

Sacrum is divided into a base, an apex and four surfaces.

Base of Sacrum

It is formed by the upper surface of 1st sacral vertebra. The first sacral vertebra is similar to the lumbar vertebra. It can be divided into following parts
1. **Body:** It articulates with L$_5$ vertebra. The anterior border is prominent and projects anteriorly. It is known as the sacral promontory.

2. **Vertebral foramen:** Is present behind the body and leads to the sacral canal below. It is triangular in shape.
3. **Pedicles**
4. **Laminae**
5. **The spine:** It forms the first spinous tubercle on posterior surface of sacrum.
6. **Transverse processes:** They are modified to form ala of sacrum on either side. Each ala is formed by fusion of transverse process and the corresponding costal element.

Apex

It is formed by inferior surface of 5th sacral vertebra and articulates with coccyx.

Pelvic/Ventral Surface

It is concave and directed downwards and forwards.

Dorsal Surface

- It is a rough, convex and irregular surface. It is directed backwards and upwards.
- A bony ridge is present in median plane called the **median sacral crest.** This bears 3 to 4 tubercles which represent the fused spines of upper 4 sacral vertebrae.
- Below the 4th tubercle is an inverted V-shaped gap called the **sacral hiatus.** The haitus is formed because the laminae of the 5th sacral vertebra fail to meet posteriorly.
- Lateral to median crest the posterior surface is formed by fused laminae of sacral vertebrae.
- The inferior articular process of 5th vertebra is free and forms **cornu** on either side of sacral hiatus.
- Four dorsal/posterior sacral foramina are present on each side of fused articular processes. These transmit the dorsal rami of upper four sacral nerves.

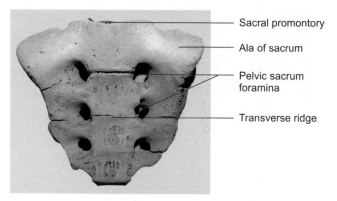

Fig. 6.35: Sacrum (pelvic surface)

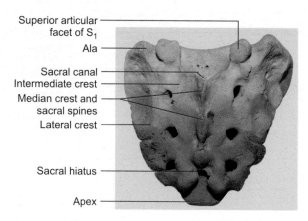

Fig. 6.36: Sacrum (Dorsal aspect)

CHAPTER-6

- Lateral most is the lateral sacral crest on each side of sacrum. It presents with transverse tubercles which are the fused transverse processes of the vertebrae.

Lateral Surfaces

- It is formed by the fused transverse processes and costal elements of sacral vertebrae.
- The upper part is wider and bears an L-shaped articular surface anteriorly. It articulates with the auricular surface of hip bone and forms the sacro-iliac joint.

Sacral Canal

- It is formed by the central foramen of fused sacral vertebrae
- It contains the cauda equina, filum terminale and spinal meninges
- Subdural and subarachnoid spaces end at the level of 2nd sacral vertebra.

COCCYX (FIG. 6.29)

It is formed by fusion of four rudimentary coccygeal vertebrae. It is a small triangular bone with the wider part above and an apex below.

Anatomical Features

It consists of
1. Base: It is formed by the upper surface of body of first coccygeal vertebra. This articulates with the apex of sacrum. Projecting up from the posterolateral

sides of the base are coccygeal cornu which represent the pedicles and superior articular surfaces. The 2nd, 3rd and 4th coccygeal vertebrae are merely bony nodules which progressively diminish in size
2. Pelvic surface: Ganglion impar is present over it.
3. Dorsal surface
4. Lateral margins
5. Apex

THORACIC CAGE

It consists of an osseo-cartilaginous framework which encloses the thoracic cavity. It is formed by twelve pairs of ribs with costal cartilages, twelve thoracic vertebrae and sternum (Fig. 6.37).

STERNUM

It is a flat bone which lies in the median part of the anterior thoracic wall (Fig. 6.38).

Anatomical Features

It has three parts
1. **Manubrium:** It is the upper part of sternum and is roughly quadrangular in shape. It lies at the level opposite to the T_3 and T_4 vertebrae. Posterior surface is related to the following important structures:
   a. Brachiocephalic artery
   b. Left common carotid artery
   c. Left subclavian artery
   d. Left brachiocephalic vein
   e. Arch of aorta, in lower part
   f. Lung and pleura, along its lateral margins

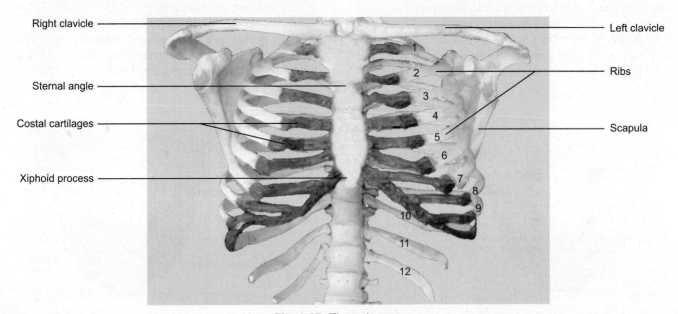

Fig. 6.37: Thoracic cage

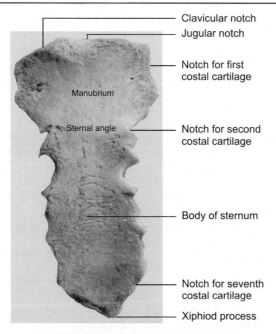

Clavicular notch
Jugular notch
Notch for first costal cartilage
Manubrium
Sternal angle
Notch for second costal cartilage
Body of sternum
Notch for seventh costal cartilage
Xiphiod process

Fig. 6.38: Sternum (anterior aspect)

2. **Body of sternum:** It lies opposite the level of bodies of T_5 to T_9 thoracic vertebrae. It is twice as long as the manubrium and is made up of four sternal segments (sternebrae). It is widest at the level of the 5th costal cartilage. Posterior surface is related to
   a. On right side: Pleura and anterior border of right lung.
   b. On left side: Pleura and left lung in upper part, pericardium and heart in lower part.
3. **Xiphoid process:** It is also known as **xiphisternum.** It is the small tapering part of the sternum which lies in the epigastric fossa. It is triangular in shape with its apex downwards. It may also be broad and flat, bifid or perforated.

RIBS

Ribs are flat bones and represent the costal elements of thoracic vertebrae. They form the largest part of the thoracic cage. There are a total of 12 pairs of ribs. These elongated, flat bones articulate posteriorly with the corresponding thoracic vertebrae. They extend up to the sternum anteriorly, (except the 11th and 12th ribs) (Figs 6.39 to 6.43). The corresponding ribs of two sides with sternum and the thoracic vertebra form an oval shaped cavity.

Classification of Ribs

1. **True ribs:** They are also called vertebrosternal ribs. These ribs articulate both with the vertebral column and the sternum. Upper seven pairs constitute true ribs.
2. **False ribs:** These ribs articulate indirectly with sternum or do not articulate with it at all. Lower

five pair of ribs are false ribs. False ribs are further divided into:
   a. **Vertebrochondral ribs:** 8th, 9th and 10th ribs articulate posteriorly with vertebrae, while anterioly their costal cartilages fuse together and then fuse with the 7th costal cartilage which joins with the sternum.
   b. **Floating ribs:** Their anterior ends do not articulate with sternum or with any costal cartilage. They lie free in abdominal wall. The 11th and 12th ribs belong to this category.
3. **Typical ribs:** They bear common features and individual identification is not possible. 3rd to 9th ribs are typical.
4. **Atypical ribs:** They have individual distinguishing features. 1st, 2nd, 10th, 11th and 12th ribs are atypical ribs.

Anatomical Features of a Typical Rib

Each typical rib presents the following three parts (Fig. 6.39):
1. **Anterior end or the sternal end:** It presents a cup shaped oval depression for articulation with the costal cartilage. This end lies at a lower level than the vertebral end.
2. **Shaft:** The shaft of a rib is thin and flat. It curves backwards and laterally from the anterior end and then turns backwards and medially. It has an upper and a lower border with an inner and an outer surface. Upper border is thick and lower border is thin inner surface is concave, smooth and is related to the pleura. The lower part has a groove known as the costal groove which contains from above downwards.
   a. Posterior intercostal vein
   b. Posterior intercostal artery
   c. Intercostal nerve
   The shaft is curved at an angle about 5 cm in front of tubercle of rib which is known as angle of rib.
3. **Posterior end or the vertebral end:** It has the following three parts:
   a. **Head:** It consists of two facets separated by a crest.
   b. **Neck:** It extends from the head to the tubercle.
   c. **Tubercle:** It is a small elevation present posteriorly at the junction of neck with shaft. It has a medial articular facet which forms the costotransverse joint with the transverse process of corresponding vertebra. The lateral part is non articular.

First Rib

It has the following peculiarities (Fig. 6.40).
   a. It is the shortest and the strongest of true ribs.
   b. It is broad and flat with upper and lower surfaces and inner and outer borders.
   c. The vertebral end has a small head with a single facet and an elongated round neck.

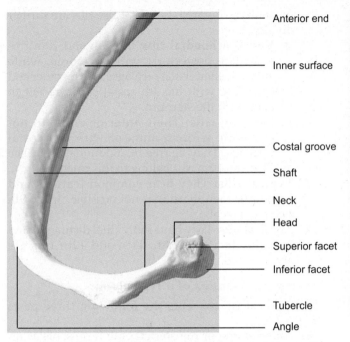

Anterior end

Inner surface

Costal groove

Shaft

Neck

Head

Superior facet

Inferior facet

Tubercle

Angle

Fig. 6.39: Typical rib of left side (seen from posterior end)

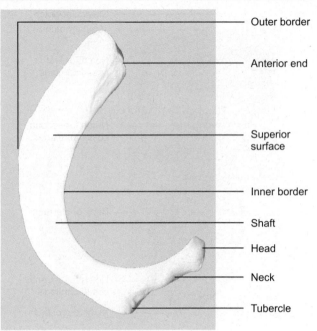

Outer border

Anterior end

Superior surface

Inner border

Shaft

Head

Neck

Tubercle

Fig. 6.40: 1st rib of left side

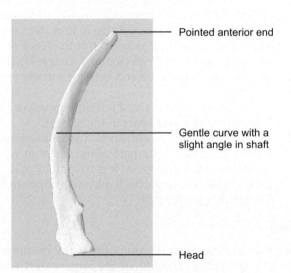

Pointed anterior end

Gentle curve with a slight angle in shaft

Head

Fig. 6.42: 11th rib of left side

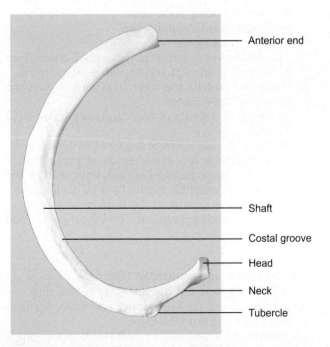

Anterior end

Shaft

Costal groove

Head

Neck

Tubercle

Fig. 6.41: 2nd rib of left side

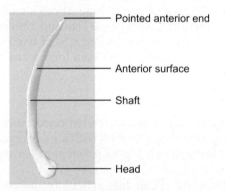

Pointed anterior end

Anterior surface

Shaft

Head

Fig. 6.43: 12th rib of left side

Second Rib

Peculiarities of 2nd rib (Fig. 6.42).
   a. It is twice as long as the 1st rib and is thinner. It is shaped more like a typical rib.
   b. Posterior angle of rib is present close to the tubercle
   c. Head presents with two facets.
   d. Costal groove, present on inner surface is short.

10th Rib

It has one single facet on its head. The rest of the features are similar to a typical rib.

11th Rib

1. **Anterior end:** It is pointed and ends midway.
2. **Posterior end:** The head has a single large facet. It does not have neck and tubercle.
3. **Shaft:** It has a gentle curve with a slight angle. A shallow costal groove is present on its inner surface.

12th Rib

It is a short floating rib attached posteriorly to T_{12} vertebra but ends anteriorly midway within the musculature (Fig. 6.43).

Costal Cartilages

- These are hyaline cartilages extending from the anterior ends of the ribs.
- These cartilages represent the unossified anterior parts of the embryonic cartilaginous ribs.
- Upper seven costal cartilages articulate with the sternum forming costosternal joints which are of the synovial variety.
- 8th to 10th costal cartilages join with each other and further join the 7th costal cartilage.

- The floating anterior ends of the 11th and 12th ribs are also capped by cartilage.
   Function: The costal cartilages provide elasticity and mobility to the thoracic column.

BONES OF UPPER LIMB

CLAVICLE

It is also known as collar bone. It connects the sternum with scapula (Figs 6.44 and 6.45).

Characteristics of Clavicle

1. It is the first bone to be ossified in the body. Ossification occurs in the 5th and 6th week of intrauterine life from two primary centres.
2. Clavicle is subcutaneous throughout.
3. It is a long bone. However, it differs from a typical long bone because of following features:
   a. It has no medullary cavity.
   b. Ossification of clavicle is membranous except at the two ends.
   c. It is placed in a horizontal position in the body.

Anatomical Features

1. The clavicle has a shaft and two ends.
2. **The medial or sternal end** is rounded and articulates with manubrium sterni forming the sternoclavicular joint. A small inferior part articulates with the first costal cartilage.
3. **The lateral end is also known as acromial end.** It is flattened and articulates with the acromian process of scapula forming acromioclavicular joint.

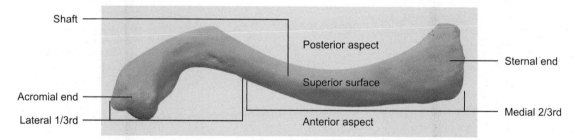

Fig. 6.44: Superior aspect of right clavicle

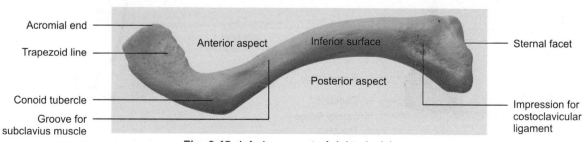

Fig. 6.45: Inferior aspect of right clavicle

4. The shaft is divided into a medial part (2/3rd) which is convex in front and a lateral part (1/3rd) which is concave in front.

HUMERUS

It is the bone of the arm (Figs 6.46 and 6.47).

Anatomical Features

It is a long bone divided into two ends (Upper and Lower) and one shaft.

Upper End of Humerus

It consists of the following parts:

1. **Head of humerus:** It is rounded and forms about 1/3rd of a sphere. It articulates with the glenoid cavity of scapula to form shoulder joint and is covered by articular cartilage.

2. **Neck of humerus**
   a. **Anatomical neck:** Is the part which surrounds the margin of head. It connects the head to the upper end of humerus.
   b. **Morphological neck:** It is the line of fusion between the epiphysis and diaphysis. It corresponds to a line passing through the lower part of greater and lesser tubercles.
   c. **Surgical neck:** Is the junction of upper end of humerus with the shaft. It is seen as a slightly constricted portion below the epiphyseal line. It is the narrowest upper part of shaft of humerus which is most likely to be fractured in case of injury to upper part of humerus.

3. **Tubercles of humerus**
   a. Lesser tubercle
   b. Greater tubercle

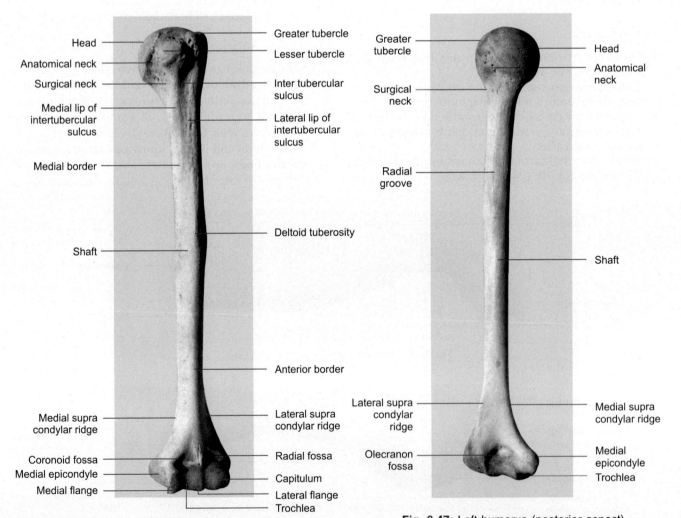

Fig. 6.46: Left humerus (anterior aspect)

Fig. 6.47: Left humerus (posterior aspect)

4. **Inter tubercular sulcus (Bicipital groove):** It is the groove present between the greater and lesser tubercles on the anterior surface of humerus below the head. It contains the following structures
   a. Tendon of long head of biceps
   b. Synovial sheath of the tendon
   c. Ascending branch of anterior circumflex humeral artery.

Shaft of Humerus

It is rounded in upper half and triangular in lower half. It presents three borders namely: anterior, medial and lateral and has three surfaces namely: anterolateral surface, anteromedial surface and posterior surface.

Lower End of Humerus

It is expanded from side to side to form the condyle and is divided into articular and nonarticular portions.
1. Articular part consists of
   a. Capitulum: It articulates with head of radius.
   b. Trochlea: It articulates with trochlear notch on ulna.
2. Non articular parts consists of two epicondyles medial epicondyle and lateral epicondyle which are felt as subcutaneous projections.

SCAPULA

It is also known as shoulder blade (Figs 6.48 and 6.49). The clavicle and scapula together form shoulder girdle. It is homologous to the ilium of hip bone.

Anatomical Features

1. It is a large, flat triangular bone situated on each side of upper part of posterolateral aspect of thorax.
2. It extends from 2nd to 7th ribs and consists of a body and three processes.
3. The body of scapula presents a costal or ventral surface and a dorsal surface. It has three borders namely: superior border, medial or vertebral border and lateral border. The borders meet at angles and form superior angle, inferior angle and lateral angle. The lateral angle presents a glenoid fossa which articulates with the head of humerus to form the shoulder joint.
4. Scapula bears three processes namely:
   a. Spinous process: It is a large process on the dorsal surface of the scapula. Its posterior border is subcutaneous.
   b. Acromion process: It is a anterior projection from the lateral most end of spinous process. It articulates with lateral end of clavicle to form acromio-clavicular joint.
   c. Coracoid process: It is a short process from upper part of glenoid cavity. It is directed anteriorly.

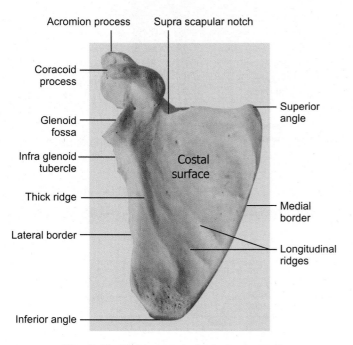

Fig. 6.48: Right scapula (anterior aspect)

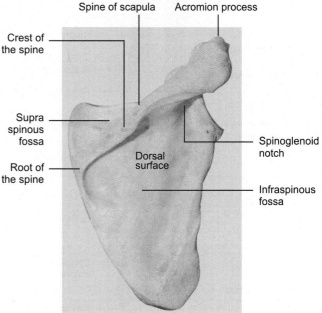

Fig. 6.49: Right scapula (posterior aspect)

CHAPTER-6

RADIUS

It is the long bone of forearm situated laterally. It is homologous with the tibia of lower limb (Figs 6.50 and 6.51).

Anatomical Features

It is divided into two ends and a shaft.

Upper End of Radius

This includes the following:
1. **Head:** It is disc shaped. The superior surface articulates with the capitulum of humerus to form elbow joint. Medial side of head articulates with ulna to form superior Radio-ulnar joint.
2. **Neck:** It is a small constricted part below the head.
3. **Radial tuberosity**

Shaft of Radius

It has three borders anterior border, medial or interosseous border and posterior border. It presents three surfaces anterior surface, posterior surface and lateral surface.

Lower End of Radius

It is the widest part of bone and has five surfaces. Medial surface articulates with head of ulna to form inferior Radio-ulnar joint. Inferior surface articulates with scaphoid laterally and lunate medially to form wrist joint.

ULNA

It is the bone of forearm placed medially and is homologous to the fibula of lower limb (Figs 6.50 and 6.51).

Anatomical Features

It has two ends and a shaft.

Upper End of Ulna

It has two processes and two articular surfaces known as notches
1. **Olecranon process:** It is an upward, hook like projection and its tip fits into the olecranon fossa of humerus when forearm is extended. Posterior surface is a smooth triangular subcutaneous area separated from skin by a bursa. This surface in its upper part forms the point of elbow, most prominent when the elbow is flexed.

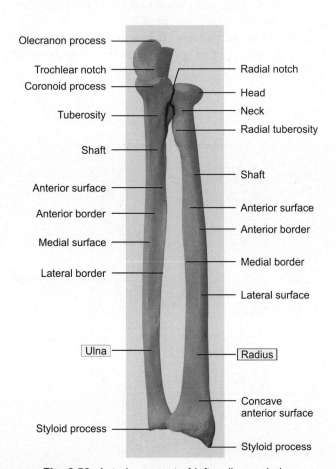

Fig. 6.50: Anterior aspect of left radius and ulna

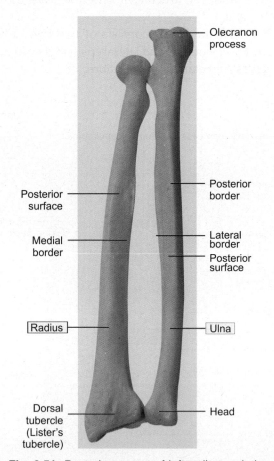

Fig. 6.51: Posterior aspect of left radius and ulna

2. **Coronoid process:** It is a bracket like forward projection from the area just below olecrenon.

3. **Trochlear notch:** It articulates with the trochlea of the humerus to form elbow joint.

4. **Radial notch:** It is situated on the lateral surface and it articulates with medial aspect of head of radius forming superior radio-ulnar joint.

Shaft of Ulna

It has three borders anterior border, lateral or interosseous border and posterior border. Posterior border is subcutaneous and can be felt on the lateral aspect of forearm, dorsally. It presents with three surfaces anterior surface, medial surface and posterior surface.

Lower End of Ulna

It consists of the following two parts

1. **Head of ulna:** It is subcutaneous posteriorly. Laterally it presents a facet for articulation with ulnar notch of radius to form inferior radio-ulnar part.

2. **Styloid process:** It projects down from the posteromedial side of lower end of ulna.

BONES OF THE HAND

Hand has twenty seven bones. These include eight carpals, five metacarpals and fourteen phalanges (Fig. 6.52).

Carpal Bones

- They are 8 short bones arranged in two rows.
- Proximal row consists of (from lateral to medial) scaphoid, lunate, triquetral and pisiform.
- Distal row consists of (from lateral to medial) trapezium, trapezoid, capitate and hamate.
- A neumonic has been designed with first letter of each bone to remember the names of the bone—She looks too pretty, try to catch her.

Metacarpals

- These are five in number and numbered from lateral to medial side (Fig. 6.52).
- The thumb is the first metacarpal and little finger the fifth metacarpal
- Each metacarpal is a miniature long bone and is divided into three parts namely, distal end which is rounded and called the head, proximal end which is expanded from side to side and named the base and shaft.

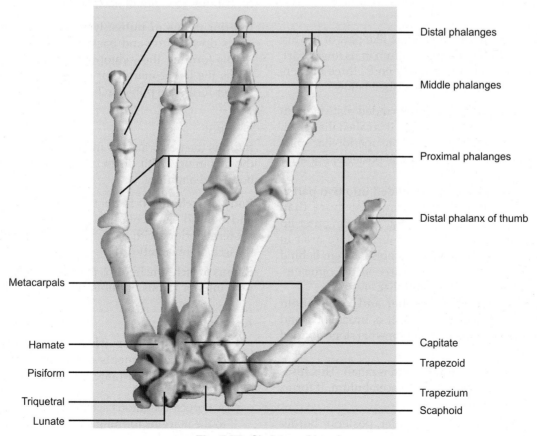

Fig. 6.52: Skeleton of hand

Phalanges

- They are fourteen phalanges in each hand.
- Two phalanges are present in thumb and rest of four fingers have three phalanges each.
- Each phalanx consists of proximal end or base, distal end or head and intermediate portion which is the shaft.

Sesamoid Bones of Upper Limb

1. Pisiform: It is ossified in the tendon of flexor carpi ulnaris.
2. Two sesamoid bones are present on the palmar aspect of 1st metacarpal bone.

BONES OF LOWER LIMB

HIP BONE

Hip bone is a large, irregular bone made up of three parts namely, ilium, pubis and ischium.The three parts are fused at a depressed area called the acetabulum. There are two hip bones in our body which meet anteriorly to form pubic symphysis. Posteriorly they articulate with sacrum to form sacroiliac joint on either side. Together they form the hip girdle (Figs 6.53 and 6.54).

The three parts of hip bone are described below:

Ilium

It forms the upper, expanded, plate like part of the hip bone. It forms 2/5th of the acetabulum in its lower part. Ilium consists of upper and lower ends, three borders and three surfaces which are described below.

Iliac crest: The upper end of the expanded plate of ilium is in the form of a long broad ridge. It is called iliac crest. The anterior end is known as anterior superior iliac spine while the posterior end is known as posterior superior iliac spine.

Morphologically iliac crest is divided into two parts:
  a. **Ventral segment:** This forms just more than anterior 2/3rd of the iliac crest. It has an outer lip and an inner lip with an intermediate area in between. A small elevation is present 5 cm behind the anterior superior iliac spine on the outer lip. This is called the **tubercle** of iliac crest.
  b. **Dorsal segment:** It is smaller and forms about posterior 1/3rd of the crest. It is broadened and consists of a lateral slope and a medial slope divided by a ridge.

Lower end: The lower end of ilium is small. This fuses with the pubis and ischium at the acetabulum. It forms 2/5th of the acetabulum.

Three borders: It has anterior border, posterior border and medial border.

Three surfaces: These are
  a. **Gluteal surface:** It is the posterior surface and is divided into four areas by three gluteal lines namely, posterior gluteal line, anterior gluteal line and inferior gluteal line.
  b. **Iliac surface or iliac fossa:** It is the anterior concave surface.
  c. **Sacropelvic surface:** It is the medial surface which articulates with sacrum. It is divided into three areas iliac tuberosity, auricular surface and pelvic surface.

Pubis

It forms the anterior and inferior part of hip bone. Anterior 1/5th of acetabulum is formed by pubis. Pubis consists of a body and two rami.

Body of pubis: It is flattened from before backwards. The upper border is known as the pubic crest. It presents with three surfaces namely, anterior surface, posterior surface and medial or symphyseal surface. The medial surface articulates with the opposite side pubis bone forming the **symphysis pubis.**

Superior ramus of pubis: It extends from the body of pubis to the acetabulum and lies above obturator foramen. It has three borders and three surfaces. It contributes to 1/5th of acetabulum.

Inferior ramus of pubis: It extends from the body of pubis downwards and backwards to meet the ischial ramus forming the ischiopubic ramus. Upper border forms the lower margin of obturator foramen. Lower border forms the pubic arch.

Ischium

It forms the posterior and inferior part of hip bone and the adjoining 2/5th of the acetabulum. Ischium has a body and a ramus.

Body of ischium: It is thick and short and lies below and behind the acetabulum. Upper end forms the posteroinferior 2/5th of acetabulum. Lower end forms the ischial tuberosity.

Ramus of ischium: It forms the ischiopubic ramus along with inferior ramus of pubis as described above.

Acetabulum

- It is a deep cup-shaped hemispherical cavity formed by all three elements of hip bone namely ilium (upper 2/5), pubis (anterior 1/5), ischium (posterior 2/5).
- A fibrocartilaginous acetabular labrum is attached to the margins forming a rim. This helps to deepen the acetabular cavity.

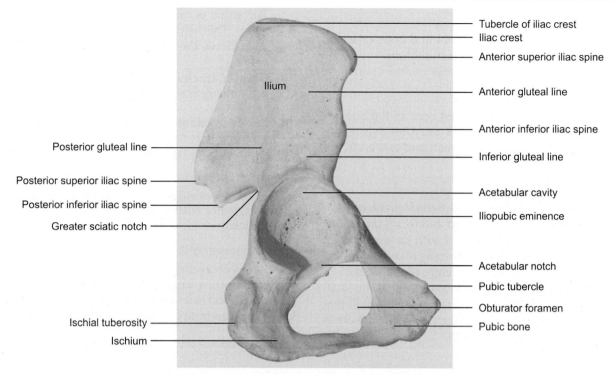

Fig. 6.53: Right hip bone (external aspect)

Labels: Tubercle of iliac crest, Iliac crest, Anterior superior iliac spine, Anterior gluteal line, Anterior inferior iliac spine, Inferior gluteal line, Acetabular cavity, Iliopubic eminence, Acetabular notch, Pubic tubercle, Obturator foramen, Pubic bone, Ilium, Posterior gluteal line, Posterior superior iliac spine, Posterior inferior iliac spine, Greater sciatic notch, Ischial tuberosity, Ischium

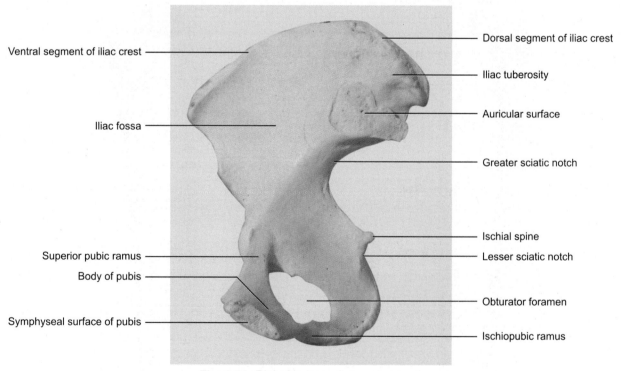

Fig. 6.54: Right hip bone (internal aspect)

Labels: Dorsal segment of iliac crest, Iliac tuberosity, Auricular surface, Greater sciatic notch, Ischial spine, Lesser sciatic notch, Obturator foramen, Ischiopubic ramus, Ventral segment of iliac crest, Iliac fossa, Superior pubic ramus, Body of pubis, Symphyseal surface of pubis

- The margin of acetabulum is deficient inferiorly and forms the acetabular notch.
- The cavity can be divided into two parts.
  a. **Nonarticular part** or the acetabular fossa.

b. **Articular part:** It is a horseshoe shaped area occupying the anterior, superior and posterior parts of acetabulum. **Acetabulum articulates with head of femur.**

Obturator Foramen

This is a large gap situated inferior and anterior to the acetabulum between the pubis and ischium

FEMUR

Femur is the longest and strongest bone of the body. It is the bone of the thigh (Figs 6.55 and 6.56). It is a long bone and can be divided into a shaft and two ends.

Upper End of Femur

This includes the head, neck and two trochanters.
1. **Head of femur:** It is globular and forms more than half of a sphere. It articulates with the acetabulum to form hip joint. A pit known as fovea is situated just below and behind the centre of the head.
2. **Neck of femur:** It connects the head to the shaft and is about 5 cm long. The neck is so inclined that it makes an angle of 165 degree with the shaft in children. This is reduced to 125 degree in adults.

The angle is more acute in females due to wider pelvis. This helps to facilitate movement at hip joint and allows the lower limb to swing clear of the pelvis.
3. **Greater trochanter:** It is a large quadrangular prominence from the upper part of junction of shaft and neck.
4. **Lesser trochanter:** It is a conical projection in the posteroinferior part of junction of neck and shaft and is directed medially

Intertrochanteric Line

It is a prominent ridge. It extends from anterosuperior angle of greater trochanter to the spiral line in front of lesser trochanter.

Intertrochanteric Crest

It is a smooth and rounded ridge which extends from posterosuperior angle of greater trochanter to the posterior aspect of lesser trochanter. A rounded elevation known as quadrate tubercle is present a little above its middle.

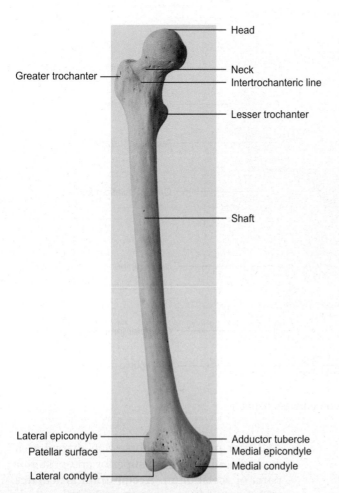

Fig. 6.55: Right femur (Anterior aspect)

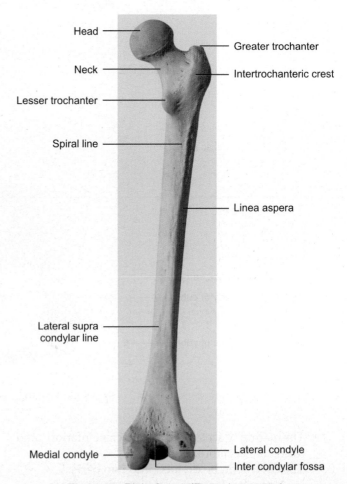

Fig. 6.56: Right femur (Posterior aspect)

Shaft of Femur

It is cylindrical in shape being narrowest in middle with expanded upper and lower parts. The shaft of femur can be divided into three parts namely, upper 1/3rd, middle 1/3rd and lower 1/3rd.

- The middle 1/3rd has 3 borders which divides the shaft into 3 surfaces. The lateral and medial borders are indistinct and extend both above and below. However the posterior border is prominent and forms a ridge known as **linea aspera.**
- The linea aspera has two lips and a central area. The two lips diverge from the upper and lower end of middle third of shaft to divide the shaft into four surfaces in the upper and lower third.
- The upward continuation of medial lip of linea aspera forms a rough line extending to the lower end of intertrochanteric line. **This is the spiral line.**
- The lateral lip continues upwards as a broad ridge posteriorly known as **gluteal tuberosity.**
- The medial and lateral lips diverge downwards to form **medial and lateral supracondylar lines.**
- The medial supracondylar line ends in the **adductor tubercle.**

Lower End of Femur

It is widely expanded and consists of two large condyles, medial and lateral. The two are united anteriorly and separated by a deep gap posteriorly, the intercondylar fossa. The two condyles are in line with shaft anteriorly but project posteriorly much beyond the plane of popliteal surface.

Articular Surfaces of Lower End of Femur

It covers both the condyles and is divided into two
1. Patellar surface: It articulates with patella.
2. Tibial surface: It articulates with upper end of tibia.

PATELLA

It is the largest sesamoid bone of body. It develops in the tendon of quadriceps femoris. It is situated in front of knee joint (Fig. 6.57). Patella is irregular in shape and is flattened anteroposteriorly. It has an apex, three borders and two surfaces namely anterior and posterior surfaces. Posterior surface articulates with the lower end of femur.

TIBIA

It is the long bone of the leg, situated medially. It is larger and stronger than fibula (Figs 6.58 and 6.59). Tibia is a long bone with two ends and one shaft.

Upper End of Tibia

It is markedly expanded and consists of the following
1. **Medial and lateral condyle:** These can be palpated by the sides of patellar tendon. Lateral surface of lateral condyle bears a facet that articulates with fibula.
2. **Intercondylar area:** It is a roughened, non articular part between the superior surfaces of the two condyles.
3. **Tuberosity of tibia.**

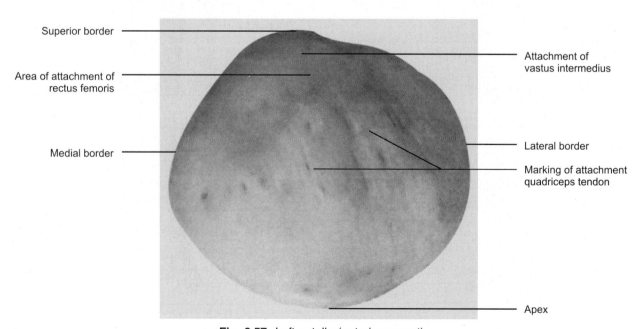

Fig. 6.57: Left patella (anterior aspect)

Shaft of Tibia

The shaft of tibia is prismoid in shape and has three borders namely anterior border, interosseous or lateral border and medial border and three surfaces namely, medial surface, lateral surface and posterior surface.

Lower End of Tibia

It is slightly expanded and quadrangular. It has five surfaces namely anterior surface, medial surface, lateral surface, inferior surface and posterior surface. The medial surface presents a short and strong bony projection extending downwards known as **medial malleolus.** The medial surface is largest and subcutaneous and forms prominence on medial side of ankle. The lateral surface articulates with talus.

FIBULA

It is the long bone of leg situated laterally. It is very slender and does not play any role in weight transmission (Figs 6.58 and 6.59). It has two ends and one shaft.

Upper End of Fibula

Is divided into
1. **Head of fibula:** It has a circular facet an anteromedial side for articulation with fibular facet of lateral condyle of tibia. Styloid process is a projection from the posterolateral aspect of head.
2. **Neck of fibula:** The head narrows down to the neck which connects it to the shaft.

Shaft of Fibula

It has three borders namely, anterior border, medial or interosseous border and posterior border and three surfaces medial or extensor surface, lateral or peroneal surface and posterior or flexor surface

Lower End of Fibula

It is also known as **lateral malleolus.** It has four surfaces anterior surface, posterior surface, lateral surface and medial surface. Lateral surface is subcutaneous. Medial surface articulates with talus. An elongated triangular area is situated above the lateral surface of lateral malleolus and is subcutaneous.

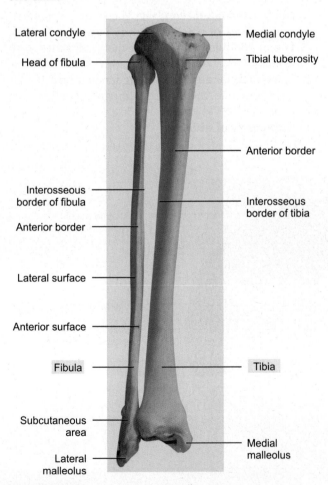

Fig. 6.58: Right tibia and fibula (anterior aspect)

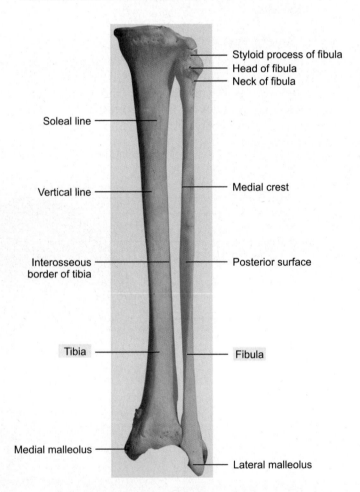

Fig. 6.59: Right tibia and fibula (posterior aspect)

BONES OF THE FOOT

They can be divided into three groups (Figs 6.60 and 6.61).

1. **Tarsal bones**
   - Tarsal bones are cubical in shape with six surfaces. These are seven in number and are arranged in two rows.
   - Proximal row consists of **talus** above and **calcaneum** below.
   - Distal row consists of four bones which lie side by side. From lateral to medial they are **cuboid, lateral cuneiform, intermediate cuneiform and medial cuneiform.**
   - The **navicular bone** lies between the two rows.

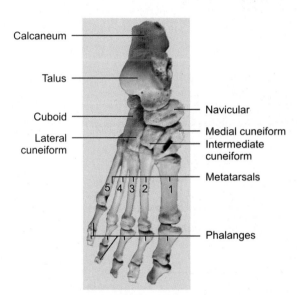

Fig. 6.60: Skeleton of foot (dorsal aspect)

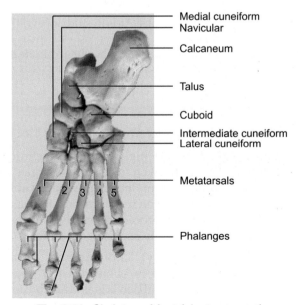

Fig. 6.61: Skeleton of foot (plantar aspect)

2. **Metatarsals:** These consist of 5 bones numbered from medial to lateral. Each metatarsal is a miniature long bone divided into a head or distal end, shaft and a base or proximal end.

3. **Phalanges:** There are fourteen phalanges in each foot with two for great toe and three each for rest of the toes. They are smaller than the phalanges of the hand.

Sesamoid Bones of Lower Limb

1. Patella–Largest sesamoid bone in the body
2. Tendon of peroneus longus has one sesamoid bone which articulates with cuboid
3. There are two small sesamoid bones in tendons of flexor hallucis brevis.
4. Sometimes there may be sesamoid bones in tendons of tibialis anterior, tibialis posterior, lateral head of gastrocnemius, gluteus maximus and psoas major.

BONY PELVIS

Pelvis means basin (Figs 6.62 and 6.63). It is formed by two hip bones sacrum and coccyx. The two hip bones are placed laterally and meet anteriorly at pubic symphysis. Posteriorly, the pelvis is completed by articulation of the two hip bones with sacrum and articulation of sacrum with coccyx. Pelvis is divided into two parts by the pelvic brim. **The pelvic brim is formed by sacral promontory, anterior border of ala of sacrum, lower ½ of medial border of ilium, pecten pubis, pubic crest and upper border of symphysis pubis.** The two parts of pelvis are false pelvis and true pelvis.

False or Greater Pelvis

It is the part of pelvis lying above the pelvic brim. It consists of lumbar vertebrae posteriorly, iliac fossae laterally and anterior abdominal wall anteriorly. The only function is to support the viscera (Fig. 10.64).

True or Lesser Pelvis

It is the part of pelvis below the pelvic brim. In the females it is adapted for childbearing The baby has to negotiate this bony passage during labour and delivery. It is further divided into three parts (Figs. 10.64 and 10.65).

1. **Pelvic inlet or pelvic brim (Fig. 10.65):** The plane of pelvic inlet makes an angle of about 55 to 60 degrees with the horizontal. Axis of inlet is a line passing through umbilicus above and the tip of coccyx below. It meets the centre of plane of inlet at right angles.

2. **Pelvic cavity:** It is a J-shaped canal curving downwards and forwards. It is bounded by pubic symphysis and body of pubis in front. On each side

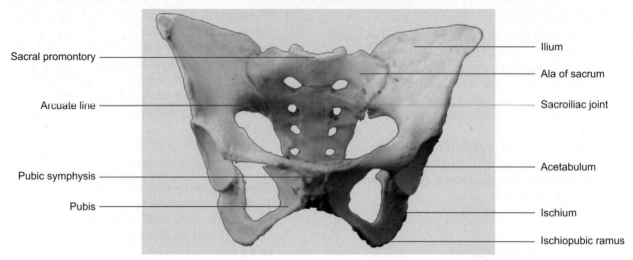

Fig. 6.62: Bony Pelvis

Sacral promontory

Arcuate line

Pubic symphysis

Pubis

Ilium

Ala of sacrum

Sacroiliac joint

Acetabulum

Ischium

Ischiopubic ramus

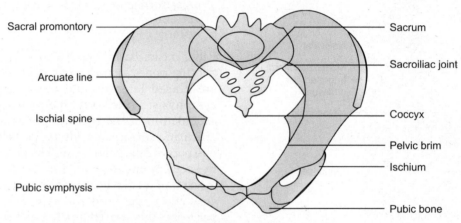

Fig. 6.63: Bony Pelvis

Sacral promontory

Arcuate line

Ischial spine

Pubic symphysis

Sacrum

Sacroiliac joint

Coccyx

Pelvic brim

Ischium

Pubic bone

is ischiopubic ramus and behind there is sacrum and coccyx.

3. **Pelvic outlet:** It is a diamond shaped inferior aperture of the pelvis. It is bounded anteriorly by subpubic arch, laterally by inferior border of ischiopubic rami and ischial tuberosities, posteriorly by sacrotuberous ligaments and tip of coccyx.

Axis of Birth Canal

It is J-shaped. At the pelvic inlet in points downwards and backwards, curves down till ischial spines. From the level of the spines it proceeds downwards and forwards to reach the outlet.

Pelvimetry

It is defined as measurement of pelvis. Pelvimetry is useful in the following studies

1. **Clinical obstetrics:** Helps in assessing the adequacy of pelvis for safe and normal delivery.

2. **Anthropological studies:** Aids in study of evolution of human being.

3 **Forensic sciences:** Helps in the determination of sex.

Methods of Pelvimetry

1. **On skeleton:** prepared from cadavers.

2. **Radiological:** It is a highly refined technique. Multiple X-rays are taken from various angles and pelvis is studied. It can detect bony pelvic abnormalities and severe pelvic contraction in selected cases. However the procedure involves exposure to radiation. This limits its use in obstetrics.

3. **Clinical pelvimetry:** This method is most commonly practiced in obstetrics–per vaginal examination is done and pelvis is assessed by noting various bony landmarks.

Diameters of Pelvis

1. Pelvic inlet

Diameter	Extent	Measurement
1. Anteroposterior		
a. Anatomic conjugate	Midpoint of sacral promontory to mid point of upper border of pubic symphysis	Male – 10 cm Female – 11.5 cm
b. Diagnonal conjugate (measured on clinical pelvimetery)	Midpoint of sacral promontory to subpubic angle	Male = 11.0 cm Female = 12.5 cm
c. Obstetric conjugate (Diagonal conjugate minus 1.5 cm)	Midpoint of sacral promontory to most prominent point on posterior surface of symphysis pubic	11.0 cm
2. Transverse	Maximum distance between two iliopectineal lines	Male = 12.5 cm Female = 13.5 cm
3. Oblique	Sacroiliac joint on one side to opposite iliopubic eminence	Male = 12 cm Female = 12.5 cm

2. Pelvic cavity

Diameter	Extent	Measurement
1. Anteroposterior diameters a. In plane of greatest dimension	Midpoint of posterior surface of pubic symphysis to junction of S_2 and S_3 vertebrae.	Male = 10.5 cm Female = 13.0 cm
b. In plane of least dimension	Lower border of symphysis pubis to junction of S_4 and S_5 vertebrae.	Male = 10 cm Female = 12 cm
2. Transverse diameters a. In planes of greatest dimension b. In plane of least dimension	Widest distance between the lateral boundaries of the plane. Between tip of two ischial spines.	Male = 11 cm Female = 12.5 cm Male = 9.5 cm Female = 10.5-11 cm

3. Pelvic outlet

Diameter	Extent	Measurement
1. Anteroposterior	Inferior margin of pubic symphysis to tip of coccyx	Male = 8 cm Female = 11.5 cm
2. Transverse	Between inner surface of two ischial tuberosities	Male = 10 cm Female = 11 cm

4. Classification of pelvis: Caldwell and Moloy classification based on shape of pelvic inlet (Figs 6.64 to 6.67).

Gynaecoid (Mesatepellic) Seen in females	Android (Brachypellic) Present in males	Anthropoid (Dolichopellic) Characteristic of apes	Platypelloid (platypellic) Flat pelvis
1. Pelvic inlet Round or oval shape with transverse diameter slightly greater than anteroposterior diameter	Triangular or heart shaped with short anteroposterior diameter, transverse diameter is widest near the promontory	Anteroposterior diameter is greater than transverse diameter	Flat type with transverse diameter much larger than anteroposterior diameter
2. Pelvic cavity a. Sciatic notches are wide b. Side walls parallel	a. Narrow b. Funnel shape	a. Wide b. Parallel	a. Wide b. Parallel (wide apart)
3. Pelvic outlet Subpubic angle Wide 85 to 90°	Narrow 70 to 75°	Wide	Very wide

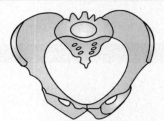

Fig. 6.64: Gynaecoid pelvis

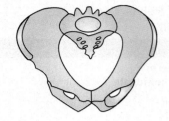

Fig. 6.65: Android pelvis

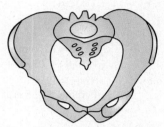

Fig. 6.66: Anthropoid pelvis

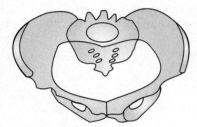

Fig. 6.67: Platypelloid pelvis

JOINTS

Joint is a junction between two or more bones and is responsible for movement, growth or transmission of forces.

Classification

Depends upon the function of the joint. They are of two types:
1. **Synarthroses:** These are solid joints without any cavity. No movement or only slight movement is possible. Synarthroses are further subdivided into
   a. Fibrous joints
   b. Cartilaginous joints
2. **Diarthroses:** They are cavitated joints and form the synovial joints in which the joint cavity is filled with synovial fluid. These joints permit free movements.

Fibrous Joints

Types of fibrous joints:
1. **Sutures (Fig. 6.68):** Sutural joints appear between those bones which ossify in membranes. The sutural membrane between the edges of two growing bones consist of osteogenic and fibrous layers. Sutural

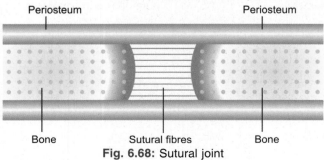

Fig. 6.68: Sutural joint

membrane connects the periosteum covering the outer and inner surfaces of bones.
Function: They provide growth and bind together the apposed margins of bones.
Example: Joints of skull are sutural joints.
2. **Syndesmosis (Fig. 6.69):** Where the surfaces of bones are united with an interosseous membrane or a ligament. The two bones lie some distance apart.
Function: Slight amount of movement is possible at these joints.
Example: Middle radio-ulnar joint, inferior tibio-fibular joint.

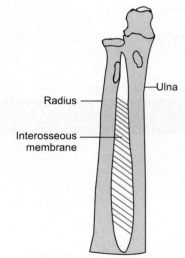

Fig. 6.69: Syndesmosis

3. **Gomphosis (Peg and socket joint) (Fig. 6.70):** Root of teeth fit in the socket of jaw and are united by fibrous tissue.

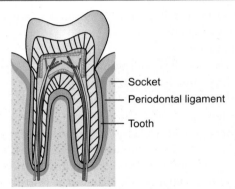

Fig. 6.70: Gomphosis

Cartilaginous Joints

Cartilaginous joints are of two types:

1. **Primary cartilaginous joint (Fig. 6.71):** It is formed when two bones are connected with the help of hyaline cartilage. This joint ultimately gets ossified. **Example:** Joint between epiphysis and diaphysis of a bone.

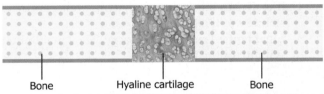

Fig. 6.71: Primary cartilaginous joint

2. **Secondary cartilaginous joint (Fig. 6.72):** All midline joints are secondary cartilaginous joints. The two bones are united with the help of fibro cartilage in the centre which is surrounded by hyaline cartilage on both the sides. Generally it doesn't get ossified. **Example:** Manubriosternal joint, symphysis pubis, intervertebral disc.

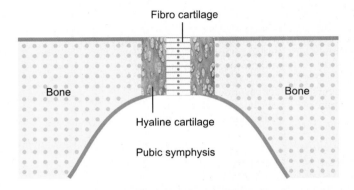

Fig. 6.72: Secondary cartilaginous joint

Formation of Intervertebral Disc

It is secondary cartilaginous joint present between body of two adjacent vertebrae. It is formed by nucleus pulposus in the centre surrounded by fibro-annulosus. Fibro-annulosus is covered by fibro cartilage which is lined by hyaline cartilage on both the sides. Intervertebral disc facilitates movement and acts as shock absorber (Figs 6.73 and 6.74).

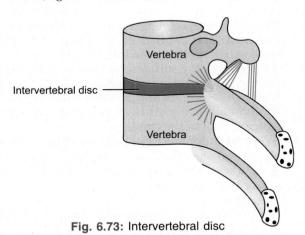

Fig. 6.73: Intervertebral disc

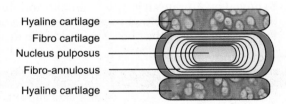

Fig. 6.74: Formation of intervertebral disc

Synovial Joint

Synovial joint permits free movement. The characteristic feature of a synovial joint is the presence of a joint cavity filled with synovial fluid and lined by the synovial membrane which is enveloped by articular capsule (Fig. 6.75).

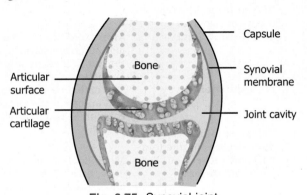

Fig. 6.75: Synovial joint

CHAPTER-6

Components of a Synovial Joint and their Function

1. **Articular surfaces:** These consist of corresponding ends of articulating bones.
2. **Articular cartilage:** Articular cartilage covers the articular surfaces of the articulating bones. It is made up of hyaline cartilage at most of the places except where the articular surfaces are ossified in membrane. In these cases articular cartilage is made up of fibrocartilage. Articular cartilage has no perichondrium and hence no regenerative power. Once it is damaged, replacement is by fibrous tissue.
   Function: The co-efficient of friction of articular cartilage is equal to 'ice on ice'. Therefore it provides a smooth gliding surface and reduces the forces of compression during weight bearing. Aricular cartilage is porous and absorbs fluid in resting condition. When joint is compressed, the fluid is squeezed out of the cartilage.
3. **Synovial fluid:** It is a clear or pale yellow, viscous slightly alkaline fluid. It is the dialysate of blood plasma with added hyaluronic acid, sulphate free glycosaminoglycans.
   Functions:
   a. It maintains the nutrition of articular cartilage.
   b. It provides lubrication to the joint cavity and helps prevent wear and tear.
4. **Synovial membrane:** It is a pink, smooth and shiny, cellular connective tissue membrane of mesenchymal origin. It lines the fibrous capsule from inside.

Articular cartilage and menisci are not lined by synovial membrane.
Functions:
a. Secretes synovial fluid
b. Liberates hyaluronic acid
c. Removes particulate matter from the synovial fluid.

5. **Joint cavity:** Formed by one of the articular surfaces. It accommodates the articular surfaces, articular cartilage, synovial fluid and synovial membrane.
6. **Articular capsule:** Consists of a fibrous capsule lined by synovial membrane on the inside. Capsule is formed by bundles of collagen fibres arranged in irregular spirals and is sensitive to changes of position of joint (Fig. 4.7).
   Function: It binds the articulating bones together.
7. **Articular disc or meniscus:** It is made up of fibrocartilage and divides the joint into two incomplete or complete joint cavities.
   Function: It helps to increase the range of movement.
8. **Labrum, if present:** It is made up of fibrocartilage. It increases the depth of cavity as well as provides stability to the joint.
9. **Ligaments:** True and accessory. They maintain the stability of the joint.

Types of Synovial Joints

	Type	Movement	Example
1.	**Plane joint**	Gliding movement is possible	Intercarpal, acromio-clavicular and intertarsal joint. Joint between 1st rib and sternum
2.	**Uniaxial joint:** Movement is possible in one axis		
	a. **Hinge joint**	Movement around transverse axis. It allows flexion and extension.	Elbow, ankle and interphalangeal joints
	b. **Pivot joint**	Movement occurs on a vertical axis. The bone acts as a pivot which is encircled by an osseo ligamentous ring.	Superior radioulnar, inferior radioulnar and median atlanto axial joints.
	c. **Condylar joint** Also known as modified hinge joint.	Movement occurs mainly on transverse axis and partly on vertical axis.	Knee joint, temporomandibular joint.
3.	**Biaxial Joint:** Movement occurs in two axes		
	a. **Ellipsoid joint**	Movement occurs around transverse and antero-posterior axes. It allows flexion, extension, adduction and abduction	Wrist joint, metacarpophalangeal, metatarsophalangeal and atlanto-occipital joints.
	b. **Saddle joint**	Movement occurs around transverse and antero-posterior axes. Conjunct rotation is also possible.	Ist carpometacarpal joint Sternoclavicular joint Calcaneo-cuboid joint
4.	**Polyaxial joints:** They have three degrees of freedom **Ball and socket (spheroidal) joint**	Movement occurs around antero-posterior, transverse and vertical axes. It allows flexion extension. adduction, abduction, rotation and cicumduction	Hip joint Shoulder joint Talo-calcaneo-navicular joint Incudo-stapedial joint.

Movements and Mechanism of Synovial Joints

There are four following types of movements taking place in synovial joints namely.

1. **Gliding:** Movement take place in plane joints where one bone slips over the other in a particular direction.
2. **Angular movements:** May be of two types:
   a. **Flexion and extension:** In flexion two ventral surfaces approximate with each other while in extension it is the opposite.
   b. **Adduction and abduction:** In adduction the body part moves towards the median plane or median axis. In abduction the body part moves away from the median plane or median axis.
3. **Circumduction:** It is a combination of flexion, extension, adduction and abduction in a successive order.
4. **Rotation:** Movement occurs around vertical axis.

Blood Supply of Joints

The articular and epiphyseal branches given off by the neighboring arteries form a periarticular arterial plexus. Numerous vessels from this plexus pierce the fibrous capsule and form a rich vascular plexus in the deeper part of synovial membrane. The blood vessels of synovial membrane terminate around the articular margin in the form of a capillary plexus. This is known as **circulus vasculosus.** It supplies the capsule, synovial membrane and epiphysis.

Lymphatic Drainage of Joints

Lymphatics form a plexus in the subintima of synovial membrane and drain into lymphatics present along the blood vessels to the corresponding regional deep nodes.

Nerve Supply of Joints

Nerve supply of a joint lies in its capsule, ligaments and synovial membrane. The capsule and ligaments have a rich nerve supply and are sensitive to pain. Articular cartilage is non sensitive because it has no nerve supply.

Articular nerves contain **sensory** and **autonomic fibres.** Some of the sensory fibres are **proprioceptive.** Autonomic fibres are **vasomotor or vasosensory.** Joint pain is often diffuse and may be associated with nausea, vomiting, slowing of pulse and fall in blood pressure. Pain commonly causes reflex contraction of muscles which fix the joint in a position of comfort. Joint pain may also referred to another uninvolved joint.

JOINTS OF UPPER LIMB

Name of Joint	Type of Joint	Movement at the joint
Sternoclavicular	Saddle type of synovial joint	Gliding and rotatory movement of scapula
Acromioclavicular	Plane synovial joint	Gliding movement of scapula
Glenohumeral (Shoulder joint)	Ball and socket type of synovial joint	Flexion, extension, adduction, abduction, circumduction, medial rotation, lateral rotation
Elbow	Hinge type of synovial joint	Flexion, extension
Superior radioulnar	Pivot type of synovial joint	Pronation, supination
Inferior radioulnar	Pivot type of synovial joint	Pronation, supination
Wrist	Ellipsoid type of synovial joint	Flexion, extension, abduction and adduction
Intercarpal and midcarpal	Plane synovial joint	Gliding and sliding
Metacarpophalangeal	Ellipsoid type of synovial	Flexion, extension, abduction and adduction
1st Carpometacarpal	Saddle type of synovial joint	Flexion, extension, abduction, adduction, opposition
Interphalangeal	Hinge type of synovial joint	Flexion, extension

Shoulder Joint

This is also known as glenohumeral joint. It is multiaxial ball and socket type of synovial joint or multiaxial spheroidal joint (Fig. 6.76).

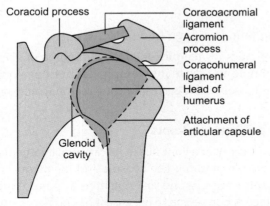

Fig. 6.76: Articular surfaces, articular capsule and ligaments of shoulder joint

Articular Surfaces
1. **Head of humerus:** It forms 1/3rd of a sphere.
2. **Glenoid cavity of scapula:** It is pear shaped, only 1/3rd of the head of humerus is accommodated in glenoid cavity.

Articular cartilage: Both articular surfaces are covered by hyaline articular cartilages. Thickness of articular cartilages are reciprocal.

Synovial membrane: It lines the joint cavity except articular cartilages. It comes out of the joint cavity along with tendon of long head of biceps.

Glenoid labrum: It is made up of fibrocartilage and is attached to the peripheral margin of glenoid cavity. It is 70% fibrous and 30% cartilagenous. It deepens the glenoid cavity.

Ligaments of Shoulder Joint
1. Fibrous capsule
2. Glenohumeral ligaments.
3. Coraco-humeral ligament.
4. Transverse ligament

Rotator cuff: Tendons of following four muscles form an expansion and attach to the fibrous capsule. This is known as the rotator cuff of shoulder joint (Fig. 6.77).
1. Supraspinatus   : Above
2. Subscapularis   : Anteriorly
3. Infraspinatus   : Posteriorly
4. Teres minor   : Posteriorly

The rotator cuff is in constant tonic contraction and keeps the head of humerus in glenoid cavity in static and kinetic state.

Coraco-acrominal arch: It acts as a secondary socket for head of humerus when the arm is raised above the head. It is formed by the coracoid process, acromion process and coraco-acromial ligament. Coraco-acromial ligament extends from the tip of acromion process to lateral border of coracoid process. Subacromial bursa lies below the arch and separates the supraspinatus from arch (Fig. 6.77).

Main Bursae in Relation to Joint
1. Subscapular bursa
2. Infraspinatus bursa
3. Subacromial bursa
4. Other bursae related to shoulder joint are bursa in relation to teres major, long head of triceps and latissimus dorsi muscles.

Arterial Supply of Shoulder Joint
1. Anterior circumflex humeral artery
2. Posterior circumflex humeral artery

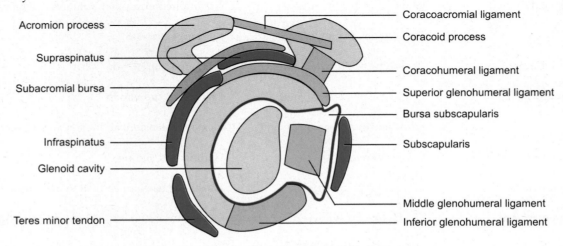

Fig. 6.77: Lateral view of shoulder joint

Movements of Shoulder Joint

Movement	Muscles involved
1. **Flexion** Axis is perpendicular to axis of abduction and adduction	• Clavicular head of pectoralis major • Anterior fibres of deltoid • Coracobrachialis and assisted by biceps brachii
2. **Extension** Axis is same as flexion	• Posterior fibres of deltoid } From pendent • Teres major } position • Latissimus dorsi } From flexed • Pectoralis major } position
3. **Abduction** Axis is parallel to plane of body of scapula	• Supraspinatus • Middle fibre of deltoid • Subscapular, infraspinatus, teres minor
4. **Adduction** Axis is same as abduction	• Anterior and posterior fibres of deltoid • Pectoralis major • Teres major • Latissimus dorsi • Coracobrachialis
5. **Medial rotation** Axis is vertical, passes from centre of humeral head to capitulum	• Pectoralis major, anterior fibres of deltoid, , teres major, latissimus dorsi, subscapularis
6. **Lateral rotation** Axis is same as medial rotation	• Infraspinatus, teres minor, posterior firbres of deltoid

3. Suprascapular artery

Nerve Supply of Shoulder Joint
1. Axillary nerve
2. Suprascapular nerve
3. Lateral pectoral nerve

Spinal cord segments supplying shoulder joint are C_5, C_6, C_7, C_8. Flexion, abduction, lateral rotation is by C_5, C_6 spinal segments. Extension, Adduction, Medial rotation is by C_6, C_7, C_8 spinal segements.

Shoulder Girdle

It consists of clavicle and scapula. Shoulder girdle connects the upper limb to axial skeleton. Clavicle articulates with the sternum at sternoclavicular joint and with scapula at acromio-clavicular joint.

Movements of shoulder girdle: It involves movement of scapula and clavicle. The clavicle moves around antero-posterior axis formed by costoclavicular ligament. Movements of scapula are tabulated below:

Movements of scapula	Muscles involved	Clavicular movements
1. **Elevation of scapula,** (Shrugging of shoulders)	• Upper part of trapezius • Levator scapulae	• Elevation of lateral end • Depression of medial end
2. **Depression of scapula** (Drooping of shoulders)	• Lower part of serratus anterior • Pectoralis minor • Weight of the limb	• Depression of lateral end • Elevation of medial end
3. **Protraction of scapula or forward movement** (As in pushing & punching movement)	• Serratus anterior • Pectoralis minor	• Forward movement of lateral end • Backward movement of medial end
4. **Retraction of scapula or backward movement** (Squaring the shoulders)	• Middle part of trapezius • Rhomboidus major and minor	• Backward movement of lateral end • Forward movement of medial end
5. **Forward rotation (Lateral rotation)** (during elevation of arm above the head)	• Upper and lower fibres of trapezius • Lower 5 digitation of serratus anterior	• Rotation of clavicle around its long axis.
6. **Backward rotation (Medial rotation)**	• Active lengthening of trapezius and serratus anterior and gravity	• Rotation of clavicle opposite to forward rotation

ELBOW JOINT

It is a hinge variety of synovial joint (Fig. 6.78). It has two parts:

1. **Humero-ulnar part:** Articular surfaces are trochlea of humerus and trochlear notch of ulna.
2. **Humero-radial part:** Structurally ball and socket, ball is capitulum of humerus and socket is superior surface of head of radius.

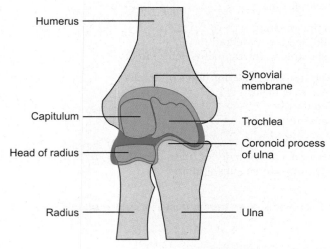

Fig. 6.78: Elbow joint

Ligaments of Elbow Joint (Fig. 6.79)

1. Capsular ligament
2. Ulnar collateral ligament
3. Radial collateral ligament

Arterial Supply of Elbow Joint

Anastomosis around elbow joint

Nerve Supply of Elbow Joint

1. Musculocutaneous nerve
2. Radial nerve
3. Ulnar nerve

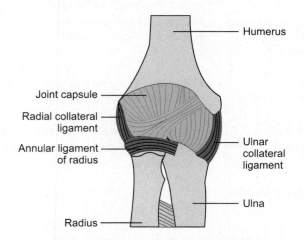

Fig. 6.79: Ligaments of elbow joint

Movements of Elbow Joint: Axis of movements of elbow joint is transverse.

Movements at elbow joint	Muscles involved
Flexion	1. Brachialis 2. Biceps brachii 3. Brachioradialis
Extension	1. Triceps 2. Anconeus 3. Gravity

Radio-ulnar Joints

Radius and ulna are joined to each other at superior and inferior radio-ulnar joints (Figs 6.80 and 6.81).

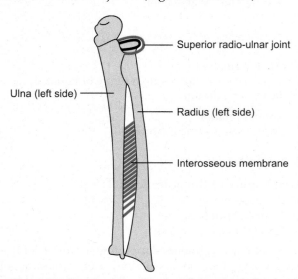

Fig. 6.80: Position of radio-ulnar joints in supination

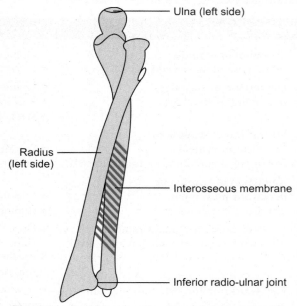

Fig. 6.81: Position of radio-ulnar joints in pronation

Superior Radio-ulnar Joint

It is pivot type of synovial joint.

Articular Surfaces
1. Head of radius.
2. Osteofibrous ring formed by annular ligament and radial notch of ulna.

Ligaments
1. Annular ligament.
2. Quadrate ligament.

Arterial Supply
Anastomosis around elbow joint.

Nerve Supply
1. Musculocutaneous nerve
2. Medial nerve
3. Radial nerve

Inferior Radio-ulnar Joint

Is a pivot type of synovial joint.

Articular Surfaces
1. Convex lateral side of head of ulna
2. Ulnar notch on radius

Ligaments
1. Fibrous capsule of joint
2. Articular disc

Arterial Supply
1. Anterior interosseous artery
2. Posterior interosseous artery

Nerve Supply
1. Anterior interosseous nerve
2. Posterior interosseous nerve

Movements of Radio-ulnar Joints

Movements	Muscles involved
Supination	• Gravity • Supinator in extension • Biceps brachii in flexion
Pronation	• Pronator quadratus • Pronator teres • Flexor carpi radialis

Supination and pronation: These movements occur at superior and inferior Radio-ulnar joints. In a semiflexed elbow rotatory movements of forearm causing supination and pronation. The turning of palm upwards is known as supination and downwards is called as pronation. The axis of movement passes from head of radius to articular disc of inferior Radio-ulnar joint. Supination is more power full than pronation because of anti-gravity movement. Pronation and supination help in picking up food and taking it to the mouth. These also help in screwing movement.

Interosseous membrane (Figs 6.80, 6.81): It connects the interosseous borders of shafts of ulna and radius. The fibres run downwards and medially. It binds the two bones and provides attachment to various muscles. It also helps in transmission of weight from radius to ulna.

Wrist Joint (Radiocarpal Joint)

It is an ellipsoid variety of synovial joint.

Articular Surfaces
1. **Superior**
   a. Inferior surface of lower end of radius
   b. Articular disc of inferior radio-ulnar joint
2. **Inferior**
   a. Scaphoid bone
   b. Lunate bone
   c. Triquetral bone

Ligaments:
1. Articular fibrous capsule
2. Radial collateral ligament
3. Ulnar collateral ligament

Arterial supply: Anterior and posterior carpal arches.

Nerve supply: Anterior and posterior interosseous nerves.

Movements

Movements	Muscles involved
1. **Flexion**	• Flexor carpi radialis • Flexor carpi ulnaris • Flexor digitorum superficialis and profundus
2. **Extension**	• Extensor carpi radialis longus • Extensor carpi radialis brevis • Extensor carpi ulnaris • Extensor long tendons
3. **Adduction**	• Simultaneous contraction of flexor and extensor carpi ulnaris
4. **Abduction**	• Abductor pollicis longus • Flexor carpi radialis • Extensor carpi radialis longus and brevis • Extensor pollicis brevis

1st CARPOMETACARPAL JOINT (FIG. 6.82)

- It is a saddle variety of synovial joint.
- It has a separate joint cavity from other carpometacarpal joint.

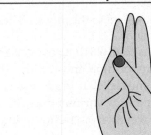

Opposition

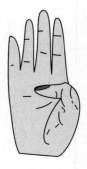

Flexion

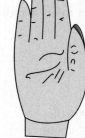

Anatomical position

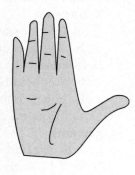

Extension

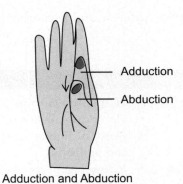

Adduction

Abduction

Adduction and Abduction

Fig. 6.82: Movements of Ist carpometacarpal joint

Articular Surfaces

- Distal articular surface of trapezium.
- Base of first metacarpal: It is convex from side to side and concave from front to back.

Ligaments

1. **Capsular ligament**
2. **Lateral ligament**
3. **Dorsal and palmar ligaments**

Movements	Muscles involved
1. **Flexion**	• Flexor pollicis brevis
	• Opponens pollicis
	• Flexor pollicis longus
2. **Extension**	• Abductor pollicis longus
	• Extensor pollicis brevis
	• Extensor pollicis longus
3. **Abduction**	• Abduction pollicis longus
	• Abductor pollicis brevis
4. **Adduction**	• Adductor pollicis
5. **Opposition**	• Abductor pollicis longus
	• Abductor pollicis brevis
	• Flexor pollicis brevis
	• Opponens pollicis

Axes of Movements of 1st Carpometacarpal Joint

- Axis of flexion and extension is along the plane of the palm.
- Axis of abduction and adduction lies perpendicular to the plane of the palm.
- Opposition is the combination of abduction flexion and medial rotation.
- Circumduction also occurs at 1st carpo metacarpal joint. Circumduction is the combination of all movements.

Arterial supply: Radial artery
Nerve supply: Median Nerve

METACARPO PHALANGEAL JOINTS

These are condylar variety of synovial joints:

Movements	Muscles involved
1. Flexion	• Interossei
	• Lumbricals
	• Flexor digitorum
2. Extension	• Extensor digitorum
3. Abduction	• Dorsal interossei
	• Extensor digitorum
4. Adduction	• Palmar interossei
	• Flexor digitorum

INTERPHALANGEAL JOINTS

- Hinge variety of synovial joints.
- Flexion is caused by **flexor digitorum superficialis** at proximal joints and **flexor digitorum profundus** at distal joints.
- Extension is caused by **interossei and lumbricals**.

JOINTS OF LOWER LIMB

Joints of lower limb are tabulated below:

Joints	Type	Movements
1. Hip joint	Multiaxial ball and socket variety of synovial joint	Flexion, extension adduction, abduction, medial rotation lateral rotation, circumduction
2. Knee joint	Complex, condylar and modified hinge joint	Flexion, extension medial rotation, lateral rotation
3. Ankle joint	Modified hinge joint	Dorsiflexion, plantar flexion
4. Superior tibiofibular	Plane synovial joint	Gliding movement during dorsiflexion of foot
5. Middle tibiofibular joint	Syndesmosis	Bind tibia and fibula
6. Inferior tibiofibular joint	Syndesmosis	Bind tibia and fibula
7. Talocalcaneonavicular joint	Ball and socket variety of synovial joint	Inversion, eversion
8. Calcaneocuboid joint	Saddle variety of synovial joint	Eversion, inversion
9. Subtalar joint	Multiaxial synovial joint	Inversion, eversion
10. Intertarsal joints	Plane synovial joint	Gliding movement
11. Tarsometatarsal joints	Plane synovial joint	Gliding movement
12. Metatarso-phalangeal joints	Ellipsoid variety of synovial joint adduction, abduction	Dorsiflexion, plantar flexion,
13. Interphalangeal joints	Hinge variety of synovial joint	Dorsiflexion, plantar flexion

Hip Joint

It is a multiaxial, ball and socket variety of synovial joint. One joint is formed on either side. It presents with
Articular surfaces: There are two articular surfaces (Figs 6.83 and 6.84).
1. Head of femur
2. Acetabulum of hip bone
Articular cartilage: It covers the articular surfaces.
Acetabular labrum:
1. It deepens the socket
2. Grasps the head of femur tightly
Synovial membrane: It lines the joint cavity except at articular surfaces.
Acetabular fat (Haversian fat): It is liquid at body temperature and fills the joint cavity.
Ligaments of Hip Joint (Figs 6.83 to 6.86)
1. **Capsular ligament:** It envelops the joint. The fibres are spirally attached. Infero medial part of capsule is the weakest.

2. **Transverse acetabular ligament (Fig. 6.83):** It extends across acetabular notch to blend with the base of ligament of head.
3. **Ligament of head of femur (ligamentum teres) (Fig. 6.84)** Triangular fibrous band ensheathed by synovial membrane. It conveys blood vessels to head of femur.
4. Ilio-femoral ligament (Fig. 6.85)
   Strongest ligament in the body.
   Function of ligament: Tension of ligament prevents hyperextension of hip joint.
5. **Pubo femoral ligament (Fig. 6.85)**
6. **Ischio femoral ligament (Fig. 6.86):** It is attached to ischium close to acetabular margin.

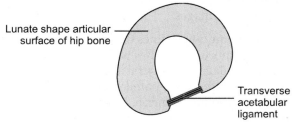

Fig. 6.83: Articular surface of hip bone

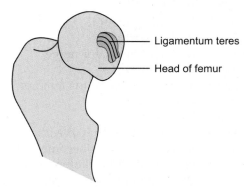

Fig. 6.84: Articular surface of femur

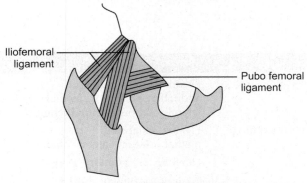

Fig. 6.85: Ligaments of hip joint

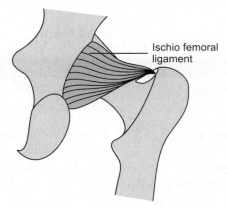

Fig. 6.86: Ligaments of hip joint

Movements occurring at hip joint and muscles involved

	Movement	*Axis*	*Muscles involved*
1.	Flexion	Transverse axis around neck of femur	Ilio-psoas, lateral part of pectineus, rectus femoris, sartorius, adductor longus. **Ilio-psoas acts as prime mover**
2.	Extension	Same as in flexion	Gluteus maximus, hamstring muscles. **Gluteus maximus acts in running and when movement is taking place against resistance. Hamstring muscles maintain extension in normal standing and walking.**
3.	Adduction	Anteroposterior axis passing through head of femur	Adductor longus, adductor brevis, adductor magnus (adductor part), pectineus, gracilis
4.	Abduction	Same as in adduction	Gluteus medius, gluteus minimus, gluteus maximus, tensor fascia lata, sartorius
5.	Medial rotation	Vertical axis passing through the centre of head of femur to lateral condyle of femur	Anterior fibres of gluteus medius, gluteus minimus, tensor fascia lata, psoas major (when foot is on the ground) **Abductors act as medial rotators**
6.	Lateral rotation	Same as in medial rotation	Gluteus maximus, piriformis, gemelli, obturator internus, obturator externus, quadratus femoris, psoas major (when foot is off the ground)

Arterial Supply of Hip Joint

It receives branches from
1. Medial and lateral circumflex arteries.
2. Superior and inferior gluteal arteries.
3. Acetabular branch of obturator artery to intra-capsular neck and head.

Nerve Supply of Hip Joint

It is supplied by spinal segment L_2, L_3, L_4, L_5
1. Nerve to rectus femoris
2. Anterior division of obturator nerve
3. Accessory obturator nerve
4. Branch from nerve to quadratus femoris
5. Sciatic nerve (occasional)
6. Superior gluteal nerve
   — Flexion is limited to 90 to 100° with an extended knee but in flexed knee it becomes 120°.
   — Extension is limited by iliofemoral ligaments. The range of extension beyond vertical line is 10° to 20°.

KNEE JOINT

It is a condylar and modified hinge synovial joint. It is called modified hinge joint because transverse axis of movement is not fixed and along with extension and flexion there is conjunct rotation of femur on tibia.

Articular surfaces (Figs 6.87 and 6.88)
1. Medial and lateral condyles of femur.
2. Medial and lateral condyles of tibia
3. **Articular surface of patella:** The entire posterior surface is articular except the apex.

Articular cartilages: All articular surfaces are covered by articular cartilages.

Synovial membrane: It lines the inner surface of fibrous capsule and portion of bones with in the capsule except articular cartilages and lateral and medial menisci. It is continuous with supra-patellar bursa and comes out along with popliteus tendon. It forms an intercondylar septum and makes anterior and posterior cruciate ligaments intracapsular and extra synovial.

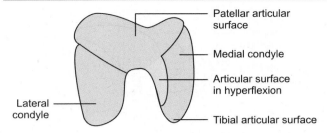

Fig. 6.87: Articular surface of femur

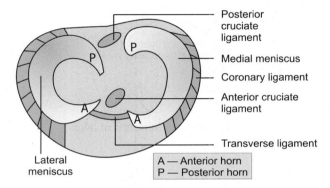

Fig. 6.88: Articular surface of tibia with ligaments

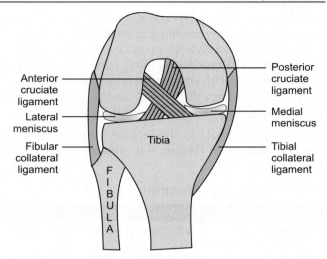

Fig. 6.89: Ligaments of knee joint

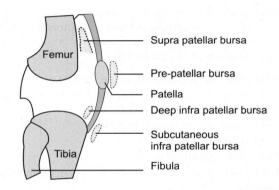

Fig. 6.90: Important bursae in relation to knee joint

Ligaments of knee joint (Figs 6.88 and 6.89)
a. Capsular ligament
b. Medial and lateral menisci
c. Ligamentum patella
d. Tibial and fibular collateral ligaments
e. Oblique popliteal ligament
f. Arcuate ligament
g. Anterior and posterior cruciate ligaments
h. Coronary ligament
i. Transverse ligament
j. Menisco-femoral ligament

Arterial Supply of Knee Joint
It is supplied by anastomosis around knee joint formed by genicular branches of following arteries:
1. Popliteal artery.
2. Femoral artery.
3. Lateral circumflex femoral artery.
4. Recurrent branch of anterior tibial artery.
5. Circumflex fibular branch of posterior tibial artery.

Nerve Supply of Knee Joint
Ten nerves supply the knee joint with root valve L_3, L_4, L_5, S_1.
1. 3 from femoral nerve
2. 3 from tibial nerve
3. 3 from common peroneal nerve
4. 1 from posterior division of obturator nerve.

Movements at knee joint: Following movements occur at the knee joint.
1. **Extension:** The range of extension is 5-10° beyond vertical line as centre of gravity falls anterior to the knee joint
2. **Flexion:** The range of flexion is 120° with extended hip, 140° with flexed hip and upto 160° when flexed passively.
3. **Medial rotation:** It is conjuct or adjunct. The range is 20° in conjunct rotation and 50 to 70° in adjunct rotation.
4. **Lateral rotation:** It is adjunct or conjunct, the range is 50 to 70° in adjunct rotation and 20° in conjunct rotation.
   Conjuct rotation occurs automatically during flexion and extension of knee.

Locking: It occurs in last 30° of extension of knee joint in which most of the ligaments are stretched except ligamentum patellae, joint is maximally congruent and extensor muscles cease active contraction.

Mechanism of locking: It occurs in last 30° of extension of knee, achieved by medial and backward rotation of medial femoral condyle in menisco-femoral compartment with simultaneous gliding forward of lateral femoral condyle with lateral meniscus in menisco-tibial compartment when the foot is on the ground. This mechanism is known as locking of the knee joint.

Unlocking: Opposite to the locking mechanism, **this occurs in first 30° of flexion.** It is initiated by popliteus muscle.

Muscles Producing Movements

Movement	Muscles involved
Extension	Quadriceps femoris, tensor fascia lata
Flexion	Semimembranosus, semitendenosus, biceps femoris Initiated by popliteus assisted by sartorius
Medial rotation	Semimembranosus, semitendienosus, sartorius, popliteus, gracilis
Lateral rotation	Biceps femoris

Important Bursae Related to Knee Joint are
There are total twelve bursae related to knee joint (Fig. 6.90).
1. Subcutaneous prepatellar bursa.
2. Suprapatellar bursa.
3. Deep infrapatellar bursa.
4. Bursa between lateral head of gastrocnemius and capsule.

Ankle Joint

It is a modified hinge variety of synovial joint.

Articular surfaces (Figs 6.91 and 6.92)
1. **Superior:** Tibio-fibular mortise which is made up of following components
   a. Lower end of tibia
   b. Medial malleolus of tibia
   c. Lateral malleolus of fibula
   Lateral malleolus is 2 cm lower than the medial malleolus
2. **Inferior:** Trochlea tali which is made up of following components
   a. Trochlear surface of body of talus
   b. Comma shaped facet on medial surface of talus
   c. Triangular shaped facet on lateral surface of talus

Articular cartilage: It covers the articular surfaces.

Synovial membrane: Synovial membrane lines the joint cavity except the articular cartilages. A synovial recess extends superiorly.

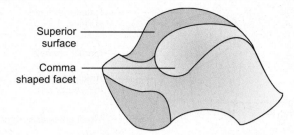

Fig. 6.91: Articular surfaces of talus

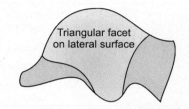

Fig. 6.92: Articular surfaces of talus

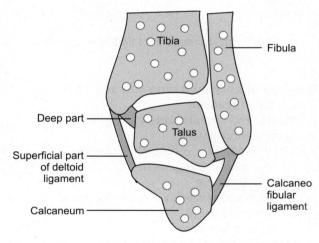

Fig. 6.93: Ankle joint, articular surfaces and ligaments

Ligaments of Ankle Joint (Fig. 6.93)
1. Capsular ligament
2. Deltoid ligament
3. Anterior talofibular ligament
4. Posterior talofibular ligament
5. Calcaneo-fibular ligament

Arterial Supply of Ankle Joint
Anterior tibial artery and peroneal arteries.

Nerve Supply of Ankle Joint
- Deep peroneal nerve, tibial nerve.
- Segmental supply: from L_4, L_5, S_1, S_2 spinal segments.

Movements: Following movements occur at the ankle joint.

1. **Dorsiflexion** upto 10°. When assisted by talar joints the range increases to 20°.
   Muscles producing dorsiflexion: Tibialis anterior, extensor digitorum longus, extensor hallucis longus, peroneus tertius.
2. **Plantar flexion:** The range of plantar flexion is 20°. It is increased to 40° when assisted by talar joints .
   Muscles producing plantar flexion: Gastrocnemius, soleus, tibialis posterior, flexor digitorum longus.

Inversion and Eversion

Inversion and eversion movements of foot occur at Talocalcaneo-navicular joint, calcaneo-cuboid joint and subtarsal joint. Subtalar joint has a major share in the movements.

Inversion: It is the raising of the medial margin of the foot above the ground so that the sole is directed downwards and medially.

Eversion: It is the raising of lateral margin of the foot above the ground so that sole faces downwards and laterally.

Features of inversion and eversion: The entire part of foot below talus moves during inversion and eversion. Movement occurs primarily at subtalar and talocalcaneo navicular joints. Inversion is accompanied by platar flexion of foot and adduction of forefoot while eversion is accompanied by dorsiflexion of foot and abduction of forefoot. Axis of movement is oblique. These movements are easily performed when the foot is off the ground. They are helpful in adjusting the foot while walking on uneven surface. Range of movement in inversion is much more than eversion. Muscles causing inversion and eversion are

Movement	Muscles involved
1. Inversion	Tibialis anterior
	Tibialis posterior
2. Eversion	Peroneus longus
	Peroneus brevis
	Peroneus tertius

JOINTS OF HEAD AND NECK

Temporomandibular Joint

It is the joint formed between the head of mandible and the articular fossa of temporal bone (Fig. 6.94).

Type: Condylar variety of synovial joint.

Articular Surfaces
1. **Upper:** Mandibular fossa or the articular eminence of the temporal bone.
2. **Lower:** Condylar process of mandible.

Articular cartilage: The articular surfaces are covered by a fibro-cartilage and not hyaline cartilage which is present in most synovial joints.

Articular disc: It is an oval fibrocartilaginous plate with a concavo-convex superior surface and a concave inferior surface. It is attached with the fibrous capsule at its periphery and divides the joint cavity into two parts
1. Upper menisco temporal compartment: Permits gliding movements
2. Lower menisco mandibular compartment: Permits rotatory as well as gliding movements.

Ligaments (Figs 6.94 and 6.95)
1. Fibrous capsule
2. Lateral temporo-mandibular ligament
3. Sphenomandibular ligament
4. Stylomandibular ligament

Movements: The lower jaw can be depressed, elevated, protruded, retracted and moved from side to side. These movements take place in both the upper and lower compartment of the joint and mostly involve both the joints simultaneously.

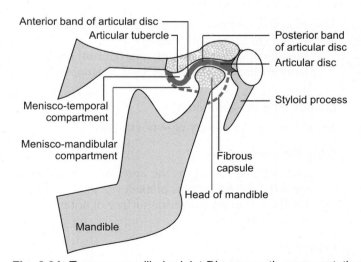

Fig. 6.94: Temporomandibular joint-Diagrammatic representation

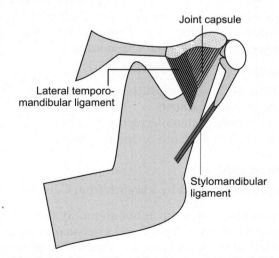

Fig. 6.95: Ligaments of temporomandibular joint

Movements	Mechanism of movement	Muscles involved
Depression	Gliding movement in menisco temporal compartment and rotatory movement in menisco mandibular compartment	• Lateral pterygoid • Geniohyoids • Mylohyoid
Elevation	Reversal of depression	• Masseter • Medial pterygoid • Temporalis (middle and anterior fibres)
Protrusion	Gliding movement in menisco temporal compartment	• Medial pterygoid • Lateral pterygoid
Retraction	Reversal of protrusion	• Posterior fibres of temporalis
Chewing	Gliding movement in menisco temporal compartment of one joint and rotatory movement in menisco mandibular compartment of other joint simultaneously	• Alternate action of medial and lateral pterygoids of each side

Nerve Supply

1. Auriculotemporal nerve
2. Masseteric nerve

Arterial Supply

1. Superficial temporal artery
2. Maxillary artery

ATLANTO-OCCIPITAL JOINTS

The first cervical vertebra, atlas articulates with the occipital condyles present on either side of the foramen magnum to form the atlanto-occipital joints.

Type: Ellipsoid variety of synovial joint

Articular Surfaces

1. **Upper:** Condyles of occipital bone of skull. These are convex both anteroposteriorly and from side to side.
2. **Lower:** Superior articular facets on the lateral mass of atlas vertebra. They are elongated and directed medially and forwards. They are reciprocal to the shape of condyles and are concave.

Ligaments

1. Fibrous capsule (capsular ligament)
2. Accessory ligaments
   a. Anterior atlanto-occipital membrane
   b. Posterior atlanto-occipital membrane

Nerve Supply

Each joint is supplied by a branch from C_1 nerve.

Movements: The main movements at the atlanto-occipital joints are of flexion and extension of the head, Slight lateral movements are also allowed but no rotation is possible.

Movement	Axis	Muscles involved
Flexion	Transverse	• Longus capitis • Rectus capitis anterior
Extension	Transverse	• Rectus capitis posterior major and minor • Semispinalis capitis • Splenius capitis • Upper part of trapezius
Lateral flexion (slight)		• Anteroposterior • Rectus capitis lateralis.

POINTS TO REMEMBER

The line of gravity of weight of the head (about 7 lbs) passes in front of the atlanto-occipital joints and hence it tends to fall forwards with gravity. The erect position of head is maintained by the traction caused by the extensor muscles particularly by semispinalis capitis and the two recti muscles.

ATLANTO-AXIAL JOINTS

The atlas (1st cervical vertebra) and axis (2nd cervical vertebra) form three joints namely

1. Median atlanto-axial joint: One, central joint
2. Lateral atlanto-axial joints: Two in number

Median Atlanto-axial Joint

Type: It is a pivot variety of synovial joint.

Articular Surfaces

1. Oval articular facet on the anterior surface of the dens (odontoid process of axis).
2. Oval facet on the posterior surface of anterior arch of the atlas.

Ligaments

1. **Fibrous capsule**

2. **Transverse ligament of atlas:** It is attached on each side to the medial surface of the lateral mass of the atlas. The transverse ligament surrounds the narrow neck of the dens posteriorly and prevents its backward dislocation. A synovial bursa is interposed between the transverse ligament and the dens. Thus the dens of axis forms the pivot which lies in a ring formed by the anterior arch of atlas and the transverse ligament. The dens divides the joint into two parts, anterior and posterior.

3. **Ligaments connecting the axis with the occipital bone**
   a. Apical ligament of dens
   b. Cruciform ligament
   c. Alar ligament
   d. Membrana tectoria

Lateral Atlanto-axial Joints

Type: Plane variety of synovial joint

Articular Surfaces
1. **Upper:** Inferior articular facet of the lateral mass of atlas. It is concave in shape
2. **Lower:** Superior articular facet of axis. It is convex, reciprocally curved to the facet on atlas.

Ligaments
1. Capsule
2. Anterior longitudinal ligament
3. Ligamentum flavum

Nerve Supply
The atlanto axial joints are supplied by rami of C_2 nerves.

Movements: The side to side movement of head is produced by rotation of the atlas along with cranium around the dens of the axis.

Muscles involved in the movement of head to one side are
a. On same side
   — Obliquus capitis inferior
   — Rectus capitis posterior major
   — Splenius capiti
b. On opposite side
   — Sternocleidomastoid

CLINICAL AND APPLIED ASPECTS

GENERAL POINTS

- **Fracture:** It is defined as break in the continuity of a bone. The most common cause of fracture is trauma or injury.
- **Osteomyelitis:** Infection of bone is known as osteomyelitis. The most common part affected is metaphysis of bone.

- **Arthritis:** It is the inflammation of joints and is characterized by pain, swelling and decrease mobility of joint involved. Common causes of arthritis are:
  1. Bacterial infections
  2. Gout
  3. Degenerative cause like osteoarthritis, is due to wear and tear of articular cartilage of the joint and is commonly associated with aging.
  4. Autoimmune causes like rheumatoid arthritis, rheumatic fever.
- **Gout** is a clinical conditions characterised by increased uric acid levels in the blood associated with recurrent attacks of acute arthiritis (the most common joint involved in arthiritis is first metatarsophalangeal joint), deposition of urate crystals in kidneys and joints. It is of two types :
  1. **Primary gout:** There is increase uric acid prodution due to enzyme abnormalities.
  2. **Secondary gout:** In this there is increase in uric acid levels in blood due to either increase destruction of nucleic acids, e.g., as seen in leukemias or defective secretion by kidneys example as seen in chronic renal failure and use of diuretics.
- **Dislocation of joint:** It is a clinical condition characterized by completed loss of apposition of the two articular surfaces of a joint. Subluxation of a joint is when the articular surfaces are partially displaced. The most common cause is injury.

SKULL

- **Clinical importance of suprameatal triangle:** Severe mastoiditis, needing surgical intervention, is treated by approaching the mastoid antrum via the supra meatal triangle. Careful anatomical delineation is important as it is related to the facial nerve posteriorly and the sigmoid sinus anteriorly.
- **Clinical significance of pterion:** Inner aspect of the pterion is related to middle meningeal vessels. In cases of an extradural haematoma due to head injury, where there is injury to middle meningeal vessels, a burr hole is drilled in the region of pterion for evacuation of blood to release the pressure.
- Fracture of anterior cranial fossa leads to damage to the cribriform plate of ethmoid bone. This can cause bleeding and/or drainage of cerebrospinal fluid (CSF) from the nose. Leaking of CSF from nose is known as rhinorrhoea.
- The usual line of fracture in injury of middle cranial fossa passes downwards from the parietal tuberosity along the squamous part of temporal bone and internally into the petrous temporal bone.

CHAPTER-6

It can cause:
— Bleeding or drainage of CSF from ear.
— Bleeding through nose.
— Vertigo due to involvement of semicircular canals.

- **Features studied in the interpretation of X-ray skull:** From clinical point of view, one should know what structures in the calvarium leave markings that are seen normally on an X-ray skull so that one can distinguish them from fractures. These structures are:
  — **Sutures:** Do not forget the occasional presence of metopic suture between two halves of the frontal bone.
  — **Middle meningeal vessels:** Their shadows are clearly seen in the lateral veiw of X-ray skull
  — **Pineal gland:** Is present near the centre of brain. It may contain small calcareous granules called corpora arenaceae or brain-sand which are radio-opaque and seen as white spots on X-ray. The position of pineal gland may be thus helpful to recognize displacements of the brain.
  — **Auricle of the ear:** It casts a semicircular shadow on lateral view of X-ray skull. Remember it is often identified as a semicircular canal by the students.
  — **Emissary foramina:** These are also seen on X-ray skull. One is usually found in the parietal bone and one in the temporal bone behind the external auditory meatus.
- The clinical importance of anterior fontanelle is due to the fact that it is easily palpated in newborns.
  — A bulging and tense anterior fontanelle is suggestive of increased intracranial tension.
  — A depressed fontanelle is a sign of dehydration in newborn.
  — The superior sagittal sinus lies below this fontanelle.
  — During labour the position of anterior fontanelle helps to identify the position of fetal head in the maternal pelvis.

BONES OF LIMBS

- Most common site of clavicle is junction of medial 2/3rd and lateral 1/3rd.
- Fracture of surgical need of humerus can damage the axillary nerve.
- Colles fracture: It is the fracture of distal end of radius. It is the most common site of fracture in elderly ladies due to osteoporosis. 2nd most common site of fracture in elderly is neck of femur.

- Fracture of pelvic bones following trauma is usually associated with severe bleeding and haemorrhagic shock due to damage to blood vessels. It is also often associated with urethral injuries.

FOOT

- Congenital talipes equinovarus is a deformity of the foot characterized by
  — Plantar flexion of foot
  — Inversion deformity of heel
  — Forefoot in various postions
- Flat foot is the flattening of the longitudinal arches. The medial border of foot touches the ground. It can be congenital or acquired. In case of congenital flat foot either achillis tendon is short or the muscle tone is poor. The cause of acquired flat foot is generally an injury to the spring ligament. The patient complains of pain in the foot due to compression of plantar nerves.
- **Pes cavus:** It is an exaggeration of the longitudinal arch. There is plantar flexion at the transverse joint so that the anterior part of the foot drops below the level of posterior part.
- Hallux valgus is a condition in which the great toe is adducted towards the midline of the foot. Primarily the defect lies in some degree of abduction of 1st metatarsal and the deviation of the great toe at proximal metatarsophalangeal joint.
- **Hammer toe:** In this deformity the metatarsophalangeal and the distal interphalangeal joints of 2nd and 3rd toe are hyperextended and proximal interphalangeal joint is acutely flexed.

SHOULDER JOINT

- Anterior dislocation of shoulder joint is more common than inferior dislocation because usually the impact of the force is from behind. Also the the joint capsule is thin anteriorly. The dislocation of head of humerus is subcoracoid.
- Axillary nerve is likely to be injured in inferior dislocation of shoulder joint.
- Chronic thickening of tendon of supraspinatus results in pain during abduction between 60 to 120°, when the tendon rubs against coraco-acromial arch. The condition is known as **painful arch syndrome.**
- Tendinitis involving rotator cuff muscles leads to restriction of all movements of the shoulder joint due to pain and adhesions. This is known as **frozen shoulder.**

ELBOW JOINT

- Partial tear of radial collateral ligament during abrupt pronation in tennis players leads to pain and tenderness over the lateral epicondyle. This condition is known as **tennis elbow.**
- Normally, in the semiflexed position olecranon and the two humeral epicondyles form an equilateral triangle. In dislocation of elbow, this relationship is disturbed.
- **Golfer's elbow:** It occurs due to partial tear of the common origin of the superficial flexor muscles of forearm and is seen more often in persons who play golf.
- Repeated pressure over olecranon process leads to inflammation of olecranon bursa and pain at elbow. This is called **student's elbow.**

WRIST JOINT

- Joints involved in movement of wrist are
  - **Radiocarpal joint:** Mainly extension and adduction.
  - **Midcarpal joint:** Mainly flexion and abduction.
- The range of movement of adduction is greater than abduction at writst joint because the styloid process of radius limits the abduction.

HIP JOINT

Trendelenburg's test is employed for testing the stability of hip joint. A positive test indicates a defect in the osseomuscular stability. It is especially used to test for abductors of hip joint. The patient with paralysis/paresis of abductor of thigh on one side has a 'lurching' gait. When the patient is asked to stand on one leg, The weak muscles will not be able to sustain the pelvis against the body weight and so pelvis tilts downwards on unsupported side.

KNEE JOINT

- Medial meniscus is more prone to injury because it is more firmly attached to the upper surface of the tibia, capsule and the tibial collateral ligament It is less able to adapt itself to sudden changes of position and tears easily. The lateral meniscus on the other hand, is drawn backwards and downwards in the groove on the posterior aspect of the lateral tibial condyle by the medial fibres of popliteus. This prevents, the lateral meniscus from being impacted between the articular surfaces of the femur and the tibia during movements of the knee joint.
- The subcutaneous prepatellar bursa may get inflamed and painful. This occurs when the knee is constantly exposed to friction as occur while washing floors in a kneel down position. This is most commonly seen in housemaids and hence, is called housemaid's knee.
- Anterior menisco femoral ligament is known as ligament of Humphrey.
- Posterior menisco-femoral ligament is called as ligament of Wrisberg.
- Iliofemoral ligament is known as ligament of Bigelow. It is the strongest ligament in the body.

TEMPOROMANDIBULAR JOINT

Dislocation usually occurs when the mouth is widely open. In this position the head of mandible glides forwards and downwards and comes to lie below the articular tubercle. The joint is highly unstable and a blow on head in this position results in forward dislocation of the head of mandible. The person will not be able to close his mouth after such an injury.

IMAGING BONES AND JOINTS IN THE BODY

- **Standard radiography:** Provides a detailed appearance of compact and cancellous bones. Their shape and extent are clearly recorded with spatial resolution of 0.1 to 0.2 mm.
- **Arthrography:** It involves introduction of iodine based contrast media or air or CO_2 into a joint cavity to assist in visualization and/or differentiating between soft tissue. In particular, joint spaces, bursae, synovial membrane, the size of menisci, intra articular ligament and articular cartilage can be studied.
- **Computerized tomography:** Useful in the study of complex joints, e.g., sacroiliac joint, ossicles with in the middle ear. Spatial resolution is 0.4 mm much less than plain radiography.
- **Ultrasonography:** Mainly useful in assessment of thickness of synovial membrane, bursae, synovial sheath of the hand.
- **Magnetic resonance imaging:** Is useful in detecting joint structures, especially vertebral joints.
- **Soft tissue radiography:** Allows the study of details of soft tissue, tendons, sheaths, ligaments, joint capsules, cartilages with the of low kilovolt X-ray unit.
- **Magnification radiography:** This technique provides the greatest details of the structural organization of bone.
- **Stero-radiography:** It provides a three dimensional evaluation of structures.
- **Radionuclide imaging:** It helps in identifying sites of bone growth and remodelling.

Chapter 7

Muscular System

INTRODUCTION

MUSCULAR TISSUE

Muscle is a contractile tissue and primarily designed for movements. The word muscle is derived from the latin word musculus which means mouse. Certain muscles resemble a mouse with their tendon representing the mouse tail.

All muscles of the body are developed from mesoderm, except the arrector pilorum, muscles of iris and myo-epithelial cells of salivary, sweat and lacrimal glands which are derived from ectoderm.

Muscle are divided into three types based on their location in relation to various body parts and on the differences in microscopic structure.
1. Skeletal muscle
2. Smooth muscle
3. Cardiac muscle

SKELETAL OR STRIATED MUSCLE

Skeletal muscles are also called voluntary muscles as they are mostly under the conscious control of central nervous system (CNS). The muscle fibres are attached to the skeletal framework of the body and help in movement of joints and bones.

Skeletal muscles are supplied by spinal and cranial nerves and are usually under voluntary control. Muscles of pharynx and diaphragm are striated but not entirely under voluntary control.

Parts of striated muscles–Each muscle presents with the following two parts
1. **Fleshy part:** It is the contractile, highly vascular part and has a higher metabolic rate.
2. **Fibrous part:** May be tendinous or aponeurotic, is non elastic, less vascular and resistant to friction.

Origin of a Muscle

The end of a muscle which is fixed during contraction is known as origin of the muscle.

Insertion of the Muscle

Movable end of a muscle is known as insertion of muscle. In limbs the distal end generally corresponds to insertions. However, in some muscles it is known that both the ends move in different conditions. Therefore, the term "attachments" of the muscle is more appropriate.

Classification of Striated Muscles

Grossly striated muscles are classified according to the direction of muscle fibres, colour of muscles and force of action.

Classification According to Direction of Muscle Fibres

1. **Parallel muscle:** Muscle fibres are parallel to the line of pull. The fibres are long, but their numbers are relatively few. (Fig. 7.1)
   Example:
   a. **Strap muscles:** Sartorius, rectus abdominus, sternohyoid.
   b. **Quadrate muscle:** Quadratus lumborum.
   c. **Fusiform muscle:** Biceps brachii, digastric. (Fig. 7.2).
   Functional characteristics: These muscles provide more range of movement but total force of contraction is less.

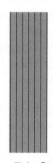
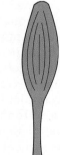

Fig. 7.1: Strap   Fig. 7.2: Fusiform

2. **Pennate muscles or oblique muscles:** Fleshy part of fibres are arranged obliquely to the line of pull. The fibres are short and a greater number of them can be accommodated. They are of the following types
   a. **Unipennate:** All fleshy fibres slope into one side of the tendon which is formed along one margin of the muscle. This gives a half feather appearance (Fig. 7.3).

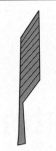
Fig. 7.3: Unipennate

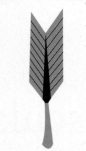
Fig. 7.4: Bipennate

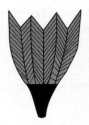
Fig. 7.5: Multipennate

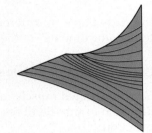
Fig. 7.6: Spiral

Example: Flexor pollicis longus, extensor digitorum, peroneus tertius

b. **Bipennate:** Tendon is formed in the central axis of the muscle and the muscle fibres slope from the two sides into the central tendon, like a feather (Fig. 7.4).

Example: Dorsal interossei of foot and hand, rectus femoris

c. **Multipennate:** A series of bipennate fibres lie side by side in one plane (Fig. 7.5).

Example: Acrominal fibres of deltoid

Fucntional characteristics: It provides for a wide range of movements.

d. **Circumpennate:** Muscle is cylindrical with a central tendon. Oblique muscle fibres converge into the central tendon from all sides.

Example: Tibialis anterior.

Functional characteristics: Total force of contraction is increased though the range of movement is less.

3. **Spiral muscle:** This type of muscle has a twisted arrangement close to its insertion (Fig. 7.6).

Example: Pectoralis major, supinator.

Functional characteristics: Spiral course imparts rotational movement.

4. **Cruciate muscle:** Muscle fibres are arranged from the superficial to deep planes in a criss cross X-shaped pattern.

Example: Masseter, sternocleido-mastoid.

Functional characteristic: This arrangement increases the range of movement.

Classification According to Force of Action

1. **Shunt muscles:** These muscles tend to draw the bone along the line of shaft towards the joint and compress the articular surfaces. Example: Brachioradialis

2. **Spurt muscles:** A swing component tends to produce angular movement of the joint. When the swing component is more powerful, the muscle is known as spurt. Example: Brachialis.

Classification According to Colour

Colour of muscle fibres depends upon the capillary density and amount of myohaemoglobin in the sarcoplasm of muscle cells. There are of two types of muscle fibres namely red muscle fibres and white muscle fibres.

Naming of Muscles

Names of the muscles are usually descriptive, that is, based on their shape, size, number of head and bellies, position, depth, attachment and action.

Nomenclature According to Shape

Shape	Example
Deltoid—Triangular	Deltoid (Fig. 7.7)
Quadratus—Square	Quadratus lumborum
Rhomboid—Diamond shape	Rhombodeus major
Teres—Round	Teres major
Gracilis—Slender	Gracilis
Rectus—Straight	Rectus femoris
Lumbrical—Worm like	Lumbricals

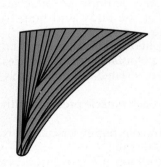
Fig. 7.7: Deltoid muscle-triangular in shape

Fig. 7.8: Digastric muscle-two bellies

Nomenclature According to Size

Size	Example
Major—Big	Pectoralis major
Minor—Small	Teres minor
Longus—Long	Adductor longus
Brevis—Short	Adductor brevis
Latissimus—Broadest	Latissimus dorsi
Longissimus—Longest	Longissimus coli

Nomenclature According to Bellies

Number of heads and bellies	Example
Biceps—2 heads	Biceps brachii
Triceps—heads	Triceps
Quadriceps—4 heads	Quadriceps femoris
Digastric—2 bellies	Digastric (Fig. 7.8)

Nomenclature According to Position

Position	Example
Anterior—in front	Tibialis anterior
Posterior—behind	Tibialis posterior
Supraspinatus—above the spine	Supraspinatus
Infraspinatus—below the spine	Infraspinatus
Dorsi—back	Lattissimus dorsi
Abdominis—of abdomen	Rectus abdominis
Pectoralis—of chest	Pectoralis minor
Brachii—of the arm	Biceps brachii
Femoris—of the thigh	Rectus femoris
Oris—of the mouth	Orbicularis oris

Nomenclature According to Depth

Depth	Example
Superficialis—Superficial	Flexor digitorum superficialis
Profundus—Deep	Flexor digitorum profundus
Externus—External	Obliquus externus
Internus—Internal	Obliquus internus

Nomenclature According to Site of Attachment

Attachment	Example
Sternum, clavicle and mastoid	Sternocleidomastoid
Coracoid process to arm	Coracobrachialis

Nomenclature According to Action

Action	Example
Extension	Extensor digitorum
Flexion	Flexor pollicis
Abduction	Abductor pollicis longus
Adduction	Adductor policis
Levator–Elevation	Levator ani
Depression	Depresser anguli oris
Supination	Supinator
Pronation	Pronator quadratus

Structure of Skeletal Muscle Fibre

- Skeletal muscle fiber is a multinucleated, elongated, cylindrical shaped cell surrounded by cell membrane named sarcolemma.

- The sarcolemma is surrounded by a basal lamina, the **endomysium.** The muscle fibers are arranged in bundles. Each bundle is covered by a layer of connective tissue, known as **perimysium.** The bundles together form a muscle which is invested by connective tissue named **epimysium** (Fig. 7.9).

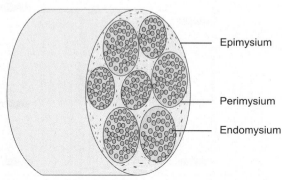

Epimysium

Perimysium

Endomysium

Fig. 7.9: Diagrammatic representation of cut section of skeletal muscle

- The cytoplasm of muscle cell is known as sarcoplasm. It contains myofibrils, well developed mitochondria and specialized sarcoplasmic reticulum. It contains a special protein complex, dystrophin—glycoprotein complex that provides strength and support to myofibrils. It also contains myoglobin, a protein that stores oxygen in muscles.
- Each fiber is made of myofibrils formed by filaments of contractile proteins. The filaments are of two types:
  — Thick filaments made up of protein, myosin
  — Thin filaments made up of proteins, actin, troponin and tropomyosin.
- The main contractile protein of the thin filaments is actin. It is arranged as a double helix and forms cross links with myosin. Tropomyosin are long filaments which have troponin units located along their length. The troponin—tropomyosin complex prevents interaction of actin and myosin.
- The arrangement of thick and thin filaments in the muscle fiber is shown in figure (Figs 7.11 and 7.12).
- The above arrangement of fibrils results in variations in the refractive index in various parts of muscle fiber. Thus, on microscopic examination of cut section of a skeletal muscle, alternate light and dark bands are seen. This gives it a characteristic appearance of **cross-striations** (Fig. 7.10). The various bands have been labeled as (Figs 7.11 and 7.12)
  1. **A-band:** It is a relatively darker band which is formed by the thick filaments made up of myosin.
  2. **I-band:** It is a relatively lighter band, formed by arrangement of thin filaments, that is actin and tropomyosin.
  3. **H-band:** It is a slightly lighter band seen in the middle of A band. This is the area of relaxed

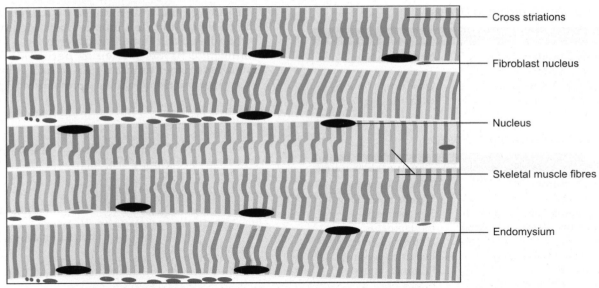

Fig. 7.10: Skeletal muscle (Stain-hematoxylin-eosin under high magnification)

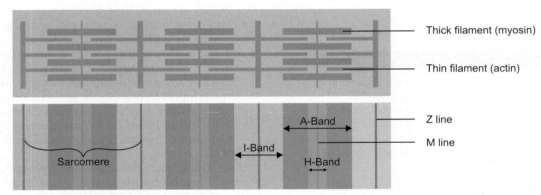

Fig. 7.11: Diagrammatic representation of striations seen on electron micrograph picture of a skeletal muscle fiber

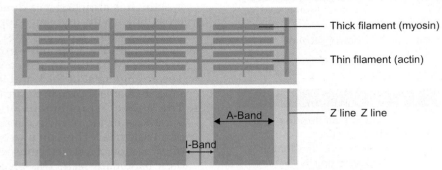

Fig. 7.12: Diagrammatic representation of striations seen on electron micrograph picture of a skeletal muscle fiber-showing changes during contraction of muscle

muscle consisting of thick filaments only, where there is no overlapping of thick and thin filaments. The width of H-band decreases during contraction of muscle.

4. **M-line:** It is the line seen in centre of H-band. Myosin filaments extend on either side from this line.

5. **Z-line:** It is a dark line seen in the centre of I-band. It appears dark due to a high refractive index. The actin filaments extend from each side of Z-line towards the myosin filaments till edge of H-zone. When muscle contracts the two adjacent Z-lines move closer.

Sarcomere: Functional unit of a muscle fiber cell is called sarcomere. It extends between the two Z-lines.

Sarcotubular System

It is a system of membrane bound vesicles and tubules that surrounds the fibrils in a muscle fiber cell. It consists of two parts:

1. **T-system:** It consists of transversely placed tubules which extend from sarcolemma to the fibrils. They transmit the action potential from cell membrane to the fibrils.
2. **Sarcoplasmic reticulum:** The tubules of sarcoplasmic reticulum are arranged longitudinally around the fibrils. They are concerned with glycogen metabolism and Ca^{2+} movement. At the junction of the sarcoplamic reticulum with T-tubules, it presents with terminal dilatations called cisterns. Two cisterns plus a T-tubule form a triad. These triads are seen at the junction of A and I – bands of the fibrils. Hence, 2 triads are present in one sarcomere.

SMOOTH OR NON-STRIATED MUSCLE

Non striated or smooth muscles are widely distributed in the wall of hollow viscera, tubular and saccular viscera, ducts of exocrine glands, blood vessels, stroma of solid organs and the tracheo-bronchial tree.

Arrangement of Smooth Muscles

*   In blood vessels smooth muscles are predominantly arranged in a circular fashion.
*   In the gastrointestinal tract smooth muscles are arranged in inner circular and outer longitudinal layers.
*   In urinary bladder, uterus and stomach smooth muscles are arranged in three layers, namely circular, longitudinal and oblique.
*   Smooth muscles are supplied by parasympathetic and sympathetic nervous system. Parasympathetic stimulation usually causes contraction while sympathetic stimulation causes relaxation of the smooth muscle.

Structure of Smooth Muscle Fiber

Smooth muscle fibers are unicellular spindle shaped cells which do not have any striations (Fig. 7.13). Each cell is surounded by cell membrane called sarcolemma. The contractile units actin and myosin are arranged irregularly. Troponin is absent. The cytoplasm contains a special calcium binding protein, calmodulin.

CARDIAC MUSCLE

Cardiac muscles are present in the heart and at the beginning of great vessels.

Structure of Cardiac Muscle Fiber

*   Cardiac muscle fibers are uninucleated, long cylindrical fibers with similar striations as seen in skeletal muscle fibers. However, since the fibers branch and interdigitate the arrangement is not linear. Each fiber is surrounded by the cell membrane or sarcolemma and has a centrally placed nucleus (Fig. 7.14).
*   Most distinctive feature of cardiac muscle fibres is the presence of interconnections between the muscle fibres in the form of side branches.
*   At the site where one muscle fiber meets the other, it shows extensive folds of sarcolemma that provides a strong union between adjacent fibers. These form **intercalated disks.** This gives the fibers an appearance of syncytium with dark lines representing the intercalated disks. Also this allows for the rapid transmission of impulses. Thus, the cardiac muscle functions as a syncytium. This is the anatomical basis for the spread of contraction over entire heart from a single point.
*   The T-system of cardiac muscle fiber is located at Z line and not at junction of A and I bands.
*   The cells are rich in mitochondria, glycogen and have a well developed capillary network.

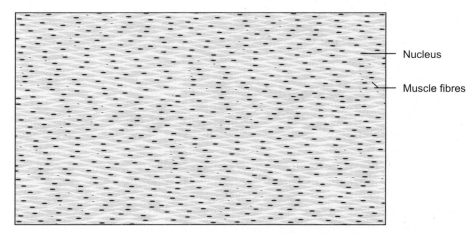

Fig. 7.13: Transverse section of smooth muscle (Stain-hematoxylin-eosin under low magnification)

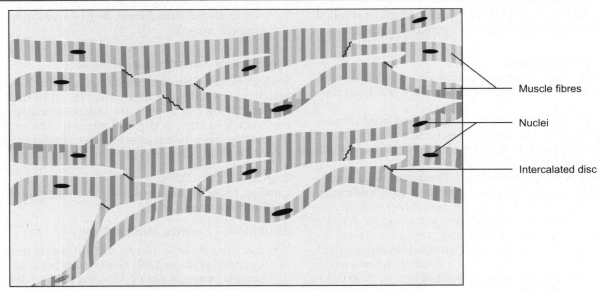

Fig. 7.14: Transverse section of cardiac muscle (Stain-hematoxylin-eosin under high magnification)

Characteristic features of skeletal, smooth and cardiac muscles.

Skeletal muscles	Smooth muscles	Cardiac muscles
1. Most abundant muscles in the body, are attached to the skeleton.	Surround the various viscera of the body.	Form myocardium of heart.
2. Supplied by spinal nerves (somatic) nerves. Are under voluntary control except pharynx and diaphragm.	Supplied by autonomic nervous system. Are mainly under involuntary control.	Supplied by autonomic nervous system, are under involuntary control. Autorhythmical activity seen.
3. Respond quickly to stimuli, undergo rapid contractions, get fatigued easily.	Respond slowly to stimuli, do not fatigue easily.	Automatic and rhythmic sustained contractions occur, do not fatigue easily.
4. Help in adjusting the individual his external environment.	Help in regulating internal environment.	Help to pump blood into circulation at regular intervals.
5. Highest control is at the cerebral cortex.	Less dependent on neuronal control.	Nervous control maintains the rhythm.

Differences in the microscopic structure of the three types of muscle fibers.

Features	Skeletal muscle (Fig. 7.10)	Smooth muscle (Fig. 7.13)	Cardiac muscle (Fig. 7.14)
1. Cell type	Cells are long, thick and cylindrical. Longest cell may be upto 30 cm in length. They are unbranched.	Cells are small and spindle shaped. They are unbranched.	Cells are cylindrical in shape. Fibres are branched.
2. Length of cell	4 to 30 cm	15 to 500 microns	80 microns
3. Number of nuclei and their position	Multinucleated. The elongated nuclei are placed peripherally.	Single nucleus which is centrally placed.	Centrally placed, single nucleus.
4. Cell arrangement	Cells lie parallel to each other and form bundles.	Cells overlap each other with distinct outlines.	Intercalated discs are present at the cell to cell junction.
5. Striations	Transverse striations are the characteristic feature and are seen as light and dark bands.	No transverse striations present but indistinct longitudinal striations may be present.	Transverse striations are present but not so clear as seen in the skeletal muscle.
6. Electron microscopic structure	T tubules are present. They form a triad and lie at the junction of A-I band.	T tubules are not present.	T tubules are present at Z lines and form dyads.

PHYSIOLOGY OF MUSCLE

Muscle cells respond to mechanical, chemical and electrical stimulie just like the nerve cells and action potentials are generated in them. These electrical changes of cell membrane further lead to production of a contractile response in muscle cell fibers. The physiology of contraction of skeletal muscle, smooth muscle and cardiac muscle is described below.

SKELETAL MUSCLE

It is also called voluntary muscle as it is mostly under conscious control by CNS. The muscle fibres are attached to the skeletal framework of the body and help in movement of joints and bones.

Excitation of Muscle Fiber (Fig. 7.15)

- Electrical activity in muscle fiber is similar to nerve fibers (for detail see page no. 206).
- Resting membrane potential of muscle fibre is maintained by Na⁺ K⁺ ATPase pumps and is about – 90mV.
- Depolarization is initiated at the neuromuscular junction by action of neurotransmitters released by terminal part of nerve fibers.
- The action potential is transmitted along the muscle fibers and to its fibrils via the T-system. Depolarization occurs due to opening of Na⁺ channels and Na⁺ influx and repolarizaiton due to closure of Na⁺ channels and opening of K⁺ channels leading to K⁺ efflux as in axons.

Contractile Response of Muscle Fibers (Fig. 7.15)

- The action potential extends to the fibrils from cell membrane via the T-system.
- This stimulates release of Ca²⁺ from cisterns of sarcoplasmic reticulum.

- Ca²⁺ binds to troponin and this results in moving away of the troponin-tropromyosin complex from actin. This allows coupling of actin and myosin.
- ATP is used to provide energy that helps in sliding of actin over myosin which causes contraction of muscle fiber.
- The cisterns now start reaccumulating Ca²⁺ from sarcoplasm by active transport, using Ca²⁺-Mg²⁺ ATPase pump and the removal of Ca²⁺ results in gradual stoppage of actin-myosin linkage and relaxation of muscle fiber.
- The contractile response to the action potential is an "all or none" phenomenan that is, either the entire muscle fiber contracts due to stimulus or there is no response. However, the action potential has a refractory period while the contractile response does not have any refractory period and repeated electrical potentials can cause repeated contractions.

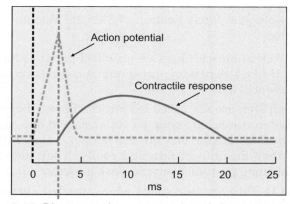

Fig. 7.15: Diagrammatic representation of electrical changes and the contractile response of a skeletal muscle fiber

Types of Contraction

Muscle can contract in two ways because besides actin and myosin it has elastic and viscous elements arranged parallel to the filaments.

Differences in electrical changes during resting phase and during action potential phase of nerve fiber and muscle

	Nerve fibre (Axon)	Muscle fiber
Resting membrane potential	– 70 mV	– 90mV
Duration of action potential	0.5 to 2 ms	2 to 4 ms
Conduction of electrical impulses	2 m/sec in thin axons to upto 120 m/sec in thick myelinated axons	5 m/sec
Absolute refractory period	0.5 to 2 ms	1 to 3 ms

1. **Isotonic contraction:** There is contraction of muscle associated with shortening of muscle fiber length. The total tension remains the same. Examples are walking, lifting objects of average weight.

2. **Isometric contraction:** The contraction of muscle is not associated with any visible change in length of muscle fiber and the tension is increased. The elastic component maintains the length. Examples are trying to lift a very heavy object, though the muscles are contracting there is no shortening and object cannot be lifted. Another example is pushing against a wall.

Tetanic Contraction

The contractile mechanism has no refractory period. Hence, repeated stimulation before end of relaxation leads to repeated contractions called as summation of contractions. If these stimulations occur before start of relaxation it leads to one prolonged contraction i.e. tetanus.

Physiological Classification of Skeletal Muscle Fibers

The skeletal muscle fibres are classified into type I and type II fibres depending on speed of contraction and ATPase activity.

Type I: They are also called red muscles fibres. They are darker in colour, are adapted for sustained and slow contractions. Hence, they are also known as slow fibres and they do not get fatigued easily. They help in maintaining posture. Example: Back muscles.

Type II: They are also called white muscles. They are adapted for short and quick contractions. Hence, they are known as fast fibres and they fatigue easily. These muscles are involved in fine skillful movements. Example: Hand and eye muscles.

Metabolism of Skeletal Muscles

The immediate energy for contraction is obtained from ATP and another energy rich phosphate compound phosphorylcreatine. At rest and during light exercise, muscles utilize free fatty acids to generate ATP while on increasing exercise, oxidation of glucose, i.e., aerobic glycolysis, generates ATP. Glucose is obtained from the store of glycogen in muscles. Part of energy is also obtained from anaerobic glycolysis, which does not require O_2.

O_2 Debt and Muscle Recovery

During strenuous exercise the blood flow to muscles is increased to provide extra O_2. If the rate of exercise exceeds the maximal O_2 consumption capacity of tissue and when glucose and fatty acid stores are depleted, fatigue sets in. This is because further energy is now provided by anaerobic metabolism that increases lactate levels and local pH. After stopping exercise extra O_2 is consumed by the tissue (above normal resting levels) for a particular duration in order to replenish the ATP and phosphyrylcreatine stores and remove lactate. This extra O_2 consumption is called O_2 debt. Once the debt is recovered, the O_2 consumtpion comes back to the normal resting levels.

Rigor: When ATP and phosphyrylcreatine stores are completely depleted without any recovery, as in death, the muscles develop a state of rigidity called rigor.

Motor Unit

Motor unit consists of a single motor neuron and the muscle fibers innervated by it.

SMOOTH MUSCLE

It is under involuntary control and mostly forms part of visceral structures in the body.

Excitation of Smooth Muscle Fiber

- The resting membrane potential is – 50 mV but it varies according to its activity which is regulated by autonomic nervous system (Fig. 7.16).
- There is spontaneous electrical activity with slow sine-wave like fluctuation of voltage. This is independent of nervous stimulation. Thus, the smooth muscle fibres are maintained in varying degrees of partial state of contraction, which is called the tone of muscle fibre.
- Action potentials occur at regular intervals over and above this waves. The tone of waves is regulated by autonomic nervous system.

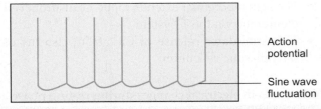

Fig. 7.16: Diagrammatic representation of electrical changes of a smooth muscle fiber

Contractile Response of Smooth Muscle

- Excitation-contraction coupling is a slow process as contraction occurs 200 ms after action potential spike and peak contraction occurs 500 ms after spike.

- Electrical changes lead to opening of Ca^{2+} channels allowing influx of ECF Ca^{2+}. Ca^{2+} binds with calmodulin and this leads to phosphorylation of myosin that activates ATP for actin-myosin coupling leading to contraction.
- Smooth muscle fibers can contract when they are simply stretched without any nerve stimulation.
- Sympathetic discharge hyperpolarizes smooth by increasing Ca^{2+} efflux and relaxes the muscle. Cholinergic (parasympathetic) discharge stimulates smooth muscle by increasing Ca^{2+} and Na^+ influx.

Metabolism of Smooth Muscle

Smooth muscles use glycogen and glucose for their energy requirements, by glycolysis.

CARDIAC MUSCLE

It is the specialised muscle of heart which is under involuntary control.

Excitation of Cardiac Muscle Fibers (Fig. 7.17)

- Resting membrane potential is – 90 mV, similar to skeletal muscle fiber.
- Stimulation leads to action potential which is longer, about 200 ms, than that of skeletal muscle fiber which is 2 ms.
- The action potential can be divided into five phases namely:
  a. **Phase 0–Rapid depolarization:** This is due to opening of Na^+ channels and Na^+ influx.
  b. **Phase 1–Rapid repolarization:** This is a short phase and occurs due to closure of Na^+ channels and opening of K^+ channels allowing efflux.
  c. **Phase 2–Plateau phase:** It is a state of sustained depolarization due to opening of Ca^{2+} channels facilitating Ca^{2+} influx. Ca^{2+} influx starts in phase 0 but continues longer.
  d. **Phase 3–Rapid final repolarization:** This occurs due to closure of Ca^{2+} channels and stoppage of Ca^{2+} and Na^+ influx and increase K^+ efflux.
  e. **Phase 4–Polarized state:** It is the restoration of resting membrane ionic composition by Na^+ K^+ ATPase pump.

It is seen that as cardiac rate increases repolarization time decreases and action potentials are shorter.

Contractile Response of Muscle Fibers

- The electrical activity leads to influx of extracellular Ca^{2+} (not from endoplasmic reticulum as in skeletal muscle). This causes actin-myosin coupling and contraction, the muscle fibers act as one unit (syncytium).
- Contraction of muscle fiber lasts 1.5 times longer than action potential. Hence, repolarization of fiber is complete only after half contraction is over. Due to this factor, absolute refractory period of the muscle is prolonged till beyond half contraction is over and even after that it is relatively refractory. Thus tetanus cannot occur in cardiac muscle.
- However, if stimulation occurs in the relative refractory period it leads to extrasystole, tachycardia and fibrillation.

Metabolism of Cardiac Muscle

About 2/3rd of energy is delivered from free fatty acids. Anaerobic metabolism plays a very small role, less than 10% in providing energy. There is a high content of myoglobin which is an O_2 storing muscle pigment.

Pacemaker in Cardiac Muscle

These are cells that discharge rhythmically on their own, that is they have automatic firing. The rate of discharge is controlled by autonomic nervous system but it is not

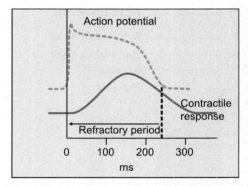

Fig. 7.17: Diagrammatic representation of electrical changes and the contractile response of cardiac muscle fiber

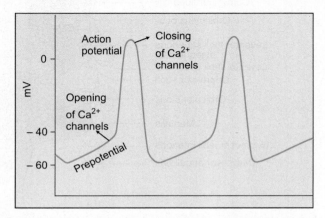

Fig. 7.18: Diagrammatic representation of electrical changes in pacemaker fibers of cardiac muscle

abolished even when nervous input is removed. Depolarization occurs due to opening of Ca^{2+} channels (for influx) and repolarization occurs due to closure of the Ca^{2+} channels and opening of K^+ channels (for efflux). The electrical potential does not have a sharp spike nor does it have a plateau. As K^+ efflux declines, Ca^{2+} channels open again starting the next wave of depolarization (Fig. 7.18).

Factors Affecting Excitability

1. **Autonomic nervous system:** On parasympathetic (Vagal) stimulation, membrane is hyperpolarized due to increased K^+ conductance (efflux). Hence, the firing rate decreases. On sympathetic stimulation however opening of Ca^{2+} channels is facilitated leading to increase firing.

2. **Extracellular K^+**
   Hyperkalemia: Repolarization is affected leading to defect in conduction of impulse which causes decrease in heart rate.

   Hypokalemia: Has no effect

3. **Extracellular Ca^{2+}**
   Hypercalcemia: It is the Ca^{2+} influx from ECF which causes action potentials and leads to contraction. Hence, rate of contractions in hypercalcemia increase, relaxation is reduced and in severe conditions the heart arrests in systole.

Hypocalcemia: Lowers contractility but does not have a significant effect.

Frank-Starling Law of Heart

According to this, under normal circumstances, the strength of contraction of cardiac muscle increases directly in proportion to the initial length or the initial stretch of muscle fibers. This means that when the end diastolic volume (see page no. 407) of heart increases, the force of contraction also will increase.

DISTRIBUTION OF VARIOUS MUSCLES IN THE BODY

This chapter gives a brief description of arrangement of the skeletal musculature of the body.

MUSCLES OF HEAD AND FACE

Muscles of Scalp

Occipito-frontalis Muscle (Fig. 7.19)

a. **Occipital bellies:** Muscular fibres arise from the lateral 2/3rd of superior nuchal lines on either side.
b. **Frontal bellies:** The fibres are attached to the skin of the eye brows and root of nose.

The fibres from both the bellies are inserted into a central fibrous layer known as the galea aponeurotica or epicranial aponeurosis.

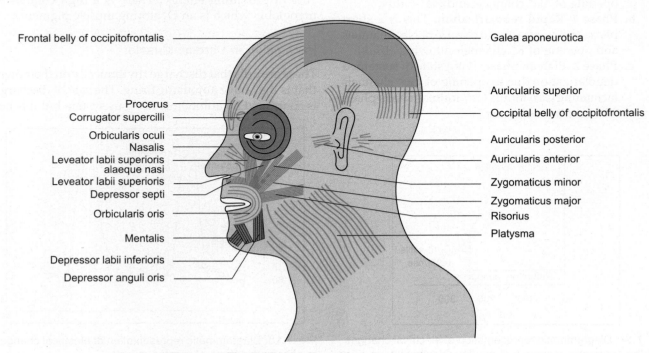

Fig. 7.19: Muscles of facial expression

Muscles of Facial Expression (Fig. 7.19)

Features of Facial Muscles

- The muscles develop from the 2nd branchial arch of the embryo.
- All are supplied by facial nerve (nerve of 2nd branchial arch) except levator palpebrae superioris which is supplied by oculomotor nerve.
- The muscles are arranged in groups around the orifices of the mouth, nose, eyes and ears. They act as dilators and constrictors of these orifices.
- These muscles are attached to the skin and their contractions are responsible for facial expressions which help in non verbal communication.
- Represent the remnants of subcutaneous muscle fibres seen in some lower animals (panniculus carnosus).

Muscles (Figs 7.19 and 7.20)

1. **Orbicularis oculi:** It surrounds the palpebral fissure. It has three parts namely palpebral, orbital, lacrimal.
   Origin: Medial palpebral ligament, adjoining frontal bone and frontal process of maxilla, lacrimal fascia and crest of lacrimal bone.
   Insertion: Subcutaneous tissue of eyebrow, lateral palpebral raphae.
   Action: It causes closure of eyelids both voluntary or while blinking. It aids in transport of lacrimal fluid by dilating lacrimal sac.
2. **Corrugator supercilli**
   Origin: Medial end of superciliary arch of frontal bone.
   Insertion: Subcutaneous tissue of eyebrow in the middle.

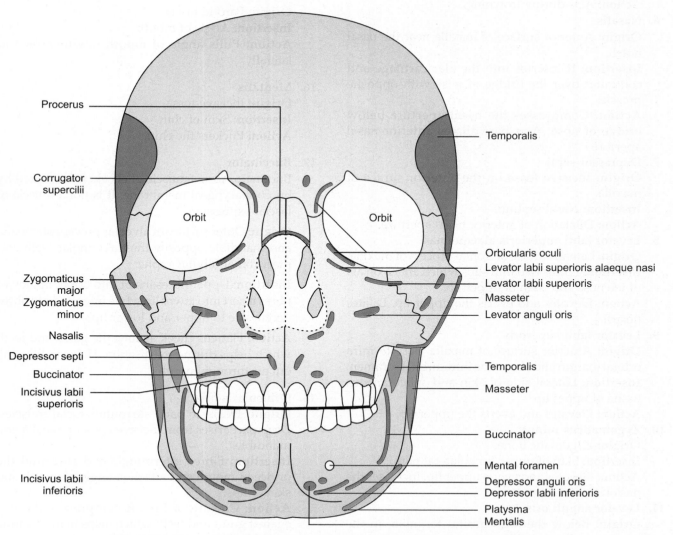

Fig. 7.20 : Norma frontalis showing attachments of muscles of facial expressions

CHAPTER-7

Action: Pulls eyebrows medially and downwards.

3. **Occipitofrontalis (Frontal part)**
   Origin: Subcutaneous tissue and skin of the eyebrow and root of nose.
   Insertion: Galea aponeurosis.
   Action: Raises eyebrows upwards.

4. **Levator palpebrae superioris:** Is like a triangular sheet.
   Origin: Inferior surface of lesser wing of sphenoid.
   Insertion: Medial margin attaches to the medial palpebral ligament. Lateral margin attaches to the Whitnall's tubercle on zygomatic bone. Central part inserts to skin of upper eyelid, anterior surface of superior tarsus, superior conjunctival fornix.
   Action: Elevates the eyelids.

5. **Procerus**
   Origin: Fascia covering nasal bone.
   Insertion: Skin between eyebrows.
   Action: Acts during frowning.

6. **Nasalis**
   Origin: Anterior surface of maxilla near the nasal notch.
   Insertion: It insertes into the alar cartilage and continues over the bridge of nose with opposite muscle.
   Action: Compresses the nasal aperture below bridge of nose. Alar part dilates anterior nasal aperture.

7. **Depressor septi**
   Origin: Incisive fossa on the anterior surace of maxilla.
   Insertion: Nasal septum.
   Action: Dilatation of anterior nasal aperture.

8. **Levator labii superioris alaeque nasi**
   Origin: Lateral surface of frontal process of maxilla.
   Insertion: Forms two thin slips which attach on ala of the nose and skin of upper lip.
   Action: Elevates and everts the upper lip. Dilates nostril

9. **Levator labii superoris**
   Origin: Anterior surface of maxilla close to infra orbital margin and above the infra-orbital foramen.
   Insertion: Lateral side of skin and subcutaneous tissue of upper lip.
   Action: Elevates and everts the upper lip.

10. **Zygomaticus minor**
    Origin: Zygomatic bone.
    Insertion: Skin of upper lip in lateral part.
    Action: Elevates and everts upper lip. Increases the nasiolabial furrow.

11. **Levator anguli oris**
    Origin: Below the infra-orbital foramen, in the cannine fossa of maxilla.
    Insertion: Angle of mouth.
    Action: Raises angle of mouth.

12. **Zygomaticus major**
    Origin: Zygomatic bone.
    Insertion: Angle of mouth
    Action: Pulls angle of mouth upwards and laterally.

13. **Depressor labii inferioris**
    Origin: Oblique line of mandible.
    Insertion: Skin of lower lip.
    Action: Pulls lower lip downwards and laterally.

14. **Depressor anguli oris**
    Origin: Posterior part of oblique line of mandible.
    Insertion: Angle of mouth.
    Action: Pulls angle of mouth downwards and laterally.

15. **Risorius**
    Origin: Parotid fascia.
    Insertion: Angle of mouth.
    Action: Pulls angle of mouth downwards and laterally.

16. **Mentalis**
    Origin: Incisive fossa.
    Insertion: Skin of chin.
    Action: Puckers the chin.

17. **Buccinator**
    Buccinator forms muscle of cheek. It is covered by buccopharyngeal membrane. It is not a muscle of fascial expression.
    Origin: Outer surface of alveolar process of maxilla and mandible opposite the three molar teeth and pterygomandibular raphe.
    Insertion: Upper fibres insert into upper lip, lower fibres insert into lower lip while intermediate fibres deccussate to upper and lower lips.
    Action: Flattens cheek against the gums and teeth which helps during mastication. Helps in blowing out air through mouth.

18. **Orbicularis oris**
    Origin: Extrinsic part surrounds facial muscles. Deep part arises from incisive fossa of maxilla and mandible.
    Insertion: Fibres intermingle and surround the orifice of mouth and attach to angle of mouth and skin of lips.
    Action: Closure of lips. It compresses the lips against gums and teeth which helps in mastication and also causes protrusion of lips.

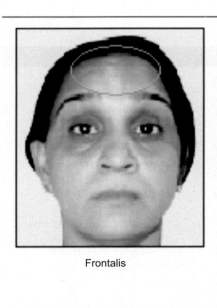

Frontalis

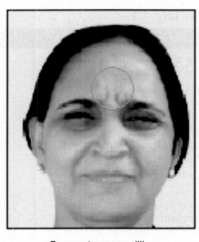

Corrugator supercilli

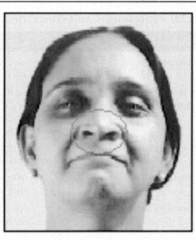

Dilator naris

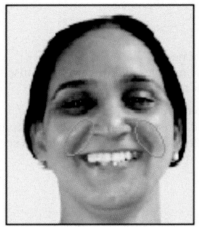

Zygomaticus major

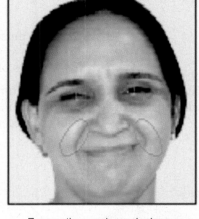

Zygomaticus major and minor

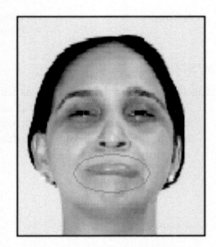

Depressor anguli oris

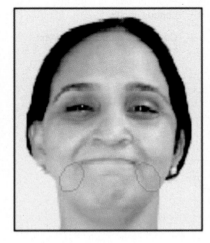

Risorius

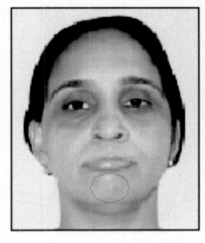

Mentalis

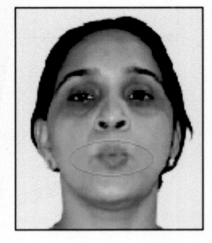

Buccinator

Fig. 7.21: Facial expressions and concerned muscles

Facial expressions and concerned muscles (Fig. 7.21)

Expression	Changes in skin of face	Muscle involved
Surprise	— Transverse wrinkles of forehead — Transverse wrinkles at bridge of nose	— Frontalis — Procerus
Frowning	Vertical wrinkles of forehead	Corrugator supercilli
Anger	— Dilatation of anterior nasal aperture — Depression of lower part of nasal septum (columella)	— Dilator naris — Depressor septi
Laughing , Smiling	Angle of mouth is drawn upwards and laterally	Zygomaticus major
Sadness	Angle of mouth drawn downwards and laterally	Depressor anguli oris
Sorrow and grief	Accentuation of nasolabial furrow with elevation and eversion of upper lip	— Levator labii superioris — Levator anguli oris — Zygomaticus minor
Grinning	Retraction of angle of mouth	Risorius
Disdain / Doubt	Puckering of skin over chin with protrusion of lower lip	Mentalis
Whistling	Pressing the cheek against gum with pursing of mouth with small opening	Buccinator

MUSCLES OF NECK

Muscles of neck can be studied as follows:
1. Muscles of anterior part and side of neck. These include sternocleidomastoid, suprahyoid muscles of anterior triangle of neck, infrahyoid muscles of anterior triangle of neck.
2. Deep muscles of neck
   a. Para-vertebral muscles, b. Pre-vertebral muscles
3. Muscles of back of neck

Sternocleidomastoid Muscle (Fig. 7.22)

Sternocleidomastoid muscle is an important, superficially placed muscle on each side of neck and is seen

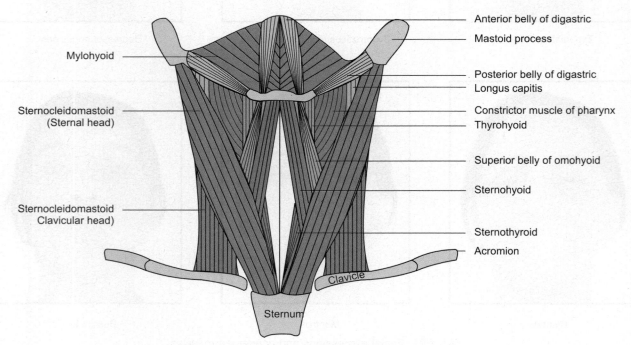

Labels: Mylohyoid; Sternocleidomastoid (Sternal head); Sternocleidomastoid (Clavicular head); Anterior belly of digastric; Mastoid process; Posterior belly of digastric; Longus capitis; Constrictor muscle of pharynx; Thyrohyoid; Superior belly of omohyoid; Sternohyoid; Sternothyroid; Acromion; Clavicle; Sternum

Fig. 7.22: Muscles of anterior part of neck

as a prominent band passing from above downwards in the neck, when the neck is turned to one side. It divides the side of neck into anterior and posterior triangles.

Origin: It arises from two heads:

1. **Sternal head:** It is attached to the upper part of anterior surface of manubrium sterni.
2. **Clavicular head:** It is attached to the upper border and anterior surface of medial 1/3rd of clavicle.

Insertion: The fibers run upwards and backwards and insert in two parts:

1. Lateral surface of mastoid, as a thick tendon.
2. Lateral half of superior nuchal line of occipital bone, as a thin aponeurosis.

Important Relations of the Muscle
Superficial relations

1. Skin, platysma
2. Superficial lamina of deep cervical fascia
3. Structures lying between superficial and deep fascia:
   a. External jugular vein
   b. Great auricular and transverse cervical nerves
4. Parotid gland, near its insertion

Deep relations

5. Near its origin it is related to:
   a. Sternoclavicular joint
   b. Sternohyoid, sternothyroid and omohyoid muscles
   c. Anterior jugular vein
   d. Carotid sheath
   e. Subclavian artery
6. Common carotid, internal carotid and external carotid arteries
7. Internal jugular, facial and lingual veins
8. Deep cervical lymph nodes
9. Vagus nerve and ansa cervicalis
10. Posterior part of muscle is related to:
    a. Splenius capitis, levator scapulae and scalene muscles.
    b. Cervical plexus, upper part of brachial plexus, phrenic nerve.
    c. Transverse cervical and suprascapular arteries
11. Occipital artery
12. Near its insertion it is related to:
    a. Mastoid process
    b. Splenius capitis, longissimus capitis and posterior belly of digastric muscle.

Nerve supply: It is supplied by spinal part of accessory nerve.

Actions

1. Acting one at a time, the muscle draws the head towards ipsilateral shoulder. This results in turning of face to the apposite side.
2. Flexion of neck is brought about when muscles of both sides act together. Along with action of longus colli, they bring about flexion of cervical part of vertebral column.
3. They aid in elevation of thorax during inspiration, when the head is fixed.

Suprahyoid Muscles of Anterior Triangle of Neck

Diagastric muscle divides suprahyoid part of neck into digastric and submental triangles. Mylohyoid muscle forms the floor of these triangles. They are tabulated below (Fig. 7.22):

Muscle	Origin	Insertion	Action
1. Digastric: It has two bellies joined by a central tendon **Nerve supply:** a. Anterior belly: Inferior alveolar nerve b. Posterior belly: Facial nerve	a. Anterior belly: Digastric fossa present lateral to the symphysis menti on the lower border of mandible b. Posterior belly: Mastoid notch on the temporal bone	Fibres from anterior belly pass downwards and backwards while from posterior belly pass downwards and forwards towards a central tendon which is connected by a fascial sling to the junction of body and greater cornu of hyoid bone	1. Depression of chin during opening of mouth 2. Draws the hyoid bone upwards during swallowing
2. Stylohyoid — Thin muscle sheet — It accompanies the posterior belly of digastric **Nerve supply:** Facial nerve	Middle of the posterior surface of styloid process	Junction of the body and greater cornu of hyoid bone anteriorly	Draws the hyoid bone upwards and backwards
3. Mylohyoid Also called diaphragma oris. Overlies the extrinsic muscles of tongue **Nerve supply:** Branch of inferior alveolar nerve	Mylohyoid line on inner surface of body of mandible	1. Body of hyoid bone 2. Median fibrous raphae which extends from the symphysis menti to centre of hyoid bone	1. Elevation of floor of mouth to push up the tongue during swallowing 2. Depression of mandible
4. Geniohyoid Ribbon shaped muscle, lies deep to mylohyoid **Nerve supply:** C_1 fibres	Inferior genial tubercle on symphysis menti	Body of hyoid bone in the centre on either side of midline	Draws the hyoid bone upwards and forwards

Infrahyoid Muscles of Anterior Triangle of Neck

These are strap like muscles which attach to the hyoid bone and thyroid cartilage. They result in the movement of these structure during speech, mastication and swallowing. The muscles are tabulated below (Fig. 7.22):

Muscle	Origin	Insertion	Action
1. **Sternohyoid** **Nerve supply:** Ansa cervicalis (C_2 and C_3 fibers)	1. Upper part of posterior surface of manubrium sterni 2. Posterior aspect of medial end of clavicle 3. Capsule of sterno-clavicular joint	Fibres of both sides converge up to the lower border of body of hyoid bone	Depression of hyoid bone
2. **Omohyoid** It consists of two bellies joined by a central tendon **Nerve supply:** a. Superior belly: C_1 fibres through hypoglossal nerve b. Inferior belly: Ansa cervicalis	1. Superior belly: Intermediate tendon beneath the sternomastoid. This tendon is anchored by a fascial sling to the clavicle 2. Inferior belly: Upper border of scapula near the suprascapular notch	1. Superior belly: Lower border of body of hyoid bone lateral to sternohyoid 2. Inferior belly: Intermediate tendon	Depression of hyoid bone
3. **Sternothyroid** **Nerve supply:** Ansa cervicalis (C_2, C_3)	1. Posterior surface of manubrium deep to sternohyoid 2. Adjoining part of medial end of 1st costal cartilage	Oblique line of thyroid cartilage below thyrohyoid	Depression of larynx
4. **Thyrohyoid** **Nerve supply:** Fibres of C_1 via hypoglossal nerve	Upper part of oblique line on thyroid cartilage	Lower border of greater cornu of hyoid bone	Depression of hyoid bone

Paravertebral Muscles of Neck

They are also called lateral vertebral muscles and include the following (Fig. 7.23)

1. Scalenus anterior
2. Scalenus medius
3. Scalenus posterior

General Features of Paravertebral Muscles

1. The scalenus medius is the largest and the scalenus posterior is the smallest of the three scalene muscles. The scalenus anterior is the 'key' muscle of the paravertebral region.

Paravertebral Muscles

Muscle	Origin	Insertion
1. **Scalenus anterior:** An elongated triangular muscle with unequal sides **Nerve supply:** Ventral rami of C_4 to C_6	Anterior tubercles of transverse processes of C_3 to C_7 vertebrae	Scalene tubercle on inner border and adjoining ridge on the superior surface of first rib between the grooves for subclavian artery and vein
2. **Scalenus medius:** A triangular muscle with unequal sides **Nerve supply:** Ventral rami of C_3 to C_8	Posterior tubercles of transverse process of C_3 to C_7 cervical vertebrae	Upper surface of first rib between the groove for subclavian artery and the tubercle of the rib
3. **Scalenus posterior:** Occasionally blends with the medius or may be absent **Nerve supply:** Ventral rami of C_6 to C_8	Posterior tubercles of the transverse processes of C_4 to C_6 vertebrae	Outer surface of the second rib behind the tuberosity for the attachment for the serratus anterior

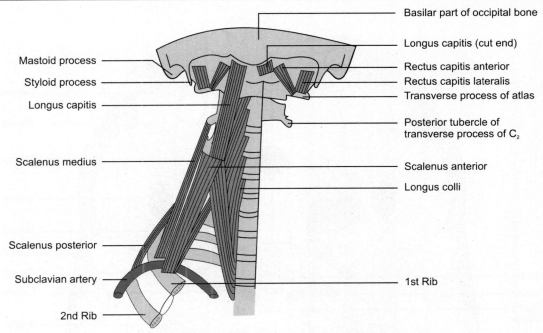

Fig. 7.23: Prevertebral and paravertebral muscles

2. The scalenus muscles extend from the transverse process of the cervical vertebrae to the first two ribs. They act to bend the cervical part of vertebral column to the same side. Acting from above they also elevate the first rib.

Prevertebral Muscles of Neck

They are also called anterior vertebral muscles and are tabulated below (Fig. 7.23):

General Features of Prevertebral Muscles

1. Lie in front of the vertebral column
2. Are covered anteriorly by a thick prevertebral fascia
3. Form the posterior boundary of retropharyngeal space
4. Extend from base of the skull to the superior mediastinum
5. Are weak flexors of the head and neck. Rectus capitis anterior causes flexion at atlanto-axial joint.

Muscle	Origin	Insertion
1. Longus colli (cervicis) It covers the anterior aspect of upper 10 vertebrae. It consists of three parts		
a. Superior oblique part	— Anterior tubercles of tansverse processes of C_3 to C_5 vertebrae	— Anterior tubercle of the anterior arch of atlas
b. Middle vertical part	— Anterior surfaces of the bodies of C_5 to T_3 vertebrae	— Anterior surface of bodies of C_2 to C_4 vertebrae
c. Inferior oblique part	— Anterior surface of bodies of T_1 to T_3 vertebrae	— Anterior tubercles of transverse processes of C_5 to C_6 vertebrae
2. Longus capitis a. Strap like muscle which appears to be continuous with scalenus anterior b. It overlaps the longus colli	Anterior tubercles of transverse processes of C_3 to C_6 vertebrae	Inferior surface of the basilar part of the occipital bone, alongside the pharyngeal tubercle
3. Rectus capitis anterior a. Very short and flat b. It lies deep to longus capitis	Anterior surface of the lateral mass of the atlas and adjoining root of transverse process	Basilar part of occipital bone in front of occipital condyle
4. Rectus capitis lateralis	Upper surface of the transverse process of atlas	Inferior surface of the jugular process of occipital bone.

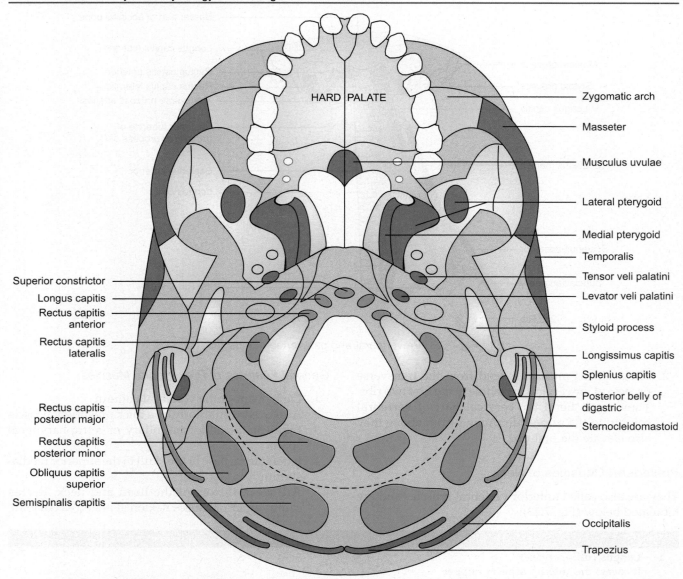

Fig. 7.24: Norma basalis showing proximal attachment of deep muscles of neck and muscles of back of neck

Longus capitis and colli cause flexion at head and neck. Rectus capitis lateralis causes lateral flexion of head and neck.

6. The muscles are supplied by branches from ventral rami of C_1 and C_2 spinal nerves except longus colli which is supplied by C_2 to C_6 spinal nerves.

Muscles of Back of Neck

The posterior aspect of neck is primarily muscular. The muscles of the back of neck are arrnaged in layers and consist of the extrinsic group and the intrinsic group of muscles.

Ligamentum nuchae: A fibrous sheath is attached to the spines of the cervical vertebrae in the median plane, beneath the deep fascia. This is the ligamentum nuchae. It is attached above to the external occipital protuberance and crest and divides the back of neck into two halves. Each half of neck is covered by muscles which lie between the deep cervical fascia and posterior aspect of cervical vertebrae.

The muscles of the back of neck are arranged in two groups on each side of the midline (Fig. 7.24)

1. **Extrinsic group:** These are placed superficially and are primarily involved in the movements of upper

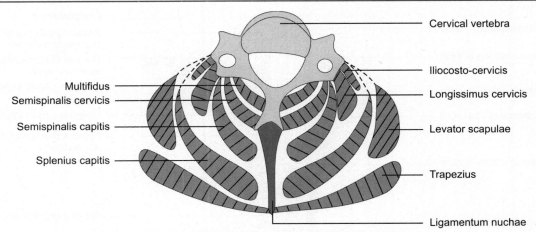

Fig. 7.25: Muscles of the back of neck (at level of C_5)

limb. They consist of the following muscles and are discussed in the respective chapter:
  a. Trapezius (see page no. 185).
  b. Levator scapulae (see page no. 185).
  c. Rhomboideus major and minor (see page no. 185).

2. **Intrinsic group:** The intrinsic group of muscles of back of neck are responsible for maintaining the upright posture of head. They are further arranged in three groups from superficial to deep:
  a. Splenius group
  b. Erector spinae
  c. Transverso-spinalis group of muscles
  d. Suboccipital muscles

MUSCLES OF THE BACK

These consist of group of muscles that are attached to the vertebral column and help in the maintenance of posture and movement of spine. They are further arranged in three groups from superficial to deep (Fig. 7.26):

a. Splenius group: This is the outermost group and consists of:
  i. Splenius capitis, it lies deep to trapezius, serratus posterior superior muscles.
  ii. Splenius cervicis, it lies deep to levator scapulae.

b. Erector spinae: It is a large muscle extending from back of the sacrum and ilium upto the skull. It lies under the splenius muscles. It consists of 3 longitudinally arranged parts:
  i. Spinalis, medially.
  ii. Longissimus, intermediate in position.
  iii. Iliocostocervicalis, laterally.

c. Transverso-spinalis group of muscles: They are the deepest group of muscles lying obliquely between the transverse processes and spines of the vertebrae. They are further divided into:
  i. Semispinalis: It is most superficial in position and consists of three parts:
    — Semispinalis thoracis
    — Semispinalis cervicis
    — Semispinalis capitis

  ii. Multifidus: This group is intermediate in position. It extends from the sacrum, ilium, transverse processes of thoracic vertebrae and articular processes of cervical vertebra as short oblique bundles of fibres.

  iii. Rotatores: They are the deepest group of muscles and are best developed in thoracic region. They consist of three parts:
    — Rotatores thoracis
    — Rotatores cervicis
    — Rotatores lumborum

d. Other deep muscles
  i. Interspinalis
  ii. Inter transversii
  iii. Suboccipital muscles

MUSCLES OF THORAX

The skeletal musculature of thoracic cage consists of intercostal muscles which are described in respiratory system (page no. 377).

Diaphragm is described in respiratory system (page no. 379).

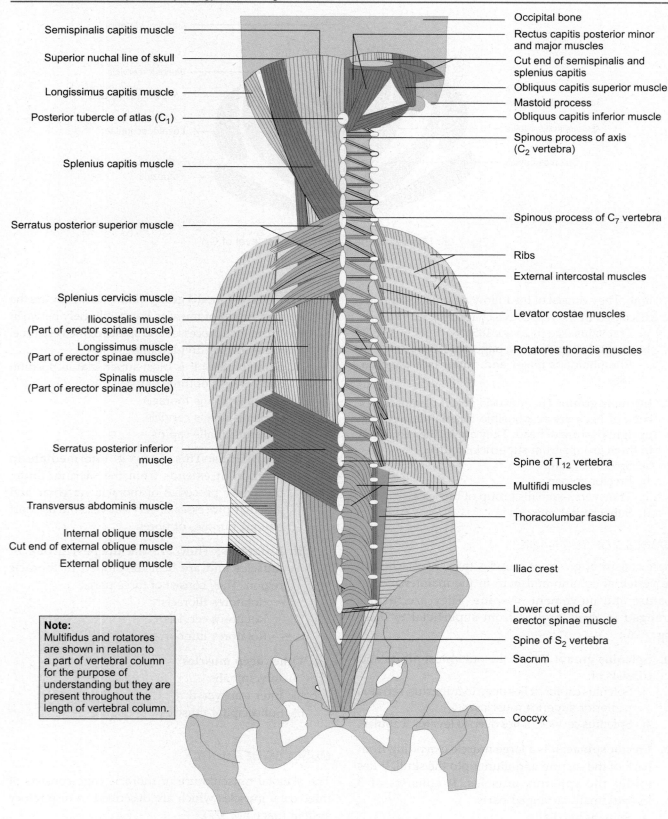

Fig. 7.26: Muscles of the back (diagrammatic representation)

MUSCLES OF ABDOMEN

They can be studied as muscles of anterior abdominal wall, muscles of posterior wall of abdomen and muscles of back of abdomen.

Muscles of Anterior Abdominal Wall (Figs 7.27 to 7.30)

Muscle	Origin	Insertion	Special features
1. **External oblique:** Direction of fibres is downward forward and medially **Nerve supply:** Ventral rami of lower six thoracic nerves	Eight fleshy slips from outer surface of lower 8 ribs	• Anterior 2/3rd of outer lip of anterior segment of iliac crest • Aponeurosis is attached to linea alba, pubic symphysis, pubic crest and pectineal line	1. Forms inguinal ligament 2. Continues as anterior wall of rectus sheath 3. Superficial inguinal ring is present in its lower part
2. **Internal oblique:** Direction of fibres is upward, forward and medially **Nerve supply:** Ventral rami of lower six thoracic nerves and L1	• Lateral 2/3rd of inguinal ligament • Intermediate lip of ventral segment of iliac crest • Thoraco-lumbar fascia	• Most posterior fibres pass vertically and are attached to lower 3 to 4 ribs and their costal cartilages • Aponeurosis is inserted into 7th, 8th, 9th costal cartilages, xiphoid process, linea alba, pubic crest and pectineal line of pubis	1. It forms the roof, anterior wall and posterior wall of inguinal canal 2. It forms the conjoint tendon 3. Forms rectus sheath
3. **Transverse abdominis:** Fibres are horizontal in direction **Nerve supply:** Ventral rami of lower six thoracic nerves and L1	• Lateral 1/3rd of upper surface of inguinal ligament • Anterior 2/3rd of inner lip of ventral segment of iliac crest • Thoraco lumbar fascia • Inner surface of lower 6 ribs and costal cartilage	• Inguinal fibres insert in pubic crest and medial part of pectin pubis • Aponeurosis is attached to linea alba.	1. It forms the roof and posterior wall of inguinal canal 2. It forms conjoint tendon 3. Forms rectus sheath
4. **Cremaster muscle** **Nerve supply:** Genital branch of genitofemoral nerve	• Middle 1/3rd of the inguinal ligament • Pubic tubercle, pubic crest conjoint tendon	Scrotum, spermatic cord tunica vaginalis	It is in the form of loops It has superficial and deep parts. It is well developed in males, while in females only few fibres are present. Insertion is by four fleshy slips
5. **Rectus abdominis** **Nerve supply:** Lower five intercostal nerves and subcosta nerve	**Medial head:** Symphysis pubis, anterior surface, **Lateral head:** Pubic crest, pubic tubercle.	Xiphoid process 5th, 6th, 7th costal cartilages	The muscle may not always be present in the body
6. **Pyramidalis** **Nerve supply:** Subcostal nerve	Symphysis pubis and pubic crest	Linea alba	

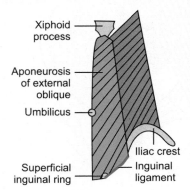
Fig. 7.27: External oblique muscle

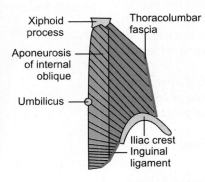
Fig. 7.28: Internal oblique muscle

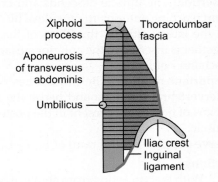
Fig. 7.29: Transversus abdominis muscle

CHAPTER-7

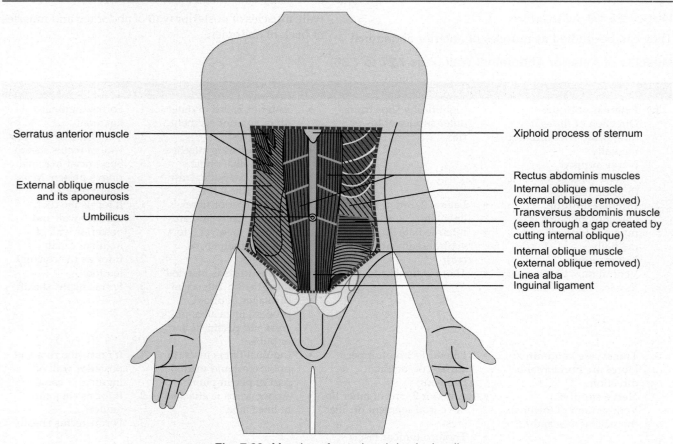

Fig. 7.30: Muscles of anterior abdominal wall

Muscles of Posterior Abdominal Wall (Fig. 7.31)
Psoas Major Muscle

Origin: It arises from the following areas:
- Anterior surface and lower border of transverse process of L_1 to L_5 vertebrae.
- In the form of 5 fleshy slips from lateral part of anterior surface of bodies of adjacent vertebrae and the corresponding intervertebral discs from T_{12} to L_5.
- From 4 tendinous arches extending between two adjacent fleshy slips.

Insertion: The muscle descends and crosses the pelvic brim reaching anterior to capsule of hip joint. It is joined on the lateral side by the fibres of iliacus muscle and together is inserted to the anterior surface of tip of lesser trochanter of femur.

Important relation: The muscle lies over upper four intervertebral foramina and hence the roots of lumbar plexus of nerves are present in the posterior mass of the muscle.

Nerve supply: Ventral rami of L_1, L_2, L_3 spinal nerves.

Actions
1. With iliacus, acting from above, it is the chief flexor of hip joint.

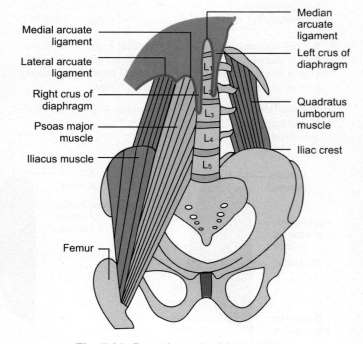

Fig. 7.31: Posterior wall of the abdomen

2. Acting from below on both sides with iliacus muscle, it flexes the trunk and pelvis forwards like in stooping.
3. It may act as a medial rotator of hip when foot is on the ground.
4. It may act as a lateral rotator of hip when foot is off the ground.

Psoas Minor Muscle

Origin: Anterior surface of bodies of T_{12} and L_1 vertebrae and intervening disc, anterior to psoas major.
Insertion: Pecten pubis and iliopubic eminence.
Nerve supply: L_1 spinal nerve.
Action: Weak flexor of trunk.

Quadratus Lumborum Muscle

Origin: Posterior 1/3rd of the inner lip of the ventral segment of the iliac crest, ilio lumbar ligament.

Insertion: Lower border of anterior surface of medial half of 12th rib, anterior surface of transverse processes of L_1 to L_4 vertebrae, by 4 small slips of tendon.

Important relations: From above downwards, subcostal nerve, iliohypogastric nerve and ilioingual nerve lie anterior to the muscle passing from medial to lateral side over it.
Nerve supply: Ventral rami of T_{12} and L_1 to L_4 spinal nerves
Action
1. Fixes last rib and aids in the inspiratory effort of diaphragm.
2. Lateral flexion of trunk-caused by contraction of muscle of one side.
3. Extension of vertebral column-Caused by contraction of muscle of both sides.

Iliacus

Origin: Upper 2/3rd of concavity of iliac fossa, inner lip of ventral part of iliac crest, ventral aspect of sacroiliac ligament, adjoining ala of sacrum.

Insertion: It joins with psoas tendon on its lateral aspect and inserts on anterior surface of lesser trochanter of femur. Few fibres may extend upto 2.5 cm below and in front of lesser trochanter over the shaft of femur.

Nerve supply: Femoral nerve (L_2, L_3).
Actions
1. With iliacus, acting from above, it is the chief flexor of hip joint.
2. Acting from below on both sides with iliacus muscle, it flexes the trunk and pelvis forwards like in stooping.

MUSCLES OF PELVIS AND PERINEUM (FIG. 7.32)

1. Muscles forming wall of pelvis. They primarily act on the lower limb.
   a. Piriformis muscle
   b. Obturator internus muscle
2. Muscles forming floor of pelvis (Fig. 7.32).
   a. Levator ani muscle
   b. Coccygeus muscle

Piriformis Muscle

Origin: Anterior surface of middle three pieces of sacrum, adjacent gluteal surface of ilium, adjacent area on capsule of sacro-iliac joint and sacrotuberous ligament.
Insertion: It passes out of pelvis via greater sciatic foramen and inserts into apex of greater trochanter of femur.
Nerve supply: Ventral ramii of S_1 and S_2.

Obturator Internus Muscle

It is covered by a well defined layer of fascia on its pelvic surface.

Origin: Pelvic surface of obturator membrane, adjacent pelvic surface of ischium, ischiopubic ramus and ilium.

Insertion: The tendon of obturator internus passes out of pelvis via lesser sciatic foramen and inserted into the medial surface of greater trochanter of femur.

Nerve Supply: Nerve to obturator internus (L_5, S_1 and S_2)

Pelvic Diaphragm

It is a gutter shaped thin sheet of muscular partition that separates the pelvic cavity from perineum. This forms floor of pelvic cavity. It is formed by two muscles namely levator ani and coccygeus and the fasciae covering them (Fig. 7.33)

Levator Ani Muscle
It has two parts
1. **Iliococcygeus**
   Origin: Posterior half of the white line from the lateral pelvic wall and from ischial spine
   Insertion: The muscle fibres pass downwards, backwards and medially to meet the muscle of opposite side forming a fibro muscular band which extends from the anus to coccyx. Few fibres pass backwards to insert into the sides of the lower 2 pieces of coccyx.
2. **Pubo-coccygeus**
   Origin: Anterior half of the white line and posterior surface of body of pubis
   Insertion: According to insertion, it can be subdivided into following parts:
   a. **Pubo-coccygeus proper:** Most posterior fibres are inserted into ano-coccygeal raphe and tip of the coccyx.
   b. **Pubo-rectalis:** Fibres wind the posterior surface of ano-rectal junction and become continuous with similar fibres of opposite side.

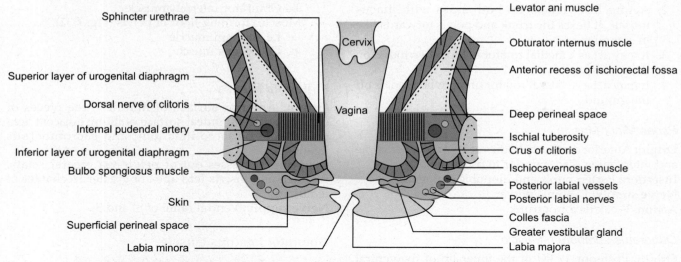

Fig. 7.32: Coronal section of urogenital triangle of female showing muscles of perineum and pelvis

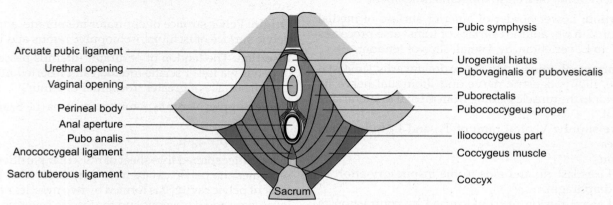

Fig. 7.33: Pelvic diaphragm

c. **Pubo-analis:** Some fibres are inserted into the wall of external and internal anal sphincter.

d. **Pubo-vesicalis or vaginalis:** These consists of most anterior fibres of pubcoccygeus muscles arising from posterior surface of pubic bone and pass by the side of prostate in male and vagina in female, where they form a sling, and are inserted into the perineal body.

Nerve supply: 4th sacral nerve and S_2, S_3 via perineal nerve

Coccygeus Muscle

It is also considered a part of levator ani known as **ischiococcygeus.**

Origin: It takes origin from the pelvic surface and tip of ischial spine.

Insertion: Fibres pass backwards and medially and insert into the margin of upper 2 pieces of coccyx and last piece of sacrum.

Nerve supply: S_4, S_5 nerves.

Fascia of Pelvic Diaphragm

1. Superior fascia of pelvic diaphragm: It covers the upper surface of levator ani.
2. Inferior fascia of pelvic diaphragm: It is present on the lower surface of levator ani.

Openings in pelvic diaphragm

1. **Hiatus urogenitalis:** It is a triangular gap between the anterior fibres of both levator ani muscles. Structures passing through this hiatus are urethra in male, urethra and vagina in female.
2. **Hiatus rectalis:** This is the aperture between the perineal body and ano-coccygeal raphe. Anorectal junction passes though it.

Functions of pelvic diaphragm

1. It supports the pelvic viscera.
2. It acts as an elevator for prostate in male and as a sphincter of vagina in female.
3. It prevents uterine prolapse.
4. Helps in maintenance of continence of faeces and urine.
5. Facilitates descent of bladder neck and anal relaxation to evacuate their contents.

Perineal Muscles (Fig. 7.32)

Muscle	Origin	Insertion
1. **Ischiocavernosus,** covers crus penis or crus clitoridis **Nerve supply:** perineal branch of pudendal nerve	Ischio pubic ramus	Sides and under surface of crus penis or clitoridis
2. **Superficial transverse perinei** **Nerve supply:** perineal branch of pudendal nerve	Medial surface of ramus of ischium	Perineal body
3. **Bulbo-spongiosus:** In males it is bipennate. In females it splits into two to cover the bulb of vestibule. **Nerve supply:** perineal branch of pudendal nerve	Perineal body and median raphae in male Perineal body in female	**In male:** Fibres embrace the bulb and corpus spongiosum and attach to median raphae **In female:** Fibres embrace corpora cavernosa and attach to median raphae
4. **Sphincter urethrae** **Nerve supply:** muscular branch of perineal nerve	**Superficial fibres:** Transverse perineal ligament and pubic arch **Deep fibres:** Ischio-pubic ramus. These encircle the urethra.	Similar fibres of the opposite side meet in midline. In female, some fibres decussate between vagina and urethra
5. **Deep transverse perinei** **Nerve supply:** muscular branch of perineal nerve	Inner (medial) surface of ramus of ischium	Perineal body

MUSCLES OF UPPER LIMB

Attachments of Muscles of Upper Limb on the Bones (Figs 7.34 to 7.43)

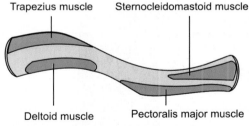

Fig. 7.34: Right clavicle (superior surface)

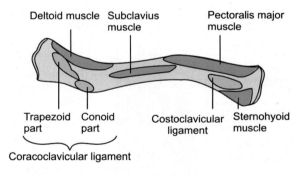

Fig. 7.35: Right clavicle (inferior surface)

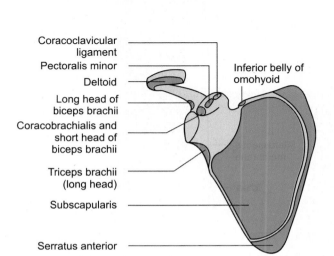

Fig. 7.36: Anterior aspect of right scapula showing muscle attachments

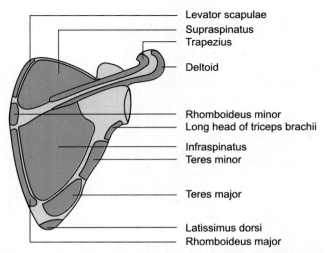

Fig. 7.37: Posterior aspect of right scapula showing muscle attachments

CHAPTER-7

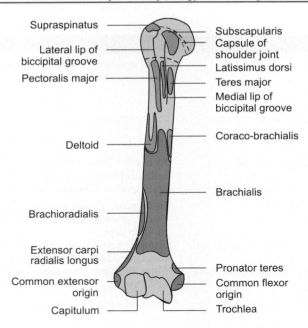

Fig. 7.38: Anterior aspect of right humerus showing muscle attachments

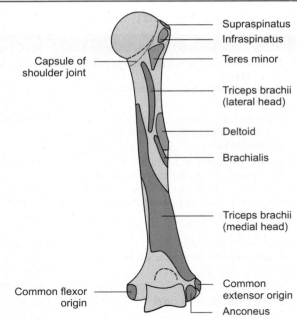

Fig. 7.39: Posterior aspect of right humerus showing muscle attachments

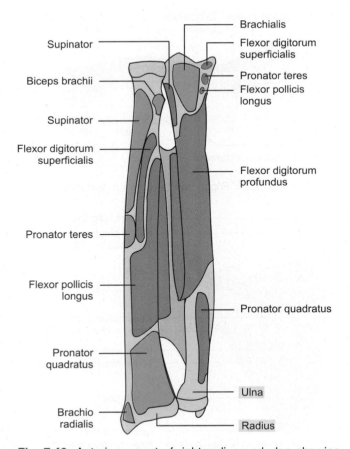

Fig. 7.40: Anterior aspect of right radius and ulna showing muscle attachments

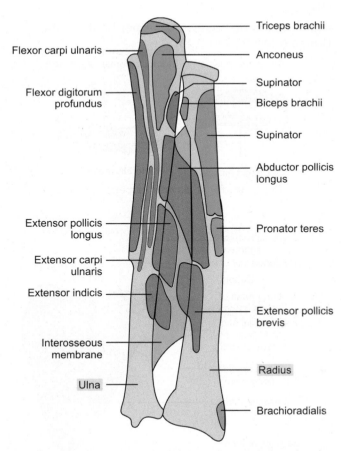

Fig. 7.41: Posterior aspect of right radius and ulna showing muscle attachments

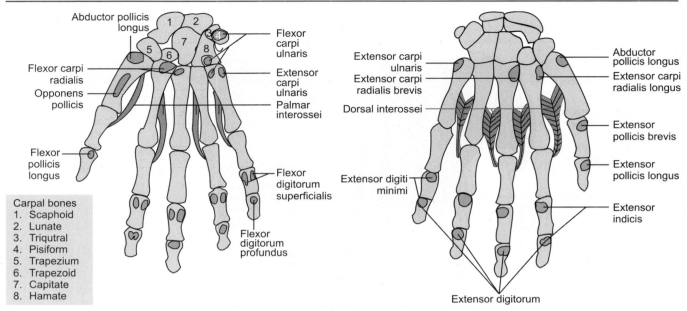

Fig. 7.42: Skeleton of right hand showing muscle attachments (anterior aspect)

Fig. 7.43: Skeleton of right hand showing muscle attachments (posterior aspect)

Muscles of Pectoral Region

Muscle	Origin	Insertion	Action
1. **Pectoralis major** (Figs 7.44, 7.51) **Nerve supply:** Medial (C_8, T_1) and lateral(C_5, C_6, C_7) pectoral nerves	1. Medial half of anterior surface of clavicle 2. Lateral part of anterior surface of sternum and medial part of costal cartilages upto 6th costal cartilages 3. Aponeurosis of external oblique muscle	Lateral lip of intertubercular sulcus of humerus as an inverted U shaped insertion	It acts on shoulder joint causing 1. Adduction 2. Medial rotation 3. Extension of flexed arm till normal pendant position 4. Accessory muscle of inspiration 5. Helps in climbing when humeral attachment is fixed
2. **Pectoralis minor** (Fig. 7.44) **Nerve supply:** Medial pectoral nerve (C_8, T_1)	1. Anterior surface of 3rd, 4th, and 5th ribs near the costo chondral junction. 2. Fascia covering inter costal muscles of corresponding spaces.	Tendon is inserted into medial border and upper surface of coracoid process of scapula	1. Draws the scapula forwards with serratus anterior 2. Helps in forced inspiration when scapula is fixed
3. **Subclavius** (Fig. 7.44) **Nerve Supply:** Nerve to subclavius ($C_5 C_6$)	As a narrow slip from anterior surface of 1st costochondral junction.	Subclavian groove on the inferior surface of middle 1/3rd of clavicle	1. Depresses clavicle 2. Steadies clavicle during movements of shoulder
4. **Serratus anterior** **Nerve supply:** Long thoracic nerve (C_5, C_6, C_7)	1. Outer surface of upper eight ribs, there are eight digitations. 2. Fascia covering corresponding intercostal muscles.	Costal surface of medial border of scapula as given below: 1. 1st digitation inserted from superior angle to root of spine. 2. 2nd and 3rd to the medial border. 3. Lower five digitations are inserted to inferior angle.	1. Protracts scapula along with pectoralis minor 2. Helps in forced inspiration

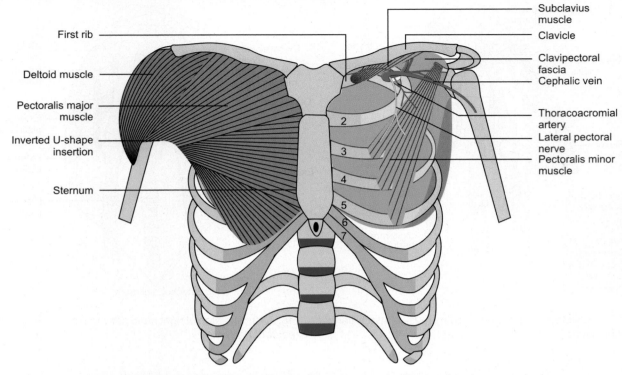

First rib

Deltoid muscle

Pectoralis major
muscle

Inverted U-shape
insertion

Sternum

Subclavius
muscle

Clavicle

Clavipectoral
fascia

Cephalic vein

Thoracoacromial
artery

Lateral pectoral
nerve

Pectoralis minor
muscle

Fig. 7.44: Clavipectoral fascia, Pectoralis major muscle, Pectoralis minor muscle

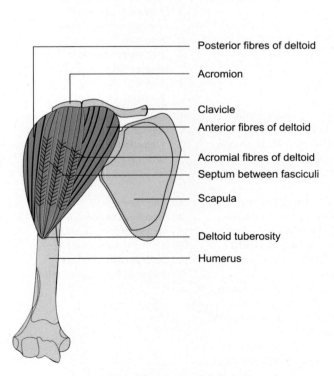

Posterior fibres of deltoid

Acromion

Clavicle

Anterior fibres of deltoid

Acromial fibres of deltoid

Septum between fasciculi

Scapula

Deltoid tuberosity

Humerus

Fig. 7.45: Attachments of deltoid muscle

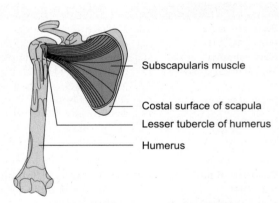

Subscapularis muscle

Costal surface of scapula

Lesser tubercle of humerus

Humerus

Fig. 7.46: Attachments of subcapularis muscle

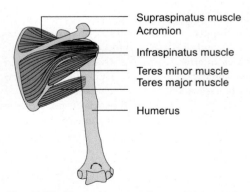

Supraspinatus muscle
Acromion
Infraspinatus muscle
Teres minor muscle
Teres major muscle

Humerus

Fig. 7.47: Posterior scapular region muscles

Muscles of Scapular Region

Muscles	Origin	Insertion	Action
1. **Deltoid (Figs 7.45 and 7.51)** **Nerve supply:** Axillary nerve $(C_{5,6})$	1. Anterior border and upper surface of lateral $1/3^{rd}$ of clavicle 2. Lateral border of acromion 3. Lower lip of crest of spine of scapula	Deltoid tuberosity-as a V shape insertion on lateral aspect of shaft of humerus Middle fibres are multi pennate	1. Abduction ⎫ acts at 2. Flexion ⎬ shoulder 3. Extension ⎭ joint Flexion and extension are caused by anterior and posterior fibres respectively
2. **Supraspinatus (Fig. 7.47)** **Nerve supply:** Suprascapular nerve (C_5)	Medial $2/3^{rd}$ of supraspinous fossa of scapula	Greater tubercle of humerus, at its upper most impression	1. Initiates abduction of shoulder joint up to $15°$ 2. Helps in stability of shoulder joint.
3. **Infraspinatus (Fig. 7.47)** **Nerve supply:** Suprascapular nerve (C_5)	Medial $2/3^{rd}$ of infra spinous fossa of scapula	Greater tubercle of humerus, below the supraspinatus	1. Lateral rotation of arm 2. Stabilization of shoulder joint
4. **Teres minor (Fig. 7.47)** **Nerve supply:** Axillary nerve $(C_{5,6})$	Dorsal aspect of upper $2/3^{rd}$ of lateral border of scapula	Greater tubercle of humerus on the lowest impression	1. Lateral rotation of arm 2. Stabilization of shoulder joint
5. **Teres major (Fig. 7.47)** **Nerve supply:** Lower subscapular nerve $(C_{6,7})$	1. Dorsal aspect of lower $1/3^{rd}$ of lateral border of scapula 2. Inferior angle of scapula	Medial lip of intertubercular sulcus on anterior aspect of humerus	1. Medial rotation of arm
6. **Subscapularis (Fig. 7.46)** **Nerve supply:** Upper and lower subscapular nerves $(C_{5,6,7})$	Medial $2/3^{rd}$ of subscapular fossa on anterior aspect of scapula	Lesser tubercle of humerus	1. Medial rotation of arm 2. Stabilization of shoulder joint

Muscles of Upper Back—Related To Upper Limb

Muscle	Origin	Insertion	Action
1. **Trapezius (Figs 7.48, 7.50)** **Nerve supply:** a. Spinal part of XI cranial nerve b. C_2 C_3 proprioceptive fibres	1. Medial $1/3^{rd}$ of superior nuchal line 2. Ligamentum Nuchae 3. Spinous process and supraspinous ligaments of all thoracic vertebrae 4. External occipital protuberance	1. Posterior border of lateral $1/3^{rd}$ of clavicle 2. Medial border of acromion 3. Spine of scapula 4. Deltoid tubercle	1. Over head abduction by facilitating rotaion of scapula 2. Elevation of scapula 3. Retraction of scapula
2. **Latissimus dorsi (Figs 7.48 to 7.50)** **Nerve supply:** Thoraco dorsal nerve $(C_{6,7,8})$	1. Spines of lower six thoracic vertebrae and their supraspinous ligaments 2. Adjoining part of posterior surface of lower four ribs 3. Inferior angle of scapula 4. Posterior layer of thoraco lumbar fascia 5. Posterior $1/3^{rd}$ of outer ribs of iliac crest	Converges as a tendon towards axilla (forms posterior fold of axilla) Inserts into floor of inter tubercular sulcus on anterior aspect of upper end of humerus.	It acts on shoulder joint and causes 1. Adduction of arm 2. Medial rotation of arm 3. Extension of arm 4. Helps in climbing by elevating trunk when arm is raised and fixed hence it is also known as climbing muscle
3 **Levator scapulae (Fig. 7.49)** **Nerve supply:** It receives branches from dorsal scapular nerve (C_5) and $C_3 + C_4$ spinal nerves	1. Transverse processes of C_1 and C_2 vertebrae 2. Posterior tubercles of transverse processes of C_3 and C_4 vertebrae	Dorsal aspect of medial border of scapula from superior angle till root of spine.	1. Elevation of scapula 2. Steadies the scapula along with rhomboideus during movement of upper limb.
4. **Rhomboideus major (Fig. 7.49)** **Nerve supply:** Dorsal scapular nerve (C_5)	Spines of T_2 to T_5 vertebrae with the intervening supra spinous ligaments	Dorsal aspect of medial border of scapula from the root of the spine to inferior angle.	1. Retraction of scapula along with rhomboideus minor 2. Also steadies scapula
5. **Rhomboideus minor (Fig. 7.49)** **Nerve supply:** Dorsal scapular nerve (C_5)	1. Lower part of ligamentum nuchae 2. Spines of C_7 and T_1 vertebrae	Dorsal aspect of medial border of scapula opposite the root of spine.	Same as above

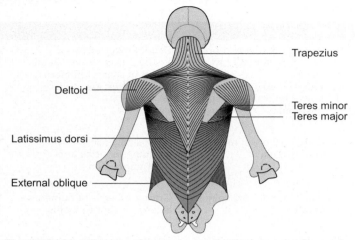

Fig. 7.48: Attachments of trapezius and latissimus dorsi muscles

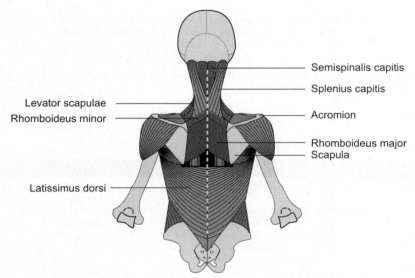

Fig. 7.49: Superficial muscles of the back

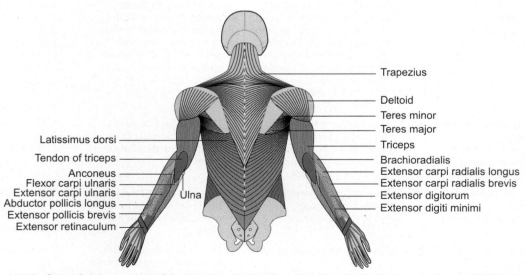

Fig. 7.50: Superficial muscles of the back and muscles of extensor compartment of arm and forearm

Muscles of Arm

Muscle	Origin	Insertion	Action
1. **Coracobrachialis (Fig. 7.51)** **Nerve supply:** It is pierced and supplied by Musculocutaneous nerve ($C_{5,6,7}$)	Tip of coracoid process	Medial border of shaft of humerus in the middle	Weak flexor of arm, acts at shoulder joint
2. **Biceps brachii (Fig. 7.51)** **Nerve supply:** Musculocutaneous nerve ($C_{5,6,7}$)	1. **Shorthead:** Tip of coracoid process 2. **Longhead:** Supraglenoid tubercle It passes through the cavity of shoulder joint	The biceps tendon is inserted on the posterior part of radial tuberosity. The tendon gives off an extension, bicipital aponeurosis which attaches to deep fascia of forearm Bicipital aponeurosis lies in the roof of cubital fossa	1. Supination in semi flexed forearm 2. Flexor of elbow joint 3. Helps in screwing movement 4. Short head causes flexion of shoulder joint 5. Long head helps in stabilisation of shoulder joint
3. **Brachialis (Fig. 7.51)** **Nerve supply:** Musculocutaneous ($C_{5,6,7}$) and Radial nerve	1. Anterior border and adjoining anteromedial and anterolateral surfaces of lower half of shaft of humerus 2. Intermuscular septa	1. Anterior surface of coronoid process of ulna 2. Tuberosity of ulna	Flexion of elbow joint. It is the main flexor of forearm
4. **Triceps brachii (Fig. 7.52)** **Nerve supply:** Radial nerve ($C_{5,6,7,8}$ T_1) Important: Branch to long head is given out in axilla by radial nerve.	**Long head:** Infraglenoid tubercle of scapula **Lateral head:** Oblique ridge along the lateral lip of spiral groove **Medial head:** Entire posterior surface of humerus below spiral groove	Posterior part of the upper surface of olecranon process of ulna	Extension of forearm, acts at elbow joint

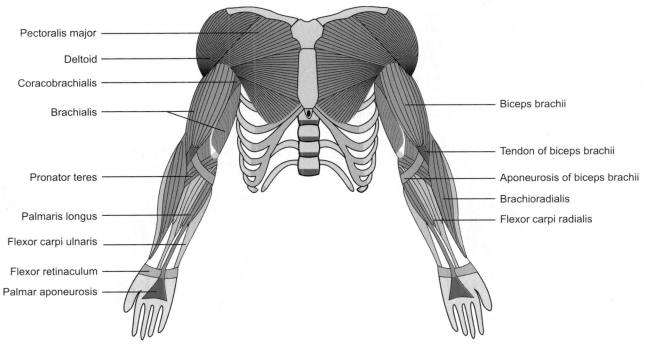

Fig. 7.51: Muscles of pectoral region, arm and forearm

Muscles of Flexor Compartment of Forearm

Muscles are arranged in three layers namely: superficial, intermediate and deep.

Superficial group: All are supplied by median nerve except flexro carpi ulnaris (Figs 7.51 and 7.52). They are tabulated below:

Muscles	Origin	Insertion	Action
1. **Pronator teres** **Nerve supply:** Median nerve, it lies between the origin of two heads	1. Humeral head a. lower part of medial supra condylar ridge b. medial epicondyle, anteriorly 2. Ulnar head: Medial border of coronoid process	Middle of lateral surface of shaft of radius, as a single flat tendon	1. Pronation 2. Weak flexor of elbow joint
2. **Flexor carpi radialis** **Nerve supply:** Median nerve	1. Medial epicondyle (common flexor origin) 2. Antebrachial fascia	Palmar surface of bases of 2nd and 3rd metacarpal bones	1. Flexor of wrist 2. Abduction of wrist along with extensor carpi radialis longus and brevis
3. **Palmaris longus** **Nerve supply:** Median nerve	Medial epicondyle (common flexor origin)	Central part of palmar aponeurosis	Weak flexor of wrist
4. **Flexor carpi ulnaris** **Nerve supply:** Ulnar nerve	1. Humeral head: Medial epicondyle, (common flexor origin) 2. Ulnar head: a. medial margin of olecranon fossa b. upper 2/3rd of posterior border of ulna	A tendinous arch connects two heads and is attached to 1. Pisiform bone 2. Hook of hamate 3. Base of 5th metacarpal bone	1. Flexion of wrist 2. Adduction of wrist with flexor and extensor carpi ulnaris

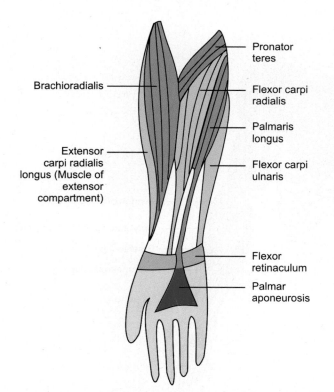

Fig. 7.52: Superficial muscles of flexor compartment of forearm

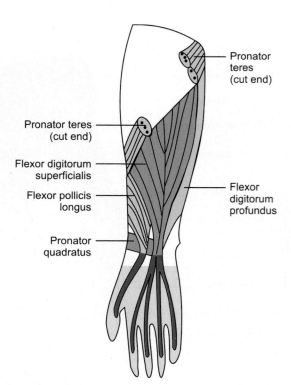

Fig. 7.53: Deep muscles of flexor compartment of forearm

Intermediate Group (Fig. 7.53)

Muscles	Origin	Insertion	Action
Flexor digitorum superficialis **Nerve supply:** Median nerve	1. Humero ulnar head: a. Medial epicondyle of humerus b. Medial margin of coronoid process 2. Radial head: anterior oblique line of radius	1. It forms four tendons arranged in one anterior and one posterior pair 2. Each digital tendon splits to allow passage of profundus tendon and then reunites 3. Each slip again divides to attach to side of shaft of middle phalanx of medial 4 digits	1. Flexion at proximal interphalangeal joints 2. Secondary flexor of metacarpophalangeal and wrist joint

Deep Group (Fig. 7.53)

Muscles	Origin	Insertion	Action
1. **Flexor pollicis longus** **Nerve supply:** Median nerve (anterior interosseous nerve)	1. Anterior surface of shaft of radius below oblique line 2. Adjacent interosseous membrane 3. Rarely, lower part of medial margin of coronoid process	Palmar surface of base of distal phalanx of thumb	Flexor of thumb
2. **Flexor digitorum profundus** **Nerve supply:** a. Medial part by ulnar nerve b. Lateral part by Median nerve (anterior interosseous nerve)	1. Upper ¾ of anterior and medial surfaces of shaft of ulna 2. Medial surface of coronoid and olecranon process 3. Adjacent interosseous membrane 4. Upper ¾ of posterior border of ulna	It forms four tendons that insert into the palmar surface of base of terminal phalanges of medial four fingers	1. Flexion of distal interphalangeal joints 2. Secondary flexors of metacarpo-phalangeal and carpal joints
3. **Pronator quadratus** **Nerve supply:** Median nerve	Bony ridge on antero-medial surface of lower ¼ of ulna	1. **Superficial fibres:** Anterior surface of lower ¼ of radius and adjoining anterior border 2. **Deep fibres:** Triangular area just above ulnar notch	Principal pronator of forearm

Muscles of Extensor Compartment of Forearm

The Muscles arranged in superficial and deep layers.

Superficial Group (Figs 7.50 and 7.54)

They are tabulated below:

Muscles	Origin	Insertion	Action
1. **Brachioradialis** **Nerve supply:** Radial nerve	Upper 2/3rd of lateral supracondylar ridge of humerus	Lateral side of radius just above the styloid process	Flexion of elbow joint (acts as shunt muscle)
2. **Extensor carpi radialis longus** **Nerve supply:** Radial nerve	Lower 1/3rd of the lateral supra condylar ridge of humerus	Base of 2nd metacarpal— dorsal surface	1. Abduction of wrist 2. Extention of wrist
3. **Extensor carpi radialis brevis** **Nerve supply:** Posterior interosseous nerve	1. Front of lateral epicondyle, common extensor origin 2. Radial collateral ligament	Dorsal surfaces of bases of 2nd and 3rd metacarpal bones	1. Extension of wrist 2. Abduction of wrist

Muscles	Origin	Insertion	Action
4. Extensor digitorum Nerve supply: Posterior interosseous nerve	Front of lateral epicondyle, common extensor origin	It forms 4 digital tendons which pass under extensor retinaculum and diverge to medial four fingers. Each tendon forms a dorsal digital expansion.	Extension at metacarpo-phalangeal joint and flexion at interphalangeal joints
5. Extensor digiti minimi Nerve supply: Posterior interosseous nerve	Front of lateral epicondyle 1. Lateral epicondyle 2. Posterior border of ulna	Joins with dorsal digital expansion of extensor tendon for the little finger	Extension of little finger
6. Extensor carpi ulnaris Nerve supply: Posterior interosseous nerve	Posterior surface of lateral epicondyle	Tubercle on medial side of base of 5th metacarpal	1. Extension of wrist 2. Adduction of wrist
7. Anconeus Nerve supply: Radial nerve		1. Lateral surface of olecranon process 2. Upper ¼th of posterior surface of shaft of ulna	1. Extension of elbow 2. Abduction of ulna during pronation

Deep group (Fig. 7.54)

Muscles	Origin	Insertion	Action
1. Supinator Nerve supply: Posterior interosseous nerve	1. Superficial fibres — radial collateral ligament 2. Deep fibres supinator crest and triangular area in front of it on ulna	1. Superficial fibres — upper 1/3rd of anterior part of lateral surface of radius 2. Deep fibres — radial bone between anterior and posterior oblique lines	Supination of forearm, in extension.
2. Abductor pollicis longus Nerve supply: Posterior interosseous nerve	1. Posterior surface of ulna below anconeus 2. Posterior surface of radius, middle 1/3rd below supinator 3. Intervening interosseous membrane	Radial side of base of 1st metacarpal	1. Abduction of thumb. 2. Extension of thumb.
3. Extensor pollicis brevis Nerve supply: Posterior interosseous nerve	1. Posterior surface of radius below abductor pollicis longus 2. Adjacent interosseous membrane	Dorsal surface of base of proximal phalanx of thumb	Extension of proximal phalanx of thumb.
4. Extensor pollicis longus Nerve supply: Posterior interosseous nerve	1. Posterior surface of shaft of ulna below abductor pollicis longus 2. Adjacent interosseous membrane	Dorsal surface of base of distal phalanx of thumb	Extension of distal phalanx of thumb.
5. Extensor indicis Nerve supply: Posterior interosseous nerve	1. Posterior surface of ulna below extensor pollicis longus 2. Adjacent interosseous membrane	Joins with index tendon of extensor digitorum and forms dorsal digital expansion	Extension of index finger.

Muscles of Hand

They consist of tendons of long flexors and extensors of forearm (described above), and intrinsic muscles of hand.

The intrinsic muscles of hand are arranged in three groups namely: thenar muscles, hypothenar muscles and deep muscles.

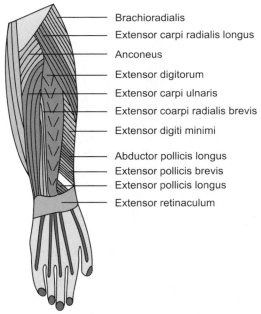

Fig. 7.54: Muscles of extensor compartment of forearm

Labels: Brachioradialis, Extensor carpi radialis longus, Anconeus, Extensor digitorum, Extensor carpi ulnaris, Extensor coarpi radialis brevis, Extensor digiti minimi, Abductor pollicis longus, Extensor pollicis brevis, Extensor pollicis longus, Extensor retinaculum

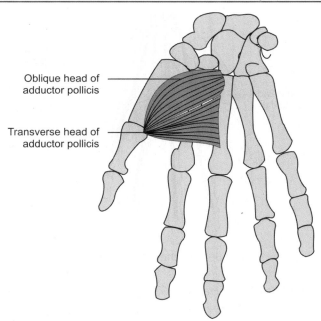

Fig. 7.55: Attachment of adductor policis

Labels: Oblique head of adductor pollicis, Transverse head of adductor pollicis

Thenar and Hypothenar Muscles

Muscles	Origin	Insertion	Action
1. **Abductor pollicis brevis (Fig. 7.55)** Nerve supply: Recurrent branch of median nerve	1. Tubercle of scaphoid and trapezium, 2. Tendon of abductor pollicis longus	Base of proximal phalanx of thumb on the radial side	1. Abduction of thumb 2. Medial rotation of thumb
2. **Flexor pollicis brevis** Nerve supply: Recurrent branch of median nerve	1. Superficial head from tubercle of trapezium 2. Deep head from trapezoid and capitate	Radial side of base of proximal phalanx	Flexion of proximal phalanx of thumb
3. **Opponens pollicis** Nerve supply: Recurrent branch of median nerve	Tubercle of trapezium	Palmar surface of shaft of 1st metacarpal	Opposition of thumb
4. **Adductor pollicis** Nerve supply: Deep branch of ulnar nerve	1. Transverse head from 3rd metacarpal bone 2. Oblique head from base of 2nd and 3rd metacarpal	Ulnar side of base of proximal phalanx of thumb	Adduction of thumb
5. **Abductor digiti minimi** Nerve supply: Deep branch of ulnar nerve	1. Pisiform bone 2. Tendon of flexor carpi ulnaris 3. Pisohamate ligament	Forms two slips and inserts on 1. Ulnar side of base of phalanx of little finger 2. Ulnar border of dorsal digital expansion of little finger	The hypothenar muscles act as a group to deeper the cup of the palm for a firm grip on a large object
6. **Flexor digiti minimi** Nerve supply: Deep branch of ulnar nerve	1. Flexor retinaculum 2. Hook of hamate	Ulnar side of bone of proximal phalanx of little finger	The hypothenar muscles act as a group to deeper the cup of the palm for a firm grip on a large object
7. **Opponens digiti minimi** Nerve supply: Deep branch of ulnar nerve	1. Flexor retinaculum 2. Hook of hamate	Ulnar side of palmar surface of shaft of 5th metacarpal bone	The hypothenar muscles act as a group to deeper the cup of the palm for a firm grip on a large object
8. **Palmaris brevis** Nerve supply: Superficial branch of ulnar nerve	1. Flexor retinaculum 2. Palmar aponeurosis	Dermis of ulnar border of palm	Protects underlying ulnar vessels and nerves

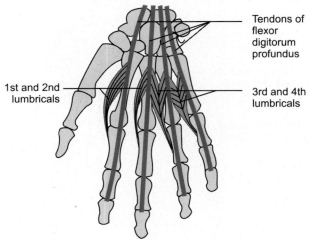

Fig. 7.56: Attachment of lumbricals

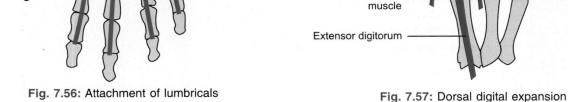

Fig. 7.57: Dorsal digital expansion

Deep Muscles of Hand

These consists of lumbricals and interossei muscles which act on fingers.

Lumbricals

They are four in number (Fig. 7.56) .

Origin

1 and 2 are unipennate: Arise from radial side of profundus tendon for index and middle finger.

Palmar Interossei

Supplied by deep branch of ulnar nerve.

3 and 4 are bipennate: Arise from adjacent sides of profundus tendons of middle and little fingers.

Insertion: Dorsal digital expansion

Nerve supply:
1. 1st and 2nd: Median nerve
2. 3rd and 4th: Ulnar nerve

Action of Lumbricals: Described below in dorsal digital expansion.

Interosseous muscles	Origin	Insertion	Action
First	Medial side of base of 1st metacarpal	Medial side of thumb	Adductor of thumb
Second	Medial half of shaft of 2nd metacarpal	Medial side of index finger	Adductor of index finger
Third	Lateral part of shaft of 4th metacarpal	Lateral side of ring finger	Adductor of ring finger
Fourth	Lateral part of shaft of 5th metacarpal	Lateral side of little finger	Adductor of little finger

Dorsal Interossei

Supplied by deep branch of ulnar nerve.

Interosseous muscles	Origin	Insertion	Action
First finger	Shaft of 1st and 2nd metacarpal	Lateral side of index finger	Abductor of index finger
Second finger	Shaft of 2nd and 3rd metacarpal	Lateral side of middle finger	Abductor of middle
Third finger	Shaft of 3rd and 4th metacarpal	Medial side of middle finger	Abductor of middle
Fourth finger	Shaft of 4th and 5th metacarpal	Medial side of 4th digit	Abductor of 4th digit

Dorsal Digital Expansion (Fig. 7.57)

Each extensor tendon of extensor digitorum becomes expanded and forms the dorsal digital expansion. It has the following parts

Base: Forms a hood over the metacarpal head and is anchored to deep transverse metacarpal ligament.

Apex: Lies close to the distal end of proximal phalanx and splits into one median and two lateral bands. Median band is inserted into the base of the middle phalanx. Lateral bands unite before insertion into the base of the distal phalanx.

Proximal wing: Formed by attachment of tendons of palmar and dorsal interossei to the dorsal digital expansion.

Distal wing: Formed by attachment of lumbricals which join the lateral band of digital expansion.

Action of Dorsal Digital Expension

Tendon of extensor digitorum: Prime mover for extension at metacarpo-phalangeal and interphalangeal joints.

Lumbricals: Flexion at metacarpo-phalangeal joint and extension at interphalangeal joints.

Dorsal intersossei: Less powerful flexor at metacarpo-phalangeal Joint, abductor of digits.

Palmar intersossei: Less powerful flexor at metacarpo-phalangeal Joint, adductor of digits.

MUSCLES OF LOWER LIMB

Attachments of Muscles of Lower Limb on the Bones (Figs 7.58 to 7.65)

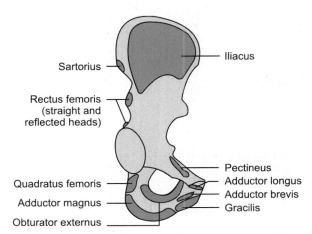

Fig. 7.58: Muscle attachments on hip bone (anterolateral aspect)

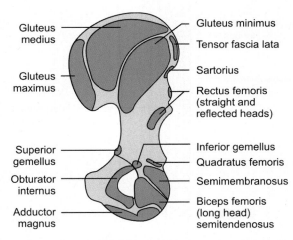

Fig. 7.59: Muscle attachments on hip bone (posterior aspect)

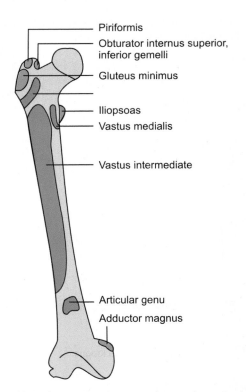

Fig. 7.60: Right femur showing muscle attachments (anterior aspect)

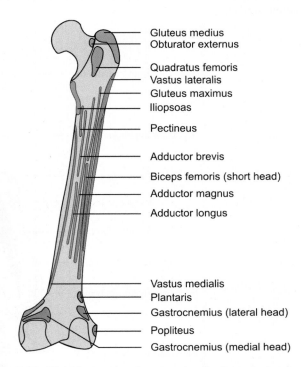

Fig. 7.61: Right femur showing muscle attachments (posterior aspect)

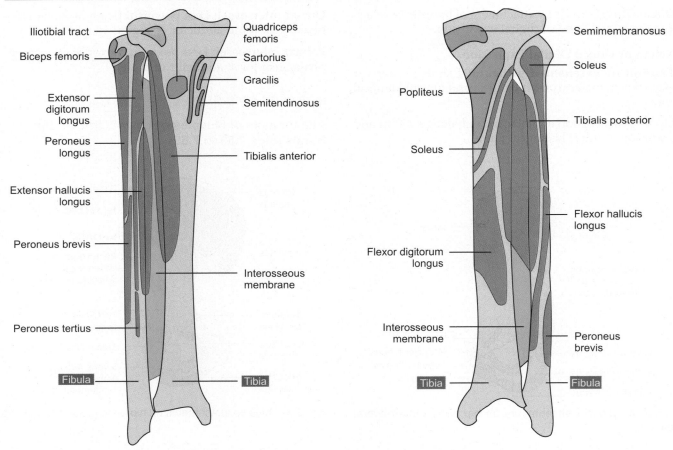

Fig. 7.62: Right tibia and fibula showing muscle attachments (anterior aspect)

Fig. 7.63: Right tibia and fibula showing muscle attachments (posterior aspect)

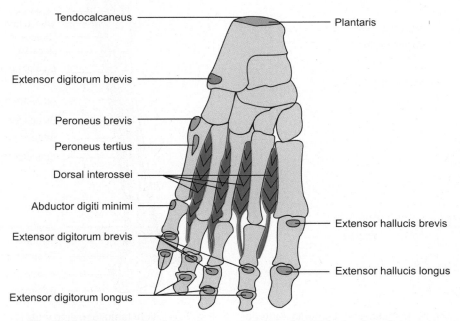

Fig. 7.64: Attachments of muscles on skeleton of right foot—dorsal aspect

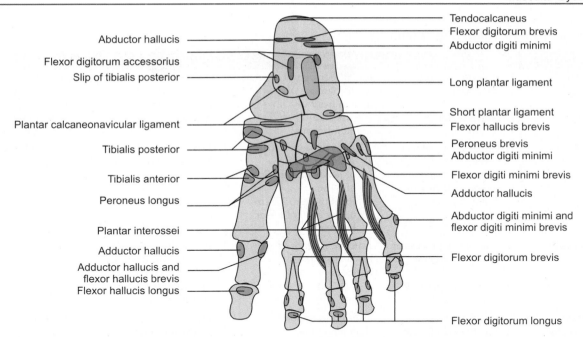

Abductor hallucis

Flexor digitorum accessorius

Slip of tibialis posterior

Plantar calcaneonavicular ligament

Tibialis posterior

Tibialis anterior

Peroneus longus

Plantar interossei

Adductor hallucis

Adductor hallucis and flexor hallucis brevis

Flexor hallucis longus

Tendocalcaneus

Flexor digitorum brevis

Abductor digiti minimi

Long plantar ligament

Short plantar ligament

Flexor hallucis brevis

Peroneus brevis

Abductor digiti minimi

Flexor digiti minimi brevis

Adductor hallucis

Abductor digiti minimi and flexor digiti minimi brevis

Flexor digitorum brevis

Flexor digitorum longus

Fig. 7.65: Attachments of muscles on skeleton of right foot—plantar aspect

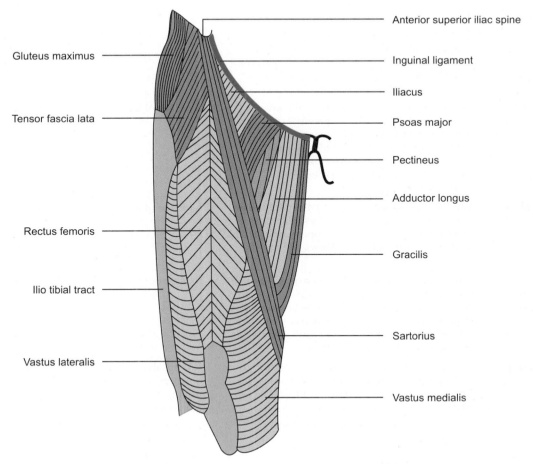

Gluteus maximus

Tensor fascia lata

Rectus femoris

Ilio tibial tract

Vastus lateralis

Anterior superior iliac spine

Inguinal ligament

Iliacus

Psoas major

Pectineus

Adductor longus

Gracilis

Sartorius

Vastus medialis

Fig. 7.66: Muscle of front and medial side of thigh

MUSCLES OF LOWER LIMB
Muscles of Front of Thigh (Fig. 7.66)

Muscle	Origin	Insertion	Action	Peculiarity
1. Sartorius (Sartor means tailor)	1. Anterior superior iliac spine 2. Notch below it	Into upper part of medial surface of tibia in front of gracilis and semitendinosus	1. Flexion of thigh and leg 2. Abduction and lateral rotation of thigh	Known as tailor muscle due to its cross legged position. Helps in formation of Guy ropes
2. Iliacus	1. Upper 2/3rd of iliac fossa 2. Ventral aspect of sacroiliac ligament 3. Adjoining ala of sacrum	1. Joins psoas tendon 2. Anterior surface of lesser trochanter of femur 3. Extends upto 2.5 cm below each of lesser trochanter	1. Flexion of hip 2. Medial rotation of femur	Joins with psoas on lateral side
3. Psoas major	1. Transverse process of L_1 to L_5 vertebrae 2. Sides of upper four lumbar vertebrae	Anterior surface of lesser trochanter of femur	1. Acting from above is the chief flexor of hip 2. Acting from below in recumbent position Raising trunk	Lies medial to iliacus
4. Pectineus Supplied by femoral and obturator nerves	1. Pectin pubis 2. Narrow area in front of it	Inserted to femoral shaft along line extending from lesser trochanter to line aspera	1. Flexor of hip 2. Adductor of hip	Posterior surface overlaps obturator externus, adductor brevis and anterior division of obturator nerve
5. Rectus femoris • Straight head • Reflected head	1. Upper part of anterior inferior iliac spine 2. Groove above acetabulum 3. Capsule of hip joint	Base of patella 1. Flexor of thigh 2. Flexes the pelvis if thigh is fixed	Extensor of leg	Two heads of origin are present
6. Vastus lateralis	1. Upper part of intertrochantric line 2. Anterior and inferior border of greater trochanter 3. Upper half of lateral lip of linea aspera	1. Lateral border of patella 2. Lateral part of base of patella 3. Fibrous capsule of knee joint	Extensor of leg	Intra muscular injection is preferred in this muscle
7. Vastus medialis	1. Intertrochantric line 2. Spiral line 3 Linea aspera 4. Medial supracondylar line	1. Medial part of base of patella 2. Upper part of medial border of patella	Extensor of leg	Prevents lateral displacement of patella
8. Vastus intermedius	1. Anterior and lateral surface of upper 2/3rd of patella of shaft of femur 2. Lower part of lateral intermuscular septum	1. Deep aspect of base 2. Lateral border of patella 3. Lateral condyle of tibia	Extensor of leg	Nerve to vastus intermedius also supplies articular genu
9. Articular genu	It arises by 3 or 4 slips from the anterior surface of the lower part of femur	Inserted into the summit of supra-patellar bursa	It keeps the suprapatellar bursa in position by pulling upwards the apex of synovial fold	It is a detached part of vastus intermedius
10. Tensor fascia lata	Anterior 5 cm of outer lip of iliac crest	Ilio tibial tract	Through ilio tibial tract 1. Extension of knee 2. Abduction and medial rotation of thigh	

Muscles of Medial Compartment of Thigh

Muscle	Origin	Insertion	Action	Peculiarity
1. **Gracilis (Fig. 7.66)** **Nerve supply:** Anterior division of Obturator nerve	Medial margin of lower part of body of pubis	Upper part of medial surface of tibia in between sartorius and semitendinosus	1. Adduction of hip 2. Flexion of knee 3. Stabilizes pelvis on tibia	Muscle may be used for grafting
2. **Adductor longus (Fig. 7.66)** **Nerve supply:** Anterior division of Obturator nerve	Circular area in the angle between the pubic crest and symphysis	Medial lip of linea aspera in the middle third of shaft of femur	1. Adduction of thigh 2. Medial rotation of thigh	Tendinous origin, May have sesamoid bone in the tendon, **rider's bone**
3. **Adductor brevis** **Nerve supply:** Anterior division of Obturator nerve	Body of pubis	Line extending from the base of lesser trochanter to upper part of linea aspera	Adduction of hip	Anterior and posterior division of obturator nerve lies vertically along the respective surfaces
4. **Adductor mangus (Fig. 7.67)** **Nerve supply:** a. **Adductor part** Posterior division of obturator nerve b. **Hamstring part** Tibial component of sciatic nerve	1. **Adductor head:** Extensor surface of ischio pubic ramus 2. **Ischial head:** Inferolateral aspect of ischial tuberosity	1. Adductor component inserts in to the femoral shaft along the line joining medial margin of gluteal tuberosity, medial lip of linea aspera and upper part of medial supracondylar line 2. Ischial fibers insert on adductor tubercle	1. Adduction of thigh 2. Medial rotation of hip	Five osseo aponeurotic openings are present in the muscle.
5. **Obtutator externus** **Nerve supply:** Posterior division of Obturator nerve	1. Outer surface of obturator membrane 2. Adjoining margin of obturator foramen	Trochanteric fossa	1. Lateral rotation of hip 2. Stabilizes the hip joint	

Muscles of Gluteal Region (Fig. 7.67)

Muscle	Origin	Insertion	Action
1. **Gluteus maximus** **Nerve supply:** Inferior gluteal (L_5, S_1, S_2)	1. Gluteal surface of ilium behind the posterior gluteal line. 2. Thoracolumbar fascia, 3. Dorsal surface of lower part of sacrum and coccyx. 4. Sacrotuberous ligament	1. 1/4th is attached to gluteal tuberosity, 2. 3/4th attached to iliotibial tract	1. Chief extensor of hip joint in running and while standing from sitting position, 2. Lateral rotator of hip joint, 3. Upper fibres cause abduction of hip joint, 4. Maintains the extended position of knee joint.
2. **Gluteus medius** **Nerve supply:** Superior gluteal nerve (L_4, L_5, S_1)	1. Outer surface of ilium between anterior and posterior gluteal line. 2. Gluteal aponeurosis	Lateral surface of greater trochanter of femur	1. Abductor of hip joint along with gluteus minimus. 2. stabilises the pelvis when opposite foot is off the ground. 3. Medial rotator of hip
3. **Gluteus minimus** **Nerve supply:** Superior gluteal nerve	Lateral surface of ilium between anterior and inferior gluteal lines	Greater trochanter of femur on lateral part of anterior surface	1. Abduction of thigh. 2. Medial rotation and flexion of thigh.
4. **Piriformis** **Nerve supply:** Ventral rami S_1, S_2	Pelvic surface of sacrum	Apex of greater trochanter of femur	1. Lateral rotation of thigh. 2. Abduction of thigh when thigh is flexed.
5. **Obturator internus** **Nerve supply:** Nerve to obturator internus (L_5, S_1)	1. Pelvic surface of obturator membrane 2. Adjoining surface of ischial tuberosity, ischiopubic ramus and ilium	Medial surface of greater trochanter of femur	1. Lateral rotation of thigh. 2. Abduction of thigh when thigh is flexed.
6. **Superior gemellus** **Nerve supply:** Nerve to obturator internus	Posterior surface of ischial spine and adjoining part of lesser sciatic notch.	Joins the superior border of tendon of obturator internus	Lateral rotation of thigh

(Contd. ......)

Muscle	Origin	Insertion	Action
7. **Inferior gemellus** **Nerve supply:** Nerve to quadratus femorus (L_5, S_1).	Upper part of ischial tuberosity and adjoining part of lesser sciatic notch.	Joins with inferior border of tendon of obturator internus.	Lateral rotation of thigh.
8. **Quadratus femoris** **Nerve supply:** Nerve to quadratus femorus.	Upper part of Lateral border of ischial tuberosity.	Quadrate tubercule on trochanteric crest of femur.	Lateral rotation and abduction of thigh.

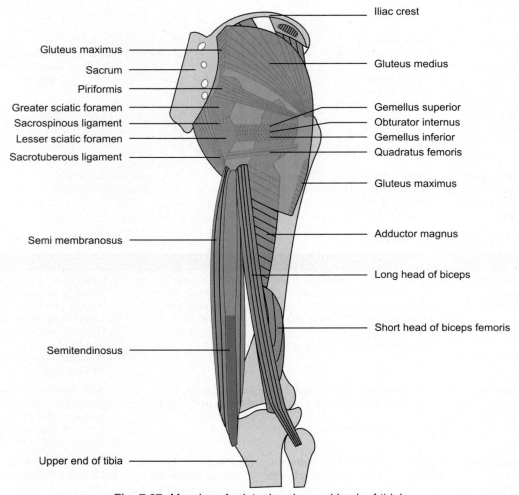

Fig. 7.67: Muscles of gluteal region and back of thigh

Muscles of Back of Thigh

They consists of hemistring muscles and short head of biceps femoris muscle.

Hamstring Muscles

They are four in number (Fig. 7.67).
1. Semimembranosus: A true hamstring muscle.
2. Semitendinosus: A true hamstring muscle.
3. Long head of biceps femoris muscle.
4. Ischial head of adductor magnus muscle.

Characteristics of hamstring muscles
1. All arise from the ischial tuberosity.
2. All are inserted beyond the knee joint to either tibia or fibula or both. Hence, they cross both hip joint and knee joint.

3. All are supplied by tibial components of sciatic nerve.
4. They act as flexors of knee and extensors of hip joint.

Semimembranosus

Origin: Upper and lateral part of ischial tuberosity. It is membranous in upper half, fleshy in lower half. It lies deep to long head of biceps and the cord like tendon of semitendinosus rests on it.

Insertion: On the horizontal groove on the posterior surface of medial condyle of tibia.

Semitendinosus

Origin: Lower and medial part of ischial tuberosity.
Insertion: Tendon pass behind medial condyle of femur upper part of medial surface of tibia.

Biceps Femoris (Fig. 7.67)
Origin:
1. Long head has origin with semitendinosus.

Muscles of Anterior Compartment of Leg and Dorsum of Foot

Nerve supply: All the muscles are supplied by deep peroneal nerve (Fig. 7.68)

2. Short head originates from
   a. lower part of lateral lip of linea aspera.
   b. Upper 2/3rd of lateral supracondylar line of femur.

Insertion: It forms a conjoint tendon which is inserted into head of fibula in front of styloid process.

Nerve Supply to Hamstring Muscles
1. Long head of biceps femoris, semitendinosus, semimembranosus and ischial head of adductor magnus are supplied by tibial component of sciatic nerve.
2. Short head of biceps is supplied by common peroneal component of sciatic nerve.

Action of Hamstring Muscles
1. Flexion of knee joint
2. Extension of hip joint especially on standing and walking
3. In semiflexed knee semimembranous and semitendinosus act as medial rotators and biceps femoris acts as a lateral rotator.

Muscle	Origin	Insertion	Action
1. **Extensor digitorum longus**	1. Upper 3/4th of medial surface of fibula 2. Interosseous membrane	It divides into four tendons for insertion into lateral 4 toes, on the base of middle and distal phalanges through dorsal digital expansion.	1. Extension of toes 2. Dorsiflexion of foot
2. **Tibialis anterior**	1. Lateral surface of shaft of tibia in upper 2/3rd 2. Interosseous membrane	1. Medial cuneiform bone, medial and plantar aspect. 2. Medial side of base of 1st metatarsal.	1. Dorsiflexion of foot 2. Inversion of foot 3. Helps to maintain arches of foot
3. **Peroneus tertius**	1. Medial surface of shaft of fibula 2. Interosseous membrane	Base of 5th metatarsal.	1. Dorsiflexion of foot 2. Eversion of foot
4. **Extensor hallucis longus**	1. Medial surface of fibula, from middle 2/4th 2. Interosseous membrane	Dorsal aspect of base of the distal phalanx of great toe.	1. Dorsiflexion of foot 2. Extension of phalaynx of great toe
5. **Extensor digitorum brevis**	1. Anterior part of upper surface of calcaneus 2. Stem of inferior extensor retinaculum	Splits into four tendons. 1. Medial most is inserted to base of proximal phalanx of great toe. 2. Rest three tendons attach to bases of middle and terminal phalanges with the dorsal digital expansions.	Dorsiflexes medial four toes in dorsiflexed ankle

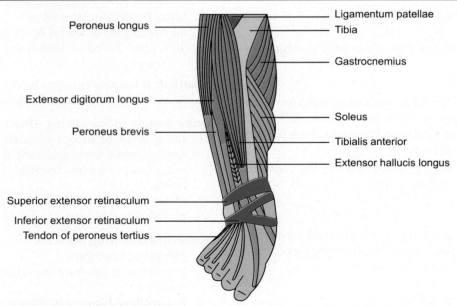

Fig. 7.68: Muscles of anterior and lateral compartment of leg

Muscles of Lateral Compartment of Leg (Fig. 7.69)

Peroneus Longus
It is bipennate in upper part
Origin
1. Head of fibula
2. Upper 2/3rd of lateral surface of fibula

Insertion: Base of 1st metatarsal and medial cuneiform bones.
Action
1. Eversion of foot
2. Steadies the leg in standing, maintaining longitudinal and transverse arches of foot.

Peroneus Brevis
Origin: Lower 2/3rd of lateral surface of shaft of fibula.
Insertion: Base of 5th metatarsal bone
Action
1. Eversion of foot
2. Helps to steady the leg

Nerve supply: The muscles are supplied by superficial peroneal nerve.

Muscles of Posterior Compartment of Leg

The muscles of posterior compartment are supplied by tibial nerve (Figs 7.69 to 7.71).

Gastrocnemius
Origin: It arises from the lateral and medial condyles of femur by two heads
Insertion: The two bellies of gastrocnemius descend down the leg and join with the soleus to form tendocalcaneous. Tendocalcaneous is inserted into the middle 1/3rd of posterior surface of calcaneum. The two heads

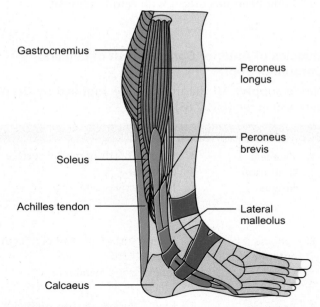

Fig. 7.69: Muscles of lateral and posterior compartment of leg

of gastrocnemius and soleus are collectively called as **triceps surae.**

Soleus
It is a **multipennate** muscle.
Origin
1. Posterior surface of head and upper ¼th of shaft of fibula
2. Soleal line and middle 1/3rd of tibia
3. Tendenous arch between tibia and fibula

Insertion: Forms tendocalcaneus with gastrocnemius.

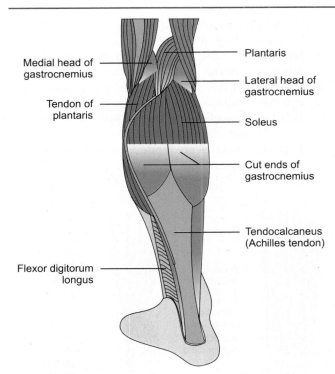

Medial head of gastrocnemius

Tendon of plantaris

Flexor digitorum longus

Plantaris

Lateral head of gastrocnemius

Soleus

Cut ends of gastrocnemius

Tendocalcaneus (Achilles tendon)

Fig. 7.70: Muscles of posterior compartment of leg

Tendocalcaneus

It is also known as Achilles tendon. It is the **strongest tendon** of the body measuring about 15 cm. it is formed by gastrocnemius and soleus muscle.

Action of tendocalcaneus: Plantar flexion of ankle joint

Action of gastrocnemius: It increases the range of movement and produces flexion of knee joint also.

Action of soleus: It is multipennate hence, increases the power of contraction. It also acts as peripheral heart. The tonic contraction of gastrocnemius and soleus prevents the anterior slipping of tibia over talus.

Popliteus

Origin: Origin is intracapsular. It arises from the anterior part of a groove on the lateral surface of lateral condyle of femur.

Insertion: On the triangular area on the posterior surface of tibia above the soleal line.

Action
Unlocking muscle of knee joint, flexion of knee joint

Tibialis Posterior

It is a **bipennate** muscle

Origin
1. Upper 2/3rd of interosseus membrane
2. Lateral part of posterior surface of shaft of tibia
3. Posterior surface of shaft of fibula

Insertion
1. Tuberosity of navicular bone
2. Sustentaculum tali of calcaneus
3. All tarsal and metatarsal bones except talus

Action
1. Inversion and adduction of foot
2. Maintenance of medial longitudinal arch
3. Plantar flexion

Flexor Hallucis Longus

Origin
1. Lower 2/3rd of posterior surface of shaft of fibula.
2. Adjacent interosseous membrane
3. Fascia covering tibialis posterior
4. Posterior intermuscular septum

Insertion: The tendon of this **bipennate** muscle lies on posterior surface of lower end of tibia beneath flexor retinaculum and lodges in the groove between posterior and medial tubercles of talus. It curves forwards to insert into the base of distal phalanx of great toe.

Action
1. Plantar flexion of great toe.
2. Secondary plantar flexion of ankle joint.
3. Maintains medial longitudinal arch of foot.

Flexor Digitorum Longus

Origin
1. Posterior surface of tibia below the soleal line, medial to vertical line.
2. Fascia covering tibialis posterior.

Insertion: The **bipennate** muscle forms the single tendon that splits into four digital tendons. Before splitting in four digital tendons it receives attachment of flexor digitorum accesorius on the lateral side. Each gives rise to a lumbrical muscle on the side and finally enters the fibrous flexor sheath, piercing the tendon of flexor digitorum brevis. It is inserted into plantar surface of base of terminal phalanx of lateral four toes.

Action
1. Plantar flexion of lateral four toes.
2. Maintains medial longitudinal arch of foot.

Plantaris

It is a small fusiform muscle.

Origin
1. Lower 1/3rd of lateral supracondylar ridge.
2. Adjoining part of popliteal surface of femur.

Insertion: It blends with the medial margin of tendocalcaneus.

Action
It is primarily a vestigeal muscle in human beings. It continues as the plantar aponeurosis in the foot.

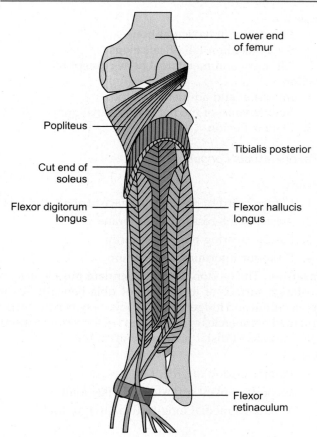

Fig. 7.71: Deep muscles of posterior compartment of leg

Layers of the Sole

Sole is divided into six layers. They are as follows (Figs 7.72 to 7.76)

1. **1st layer:** It lies beneath the plantar aponeurosis. It has three short muscles, all are intrinsic muscles of the foot. These muscles are
   a. Abductor hallucis
   b. Flexor digitorum brevis
   c. Abductor digit minimi
2. **2nd layer:** It contains medial and lateral plantar nerves and vessels.
3. **3rd layer:** It has two extrinsic tendons and two intrinsic muscles.

   Extrinsic muscles are
   a. Tendon of flexor hallucis longus
   b. Tendon of flexor digitorum longus
   Intrinsic muscles are
   a. Flexor digitorum accessorius
   b. Lumbricals are four in number
4. **4th layer:** It contains three intrinsic muscles of foot which are limited to region of metatarsals. These muscles are
   a. Flexor hallucis brevis
   b. Adductor hallucis
   c. Flexor digiti minimi brevis
5. **5th layer:** It contains deep part of lateral plantar artery and nerve.
6. **6th layer:** It has seven intrinsic muscles and two extrinsic tendons.
   Intrinsic muscles are four dorsal interossei and three plantar interossei.
   Extrinsic muscles are tendons of peroneus longus and tibialis posterior.

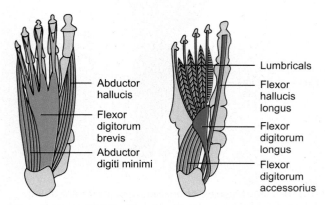

Figs 7.72 and 7.73: Muscles of 1st and 3rd layer of sole

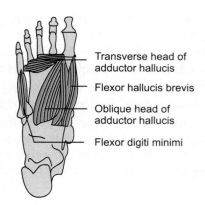

Fig. 7.74: Muscles of 4th layer of sole

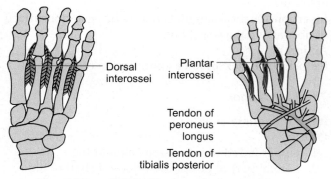

Figs 7.75 and 7.76: Muscles of 6th layer of sole

Chapter 8

Anatomical and Functional Organization of Nervous System

INTRODUCTION

Nervous system is the system which responds to the internal and external environments in order to maintain the internal environment and manipulate the external environment for survival and existence. Nervous system regulates all functions of the body.

Parts of Nervous System

1. **Central nervous system (CNS):** It consists of brain and spinal cord (Fig. 8.1).
   Brain: It is also known as encephalon. It lies in the cranial cavity and continues as the spinal cord. It consists of following parts:
   a. **Prosencephalon or forebrain:** It is further subdivided into telencephalon (cerebral hemispheres) and diencephalon (thalamus proper and its related neuronal masses).
   b. **Mesencephalon or midbrain:** It is made up of cerebral peduncles.
   c. **Rhombencephalon or hind brain:** Hind brain is made up of pons and medulla oblongata, ventrally and cerebellum, dorsally.
   Spinal cord: It is also known as spinal medulla. It is the caudal, elongated part of central nervous system which occupies the upper 2/3rd of the vertebral canal.
   Functions of CNS: Perception, integration and analysis of all types of sensory input and initiation of motor activity.
2. **Peripheral nervous system (PNS):** It includes those parts of nervous system which lie outside the central nervous system. It consists of twelve pairs of cranial nerves, thirty one pairs of spinal nerves, somatic and special sense receptors and the autonomic nervous system.
   Cranial nerves: All are attached to the ventral surface of the brain except 4th cranial nerve (trochlear nerve) which arises from its dorsal surface.
   Spinal nerves: Each pair of spinal nerves are attached to the sides of the spinal cord by two roots.

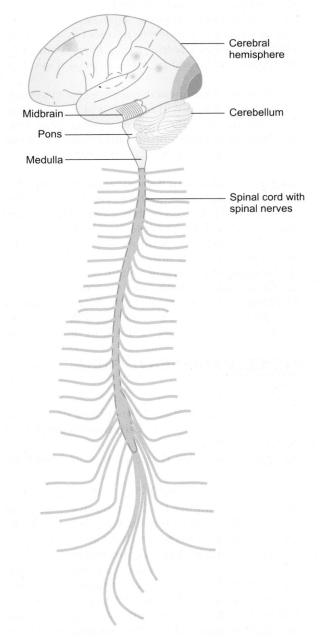

Fig. 8.1: Parts of brain with spinal cord

Autonomic nervous system: It has two components namely:
   a. Sympathetic nervous system
   b. Parasympathetic nervous system
Functions of PNS: It carries impulses from peripheral sensory receptors and sense organs to the central nervous system and back from the central nervous system to the effector organs, e.g., muscles and glands.

Functional Subdivision of Nervous System

Nervous system is classified into the following two types according to the functional differences:
1. **Somatic nervous system:** This deals with t he changes in the external environment and has both afferent and efferent components. It has connections with both central and peripheral nervous systems.
   Function:
   a . **Afferent component or somatosensory system:** It is concerned with carrying and processing conscious and unconscious sensory impulses.
   b. **Efferent component or somatomotor system:** It is concerned with the voluntary control of muscles.
2. **Visceral or autonomic nervous system:** It responds to the various changes in the internal environment of the body. It also has both sensory (afferent) and motor (efferent) components. It is derived from the central as well as the peripheral nervous system.
   It is further divided into:
   1. **Sympathetic nervous system**
   2. **Parasympathetic nervous system**
   Function: It is concerned with the regulation of visceral functions that maintain the internal homeostasis and works mostly at the unconscious level.

NERVE CELL AND NERVE FIBRE

NEURON

Neuron is the structural and functional unit of the nervous system (Figs 8.2 to 8.4). **Each neuron consists of**
   a. Soma or cell body
   b. Neurites or processes: They are, axons and dendrites

Soma or Cell Body (Perikaryon)

Cell body is surrounded by a plasma membrane or neurolemma. The plasma membrane contains various integral, membrane proteins which act as Na^+, K^+, Ca^{++}, Cl^- ion channels. It also has receptor proteins.

The shape of cell body can vary from stellate, fusiform, basket shape, flask or pyramidal shape. Soma is made up of the following two components:
1. **Cytoplasm:** It contains numerous organelles and inclusion bodies. Cytoplasm is surrounded by the plasma membrane.

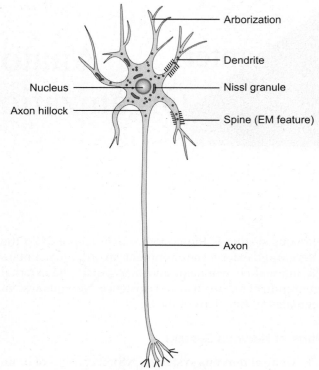

Fig. 8.2: Multipolar neuron

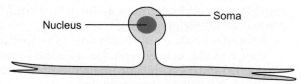

Fig. 8.3: Unipolar neuron

2. **Nucleus:** It is large, vesicular and contains a prominent nucleolus.

Cytoplasmic Organelles and Inclusions

a. **Nissl bodies:** These are made up of rough endoplasmic reticulum with ribosomes. They are basophilic in nature. Nissl bodies are present in cell body and dendrites. They are absent in axons. These bodies disappear, when the neuron is injured and this phenomenon is known as **chromatolysis.**
   Functions: Synthesis of new proteins and enzymes.
b. **Smooth endoplasmic reticulum**
   Functions: It helps in transmission of neurochemical substances by forming synaptic vesicles.
c. **Golgi apparatus:** It is present close to the nucleus and is absent in axon and dendrites.
   Functions: Is responsible for the packaging of neurosecretions.
d. **Mitochondria:** These are rod like structure with double membrane, present in soma, dendrites and axons.
   Functions: Mitochondria are the site of production of energy molecules for the cell.

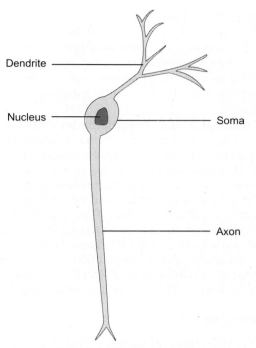

Fig. 8.4: Bipolar neuron

e. **Lysosomes:** They are thick walled membranous vesicles containing hydrolytic enzymes.
   Functions: Phagocytosis, hydrolysis of Nissl bodies.
f. **Neurofilaments and Microtubules:** These are aggregated at the axon hillock. They form the cytoskeleton of the neuron.
   Functions: Are responsible for the shape and mobility of the neuron. Microtubules provide contractility to the neuron.
g. **Centrioles:** These are present in soma.
   Functions: They help in regeneration of the cytoplasmic microtubules.
h. **Pigments and mineral containing granules:**
   — **Old age pigments:** Lipofuscin, Lipochrome.
   — **Neuromelanin:** Present in substantia nigra.
     Functions: Synthesis of dopamine.
   — **Zn (zinc):** Present in hippocampus.
   — **Fe (Iron):** Present in oculomotor nucleus.
   — **Cu (copper):** Present in locus ceruleus.

Axons and Dendrites

These are processes which arise from the cell body.
1. **Dendrites:** These are 5 to 7 small processes which branch repeatedly and end in terminal arborization. The ends form dendritic spines. They contain Nissl bodies, mitochondria and neuro filaments. They receive and transmit impulses towards the cell body.
2. **Axons:** These are generally single and they terminate away from the cell body. Collateral

branches may be present at right angles. Nissl bodies are absent. Spines are absent. They carry impulses away from the cell body. The terminal portion of axons usually branch and end in dilated ends called as synaptic knobs.

Axons are surrounded by myelin sheath (Fig. 8.5). Myelin sheath consists of a protein—lipid complex which is produced by Schwann cells. Schwann cells surround the axons and are present along the length of the axons. The myelin sheath is deficient at regular intervals of around 1 mm. These points are known as nodes of Ranvier.

PHYSIOLOGY OF NERVE CELL

Functions of Each Part of Neuron

1. **Cell body:** It houses the various cell organelles that help in protein synthesis and maintain the function of metabolism of neurons.
2. **Dendrites:** These receive impulses and transmit them to cell body.
3. **Axon:** It generates and transmits nerve impulses, as action potentials, away from cell body.
4. **Myelin sheath:** It helps in insulating the nerve impulses from surrounding cells. Hence, it facilitates transmission of impulses.
5. **Synaptic knobs:** These contain vesicles which store various neurotransmitters. The neuro-transmitters

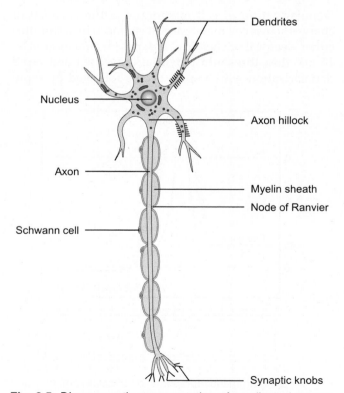

Fig. 8.5: Diagrammatic representation of myelinated neuron

are chemical molecules that released in response to action potential changes reaching the synaptic knobs (Fig. 8.8).

Nerve Excitation and Conduction of Impulse

Nerve cells can be stimulated by mechanical, electrical and chemical stimuli. The stimulation leads to production of two types of responses:
1. Action potentials or propagated disturbances.
2. Electrotonic potentials or local, non propagative responses.

Resting Membrane Potential

This is the potential difference present across the neuronal cell membrane (neurilemma in this case). It is equal to –70 mV.

Mechanism of resting membrane potential: The intracellular Na^+ is actively pumped out of the cell and K^+ is actively transported into the cell by basolateral Na^+, K^+ ATPase pump. Na^+ diffuses back and K^+ diffuses out along their respective concentration gradients. However, K^+ channel permeability is higher giving rise to a positive charge that is maintained on outer aspect of membrane with respect to inner aspect. The membrane in resting membrane potential is said to be polarized.

Action Potential

Depolarization of cell membrane is the reversal of charges across cell membrane. It is caused by a stimulus either electrical or chemical. If depolarization occurs by 15 mV then **threshold potential** is reached and rapid depolarization with a spike occurs followed by rapid

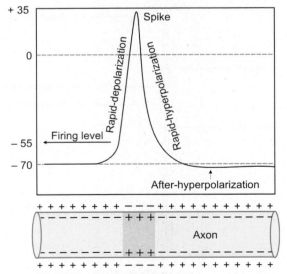

Fig. 8.6: Diagrammatic representation of action potential and electrical changes across neuronal cell membrane

repolarization. This is action potential. The action potential is an 'all or none' phenomenon, that means either the stimulus will elicit no response or will cause action potential upto the maximum capacity of the nerve fibre. The intensity of action potential does not increase any further with the increase in intensity of stimulus (Fig. 8.6).

Ionic Basis of Action Potential: Stimulation of nerve cells by a neurotransmitter or by the mechanical stretch of axons or by an electrical impulse leads to opening up of Na^+ channels that allow influx of Na^+. This leads to depolarization. As the depolarization becomes more than 7mV, voltage gated Na^+ channels also open leading to a further rapid influx of Na^+. There is a sharp spike of depolarization now. These channels however, close within one second and the K^+ channels open. Opening of K^+ channels allows rapid efflux of K^+ ions. The stoppage of Na^+ influx and rapid K^+ efflux corrects the electrical charges. This is called repolarization.

Refractory Period

It is the time interval during which the nerve once stimulated, does not respond to a second stimulus even if it is stronger than 1st. As the resting membrane potential is reached, the nerve can be excited again.

Propogation and Conduction of Electric Impulses

- When depolarization reaches the firing level or threshold potential, the rapid electrical changes of action potential lead to self propagation of the depolarization wave to the membrane ahead of action potential. The currents are setup in a circular circuit like fashion depolarizing successively the part of membrane ahead of the site of original action potential.
- In myelinated fibers the current flow occurs between two nodes of Ranvier as myelin acts as an insulator. This is called **saltatory conduction** and is responsible for rapid conduction of impulses.
- The conduction usually occurs in one direction in axons which is towards their terminal ends. This is called **orthodromic conduction.** Conduction also occurs in opposite direction and is known as **antidromic conduction.**
- Since at synapses, electrical conduction is only one way, the antidromic impulses die out at that point.

Compound Action Potentials

Peripheral nerves are made of multiple axon fibers bound by a fibrous envelope, the epineurium. The fibers have various speeds of conduction. Thus, when an electrical stimulation is applied to the nerves, multiple electrical potentials can be recorded by electrodes placed on the nerve. This is called compound action potential.

Electrotonic Potential/Graded Potential

It is seen that a subthreshold stimulus causes mild depolarization. However, this gets corrected due to opening up of K^+ channels allowing effusion of anions and opening of Cl^- channels allowing influx of cations. This decays the potential. Hence, graded potentials are limited to a small region of axon which is stimulated and are not propagated. When the depolarization occurs by more than 15mV or resting membrane potential reaches –55mV, action potential is propagated.

NERVE

Structure of Nerve Fiber and Nerve Trunk

Nerve fiber: It is primarily made up of axon of a neuron (occasionally dendrites also) which is covered by neurilemma. Neurilemma is made up of Schwann cells. Schwann cells lay down the myelin sheath around the axon under the neurilemma. A thin layer of connective tissue named endoneurium is pesent between two adjacent nerve fibers.

Nerve trunk: It is made up of a number of bundles of nerve fibres. Nerve fibres are arranged in fascicles which are surrounded by a thin layer of connective tissue known as perineurium. A number of fascicles together form a nerve trunk. The outer most covering of nerve trunk is a connective tissue layer named epineurium (Fig. 8.7).

Type of Nerve Fibers and their Functions

General facts about nerve fibres and conduction:
1. Myelinated nerves conduct impulses faster than unmyelinated nerves.
2. Nerves with larger diameter have greater speed of conduction of impulses.
3. Large nerve axons usually respond to touch, pressure and proprioception while smaller nerves usually respond to temperature, pain and autonomic functions.

Nerve fibers are classified as A, B and C according to the diameter of the fibers. The diameter and speed of conduction of impulses in A fibers is higest and lowest in C group. A-group is further divided into α, β, γ, δ. The fiber size decreases from α to γ. The functions of each one is given below:

Type of nerve fibers	Function
A-α	Proprioception, somatic motor
A-β	Touch, pressure
A-γ	Motor to muscle spindles
A-δ	Pain, temperature
B	Preganglionic autonomic nerve fibers
C-Dorsal root ganglion fiber	Pain, touch, reflex response
C-Sympathetic component	Postganglionic sympathetic nerve fibers

B fibers are most susceptible to hypoxia while A are most susceptible to pressure and C to action of local anaesthetics.

SYNAPSES AND NEUROMUSCULAR JUNCTION

Synapse

Synapses are specialized junctions between two or more neurons. The axon of one neuron divides into terminal buttons known as synaptic knobs which come in contact with soma or dendrites of another neuron (Fig. 8.8).

Components of a Synapse

1. **Presynaptic membrane:** It is the axolemma of the presynaptic neuron.
2. **Postsynaptic membrane:** It is the cell membrane of the postsynaptic neuron.
3. **Synaptic cleft:** A 20 to 30 nm wide cleft is present between the two membranes.

Types of Synapses

1. **Axo-dendritic:** Synapse between axon of one neuron with the dendrite of other neuron.
2. **Axo-somatic:** Synapse between axon of one neuron with the soma of other neuron.
3. **Axo-axonic:** Synapse between axon of one neuron with the axon of other neuron.
4. **Dendo-dendritic:** When dendrites of two different neurons make a synapse.

General Features of a Synapse

- The terminal portion of axons usually branch and end in terminal dilated ends named synaptic knobs.

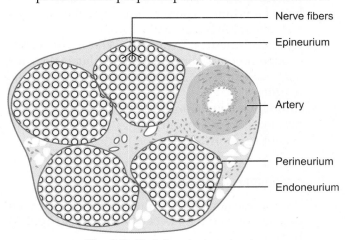

Fig. 8.7: Peripheral nerve trunk

Nerve fibers
Epineurium
Artery
Perineurium
Endoneurium

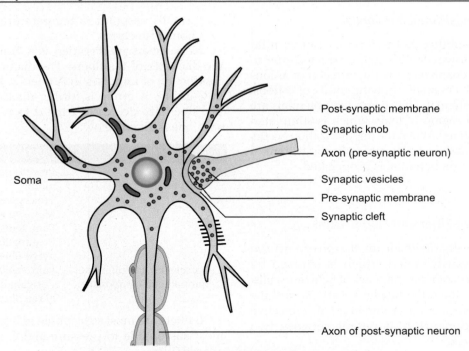

Fig. 8.8: Diagrammatic representation of a synapse

These knobs contain neurotransmitters bound in vesicles. These synaptic knobs form synapses with dendritic spines, proximal part of dendrites, cell bodies or end on axons of post synaptic neurons.

- The presynaptic terminal is seperated by a synaptic cleft from the postsynaptic neuron. It contains extra cellular fluid.
- The action potential on reaching the terminal end of an axon stimulates release of the neurotransmitter.
- Neurotransmitters are chemical mediators that bind to receptors present on the postsynaptic membrane. This interaction leads to opening or closing of ion channels. This means it can lead to excitation or inhibition of the postsynaptic neuron.
- Postsynaptic neurons receive inputs from axonal endings of a number of neurons. This is known as convergence. Also, axons may divide into branches and end on various post synaptic neurons. This is known as divergence.

Transmission of Impulses at Synapses

- Electrical changes at the presynaptic end cause influx of Ca^{2+} ions. This triggers release of the neurotransmitter substances.
- The neurotransmitters bind to receptors on postsynaptic neurons and can produce depolarization leading to excitatory post synaptic potentials or hyperpolarization leading to inhibitory postsynaptic potentials.

- The summation of stimulatory and excitatory potentials results in action potential if firing level is reached. The usual site of initiation of an impulse is the postsynaptic neuron is the initial segment of axon, just beyond its origin from cell body.
- There is a delay of about 0.5 ms between the impulse reaching the presynaptic terminal and response obtained in the postsynaptic neuron. This is known as **synaptic delay** and it covers the time taken for neurotransmitter release and action.
- Since the transmission of impulses is dependant on the action of neurotransmitters, synaptic junctions ensure one-way conduction. Any impulse generated in axon travels towards its terminal end (orthodromic conduction) and also towards the cell body (antidromic conduction). Thus, the impulses arriving at cell bodies will eventually decay.
- Excitatory neurotransmitters: These are acetylcholine, norepinephrine, aspartate, glutamate. They act by opening Na^+, Ca^{2+} channels in postsynaptic neurons.
- Inhibitory neurotransmitters: These are GABA, glycine. They act by opening Cl^- channels in postsynaptic neurons.

Neuromuscular Junction

- It is the junction between the terminal part of axon of a neuron and the skeletal muscle fiber supplied by it.

- The terminal part of axon is unmyelinated and divides into terminal synaptic button like endings. This is the presynaptic membrane.
- The part of muscle fiber coming in contact with axon is thickened and the sarcolemma is thrown into number of folds. This forms the postsynaptic membrane also named **motor-end plate**.
- The action potential at nerve endings increases Ca^{2+} influx which stimulates release of acetylcholine. Acetylcholine is the neurotransmitter at neuro-muscular junctions.
- Skeletal muscle membrane has N-receptors (nicotinic receptors) for acetylcholine. Activation of these receptors results in opening of Na^+ channels. The influx of Na^+ leads to depolarization of muscle fibers. The endplate potentials thus developed lead to formation of action potentials.

GLIAL CELLS

These consist of supporting cells present along the nerves in the nervous system. They are numerous in central nervous system (CNS) where they can be classified into four types:

1. **Microglia:** They are phagocytic cells similar to tissue macrophages and are derived from blood vessels.
2. **Oligodendrogliocytes:** These are rounded cells arranged in clusters. They synthesize and maintain myelin around axons of nerve fibers in CNS.
3. **Astrocytes:** They are relatively larger, star shaped cells which have membranous processes extending from the cell body called foot processes. They act as supporting cells and provide for **neurotropins** the growth factors to the nerve. They also form the blood brain barrier with capillary endothelium. They help in providing nutrition to the neurons.
4. **Ependymal cells:** Ependymal cells form blood CSF barrier and secrete CSF. These cells are present in ventricles of brain and central canal of spinal cord.

In the peripheral nervous system, Schwann cells are considered as glial cells.

GREY AND WHITE MATTER

The nervous tissue is made up of neurons, nerve fibers and the supporting neuroglial cells. Arrangement of nervous tissue in central nervous system is of two types:

1. **Grey matter:** These are areas primarily made up of neuronal cell bodies with dendrites and mostly unmyelinated axons with neuroglial cells. For example, various nuclei in the brain.
2. **White matter:** These are areas which consist primarily of nerve fibres or axons. The myelinated nerve fibres predominate in these areas which gives it a relatively pale or white colour.

CENTRAL NERVOUS SYSTEM

Cavity present in cranium of skull is known as cranial cavity. It lodges brain, meninges, CSF and blood supply of brain.

MENINGES

The brain is enclosed in three protective membranes called meninges (Figs 8.9, 8.10). From without inwards these are:

1. **Duramater (outermost):** pachymeninx
2. **Arachnoid mater (middle)**
3. **Pia mater (innermost)**

The three membranes are separated from each other by two spaces

1. **Subdural space:** It is a potential space present between the duramater and the arachnoid mater. It usually has a thin capillary layer of fluid in it.
2. **Subarachnoid space:** It lies between the arachnoid mater and the pia mater. Subarachnoid space contains cerebrospinal fluid (CSF).

The three meninges continue over the caudal extension of brain, i.e., spinal cord.

Dura Mater

Cranial dura is the thickest and the toughest membrane in our body. It consists of two layers:

1. **Outer endosteal layer:** It serves as the inner periosteum (endocranium). It lines the inner aspect of cranial cavity and becomes continuous with the periosteum (pericranium) over the skull at the sutures and foramina. This layer provides sheaths for various cranial nerves.
2. **Inner meningeal layer:** This layer encloses the brain. It continues as the spinal dura over the spinal cord, at the foramen magnum. It is mostly fused with the endosteal layer except, at places where venous sinuses are enclosed between the two layers.

Folds of Duramater

At places, the meningeal layer is folded on itself to form folds which serve as partitions that divide the cranial cavity into compartments (Fig. 8.9). These are:

1. **Falx cerebri:** It is a large sickle-shaped fold of duramater occupying the median longitudinal fissure between the two cerebral hemispheres. Various venous sinuses enclosed in the falx cerebri are:
   a. **Superior sagittal sinus:** It lies within the convex upper border.
   b. **Inferior sagittal sinus:** Is enclosed within the lower concave margin.
   c. **Straight sinus:** Lies along the line of attachment of the falx cerebri with the tentorium cerebelli.

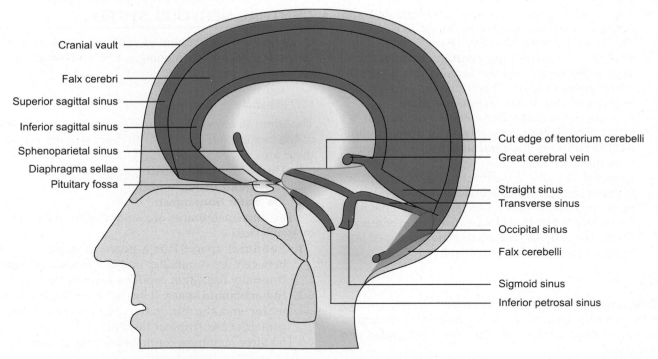

Fig. 8.9: Folds of duramater and dural venous sinuses (sagittal section of head and neck)

2. **Tentorium cerebelli:** It is a tent-shaped fold of duramater which forms the roof of posterior cranial fossa. It separates the cerebellum from the occipital lobes of cerebrum. Venous sinuses enclosed in the tentorium cerebelli on each side are
   a. **Transverse sinus:** Lies within the posterior part of the attached margin.
   b. **Superior petrosal sinus:** Present within the anterolateral part of the attached margin.
3. **Falx cerebelli:** It is a small sickle shaped fold of dura mater in the sagittal plane projecting forwards into the posterior cerebellar notch. Occipital sinus is enclosed within falx cerebelli, along its posterior attached part.
4 **Diaphragma sellae:** It is a small, circular, horizontally placed fold of dura mater that forms the roof of the hypophyseal fossa. It has a central aperture which provides passage to the stalk of the hypophysis cerebri.

Arterial Supply of Duramater

The outer layer is richly vascular but the inner layer, being more fibrous has little vascular supply. The cranial dura is supplied by branches of the following arteries:
1. Middle meningeal artery
2. Anterior ethmoidal artery
3. Posterior ethmoidal artery
4. Ophthalmic artery
5. Accessory meningeal artery

6. Internal carotid artery
7. Meningeal branch of ascending pharyngeal artery
8. Vertebral artery
9. Occipital artery

Nerve Supply of Duramater

The dura lining the floor of cranial cavity has a rich nerve supply and is quite sensitive to pain. It is supplied by the following nerves.
1. In the region of anterior cranial fossa, by anterior ethmoidal nerve and maxillary nerve.
2. In the middle cranial fossa, by maxillary nerve, mandibular nerve and trigeminal ganglion.
3. In the posterior cranial fossa, by recurrent branches from $C_{1,2,3}$ spinal nerves and meningeal branches from 9th, 10th and 12th cranial nerves.

Intracranial Dural Venous Sinuses (Fig. 8.9)

There are various venous channels enclosed within the cranial dura and they are present either between the two layers of cranial dura or between the reduplicated meningeal layer of dura. They are lined by endothelium only (muscular coat is absent) and do not have valves. They receive venous blood from cranial cavity and brain. CSF also drains into these sinuses. They receive valveless emissary veins which regulate the intracranial blood flow and maintain equilibrium of venous pressure within and outside the skull. There are seven paired and

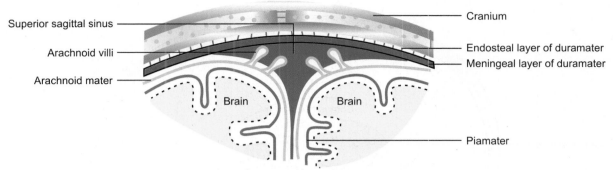

Fig. 8.10: Meninges of brain

seven unpaired sinuses. Unpaired sinuses are superior sagittal sinus, inferior sagittal sinus, straight sinus, occipital sinus, anterior intercavernous sinus, posterior intercavernous sinus, basilar venous plexus sinus. Paired sinuses are cavernous sinus, superior petrosal sinus, inferior petrosal sinus, transverse sinus, sigmoid sinus, spheno-parietal sinus and petro-squamous sinus.

Arachnoid Mater (Fig. 8.10)

It is a delicate membrane present between the dura mater and piamater. It is made up of mesothelial cells resting on a network of connective tissue. It covers the entire brain and provides a tubular sheath to the cranial nerves upto their exit from the skull. It presents with two special features namely,

1. **Subarachnoid cisternae (Fig. 8.11):** These are dilated subarachnoid spaces present in relation to the brain. There are six main cisternae, three in relation to the ventral surface of brain stem, two in relation to its dorsal surface and one within the brain. They are
   a. Pontine cistern
   b. Interpeduncular cistern
   c. Chiasmatic cistern
   d. Cisterna magna or cerebello-medullary cistern
   e. Cisterna ambiens or superior cistern
   f. Cistern of lateral fossa
   g. Cistern of lamina terminalis
   h. Callosal cistern
2. **Arachnoid villi and granulations (Figs 8.10, 8.11):** These are extentions of arachnoid mater along with subarachnoid space into the wall of dural venous sinuses.

Pia Mater (Fig. 8.10)

It is a thin, vascular membrane which intimately invests the surfaces of brain. It dips down in the cranial sulci and fissures.

Tela choroidea: These are bilaminar folds of pia mater present in relation to the 3rd ventricle and lower part of the roof of 4th ventricle. Tela choroidea provides for the vascular tufts of choroid plexuses.

Choroid Plexus

It is made up of numerous villi like projections on the ventricular aspect of the ependyma. Each villus consists of the following:
1. Capillary plexus, consisting of afferent and efferent vessels
2. Connective tissue stroma derived from pia mater
3. Cuboidal ependymal cells resting on basement with tight junctions.

Choroid plexus is present in following sites
1. C-shaped choroidal fissure of lateral ventricles
2. Roof of 3rd ventricle
3. Roof of 4th ventricle

Function of choroid plexus: It secretes the cerebrospinal fluid.

CEREBROSPINAL FLUID (CSF)

Cerebrospinal fluid is a clear, colourless and odourless fluid which fills the subarachnoid space and surrounds the brain and spinal cord. Biochemical studies have shown a higher concentration of Na^+, Cl^- and Mg^{2+}ions and a lower level of K^+, Ca^{2+} and glucose in CSF as compared to the plasma. It is considered to be actively secreted by the choroid plexus instead of the previous belief that it is an ultrafiltrate of the plasma.

Secretion of CSF: Cerebrospinal fluid is secreted by the choroid plexus of the lateral, 3rd and 4th ventricles. A small amount of CSF is also secreted by the ependymal cells of the central canal of spinal cord.

Characteristics of CSF

1. **Total volume:** It is about 130 to 150 ml. Out of this 25 ml lies in the ventricles and the rest is in the subarachnoid space.
2. Daily rate of production: 600 to 700 ml.
3. Rate of CSF formation per minute: 0.3 ml/min.
4. Normal CSF pressure: 80 to 180 mm of water or 60 to 150 mm of CSF.

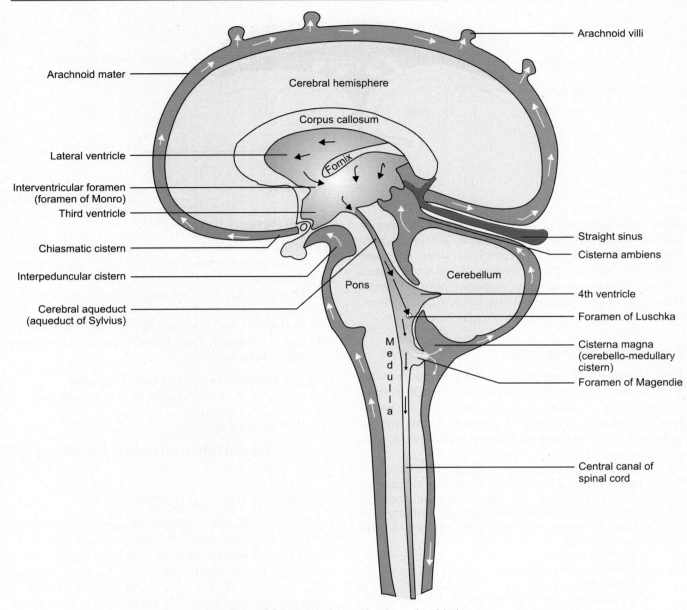

Fig. 8.11: CSF circulation and subarachnoid cisterns

5. PH: 7.35
6. Specific gravity: 1007.

Circulation of CSF (Fig. 8.11)

- CSF is produced in the lateral ventricles.
- It passes into the 3rd ventricle via the two interventricular formamina (foramen of Monro).
- Then it flows into the 4th ventricle through the aqueduct of Sylvius.
- From here, it enters the cerebello-medullary cistern through the foramen of Lusckha and Magendie.

- Finally, it fills the entire subarachnoid space.
- The CSF is absorbed back into circulation via the arachnoid villi from where it enters the superior sagittal sinus.

Absorption of CSF

1. CSF drains into the superior sagittal sinus through arachnoid granulations.
2. A small amount of fluid is absorbed into the cervical lymphatic system through the sheaths over the cranial nerves.
3. CSF flows from higher to lower pressures, from choroid plexus to arachnoid granulations.

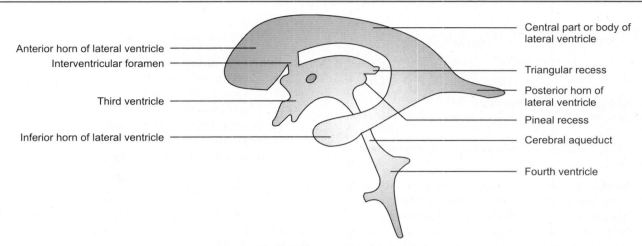

Fig. 8.12: Ventricular system of brain

Functions of CSF

1. Acts as a hydraulic shock absorber by providing a fluid filled jacket to the brain and spinal cord.
2. Provides a constant environment to neurons as they are highly sensitive and specialized cells.
3. Helps in the reduction of weight of brain due to forces of buoancy.
4. It conveys nutritive material to the central nervous system and helps in removal of waste products.

Ventricular System

It consists of a series of interconnecting spaces and channels within the brain. It contains the cerebrospinal fluid secreted by the choroid plexuses. There are a total of five ventricles present in the central nervous system (Fig. 8.12). These are

In Brain
1. 2 lateral ventricles
2. One 3rd ventricle
3. One 4th ventricle

In Spinal Cord
4. Terminal ventricle

Lateral ventricles: One lateral ventricle is present in each of the cerebral hemispheres. It is a C-shaped cavity lined by ependyma and filled with cerebrospinal fluid.

Third ventricle: It is a midline space present between the two thalami. It is lined by ependyma and represents the primitive cavity of forebrain vesicle.

Fourth ventricle: 4th ventricle is the cavity of the hind brain. It lies between the cerebellum dorsally and the pons and upper open part of medulla ventrally. It is almost shaped like a diamond. Three formina connect the forth ventricle to the sub arachnoid space of brain. These are, two formina of Luschka and one foramen of magendie which lie in the lower part of roof of 4th ventricle.

Terminal ventricle: It lies at the level of conus medullaris of spinal cord.

CEREBRAL HEMISPHERES

There are two cerebral hemispheres, each made up of cortical grey matter on the surface and white matter in the core. The cerebral hemispheres are separated from each other by a median longitudinal fissure. This fissure is incomplete. Corpus callosum obliterates the fissure in its middle part and connects the two hemispheres. A sickle shaped fold of meningeal layer of duramater, falx cerebri, occupies the median longitudinal fissure above the corpus callosum. A cavity is present in each cerebral hemisphere known as the lateral ventricle.

The nuclear masses of grey matter embedded in the white matter are known as the basal nuclei. Till the 3rd month of intra-uterine life each cerebral hemisphere remains smooth. Later sulci appear on them to accommodate more and more number of neurons. The surface of each cerebral hemisphere becomes convoluted to form gyri and sulci.

Each cerebral hemisphere presents with three borders, three poles and three surfaces (Fig. 8.13).

Borders of Cerebral Hemisphere
1. Superomedial border
2. Inferomedial border
3. Inferolateral border

Three poles
1. **Frontal pole:** It is the anterior end of the cerebral hemisphere which is blunt and rounded.
2. **Occipital pole:** It is the posterior end of the cerebral hemisphere. It is more pointed.
3. **Temporal pole:** It lies below and in front and is blunt and rounded.

Three surfaces
1. **Superolateral surface:** It is convex and takes the shape of the inner surface of vault of the skull.

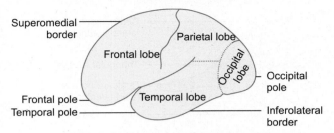

Fig. 8.13: Lobes and poles of cerebral hemisphere

2. **Medial surface:** It is flat, vertical and separated from the medial surface of the opposite cerebral hemisphere by the median longitudinal fissure.
3. **Inferior surface:** It is irregular and can be divided into anterior orbital and posterior tentorial parts.

Each hemisphere presents classically with six lobes. They are

1. Frontal lobe
2. Parietal lobe
3. Temporal lobe
4. Occipital lobe
5. Insular lobe
6. Limbic lobe

Functions of Cerebral Hemispheres

The cerebral hemispheres contain motor and sensory areas. Cerebral cortex is the highest level of control of motor activities both voluntary and involuntary. It is also the highest integration of various afferent inputs from the general and special sensory system.

Left cerebral hemisphere predominates in right handed person and the right cerebral hemisphere predominates in left handed person.

1. **Functions of right cerebral hemisphere**
   a. Non verbal commnication
   b. Musical skill
   c. Geometrical comprehension
   d. Spatial comprehension
   e. Temporal synthesis
2. **Functions of left cerebral hemisphere**
   a. Verbal communication
   b. Linguistic function
   c. Mathematical analysis
   d. Sequential comprehension
   e. Analytical function
   f. Direct link to consciousness

Functional Areas of Cerebral Cortex

Cortical areas have been divided into different functional areas by different neurobiologists namely Campbell Brodmann and Vogt. The most widely used classification is the Brodmann's classification (Figs 8.14 and 8.15).

Primary Motor Area – Area no. 4

- It lies in the precentral gyrus on the superolateral surface and in the anterior part of the paracentral lobe on the medial surface of cerebral hemisphere. It is structurally made up of agranular cortex.
- **Body representation in primary motor area:** The body is represented in upside down manner starting from the superolateral surface going to the medial surface of cerebral hemisphere.
  a. **Representations on superolateral surface (from below upwards):** Lip, tongue, larynx, pharynx, face, head and neck, upper extremity with extensive area for fingers and hand, trunk and lower extremity above the knee.
  b. **Representations on medial surface:** Lower extremity below knee, urinary bladder (micturition), anal canal (defecation) (Fig. 8.16).

The extent of representation of a body part depends upon the activity and skill of movements of that body part and not its size.

Cortical areas are divided into motor, sensory and psychical areas.

Sensory areas	Motor areas	Psychical cortex and area related to limbic system
Primary somesthetic area: 3, 1, 2 Secondary somesthetic area: below 4, 3, 1, 2 Somesthetic association area: 5, 7, 40 Primary visual area: 17 Association visual area: 18, 19 High visual association area: 39 Primary auditory area: 41 Auditory association area: 42 Wernicks area: 22 Area for smell: 28 Area for taste: 43	Motor area: 4 Premotor area: 6, 8 Frontal eye field: 8 Prefrontal speech area: 44, 45 Supplementary motor area: Posterior part of medial frontal gyrus Second motor area: Superior lip of posterior ramus of lateral sulcus	Anterior part of temporal lobe and temporal pole Areas related to limbic lobe: 23, 27, 36, 28, 38

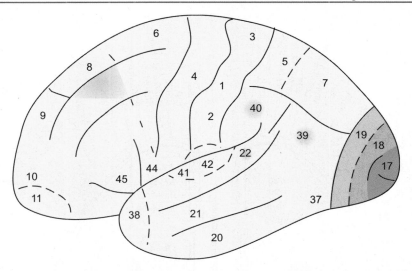

Fig. 8.14: Brodmann's functional areas of left cerebral cortex on supero-lateral surface

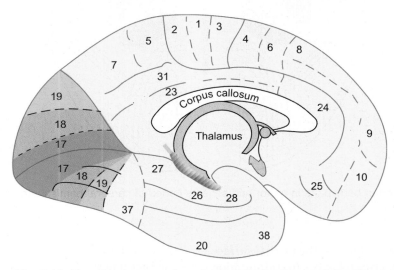

Fig. 8.15: Functional areas of cerebral cortex on the medial surface

Functions of Primary Motor Area

1. This area is responsible for the control of voluntary movements of contralateral side of the body.
2. It also controls micturition and defecation.

Premotor Area: Area no. 6 and 8

Area no. 6

It includes posterior part of superior, middle and inferior frontal gyri. It extends on the medial surface of the frontal lobe with supplementary frontal area.

Functions

1. It is responsible for control of skillful voluntary movements specially programming of movements.

2. Upper part of area no. 6 in dominant hemisphere is considered as the writing centre.
3. Lower part of area no. 6 which continues with area no. 44, 45, in frontal gyrus, controls the movement of lip, tongue, larynx, pharynx and palate.

Broca's Speech Area

It is area no. 44, 45. It is the motor speech area and lies in left cerebral hemisphere in a right handed person.

Area no. 8

It lies in front of area no. 6 and in posterior part of middle frontal gyrus. It is also known as frontal eye field.

Function: It regulates the voluntary conjugate movements of eyes.

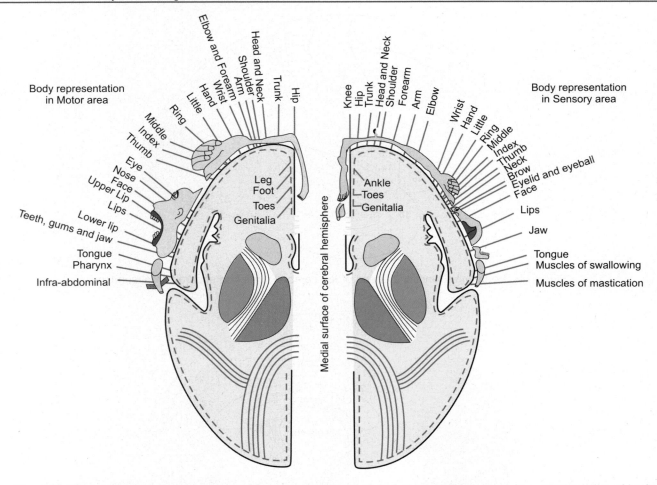

Fig. 8.16: Representation of body parts in motor and sensory cortex of cerebral hemisphere in coronal section of brain

Supplementary motor area: It lies on the medial surface in posterior part of medial frontal gyrus in continuation of area no. 6. Experimental evidences show that stimulation of this area leads to bilateral synergistic movements of postural nature.

Second motor area: It lies in the superior lip of posterior ramus of lateral sulcus just below area no. 4, 3, 1 and 2. Experimental evidence has shown that loss of second motor area leads to spasticity of muscles.

Prefrontal Cortex or Prefrontal Area (Fig. 8.14)

It lies in the frontal lobe. The area rostal to premotor area constitutes the prefrontal cortex. It is area no. 9 to 12.

Functions of prefrontal cortex: It is mainly related to the following functions of the individual.

1. Abstract thinking
2. Depth of feeling
3. Mature judgement
4. Foresight
5. Tactfulness
6. Pleasure and displeasure

Primary Somesthetic Area or Sensory Area

- **It is area no. 3, 1 and 2:** It is located on the post-central gyrus, on superolateral surface and extends to posterior part of paracentral lobule on medial cerebral surface. It is made up of granular cortex.
- **Body representation in primary somesthetic area:** It is again upside down as in the case of primary motor area. Lower limb, micturition and defecation functions are represented on the medial surface in posterior part of the paracentral lobule. It represents the contralateral side of the body (Fig. 8.16).

Functions of Primary Somesthetic Area

1. It is responsible for the localization, analysis and discrimination of cutaneous and proprioceptive impulses.

2. The lowest part of the post central gyrus acts as receptive centre for taste sensation.
3. Few motor fibres also arise from this area which modulate the sensory impulses.

Area	Functions
Area no. 3	It is responsible for cutaneous sensations of touch, pressure, position, vibration, pain and temperature.
Area no. 1	It is responsible for cutaneous and joint sense
Area no. 2	Deep proprioceptive senses from muscle and joints

Secondary Somesthetic Area

It lies in the upper lip of posterior ramus of lateral sulcus below area no. 4, 3, 1, 2. In this area the body is represented as face in front and leg behind.

Function: It is responsible perception of pain from the contralateral side of the body.

Somesthetic Association Area

It is the area no. 5, 7 lies in superior parietal lobule.
Function: It is responsible for processing for perception or recognition of general senses.

Higher Association Somesthetic Area

It is the area no. 40 which and lies in supramarginal gyrus. It is connected with area no. 5, 7. There are reciprocal connections with pulvinar also.
Function: It is responsible for sense of stereognosis.

Primary Visual Area

It is the area no. 17. It lies along the lips and wall of calcarine sulcus and includes the cuneus and lingual gyrus. This area is limited by the lunate sulcus and is also known as the **striate cortex.**
Function: This area is responsible for simple visual impression. Detail analysis and discrimination is not done in this area.

Visual Association Area

Area no. 18, 19 are known as visual association area. They surround area no. 17 on medial and lateral surfaces of occipital lobe area no. 18 responds to linear stimuli where as area no.19 to angular stimuli. This area is also known as the parastriate cortex.
Function: It helps in recognition of objects. It is also responsible for producing conjugate eye movements in opposite direction. Therefore is also known as the **occipital eye field.**

Higher Visual Association Area

Area no. 39, it is located in angular gyrus of parietal lobe.
Function: Its function is to comprehend the various objects and symbols of language by vision.

Primary Auditory Area

It is area no. 41 and lies in the anterior transverse temporal gyrus. It has bilateral representation.
Functions: It is responsible for detection of frequency of sound and direction from where a sound is originated. Low frequency sound is detected in antero-lateral part and high frequency sounds are detected in postero-medial part of anterior transverse temporal gyrus.

Auditory Association Area

Area no. 42. It lies in posterior transverse gyrus.
Function: It correlates the present auditory information with the past experience.

Higher Auditory Association Area

It is the area no. 22 which lies in posterior transverse temporal gyrus. It is also known as Wernicke's area.
Function: It is concerned with comprehension of spoken language and interpretation of sound.

Vestibular Area

It lies in the lower part of postcentral gyrus.
Functions: It helps in motor regulation and conscious spatial orientation that maintains equilibrium of the body.

Area for Taste

It is area no. 43. It lies in the superior wall of the posterior ramus of lateral sulcus adjacent to the lower part of the somesthetic area.
Function: Responsible for perception of taste sensations.

Psychical Cortex

It is the region of anterior part of the temporal lobe. It is responsible for recall of seen, music heard and other experience of recent past when electrically stimulated.

White Matter of Cerebrum

White matter of cerebrum is arranged in the following three types (Fig. 8.17):
1. Association fibres
2. Projection fibres
3. Commissural fibres

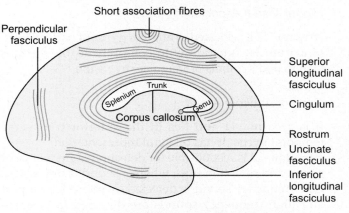

Fig. 8.17: Bundles of fibres in cerebral hemisphere

Association Fibres

These fibres connect one functional area of the cerebral cortex to the other of the same cerebral hemisphere. The various association fibres are described below:

1. Cingulum

2. Superior longitudinal fasciculus
3. Inferior longitudinal bundle
4. Uncinate fasciculus
5. Fronto-occipital fasciculus

Projection Fibres

These fibres connect cerebral cortex to other parts of brain and spinal cord. They include to and fro fibres from the cerebral cortex. These are:

1. Fimbria
2. Fornix
3. Corona radiata
4. **Internal capsule:** It is a compact V shaped band of neocortical projection fibres. It lies in the deep substance of each cerebral hemisphere.

Commissural Fibres

These fibres connect functional area between the two cerebral hemispheres. The various commissural fibres are described below:

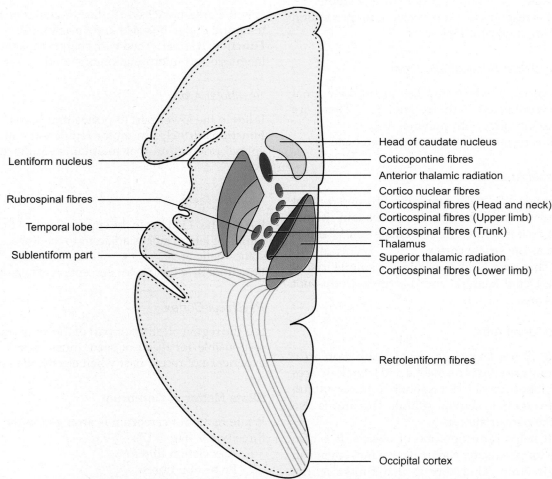

Fig. 8.18: Internal capsule (horizontal section of left cerebral hemisphere)

1. Anterior commissure
2. Hippocampal commissure
3. Habenular commissure
4. Posterior commissure
5. Corpus callosum

Corpus Callosum

It is the largest band of commissural fibres of the neocortex which connects most of the functional areas of the cerebral hemisphere. It is an arched band of fibres with convexity directed upwards. It can be divided into following parts from before backwards

1. Rostrum
2. Genu
3. Trunk
4. Splenium

Functions of Corpus Callosum

1. Transfer of learning process from one hemisphere to another.
2. Transfer of speech function from one hemisphere to another.

Internal Capsule

It lies in the deep substance of each cerebral hemisphere. It is a compact bundle of fibres which consists of afferent and efferent fibres of the neocortex. It is V-shaped on cross section with the concavity directed laterally (Fig. 8.18).

Extent

Superiorly	:	It is continuous with the corona radiata.
Inferiorly	:	It is continuous with the crus cerebrum of the midbrain.
Medially	:	It is bounded by head of caudate nucleus and thalamus.
Laterally	:	It is bounded by lentiform nucleus.

Fibres passing through internal capsule are shown in (Fig. 8.18)

BASAL GANGLIA

Basal ganglia are primarily masses of grey matter which lie in the white core of each cerebral hemisphere. The basal ganglia receive inputs from thalamus and cerebral cortex (corticostriate projection) to thalamus and then on to cerebral cortex. Their exact function is unclear but they are responsible for planning and programming of movement. They comprise of the following (Figs 8.19, 8.20):

1. Corpus striatum
2. Claustrum
3. Amygdaloid body

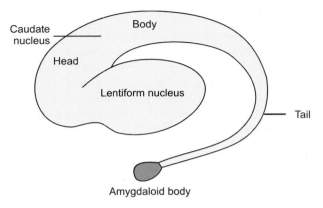

Fig. 8.19: Components of basal ganglia

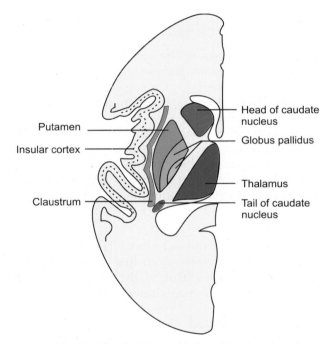

Fig. 8.20: Components of basal ganglia

Corpus Striatum

It is divided into two parts by the fibres of internal capsule.

1. **Caudate nucleus:** It is the medial band of grey matter.
2. **Lentiform nucleus:** It consists of a biconvex mass of grey matter that lies lateral to the caudate nucleus. It is further divided into two parts by the external medullary lamina.
   a. **Putamen:** The outer larger part which is dark in colour.
   b. **Globus pallidus:** The inner pale part. An internal lamina further divides it into outer and inner segments.

Claustrum

It is a thin sheet of grey matter present between the putamen and the insular cortex. It is separated from the putamen by a thin sheet of white matter called the external capsule. The white matter of insula (extreme capsule) separates it from the insular cortex. Antero-inferiorly, it is continuous with the anterior perforated substance and amygdaloid body.

Amygdaloid Body

It is continuous with the tail of caudate nucleus but structurally and functionally it is related to the limbic system.

Functions of Basal Ganglia

Basal ganglia belong to the extra pyramidal system. Following functions are assigned to them.
1. Help in regulation of muscle tone through its connections with substantia nigra, thalamus and cerebral cortex.
2. Suppress abnormal involuntary movements by acting on the descending pathways to spinal cord.
3. Play an important role in controlling the axial and girdle movements of the body and positioning of proximal parts of the limbs.

DIENCEPHALON

It is also known as the interbrain. The diencephalon consists of grey matter which lies between the two cerebral hemispheres around the cavity of the 3rd ventricle. Inferiorly, it is continuous with the midbrain.

Parts of Diencephalon

Diencephalon is made up of the following parts (Fig. 8.21)
1. **Thalamus (dorsal thalamus):** It lies in the dorsal part of the diencephalon.
2. **Epithalamus:** It lies dorsomedial to the dorsal thalamus. It consists of pineal gland, habenular nucleus, habenular commissure and posterior commissure.
3. **Metathalamus:** It is formed by the medial and lateral geniculate bodies which are incorported into the caudal part of thalamus.
4. **Subthalamus (ventral thalamus):** It lies lateral to the hypothalamus and consists of the subthalamic nuclei and rostral extension of red nucleus and substantia nigra.
5. **Hypothalamus:** It lies below the hypothalamic sulcus and forms the most ventral part of the diencephalon.

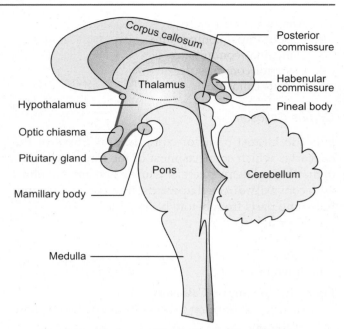

Fig. 8.21: Thalamus, Epithalamus, Hypothalamus

Dorsal Thalamus (Thalamus) (Fig. 8.22)

There are two thalami. Each thalamus is an ovoid mass of grey matter present on each side in relation to the lateral walls of the 3rd ventricle, dorsal to hypothalamic sulcus. **Both thalami act as the highest relay centre for all sensations except olfaction.**

Measurements

Antero-posterioly	:	4 cm
Vertically	:	1.5 cm
Transversely	:	1.5 cm

Presenting Parts

It has two ends and four surfaces (Fig. 8.22).

Anterior end: It is narrow and forms the posterior boundary of interventricular foramen.

Posterior end: It is broad and overlaps the superior colliculus of midbrain. This end is also known as the pulvinar. It presents caudally with the lateral and medial geniculate bodies.

Superior surface: It is convex. Lateral part of the upper surface of the thalamus forms the floor of the central part of lateral ventricle. The medial area of the upper surface is separated from the body of the fornix by the tela choroidea of the 3rd ventricle.

Inferior surface: It is related to zona incerta and the subthalamic nuclei.

Medial surface: It forms a major part of the lateral wall of the 3rd ventricle and is lined by ependyma.

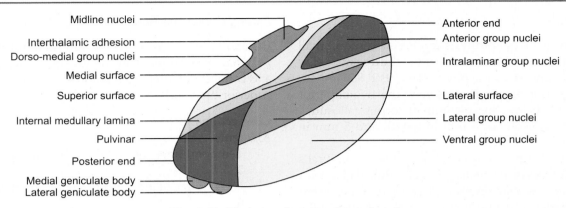

Fig. 8.22: Thalamus (as seen from above)

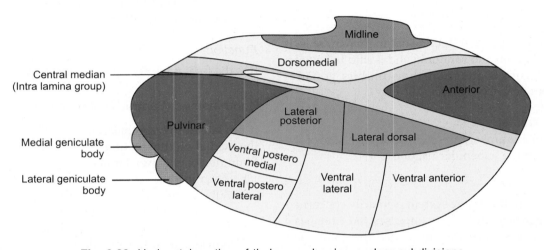

Fig. 8.23: Horizontal section of thalamus showing nuclear subdivisions

Lateral surface: It is related to posterior limb of internal capsule which separates it from the lentiform nucleus.

Nuclear Subdivisions of Thalamus

Six groups of nuclei are identified in the thalamus. All the nuclei are connected to the cerebral cortex and also to other parts of the brain. These nuclei are (Fig. 8.23):

1. Anterior nuclei
2. Lateral nuclei
3. Dorsomedial nuclei
4. Midline nuclei
5. Intralaminar nuclei
6. Reticular thalamic nuclei

Functions of Thalamus

1. The thalamus is the major relay station for sensory inputs from all over the body It receives impulses from somatic afferents, special afferents (except smell) and reticular afferents. It integrates and relays inputs to cerebral cortex. Processing and integration of various impulses is also done in thalamus.
2. It has a significant role in arousal and alertness, with the help of intra-laminar, midline, dorsolateral and anterior group of nuclei.
3. It regulates the activities of motor pathway by connecting the cerebellum and globus pallidus with motor cerebral cortex.
4. It is associated with the autonomic control of viscera through its connections with the hypothalamus
5. It plays a role in an individual's personality and intellect through the frontal lobe connections.
6. Thalamus helps in appreciating the pain and temperature sense.
7. The integration of various inputs is responsible for the emotional response that occurs on the basis of information processed by thalamus.

Pineal Body

- Pineal gland or **epiphysis cerebri** is a conical, small organ attached to the roof of the third ventricle by a stalk known as the pineal stalk (Fig. 8.21).
- It lies in a depression between the two superior colliculi, below the splenium of corpus callosum.
- It measures about 8 mm in length and 5 mm in width.
- It is made up of pinealocytes or parenchymal cells and astrocyte like neuroglial cells. Pineal gland is a highly vascular organ and contains fenestrated capillaries. Calcium granules get deposited in the gland after puberty.

Function

Pineal gland is a neuro-endocrine organ in mammals. It is rich in melatonin and seretonin and is said to have an antigonadotrophic function that inhibits gonadal development before puberty.

Habenular Nuclei

They are two in number, present one on each side of the pineal stalk in the habenular trigone.

Function

It forms a part of the limbic system primarily concerned with the integration of olfactory impulses and other basic emotional drives to further influence the concerned viscera.

Metathalamus

It is the dorsal part of thalamus and consists of following two parts:

Medial Geniculate Body

It is an oval shaped elevation on the inferior aspect of pulvinar with the long axis directed anterolaterally.

Connections
Afferents
1. Mostly from the inferior colliculus of the same side. A few fibres come from opposite side
2. Lateral lemniscus
Efferents
1. Form the auditory radiation which terminates in the auditory area of temporal lobe, area no. 42, 41.

Function

It is the final relay centre for hearing.

Lateral Geniculate Body

It is an oval elevation in the inferolateral aspect of pulvinar. It is larger than the medial geniculate body and connected with the superior colliculus through the superior brachium.

Connections
Afferents
1. Temporal fibres of the retina of same side in layer 2, 3, 5.
2. Nasal fibres of the opposite retina end in layer 1, 4, 6
Efferents
1. Efferent fibres form the optic radiation which terminates in the occipital cortex or visual cortex area no. 17, 18, 19.

Function

It is the final relay centre in the visual pathway.

Subthalamus (Ventral Thalamus)

It lies lateral to hypothalamus and hence is not seen in the medial sagittal section.
Main nuclei of subthalamus
1. Zona incerta
2. Subthalamic nucleus
3. Cranial extension of substantia nigra.
4. Cranial extension of red nucleus.
5. Nucleus of ansa lenticularis.

Hypothalamus

Hypothalamus lies in the ventral part of the diencephalon and consists of collection of nerve cells in a matrix of neuroglial tissue (Figs 8.21 and 8.24).

Extent

Dorsally	:	Hypothalamic sulcus, thalamus
Ventrally	:	Lamina terminalis
Superiorly	:	Lamina terminalis
Inferiorly	:	Upto the vertical plane just caudal to the mamillary bodies
Medially	:	Ependymal lining of 3rd ventricle
Laterally	:	Upto the subthalamus and internal capsule.

Nuclei of Hypothalamus

Hypothalamus is divided into lateral and medial areas by a column of fornix, mamillo-thalamic tract and fasciculus-retroflexus. The nuclei are arranged in four regions and are tabulated below:

Preoptic region	Supra-optic region	Tuberal-infundibular region	Mamillary region
Preoptic nucleus: Lies in the anterior wall of the 3rd ventricle, between the supraoptic nucleus below and the anterior commissure above.	It lies above the level of optic chiasma and consists of 1. Ventromedial nucleus 2. Suprachiasmatic nucleus 3. Anterior nucleus 4. Paraventricular nucleus	Is the widest part which lies above the tuber cinereum and has the following nuclei 1. Medial nucleus 2. Dorsomedial nucleus 3. Arcuate nucleus 4. Posterior hypothalamic nucleus 5. Lateral hypothalamic nucleus	Consists of the mamillary bodies with the following nuclei 1. Supraoptic nucleus 2. Lateral nucleus 3. Intercalated nucleus

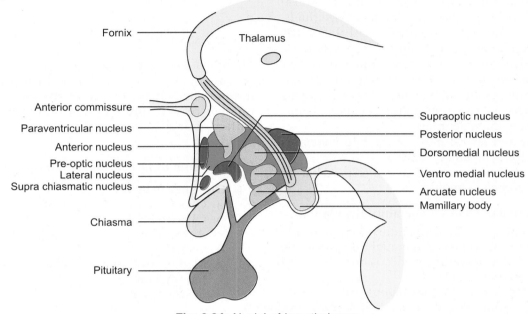

Fig. 8.24: Nuclei of hypothalamus

Connections of Hypothalamus

- The hypothalamus receives afferents from limbic system (hippocampus and amygdaloid nucleus) midbrain, pons, retina, thalamus and basal ganglia
- The hypothalamus sends efferents to limbic system, thalamus and cingulated gyrus in cerebrum, reticular formation of midbrain which projects to spinal motro neurons and posterior pituitary.

Functions of Hypothalamus

1. **Neuro-endocrine control:** It secretes following hormones:
   a. CRH: Corticotropin releasing hormone
   b. GnRH: Gonadotrophin releasing hormone
   c. Prolactin releasing hormone
   d. Prolactin inhibitory hormone (identified as neurotransmitter dopamine)
   e. Growth hormone releasing hormone
   f. TRH: Thyrotropin releasing hormone
   g. ADH
   h. Oxytocin
2. Regulates body temperature
3. Regulates circadian (day-night) rhythm of various activity eg. sleep, appetite
4. Controls emotional behaviour, e.g., fear and anger etc. It integrates autonomic motor and endocrinal responses to various afferent stimuli.
5. Regulates various functions for body preservation
   a. Hunger and satiety
   b. Thirst
   c. Sexual behaviour
6. Regulates autonomic nervous system activity.
   a. Posterior and lateral parts of the hypothalamus regulate the sympathetic activity.
   b. Preoptic and supraoptic areas are responsible for parasympathetic activity.

Role of hypothalamus on hunger and satiety

- Hypothalamus has a hunger centre, located laterally. This is continuously active and responsible for appetite.
- It also has a satiety centre, located venteromedially. This acts to inhibit function of hunger centre.

- Satiety centre is stimulated by:
  1. Food in GIT: Via action of peptide hormone
  2. Blood glucose levels: hyperglycemia increases uptake of glucose by hypothalamus
  3. Hormonal stimuli: From adipose tissue, insulin and glucagon levels
  4. Temperature of body: Rise in temperature inhibits appetite.

Role of Hypothalamus in Thirst

- Hypothalamus has osmoreceptors in lateral preoptic area that sence osmolality of body fluids. Increase plasma osmolality stimulates the osmoreceptors responsible for thrist sensation.
- Fall in ECF volume as seen in hemorrhage and dehydration due to diarrhea activates renin-angiotensin system. Angiotensin II thus produced acts on specialized receptor area of hypothalamus to stimulate thirst neurons.
  Posterior and lateral parts of the hypothalamus regulate the sympathetic activity.
  Preoptic and supraoptic areas are responsible for parasympathetic activity.

Role of Hypothalamus in Temperature Regulation

- The normal oral body temperature is traditionally said to be 37°C. There is a day-night fluctuation of 0.5 to 0.7°C. Temperature of body is lowest at 6 AM and highest in evening.
- The hypothalamus integrates inputs from sensory receptors from skin, deep tissues, spinal cord, cerebral cortex and hypothalamus itself.
- The posterior hypothalamus is responsible for initiating the following responses to cold like:
  a. Shivering (at 35.5°C), increase hunger, increase motor activity and stimulation of adrenergic activity that helps to increase heat production.

b. Vasoconstriction (starts at 36.8°C) in cutaneous circulation helps to conserve heat.
c. Reflex curling up of the body helps to decrease surface area and reduce heat loss.
- The anterior hypothalamus is responsible for initiatating response to warmth like:
  a. Cutaneous vasodilatation (starts above 37°C), sweating, and increase respiration to increase heat loss.
  b. Decrease appetite and activity to decrease heat production.

LIMBIC SYSTEM

The term limbic system was introduced by Broca in 1878. Its functions are concerned with preservation of individuals and furthering of species. It includes a number of structures present on the infero-medial surface of cerebral hemispheres.

Components of Limbic System (Fig. 8.25)

1. **Olfactory pathway**
   a. Olfactory nerve
   b. Olfactory bulb
   c. Anterior olfactory nucleus
   d. Olfactory tract
   e. Medial and lateral olfactory stria and their termination
   f. Olfactory cortex

2. **Pyriform lobe**
   a. Pre-pyriform region: It includes lateral olfactory gyrus and gyrus ambiens
   b. Para-amygdaloid region: It includes gyrus semilunaris
   c. Entorhinal area: Area no. 28.

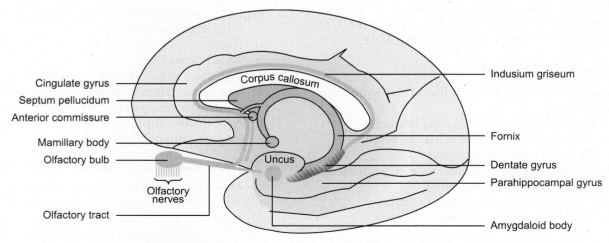

Fig. 8.25: Components of limbic system (medial and inferior surface of right cerebral hemisphere)

3. **Amygdaloid body and its efferent pathways**
   a. Amygdaloid body
   b. Stria terminalis
4. **Hippocampus formation**
   a. Indusium griseum
   b. Longitudinal stria
   c. Gyrus fasiolaris
   d. Dentate gyrus
   e. Hippocampus
   f. Alveus
   g. Fimbria
   h. Fornix
5. **Limbic lobe**
   a. Septal area
   b. Cingulate gyrus
   c. Parahippocampal gyrus
6. **Other structures related to limbic system**
   a. Hypothalamus
   b. Habenular nucleus
   c. Anterior nucleus of thalamus
   d. Midbrain
   e. Stria medullaris thalami
   f. Fasciculus retroflexus
   g. Medial longitudinal bundle
   h. Interpeduncular nucleus

Olfactory nerves: These are the central processes of the bipolar olfactory neurons present in the olfactory epithelium which lie in relation to the roof, adjoining septum and lateral wall of nasal cavity. The olfactory mucosa covers an area of 2.5 cm^2. There are almost 10 million olfactory neurons present in man. Olfactory nerves consist of 15 to 20 bundles of fibres which pass through the cribriform plate of ethmoid bone and terminate in the olfactory bulb.

Olfactory bulb: These are two in number, present one on each side of midline in the orbital surface of the frontal lobe of cerebral hemisphere.

Olfactory cortex: It is divided into
   a. Primary olfactory cortex
   b. Secondary olfactory cortex–Entorhinal area no. 28.

Functions of Limbic System

It is primarily concerned with the following
1. **Preservation of individual:** Searching for food and drink, defense mechanisms .
2. **Preservation of species:** Sexual and mating behavior, rearing of new born, social behavior.
3. **Emotional behavior:** Mood, fear, anger, pleasure, physical expression of emotions.
4. **Recent memory:** Storage of events, sense of time.

Parts of limbic system and their functions

Parts of limbic system	Functions
1. Olfactory pathway	• Highly developed in lower vertebrates • Concerned with sensation of smell • Integration of various impulses with smell and activation of other neuronal pathways responsible for emotional behaviour, salivation, gastrointestinal motility and sexual urge (in lower vertebrates)
2. Hippocampus formation	Arousal response
3. Amygdaloid body	Sexual behavior, aggression and fear response
4. Amygdaloid body, hippocampus, mamillary body, cingulate gyrus	Recent memory
5. Septal area	Pleasure
6. Septal area, hippocampus, hypothalamus	Removal centre

RETICULAR FORMATION

It is a diffuse network of nerve fibres and neurons which occupy the ventral part of the entire brain stem (midbrain, pons and medulla). It occupies the area between the cranial nerve nuclei, sensory and motor nuclei and the named long and short white tracts. It is considered as the most ancient part of the central nervous system in vertebrate phylogeny. However, now it is believed that the highly specific pyramidal and extrapyramidal systems and the non-specific network of reticular formation are both indispensable and have evolved as interdependant paths which contribute to the total response of the organism (Fig. 8.26).

Characteristics of Reticular Formation

Reticular formation consists of deeply placed ill-defined collection of neurons and fibres. It has diffuse connections. This system contains serotonergic, cholinergic and catecholamine group of neurons. It consists of two pathways:

1. **Ascending reticular pathway**
   • It is also called reticular activating system. It receives inputs from all sensory pathways, visceral afferents and from autditory and visual pathway.

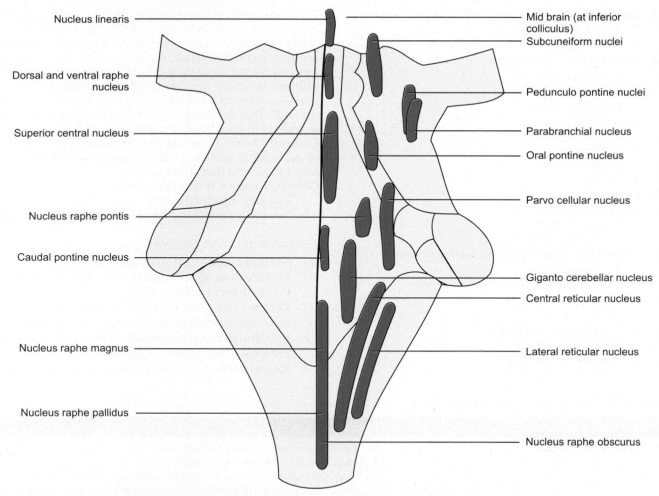

Nucleus linearis

Dorsal and ventral raphe nucleus

Superior central nucleus

Nucleus raphe pontis

Caudal pontine nucleus

Nucleus raphe magnus

Nucleus raphe pallidus

Mid brain (at inferior colliculus)

Subcuneiform nuclei

Pedunculo pontine nuclei

Parabranchial nucleus

Oral pontine nucleus

Parvo cellular nucleus

Giganto cerebellar nucleus

Central reticular nucleus

Lateral reticular nucleus

Nucleus raphe obscurus

Fig. 8.26: Location of various reticular nuclei in the brain stem (dorsal view)

- The fibers ascend from pons to thalamus and have multisynaptic connections with cerebral cortex.
- It is the pathway for alertness and conscious state of body.

2. Descending reticular pathway
- It is both inhibitory and facilitatory
- The inhibitory fibers project to motor cortex, cerebellum, medulla and via reticulospinal tract to spinal neurons. They inhibit movements.
- The facilitatory fibers descend on spinal neurons and produced movements.

Extent

Rostral   :   Diencephalon. It includes the intralaminar and ventral anterior nuclei of thalamus, hypothalamus, zona incerta of subthalamus.

Caudal   :   It is considered to extend till the neurons of lamina VII of spinal grey matter as the spinoreticular and reticulospinal tracts.

Functions of Reticular Formation

It forms an important component of the somatic and visceral functions of the body. Unilateral stimulation of the reticular pathway often leads to a bilateral response.

1. It is essential for life. The neurons of reticular formation are grouped in medulla forming centres for respiration, cardiovascular function etc.
2. It is responsible for conscious perception of surroundings at each time.
3. Control of the stretch reflexes, movement and posture of body.

MID BRAIN

Midbrain is the shortest segment of the brain stem (only 2 cm long). It extends ventro-rostrally from the pons to the diencephalon and lies in the posterior cranial fossa between the dorsum sellae of sphenoid bone in front and the notch of tentorium cerebelli behind (Fig. 8.33).

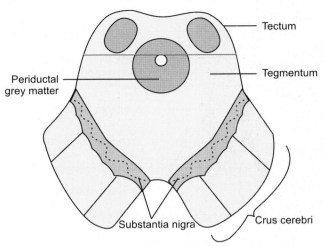

Fig. 8.27: Parts of mid brain (in transverse section)

Components

The mid brain can be divided into two cerebral peduncles, one on each side of midline which enclose the cerebral aqueduct. Each cerebral peduncle further consists of four parts arranged venterodorsally. These are (Fig. 8.27):

1. **Crus cerebri:** Extends from the cranial border of pons to undersurface of the cerebral hemispheres
2. **Substantia nigra:** A pigmented nerve cell zone present between the crus cerebri and the tegmentum.
3. **Tegmentum:** Tegmentum is the part which lies ventral to an imaginary coronal plane passing through the cerebral aqueduct and dorsal to substantia nigra.
4. **Tectum:** Dorsal part of midbrain present posterior to the line passing through cerebral aqueduct. It is made up of a pair of superior and inferior colliculi.

External Features

Crus cerebri: The ventral surface of midbrain presents two crura cerebri which extend rostrally from the cranial border of pons. They diverge on each side of the interpeduncular fossa as they ascend up to disappear under the cerebral hemispheres. Superficial surface of each crus cerebri is corrugated and is crossed from above downwards by

1. Optic tract
2. Posterior cerebral artery
3. Superior cerebellar artery

The oculomotor nerve arises from a medial sulcus present on each crus. The trochlear nerve winds around the lateral side of each crus.

Tectum: The dorsal surface of midbrain presents with four rounded elevations, a pair of superior colliculi and a pair of inferior colliculi, one on each side of midline. The two superior colliculi are separated from each other by a median vertical sulcus or the cruciform sulcus. A horizontal sulcus is seen between the two superior and the two inferior colliculi. The dorsal surface of midbrain is demarcated from the pons by the trochlear nerves which emerge by the side of the frenulum veli and pass ventrally.

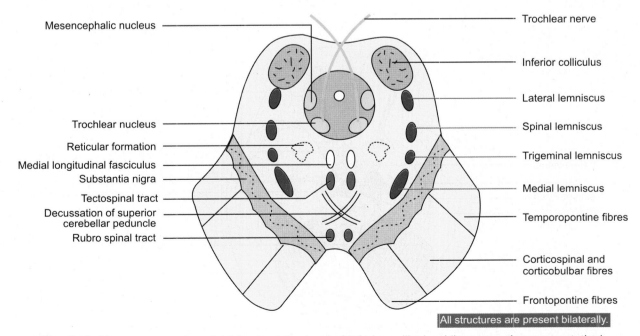

Fig. 8.28: Transverse section of midbrain at the level of inferior colliculus (diagrammatic representation)

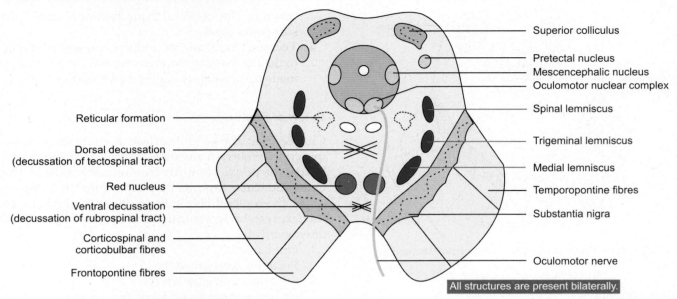

Fig. 8.29: Transverse section of midbrain at the level of superior colliculus (diagrammatic representation)

Internal Structure of Mid Brain

- The mid brain is studied in two transverse sections, one at the level of inferior colliculus and the second at the level of superior colliculus (Figs 8.28 and 8.29).
- Venterodorsally both sections present with
  a. Cura cerebri
  b. Substantia nigra
  c. Tegmentum with cerebral aqueduct and periaqueductal grey matter.
  d. Tectum

Interpeduncular Fossa

This fossa is present in relation to base of brain between optic chiasma and crus cerebri (Fig. 8.30).

Boundaries

Anterior	:	Caudal border of optic chiasma
Anterolateral	:	Optic tract on each side
Posterolateral	:	Crus cerebri on each side
Posterior	:	Cranial border of pons

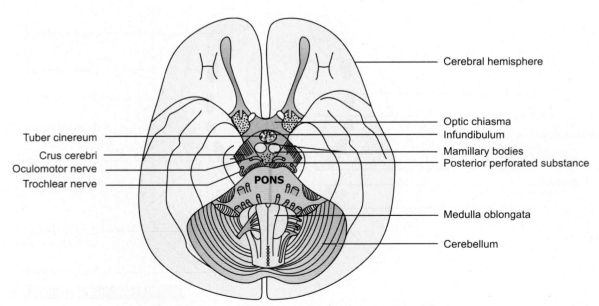

Fig. 8.30: Base of brain showing interpeduncular fossa

Structures present in the floor of the interpeduncular fossa (from before backwards)
  a. Infundibular stem
  b. Tuber cinereum
  c. Median eminence
  d. A pair of mamillary bodies
  e. Posterior perforated substace – It is the area of grey matter which is pierced by the central branches of posterior cerebral arteries.

PONS

Pons means bridge. It is that part of brain stem which connects the midbrain to medulla and is also known as the metencephalon. Ventrally, it is related to clivus and dorsally, to the 4th ventricle and cerebellum. Laterally, on each side, are present the middle cerebellar peduncles which connect it to the corresponding lobes of cerebellum (Fig. 8.33).

Extent : Upper end of medulla oblongata to the cerebral peduncles of midbrain.

External Features

It has ventral and dorsal surfaces.

Ventral Surface

- It rests on the clivus and is convex from side to side and from above downwards.
- It presents a longitudinal sulcus in the middle known as sulcus basilaris which lodges the basilar artery.
- Ventral surface is continuous on each side with the middle cerebellar peduncle.
- The two roots of trigeminal nerve (sensory and motor) are attached about the mid pontine level at its junction with the middle cerebellar peduncle.

- This surface shows numerous transverse ridges and grooves.
- A horizontal sulcus is present between the medulla and pons. This gives attachment to the VI, VII and VIII cranial nerves from medial to lateral direction.
- Peripheral end of the horizontal sulcus on each side forms the cerebello-pontine angle.

Dorsal Surface

- The dorsal surface of pons forms the upper part of floor of 4th ventricle.
- It lies rostral to the stria medullaris and is overlapped by the superior cerebellar peduncles on lateral side.
- The median sulcus continues up from medulla and divides the dorsal surface into 2 equal halves.
- Each half is further divided into a medial and a lateral part by the sulcus limitans. This sulcus presents with a deep depression known as superior fovea at the lower end of pons where the floor of 4th ventricle is widest.
- The medial area presents with a rounded elevation next to the superior fovea called the facial colliculus. It is formed by the internal genu of motor fibres of facial nerve which wind around the abducent nerve nucleus
- The lateral area forms the vestibular area overlying the four groups of vestibular nuclei.

Internal Structure

On cross section the pons is studied in two parts (Figs 8.31 and 8.32):
  1. Ventral or basilar part
  2. Dorsal or tegmental part

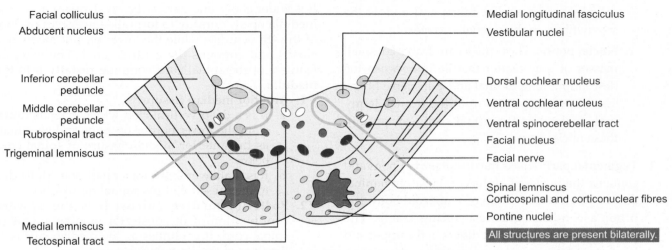

Facial colliculus
Abducent nucleus

Inferior cerebellar peduncle
Middle cerebellar peduncle
Rubrospinal tract
Trigeminal lemniscus

Medial lemniscus
Tectospinal tract

Medial longitudinal fasciculus
Vestibular nuclei

Dorsal cochlear nucleus
Ventral cochlear nucleus
Ventral spinocerebellar tract
Facial nucleus
Facial nerve

Spinal lemniscus
Corticospinal and corticonuclear fibres
Pontine nuclei

All structures are present bilaterally.

Fig. 8.31: Transverse section of pons at the level of facial colliculus (diagrammatic representation)

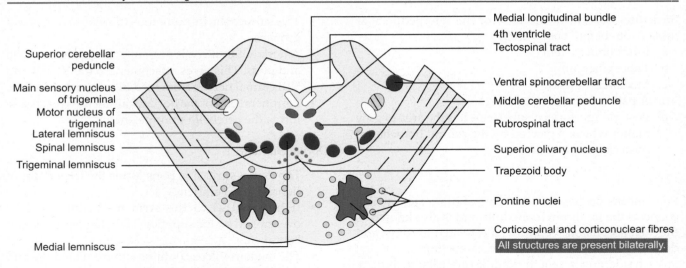

Fig. 8.32: Transverse section of pons at its upper part (diagrammatic representation)

1. **The basilar part:** It is occupied by the descending longitudinal and transverse fibres and the nuclei pontis.

   a. The following **longitudinal fibres** descend from the basis pedunculi of midbrain.
   — **Corticospinal fibres:** These continue downward and form the pyramids in the medulla oblongata.
   — **Corticonuclear fibres:** These end in the nuclei of cranial nerves in the pons.
   — **Corticopontine fibres:** They synapse in the nuclei pontis.

   b. **Transverse fibres:** These are axons of the nuclei pontis which cross to the opposite side and run in the middle cerebellar peduncle. They are called pontocerebellar fibres and end as the mossy fibres in the cerebellar cortex.

   c. **Nuclei pontis:** These nuclei are scattered, small masses of grey matter that lie in between the descending longitudinal and transverse fibres. The descending fibres from the frontal, temporal, parietal and occipital cortex synapse in these nuclei pontis.

2. **Tegmental part:** This is the dorsal part of pons and contains the nuclei of abducent, facial, trigeminal and vestibulocochlear nerves, trapezoid body and other ascending and descending tracts. The structure of tegmental part differs in the upper and lower (caudal) segments.

MEDULLA OBLONGATA

Medulla oblongata is the caudal and ventral part of the hind brain. It is lodged in the inferior cerebellar notch and lies on the basi-occiput (Fig. 8.33).

Extent: It extends from the lower border of pons (ponto medullary sulcus) to an imaginary horizontal plane which passes just above the attachment of first pair of cervical nerves on the spinal cord. This plane corresponds with the upper border of atlas and cuts the middle of the odontoid process of axis vertebra.

Shape: It is piriform in shape

Dimensions:

Length	:	3 cm
Width	:	2 cm
Thickness	:	1.3 cm

External Features

It is wider above and narrow below. Upper part of the medulla opens dorsally to form the lower part of floor of the 4th ventricle while the lower part of medulla is closed and contains the central canal. The external features of the spinal cord continue **rostally into the medulla.**

1. **Anterior median fissure**
   a. It is a deep vertical cleft which extends down from the lower border of pons and continues as the anterior median fissure of spinal cord below.
   b. It is shallower in the lower part of medulla due to the presence of pyramidal decussation.

2. **Posterior median sulcus:** It is the upward continuation of the posterior median sulcus of spinal cord. It continues as the median sulcus of the floor of the 4th ventricle.

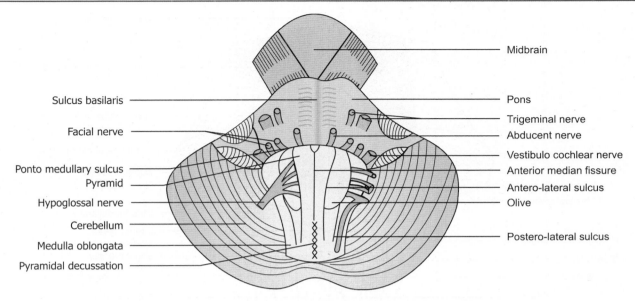

Fig. 8.33: Ventral surface of medulla, pons, cerebellum, midbrain

3. **Anterolateral sulcus:** Each sulcus is present between anterior and lateral areas. Hypoglossal nerve rootlets emerge out from this sulcus on each side.
4. **Posterolateral sulcus:** Posterolateral sulci separate the lateral areas from posterior areas. From above downwards the glossopharyngeal, vagus and cranial part of accessory nerves emerge from this sulcus.

The anterior fissure and the sulci divide the medulla into the following regions
1. **Anterior region**
   — It is the area present between the anteromedian fissure and the anterolateral sulcus on each side.
   — It presents a bulge known as the pyramid on each side of midline. Each pyramid contains corticobulbar, corticonuclear and corticopontine fibres. Venteromedially over the pyramids, are present neurons of the arcuate nuclei.
   — Abducent nerve emerges at upper end of pyramid where it joins the lower border of pons.
2. **Lateral region**
   — It is present between the anterolateral and posterolateral sulcus on each side.
   — An oval elevation is present in the upper part of lateral region known as olive. Inferior olivary nucleus lies under it.
   — Two roots of the facial nerve emerge out from the area between the lower border of pons and upper end of olive.
   — The lateral area is occupied by posterior and anterior spinocerebellar tracts, lateral spinothalamic tract, spino-olivary and olivospinal tracts.

3. **Posterior region**
   — This area of medulla lies between posterolateral sulcus and posterior median sulcus on each side of midline.
   — It is studied in two parts
   a. **Caudal part: Is closed and inferolateral in position**
      – The caudal part lies outside the floor of 4th ventricle.
      – It presents two rounded elevations in the upper part. These are, the gracile tubercle medially and the cuneate tubercle laterally which overlie the nucleus gracilis and nucleus cuneatus respectively.
      – Further below, it presents longitudinal elevations over the fasciculus gracilis and fasciculus cuneatus. These continue downwards into the spinal cord.
      – Lateral to the fasciculus cuneatus lies another slight elevation known as tuberculum cinereum. This overlies the nucleus and spinal tract of the trigeminal nerve.
   b. **Rostral part: Is open and superomedial in position (Fig. 8.34).**
      – Rostral part of the posterior area of medulla forms the floor of the 4th ventricle. It is limited superiorly by the stria medullaris.
      – It is bounded laterally at its upper end by the inferior cerebellar peduncles which connect the medulla to the cerebellum.
      – On each side, this posterior part is divided further into medial and lateral areas by a sulcus known as sulcus limitans.

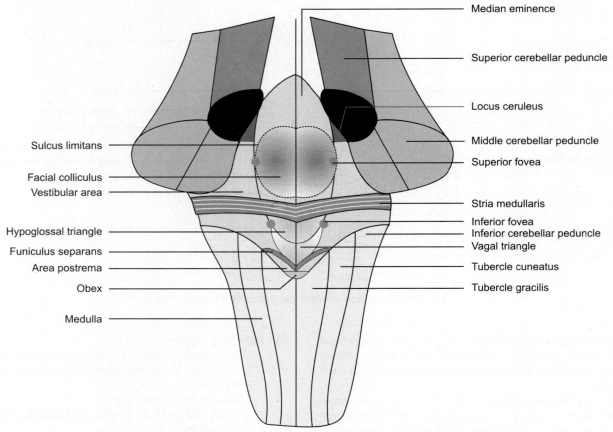

Fig. 8.34: Floor of fourth ventricle showing the rostral part of medulla

- The medial area below stria medullaris presents with a triangular elevation overlying the hypoglossal nucleus.
- The lateral area overlies the four vestibular nuclei and is called the vestibular area.
- A depression called inferior fovea is seen in lower part of sulcus limitans.
- Caudal to inferior fovea and between the medial hypoglossal area and lateral vestibular area lies the vagal trigone which overlies the dorsal nucleus of vagus nerve.
- The lowest part of lateral area presents with area postrema. This is separated from the vagal trigone by an ependymal thickening named funiculus separans.

INTERNAL FEATURES OF MEDULLA OBLONGATA

It is studied in transverse sections taken at three different levels. These sections are described from caudal to rostral side as follows (Figs 8.35 to 8.37):

1. **Transverse section at the level of pyramidal decussation.**
   Features:
   a. Central canal of spinal cord continues up in this section.

   b. Fasciculus gracilis and fasciculus cuneatus are present.
   c. Nucleus of spinal tract of trigeminal is seen.
   d. All ascending tracts of spinal cord continue as it is. Spinotectal tract, posterior spino cerebellar tract, anterior spinocerebellar tract.
   e. Pyramidal decussation is seen.
   f. Lateral corticospinal tract, reticular formation, rubrospinal tract, vestibulo spinal tract, olivo-spinal tract are present.

2. **Transverse section at the level of nucleus gracilis and nucleus cuneatus.**
   Features:
   a. Central canal is present which continues above into the fourth ventricle.
   b. Nucleus gracilis and nucleus cuneatus are present.
   c. Sensory decussation seen.
   d. Accessory cuneate nucleus and inferior olivary nucleus is seen.
   e. Nucleus of hypoglossal nerve is present.

3. **Transverse section at the level of olive**
   Features:
   a. This section passes through open part of medulla and cavity of 4th ventricle is seen.

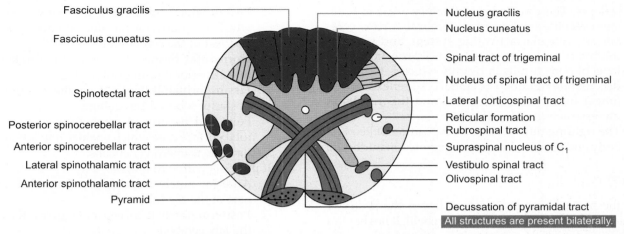

Fig. 8.35: Transverse section of lower part of medulla at the level of pyramidal decussation (diagrammatic representation)

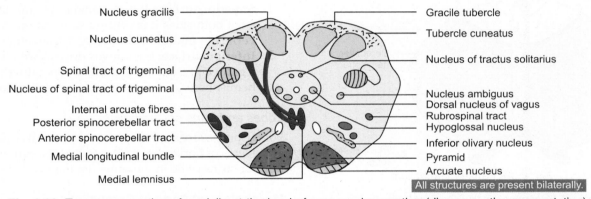

Fig. 8.36: Transverse section of medulla at the level of sensory decussation (diagrammatic representation)

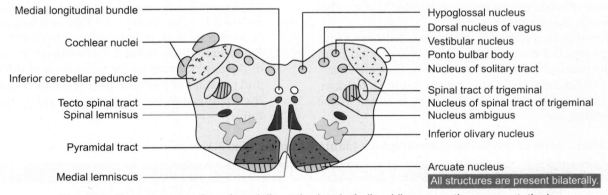

Fig. 8.37: Transverse section of medulla at the level of olive (diagrammatic representation)

b. Nucleus of hypoglossal nerve, dorsal nucleus of vagus, nucleus ambiguus, nucleus of tractus solitarius are present.

c. Inferior and medial vestibular nuclei are present.

d. Inferior olivary nucleus is present.

Physiology of Brain Stem

- Brain stem is formed by midbrain, pons and medulla. It houses many vital centers of the body like respiratory center, cardiovascular center etc.
- The reticular formation of medulla and pons control the muscle spindle sensitivity and the stretch

reflexes. These reticular facilitatory areas in brain stem receive imputs from cerebral cortex, cerebellum, reticular activating system, and reticular inhibitory area of basal ganglia. Transection at the level of pons results in rigidity which is termed as decerebrate rigidity. The spinal cord reflexes are no longer under cerebral control and this results in increase activity of γ-efferents.

- The righting reflexes to correct position of head on body and body on body are integrated in midbrain.

CEREBELLUM

It is the part of hind brain which lies in the posterior cranial fossa below the tentorium cerebelli. It lies behind the pons and medulla, separated from them by the cavity of 4th ventricle (Figs 8.34).

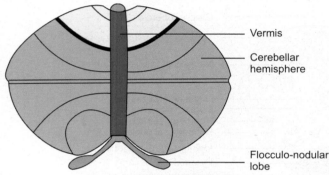

Fig. 8.38: Parts of cerebellum

Anatomical Features of the Cerebellum

- Cerebellum is oval in shape, flattened from above downwards. It is made up of two laterally placed hemispheres, connected to each other by a median worm like vermis (Fig. 8.38).
- The superior vermis is continuous with the hemispheres but the inferior vermis is separated from the hemispheres by a deep furrow, the vallecula.
- Both cerebellar hemispheres are thrown into transverse folds or folia separated by fissures. These fissures are

1. **Posterolateral fissure:** It is the primary fissure which lies between the flocculo-nodular lobe and rest of the cerebellum.
2. **Horizontal fissure:** It divides the cerebellum into superior and inferior surfaces.
3. **Fissura prima:** It lies between the anterior and posterior lobes of cerebellum.
   Folia and fissures of cerebellum increase the total surface area which enables it to accommodate the numerous neurons.
- It presents with two notches
  1. **Anterior notch:** It lodges the pons and upper part of the medulla.
  2. **Posterior notch:** It is deep and narrow. It lodges the falx cerebelli.

Surfaces of Cerebellum

1. **Superior surface:** It is elevated in the midline and from both sides it is continuous with the superior vermis in middle without any demarcation.
2. **Inferior surface:** It is convex downwards. There is a groove present in the midline separating the two hemispheres. Inferior vermis lies in this groove.

Lobes and Parts of Cerebellum

For the purpose of studying the cerebellum, it is unfolded at the level of horizontal fissure so that the superior and inferior surfaces lie in the same flat plane (Fig. 8.39).

Morphological Parts of Cerebellum

Based on physiological criteria it is divided into:
1. **Archicerebellum (vestibular cerebellum):** It is phylogenetically, the old part of cerebellum. It includes the flocculonodular lobe and lingula and is concerned with maintenance of equilibrium.
2. **Paleocerebellum (spinal cerebellum):** It consists of the anterior lobe (except lingula) and the uvula and pyramid of posterior lobe. It is concerned with the maintenance of muscle tone and posture of limbs.

The various parts of cerebellum identified are tabulated below (Fig. 8.39):

Lobe	Parts of cerebellar hemisphere (on each side of vermis)	Parts of vermis
1. Anterior lobe	1. Ala 2. Quadrangular lobe	1. Lingula 2. Central lobule 3. Culman
2. Posterior lobe	1. Lobulus simplex 2. Superior semilunar lobule 3. Inferior semilunar lobule 4. Biventral lobule 5. Tonsil	1. Declive 2. Folium 3. Tuber 4. Pyramid 5. Uvula
3. Flocculo-nodular lobe	Flocculus	Nodule

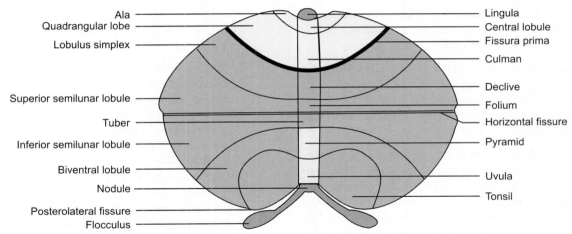

Fig. 8.39: Anatomical and morphological subdivisions of cerebellum

3. **Neocerebellum (cerebro-pontine cerebellum):** It is the newest part of cerebellum which is maximally developed in mammals and consists of most of the posterior lobe. This part of the cerebellum is concerned with coordination and smooth movements.

Internal Structure of Cerebellum

Structurally the cerebellum has three components
1. **Cerebellar cortex:** Present on the surface.
2. **White matter:** Present in medullary core.
3. **Cerebellar nuclei:** Deeply embedded in medullary core.

Cerebellar cortex (Fig. 8.40): It is the grey matter present on the surface of cerebellum and is uniform all through.

It consists of three layers with five types of neurons, termination of afferent fibres, neuroglia and blood vessels.

1. **Molecular layer:** It is the outermost layer and consists of stellate cells and basket cells.
2. **Purkinje cell layer:** It is the intermediate layer and consists of a single stratum of Purkinje cells.
3. **Granular layer:** It is the innermost layer and consists of granule cells and golgi cells.

White matter of cerebellum: It forms the central core of cerebellum. In a sagittal section, it presents with a characteristic branching pattern, resembling branches of a tree, which is termed as **arbor vitae.**

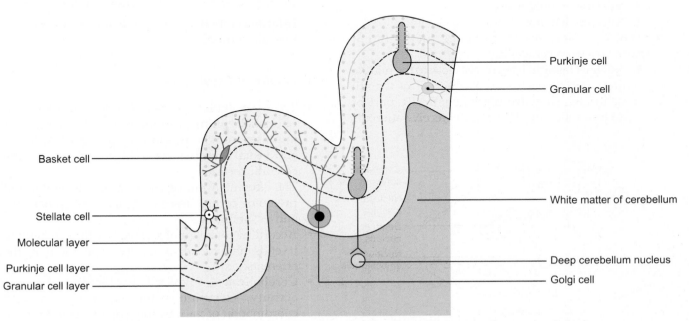

Fig. 8.40: Layers and cells of cerebellar cortex and its fibres (Diagrammatic representation)

The white matter consists of afferent and efferent fibres the afferent fibres are climbing and mossy fibres. These are arranged in two types:

1. **Intrinsic fibres:** These fibres are limited within the cerebellum. They connect its various parts with each other and consists of the association fibres, commissural fibres and myelinated axons of the Purkinje cells.

2. **Extrinsic fibres:** These fibres connect the cerebellum with various parts of the brain stem. They are conveyed by three pairs of peduncles namely,

   a. **Inferior cerebellar peduncle:** Also known as the **restiform body**. Each of the peduncles lies between the dorso-lateral aspect of medulla oblongata and the cerebellum. They mainly conveys afferent fibres to the cerebellum.

   b. **Middle cerebellar peduncles:** Also known as **brachium pontis**. They mainly convey afferent fibres and connect the cerebellum to the pons.

   c. **Superior cerebellar peduncles:** Also called as **brachium conjunctivum.** They convey predominantly, efferent fibres from cerebellum to the midbrain below the level of inferior colliculus.

Cerebellar Nuclei

- There are four pairs of deep nuclei that lie in the medullary core of the cerebellum.
- These nuclei are arranged in each hemisphere from medial to lateral side as follows (Fig. 8.41):
  1. Nucleus fastigii
  2. Nucleus globosus
  3. Nucleus emboliformis
  4. Nucleus dentatus
- Axons of these nuclei form the final efferent pathways from cerebellum.
  1. **Nucleus fastigii:** It is present close to the middle line, one on each side, in the roof of the 4th ventricle. They are phylogenetically part of archi-cerebellum. These nuclei receive afferents

from the vermal cortex. The efferents pass via inferior cerebellar peduncles to vestibular and medullary reticular nuclei.

2. **Nucleus globosus**
3. **Nucleus emboliformis:** The nucleus emboliformis and globosus are together known as **nucleus interpositus** and form part of the paleo-cerebellum. They both receive afferents from paravermal cortex. Efferents are given to the contralateral red nucleus, brain stem reticular nuclei and inferior olivary nucleus via superior cerebellar peduncles.

4. **Dentate nucleus:** It is part of the neo-cerebellum. It presents as crenated nuclear mass. It receives afferents from the lateral cortex of cerebellum. Efferents form the cerebello-rubro-thalamic fibres and pass via the superior cerebellar peduncles.

Arterial Supply of Cerebellum

Cerebellum is supplied by following arteries:
1. Superior cerebellar artery, branch of basilar artery
2. Anterior inferior cerebellar artery, branch of basilar artery
3. Posterior inferior cerebellar artery, branch of vertebral artery.

Venous Drainage of Cerebellum

It is through the following veins:

1. **Superior cerebellar veins:** Drain into straight, transverse and superior petrosal sinuses.

2. **Inferior cerebellar veins:** Drain into transverse and inferior petrosal sinuses.

Physiology of Cerebellum

- The cerebellum receives afferents from vestibular nuclei (labyrinth), proprioceptive and exteroceptor impulses from body and head and neck, auditory and visual impulses via colliculi and inputs from cerebral cortex.
- The efferents from cerebellum pass to motor and premotor cortex, descending tracts of spinal cord and vestibular nuclei.
- According to the input received by the cerebellum, it sends inhibitory or excitatory responses along the efferents.
- Cerebellum is involved in planning of motor activity, execution of the motor activity with coordination of various movements including eye coordination. It is involved with learning of

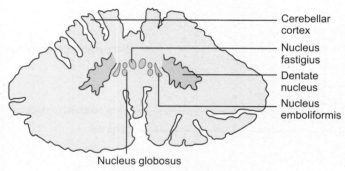

Fig. 8.41: Deep nuclei of cerebellum

adjustments to eventually allow coordination of movements.

- Lesions of cerebellum lead to ataxia. Ataxia is incoordinated movements with loss of rate, range, force and direction, example drunken gait, stressed speed, intension tremors.

Functions of Cerebellum

1. **Controls body posture and equilibrium**
   — It is by the flocculonodular lobe of cerebellum.
   — Afferents from vestibular nuclei and vestibular apparatus of ear.
   — Efferents to vestibular nuclei which connect to vestibulospinal tracts.

2. **Controls muscle tone and stretch reflexes**
   — It is by anterior lobe of cerebellum.
   — Inhibits the γ-efferent discharge to muscle spindles.

3. **Responsible for coordination of movements both voluntary and involuntary.**
   a. Control of voluntary movements
   — All three lobes of cerebellum are involved.
   — Afferent input is from cerebral cortex, eye and ear tactile receptors.
   — Efferent are sent along cerebello cortical tract to effect motor activity in corticospinal tracts.
   b. Control of involuntary movements, e.g., neck tighting movements to motion.
   — Involves activity in deep cerebellar nuclei.
   — Afferents are from proprioceptive, and sensory pathways from all over body. It also receives input from motor cortex, basal ganglia and reticular formation.
   — Efferents are sent back to cerebral motor cortex, basal ganglia and reticular formation to integrate body movements.

4. **Controls eye movements:** Integrates inputs to coordinate eye movements with body movements, helps in judgment of distance and focusing on one object.

SPINAL CORD

Spinal cord is the caudal, elongated and cylindrical part of the central nervous system which lies in the vertebral canal.

Anatomical Features (Fig. 8.42)

Extent: It extends from the medulla oblongata above to the conus medullaris below.

In adults: It extends from the upper border of C_1 vertebra just above the origin of 1st cervical nerve to lower border of L_1 vertebra.

In infants: it extends from the upper border of C_1 vertebra to lower border of L_3 vertebra.

In intrauterine life (upto 3 months): In the intrauterine life the spinal cord occupies the entire length of vertebral canal. Eventually, with the rapid growth of vertebral column the cord comes to occupy only the upper 2/3rd of the vertebral canal. Thus, any particular spinal segment lies at a higher level that the corresponding vertebra of the same number.

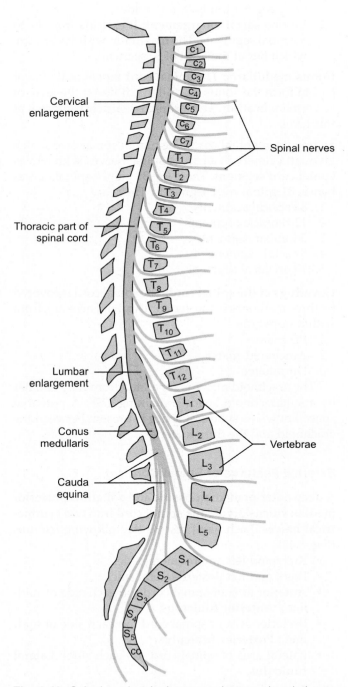

Fig. 8.42: Spinal cord, spinal roots and nerves in relation to vertebral column

Length: 45 cm in adult male and 42 cm in adult female.

Weight: 30 gms.

Enlargements: There are two fusiform enlargements present in the spinal cord to accommodate more number of neurons which supply the muscles of upper and lower limbs.

1. **Cervical enlargement:** It extends from C_4 to T_2 spinal segments. The maximum width is at the level of C_6 segment. It is 38 mm wide.
2. **Lumbo-sacral enlargement:** It extends from L_2 to S_3 spinal segments. The maximum width is 35 mm. which lies at the level of S_1 segment.

Conus medullaris: The spinal cord tapers at its lower end to form the conus medullaris. It lies at the level of L_1 vertebra in adult. The terminal ventricle is present at this level.

Segments of spinal cord: The part of spinal cord which gives attachment to a pair of spinal nerves is known as **spinal cord segment.** There are 31 pair of spinal nerves hence, 31 spinal cord segments. These are

1. 8 cervical segments
2. 12 thoracic segments
3. 5 lumbar segments
4. 5 sacral segments
5. 1 coccygeal segment

Coverings of the spinal cord: The spinal cord is covered by three meninges in the vertebral canal. These are, from within outwards

1. Pia mater
2. Arachnoid mater
3. Duramater

The arachnoid mater is separated from the piamater by a subarachnoid space containing CSF. A potential space known as subdural space is present between the arachnoid and the dura mater.

External Features of Spinal Cord

A deep anterior median fissure and a shallow posterior median sulcus divide the spinal cord into two symmetrical halves. Each half presents the following features (Fig. 8.42):

- Right and left antero-lateral sulci.
- Right and left postero-lateral sulci.
- Anterior area of spinal cord (on each side of midline): **Anterior funiculus.**
- Posterior area of spinal cord (on each side of midline): **Posterior funiculus.**
- Lateral area of spinal cord (on each side): **Lateral funiculus.**

Cauda equina: The spinal cord ends as the conus medullaris at lower border of L_1 vertebra. Below this,

the dorsal and ventral roots of the spinal segments from L_2 to coccygeal segment lie free in the vertebral canal as they pass towards their corresponding intervertebral foramina. The nerve roots are arranged around the filum terminale in a fashion that resembles a horse tail and hence the term cauda equina.

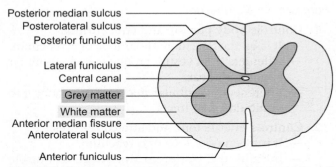

Fig. 8.43: Transverse section showing features of spinal cord (Diagrammatic representation)

Internal Features of Spinal Cord

On transverse section, the spinal cord consists of a central canal surrounded by the grey matter. The white matter lies in the periphery outside the grey matter (Fig. 8.43).

Grey Matter

It is made up of neuronal cell bodies, neuroglial cells, nonmyelinated processes of neurons and blood vessels. The grey matter is arranged around the central canal in the form of the english letter 'H'.

Organisation of Grey Matter of Spinal Cord

The grey matter is organised into three columns namely (Fig. 8.44):

1. Anterior grey column
2. Posterior grey column
3. Intermediate region of grey matter.

Anterior grey column: It consists of lower motor neurons of three types:

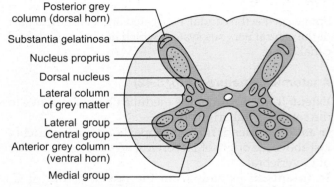

Fig. 8.44: Organization of grey matter of spinal cord

1. **α-motor neurons:** They are thickly myelinated and 25mm or more in length. They supply the extra fusal fibres of muscle.
2. **γ-motor neurons:** They are smaller, 15 to 25 mm in length with thin myelination. They supply the intrafusal fibres of muscle.
3. **β-motor neurons:** They are intermediate in size with thin myelination. They supply both extrafusal and intrafusal fibres of muscle spindle.

The neurons are arranged in three groups of longitudinal columns

1. **Medial group:** Present along the entire length of the cord. It controls axial (muscles of trunk) and proximal limb muscles.
2. **Lateral group:** Present only in cervical and lumbosacral enlargements. It supplies the distal limb muscles which are concerned with skillful movements.
3. **Central group:** Mainly present in cervical region from C_3 to C_5 and in lumbosacral region of cord. It forms the phrenic nerve nucleus ($C_{3,4,5}$). It also has interneurons

Posterior grey column: It consists of two types of nerve cells.

1. **Interneurons:** They are small neurons that interconnect a sensory neuron to a motor neuron to elicit a reflex response. Some neurons receive inputs from the descending pathways also.
2. **Tract cells:** The axons arising from these tract cells form ascending (sensory) tracts.

There are four sets of longitudinal neuronal columns present in posterior grey column (Fig. 8.44). These are

1. **Substantia gelatinosa:** Receives sensation of pain and temperature.
2. **Nucleus proprius:** Cells carry sensation of touch, pressure, pain and temperature.
3. **Nucleus dorsalis (Clarke's nucleus):** Receives sensation of touch and pressure.
4. **Nucleus of visceral afferent:** Receives afferents from the viscera and projects to the efferent nuclei of the autonomic nervous system.

Intermediate region of grey matter: It forms the lateral horn which is characteristically seen in T_1 to L_2 spinal segments. These contain cells which are the preganglionic neurons of the sympathetic outflow. These cells give rise to thinly myelinated axons that terminate in the corresponding ganglia of the sympathetic trunk.

The intermedio-medial column is also present in S_2 to S_4 spinal segments and consists of preganglionic neurons of the parasympathetic (sacral) outflow.

Central Canal

It is present longitudinally along the entire length of spinal cord surrounded by the grey matter (central commissure). It is the downward continuation of the 4th ventricle. This canal is dilated in the region of conus medullaris and forms the terminal ventricle. It is lined by ependymal cells and contains CSF.

White Matter

It surrounds the H-shaped grey matter of the spinal cord. White matter occupies the peripheral part of the spinal cord. It consists of myelinated nerve fibres, neuroglial cells and blood vessels. The white colour is due to the myelinated nerve fibres.

Organization of White Matter in Spinal Cord

It is arranged into the following parts in each of the two halves of the cord.

1. **Anterior funiculus:** It extends from the anterior median fissure to the lateral most fibers of the ventral roots of the spinal nerve.
2. **Lateral funiculus:** It lies between the emergence of ventral roots of spinal nerve and the postero-lateral sulcus.
3. **Posterior funiculus:** It extends from the postero-lateral sulcus to the posterior median sulcus (septum).

Tract or fasciculus: The fibres of white matter of spinal cord are grouped into different tracts. Tract is a bundle of nerve fibres within the central nervous system having specific cells of origin, identical site of termination with a definite location in the spinal cord. The fibres of one tract have similar function and are arranged somatotopically.

Tracts of spinal cord: The tracts are of two types

1. **Ascending tracts:** These consist of fibres (sensory) arising from a somatic or a visceral receptor which ascend to the brain via spinal cord.
2. **Descending tracts:** These consist of fibres (motor) descending down from various parts of brain to spinal cord for distribution to the body.

Five groups of nerve fibres are encountered in the white matter. These are:

1. Sensory fibres from dorsal roots of spinal nerve. These provide input to the segmental interneurons and tract cells of posterior grey column.
2. Long ascending fibres from tract cells of spinal grey columns.
3. Long descending fibres from cerebral cortex and other supra-spinal nuclei. These terminate on the posterior grey column of spinal cord.
4. Short intersegmental fibres: Consist of ascending and descending fibres connecting adjacent spinal cord segments.
5. Ventral roots of spinal nerves consisting of fibres from anterior and lateral spinal grey columns.

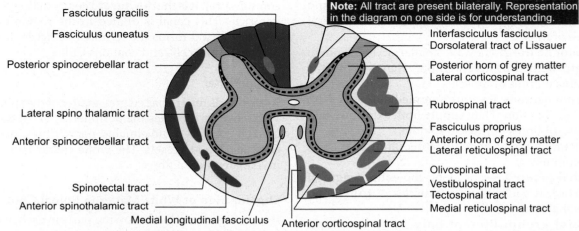

Fig. 8.45: Transverse section of spinal cord showing grey matter and main fibre tracts of spinal cord (Diagrammatic representation)

The various tracts of spinal cord are tabulated below (Fig. 8.45):

Funiculus	Ascending tracts	Descending tracts
Anterior	1. Anterior spinothalamic	1. Anterior corticospinal
		2. Tectospinal
		3. Vestibulospinal
		4. Medial reticulospinal
Lateral	2. Posterior spino-cerebellar	5. Lateral corticospinal
	3. Anterior spino-cerebellar	6. Rubrospinal
	4. Lateral spinothalamic	7. Lateral reticulospinal
	5. spino-tectal tract	
	6. Dorsolateral tract of Lissauer	8. Olivo spinal
Posterior	7. Fasciculus gracilis or tract of Gall	9. Fasciculus septomarginalis
	8. Fasciculus cuneatus or tract of Burdach	10. Fasciculus interfasciculus

Description of ascending tracts–salient features

Tract	Origin	Termination	Crossing over	Sensations carried
1. Anterior spinothalamic tract (Axons of second order sensory neurons)	Lamina I to IV of spinal grey matter	Joins with medial lemniscus in lower medulla and then to terminates in the ventroposterolateral nucleus of the thalamus	Ascends 2 to 3 spinal segments and then crosses to the opposite side	• Non-discriminative touch • pressure
2. Lateral spinothalamic tract (Axons of second order sensory neurons)	Lamina I to IV of spinal grey matter	Forms the spinal lemniscus in the medulla and ends in the ventro-postero-lateral (VPL) nucleus and intra laminar nuclei of thalamus	Crosses to opposite side in the same spinal cord segment	• Pain • Temperature
3. Anterior spino-cerebellar tract or ventral spino-cerebellar tract (Axons of second order sensory neurons)	Lamina V to VII of spinal grey matter (T_1-L_2)	Ipsilateral anterior cerebellar vermis	It crosses twice a. 1st it crosses to opposite side in the same spinal segment b. Crosses back to same side at the level of midbrain through the superior cerebellar peduncle	• Unconscious proprioception and exteroceptive information from the lower part of the body and lower limbs • Responsible for maintaining posture and gross movement of entire lower limb.

Tract	Origin	Termination	Crossing over	Sensations carried
4. Posterior spino-cerebellar tract or dorsal spino-cerebellar tract (Axons of second order senosry neurons)	Lamina VII of spinal grey matter or Clarke's column (T_1 to L_2)	The fibres pass via the ipsilateral inferior cerebellar peduncle to terminate in rostral and caudal part of cerebellar vermis	No crossing over. The fibres ascend ipsilaterally.	• Unconscious proprioception and touch and pressure from lower half of the body and lower extremity • Responsible for the fine coordination between movements of various muscles of lower limb.
5. Dorsal column of white matter (Axons of first order sensory neurons)				Conscious kinetic and static proprioception, vibration sense, discriminatory touch and pressure from lower limb and lower half the body is carried by fasciculus gracilis and from upper limb and upper half of the body by fasciculus cuneatus
a. Fasciculus gracilis	Sensory neurons in dorsal root ganglia	Nucleus gracilis in lower medulla	Uncrossed	
b. Fasciculus cuneatus	Sensory neurons in dorsal root ganglia	Nucleus cuneatus in medulla	Uncrossed	
6. Dorso-lateral tract	Lateral division of dorsal nerve root	Lamina I to IV	Uncrossed	Pain and temperature

Description of descending tracts–salient features

Tracts	Origin	Termination	Crossing over	Function
1. Corticospinal or pyramidal tract Occupies the pyramid of medulla	Area no.4, 6, 3, 1, 2 of cerebral cortex	Lamina of IV to VII of spinal grey matter interneurons and then to lamina IX	a. Lateral corticospinal tract crosses over in lower part of medulla b. Anterior corticospinal tract crosses to opposite side in the corresponding spinal segment	— Responsible for skillfull voluntary movements — Facilitates flexors and is inhibitory to extensors
2. Rubrospinal tract	Red nucleus of midbrain	Lamina V to VII and then to IX of spinal grey matter	Midbrain at the level of superior colliculus	Same as corticospinal tract
3. Tectospinal tract	Superior colliculus	Lamina VI and VII of spinal grey matter	Midbrain at the level of superior colliculus	Reflex pathway for turning head and moving arm in response to visual and hearing stimuli
4. Vestibulo-spinal tract				
a. Lateral vestibulo-spinal tract	Lateral vestibular nucleus in upper medulla	Lamina VII, VIII and IX of spinal grey matter	Uncrossed	Facilitates extensor motor neurons and is inhibitory to flexors
b. Medial vestibulo-spinal tract	Medial vestibular nucleus in upper medulla	Lamina VII, VIII and IX of spinal grey matter	Uncrossed (few fibres cross)	No definite function is defined, probably is same as the lateral tract.

Tracts	Origin	Termination	Crossing over	Function
5. **Reticulo-spinal tract**				
a. Medial	Pontine reticular formation	Lamina VII, VIII, IX of spinal grey matter	Uncrossed	a. Facilitates extensor motor neurons and is inhibitory to flexors.
b. Lateral	Giganto-cellular component of medullary reticular formation of medulla	Lamina VII, VIII and IX of spinal grey matter	Uncrossed	b. Inhibit extensor motor neurons and is facilitatory to flexors
6. **Olivo-spinal tract**	Inferior olivary nucleus	Anterior grey column	Uncrossed	Uncertain

CLINICAL AND APPLIED ASPECT

NEURONS AND NEUROGLIA

- **Nerve injury:** Injury to nerve can be caused by trauma, ischemia, toxic substances or high temperature > 104°F. The changes after any injury occur in the following sequence:
  - **Retrograde degeneration:** Changes begin in the cell body of the damaged nerve fiber. There is disintegration of Nissl's granules along with disruption of golgi apparatus, mitochondria and neurofibrils. Cells allow entry of fluid and become round and nucleus is pushed to one side.
  - **Antegrade degeneration:** The changes in the segment distal to the site of injury are termed as **Wallerian degeneration.** Cylinder of axon distal to injury breaks up and disappears. The myelin sheath also gradually disintegrates. Schwann cells start multiplying and form cords to fill the endoneural tubes.
  - **Degeneration at site of injury:** Schwann cells elongate to fill the gap at site of injury. If gap is > 3 cm then the space cannot be filled completely.
  - **Regenerative changes:** They start by 3rd week or 20 days. Nissl's granules and organelles reappear. The axon from the proximal stump grows fibrils which are guided by Schwann cells towards the distal end. One of the fibrils enlarges and bridges the gap to complete the axon tube while the rest degenerate. If gap is > 3 cm regenerating fibrils intermingle and form a collection of fibers called **neuroma.** This appears as a lump and may be painful.
- **Gliosis:** It is the proliferation of astrocytes leading to formation of local fibrosis which acts as a space occupying lesion in the brain.
- In demyelinating conditions like multiple sclerosis, oligodendroglia, cells responsible for laying down myelin sheath of neurons of CNS, are destroyed by presence of autoimmune antibodies.

NEUROMUSCULAR JUNCTION

- **Myasthenia gravis:** It is an autoimmune disease which results in formation of antibodies to N-acetylcholine receptors at the neuromuscular junction. The distruction of these receptors results in weakness and fatigue of muscles. It mainly affects eye muscles, facial muscles and muscle for chewing and swallowing.
- **Drugs affecting neuromuscular trans-mission**
  - **Botulin toxin:** It blocks the release of acetylcholine from presynaptic membranes. This leads to relaxation of muscles.
  - **Acetylcholine receptor antagonists:** Tubocurare and gallamine act as competitive inhibitors of N-acetylcholine receptors while succinylcholine acts by persistent depolarization and exhaustion of ATP. The ultimate result is muscle relaxation.
  - **Anti-choline esterases:** Neostigmine, edrophonium are drugs that prevent destruction of acetylcholine by binding to acetylcholine esterases. Acetylcholine levels are increased leading to muscle stimulation. They are used to reverse the block by tubocurare but cannot reverse succinylcholine block.

FUNCTIONAL AREAS OF CEREBRAL HEMISPHERE

- Brodmann's classification divides the cerebral cortex into 52 areas.
- The effects of any lesion of area no. 4 or motor area are as follows:
  Initially there will be flaccid paralysis of contralateral side. Generally there is no isolated lesion of area 4. It is usually associated with lesion of area no. 6 and 8. In such cases there is an upper motor neuron paralysis.
- The effect of lesion of prefrontal cortex :
  It usually occur due to a tumor of frontal lobe where patient presents with the following
  a. Lack of self responsibility
  b. Vulgarity in speech
  c. Clownish behavior
  d. Feeling of euphoria
- Prefrontal leucotomy is not preferred in a terminally ill cancer patient to relieve pain because the patient may not feel pain but he looses responsibility towards self. He does not bother about himself.
- The effect of lesion of area no. 40 is astereognosis and tactile aphasia.

- When patient is unable to recognise the written words even when written by the patient himself. This is known as word blindness. It is seen in lesion of area no. 39.
- In the lesion of area no. 22, patient will develop sensory aphasia or word deafness. Patient cannot interpret words spoken by himself or others. Fluency of speech is maintained but patient speaks nonsense words in between.
- Following are the four speech centres interconnected with each other which help in the development of speech in a child.
  Area no. 39, 40 and 22 are interconnected with each other. The child starts learning speech with the help of these areas. Area no. 22 is further connected to the area no. 45, 44 with the help of arcuate fasciculus. Area 45, 44 is the motor speech area that controls the movement of muscles involved in all three components of speech.
  — **Area no. 22:** Comprehension of spoken language and recognition of familiar sounds and words.
  — **Area no. 39:** Recognition of object by sight and storage of visual images
  — **Area no. 40:** Recognition of object by touch and proprioception
  — **Area no. 45, 44:** Is the motors speech area and controls movement of lips, tongue, larynx, pharynx and palate.
- The lesion of area no. 45, 44 will lead to loss of fluency of speech or motor aphasia.
- In the involvement of posterior cerebral artery, the part of the visual cortex which represents macula will be spared as this part is supplied by both posterior cerebral and middle cerebral artery.
- In the involvement of anterior cerebral artery there is incontinence of urine and feaces due to damage to paracentral lobule of cerebral cotex.

INTERNAL CAPSULE

A small lesion of internal capsule produces wide spread paralysis because of the compact arrangement of fibres in it. The usual clinical presentation of a lesion in internal capsule is contralateral cranial nerve palsy with contralateral hemiplegia.

BASAL GANGLIA

Lesions in basal ganglia lead to following conditions
- **Parkinsonism** (Paralysis agitans)
  — Increased muscular rigidity
  — Lead pipe rigidity
  — Mask like face
  — Pill rolling movements of fingers
- **Chorea**
  — Brisk, jerky purposeless movements of distal parts of the extremities
  — Twitching of facial muscles

- **Athetosis:** Slow worm like writhing movements of the extremities mainly affecting wrists and fingers.
- **Wilson's disease**
  — Muscular rigidity
  — Tremors

MID BRAIN

- Perinaud's syndrome results from a lesion in the superior colliculus this occurs when this area is compressed by a tumor of the pineal body. The characteristic feature of Perinaud's syndrome is the paralysis of upward gaze without any affect on other eye movements. The anatomical basis for this is obscure but experiments indicate that this area may contain a "centre" for upward movement of the eyes.
- Benedikt's syndrome results from a lesion in the tegmentum of midbrain. This destroys the medial lemniscus, red nucleus and fibres of oculomotor nerve and superior cerebellar peduncle (brachium conjuctivum).

Characteristic features of Benedikt's syndrome (Fig. 25.8)
1. External strabismus (lateral squint) and ptosis on the same side. This is due to involvement of oculomotor nerve fibres
2. Loss of tactile, muscle, joint position, vibratory, pain and temperature sense in the opposite of the body including face. This is due to involvement of medial lemniscus which at this level has been joined on its lateral side by lateral spino-thalamic tract.
3. Tremor and irregular twitching movements of opposite arm and leg. This is due to involvement of red nucleus and superior cerebellar peduncle, which contain afferent fibres from the opposite cerebellar hemisphere.

- Weber's syndrome occurs mostly due to a vascular lesion of the midbrain involving third cranial nerve nucleus and corticospinal tract.

Characteristic Features
1. Ipsilateral divergent strabismus (squint), due to involvement of third cranial nerve.
2. Contra-lateral hemiplegia, due to involvement of cortico-spinal tract.

PONS

- A tumour in the cerebello-pontine angle, where the cerebellum, pons and medulla meet, causes the cerebello-pontine syndrome. It affects the 7th and 8th cranial nerves which are attached here and gives rise to following symptoms.
  — There is ringing in ears or loss of hearing on the affected side due to the involvement of VIII cranial nerve.

— Pressure on the cerebellum results in ataxia and tremors on the side of lesion.
— Pressure on the facial nerve leads to
  i. Paralysis of the muscles of the face
  ii. Hyperacusia due to paralysis of stapedius
  iii. Loss of taste sensation in the anterior two-thirds of the tongue on the same side.
- Thrombosis of pontine branches of basilar artery generally affects the **medial part of pons and this causes**
  — Hemiplegia of the opposite side (involvement corticospinal fibres).
  — Paralysis of lateral rectus of the same side due to involvement of VI nerve produces convergent squint.
  Lesion of lateral part of pons will produce
  — Loss of all general sensations of face and forehead due to involvement of spinal tract of trigeminal nerve.
  — Lower motor neuron paralysis of muscles of mastication of the same side due to the involvement of motor nucleus of V nerve.

MEDULLA

- **Medial medullary syndrome** is also known as alternating hypoglossal hemiplegia. It results from the occlusion of anterior spinal artery and its paramedian branches which supply the symmetrical halves of medial zone of the medulla on each side of midline. Characteristic features are (Fig. 25.2).
  — Ipsilateral lower motor neuron paralysis of. tongue muscles with atrophy.
  — Contralateral upper motor neuron hemiplegia
  — Loss of discriminative sense of position and vibration of the body.
- **Lateral medullary syndrome** is also known as Wallenberg's syndrome. It is usually due to the thrombosis of posterior inferior cerebellar artery that produces damage to the dorsolateral part of the medulla. Characteristic features are: (Fig. 25.2)
  — Loss of pain and temperature on the opposite half of the body below the neck
  — Loss of pain and temperature on the same side of the face
  — psilateral paralysis of the muscles of the soft palate, pharynx and larynx
  — Ipsilateral ataxia
  — Giddiness, nystagmus
- Following arteries supply the medulla oblongata
  — Vertebral artery
  — Anterior spinal arteries
  — Posterior spinal arteries
  — Posterior inferior cerebellar artery
  — Branches from basilar artery

CEREBELLUM

- **Archicerebellar syndrome** is caused by the involvement of flocculo-nodular lobe. Patients presents with
  1. Disturbance of equilibrium
  2. Wide base walk
  3. Inability to maintain an upright posture and swaying from side to side.
- **Lateral cerebellar syndrome** is also known as the neocerebellar syndrome. It affects the neocerebellar part of the cerebellum and presents as follows:
  1. **Disturbance of posture**
     — Atonia or hypotonia: The muscle tone is either completely lost (atonia) or markedly decreased (hypotonia) on the affected side leading to abnormalities like the face is rotated towards the opposite side, the leg is abducted and rotated outwards.
     — Nystagmus: Involuntary movement of the eyeballs which occurs when the patient attempts to fix his eyes on an object.
     — Tendon reflexes become weak and pendular.
  2. **Disturbances of voluntary movement**
     — **Asthenia:** There is feebleness of movement.
     — **Ataxia:** It is the incoordination of movements. Ataxia is marked in cerebellar lesions.
     — **Decomposition of the movement:** The movement seems to occur in stages.
     — **Asynergia:** Lack of coordination between protagonists, antagonists and synergists.
     — **Dysmetria:** The movement loses direction, range and force, therefore, the movements overshoot their intended mark, i.e., past pointing (hypermetria) or fall short of it (hypometria).
     — **Intention tremors:** These tremors are coarse and are clearly be seen when the part is used in a voluntary movement.
  3. **Disturbances in gait:** The patient has an unsteady gait with the feet kept apart while walking.
  4. **Effect on speech (Dysarthria or scanning speech):** It is slow, imperfect due to incoordination.

The cerebellar lesion of one hemisphere produces dysfunction on the same side of the body whereas the lesions of the vermis affect both the sides.

Chapter 9
Peripheral Nervous System

It includes those parts of nervous system which lie outside the central nervous system. It consists of twelve pairs of cranial nerves, thirty one pairs of spinal nerves, somatic and special sense receptors and the autonomic nervous system.

SPINAL NERVES AND PERIPHERAL NERVES

SPINAL NERVES (FIG. 9.1)

Each spinal nerve is formed by a ventral root and a dorsal root attached to the spinal cord. These two roots unite in the intervertebral foramina to form spinal nerve.

Ventral root: It contains the axons of neurons in anterior and lateral spinal grey column. Thus, it is made up of motor nerve fibres.

Dorsal root: It contains central processes of neurons situated in the dorsal root ganglion (spinal ganglion). Thus, it is made up of sensory nerve fibres.

Spinal ganglion (Dorsal root ganglion): It is the collection of neurons enclosed in a fibrous tissue capsule with satellite cells. Spinal ganglion is present on the dorsal root of each spinal nerve. It contains unipolar neurons which divide into peripheral and central processes. 1st cervical ganglion may be absent.

Each spinal nerve contains motor and sensory fibres and divides into a ventral ramus and a dorsal ramus. Dorsal rami of spinal nerves divide into medial and lateral branches which supply the muscles and skin of the back. Each ventral ramus of spinal nerves divides into divisions which join to form plexuses that further

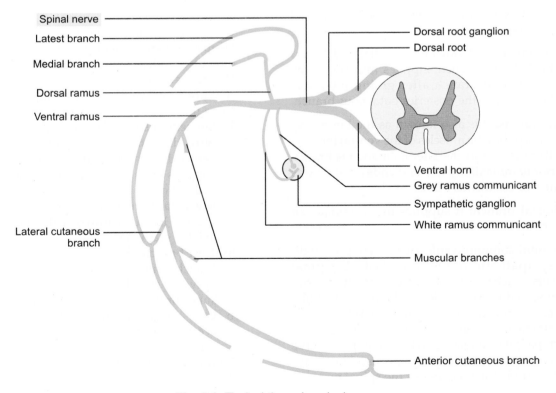

Spinal nerve
Latest branch
Medial branch
Dorsal ramus
Ventral ramus
Lateral cutaneous branch

Dorsal root ganglion
Dorsal root
Ventral horn
Grey ramus communicant
Sympathetic ganglion
White ramus communicant
Muscular branches
Anterior cutaneous branch

Fig. 9.1: Typical thoracic spinal nerve

give branches to supply skin and muscles of upper limb, lower limb and body wall.

There are 31 pairs of spinal nerves. These are:
- 8 Cervical spinal nerves
- 12 Thoracic spinal nerves
- 5 Lumbar spinal nerves
- 5 Sacral spinal nerves
- 1 Coccygeal spinal nerve

Functional Components of a Spinal Nerve

There are two functional components of a spinal nerve:

1. **Somatic component:** It contains both efferent (motor) and afferent (sensory) fibres.

2. **Visceral component:** It constitutes the autonomic nervous system. There are again efferent and afferent components of this nervous system.

Typical Thoracic Spinal Nerve (Fig. 9.1)

Typical thoracic spinal nerves in general do not form any plexus and are limited to supplying the thoracic wall. The dorsal rami of thoracic spinal nerves give branches to supply the skin and muscles of the back of the corresponding region. The ventral rami supply the antero-lateral surfaces of lower part of neck, thorax and abdomen.

Branches: Following are the branches of a typical thoracic spinal nerve:

1. **Dorsal ramus:** It divides into medial and lateral branches. Medial branch supplies muscles of the back and lateral branch after giving muscular branches becomes the posterior cutaneous branch.

2. **Ventral ramus:** It is also known as the intercostal nerve. It supplies the muscles of the ventral thoracic wall. It gives rise to the lateral cutaneous branch posterior to midaxillary line and ends anteriorly as the anterior cutaneous branch.

3. **Meningeal branch:** It supplies the duramater of spinal cord.

4. **White rami communicantes:** These are preganglionic sympathetic fibres from T_1 to L_2 spinal segments which pass through the respective ventral root of spinal nerve and leave the nerve as white rami communicantes. They further relay in the sympathetic ganglion. Post ganglionic fibres from the sympathetic ganglion join the same spinal nerve as the grey rami communicantes. These are distributed via the branches of the spinal nerve.

PERIPHERAL NERVES

Interconnection of ventral rami of two or more spinal nerves gives rise to a plexus. The plexus further gives rise to nerves which supply skin and muscles of body wall and limbs. These nerves are known as peripheral nerves.

The various plexuses that supply different regions of the body are:
1. Cervical plexus
2. Brachial plexus
3. Lumbar Plexus
4. Sacral and coccygeal plexus

CERVICAL PLEXUS

Cervical plexus is formed by interconnection of ventral primary rami of upper four cervical nerves (C_1 to C_4) (Fig. 9.2). It supplies muscles and skin of head and neck region, upper part of trunk and shoulder region. It also supplies diaphragm through phrenic nerve.

Branches of Cervical Plexus

1. **Superficial cutaneous branches:** These branches supply the skin over back of scalp front of face, front of neck and shoulder region.
   a. Lesser occipital nerve: C_2
   b. Great auricular nerve: $C_{2,3}$
   c. Transverse cervical nerve: $C_{2,3}$
   d. Supraclavicular nerve: $C_{3,4}$
2. **Deep muscular branches:** They supply the muscles directly or indirectly via communicating branches.
   Direct branches
   a. **Phrenic nerve:** $C_{3,4,5}$—This supplies the diaphragm.
   b. **Descendens cervicalis nerve:** $C_{2,3}$—**This joins with descendans hypoglossi to form ansa cervicalis in front of the carotid sheath.** It supplies sternohyoid, sternothyroid and inferior belly of omohyoid.
   c. **Muscular branches:** These are nerve to rectus capitis, longus capitis, scalenus medius and levator scapulae.
   Indirect branches:
   a. Branch from C_1 communicates with hypoglossal nerve to supply thyrohyoid, geniohyoid and superior belly of omohyoid.
   b. $C_{2,3,4}$ communicates with the spinal root of accessory nerve to supply sternocleidomastoid muscle (C_2).
3. **Communicating branches:** Each ventral ramus of the cervical nerve receives a grey rami communi-

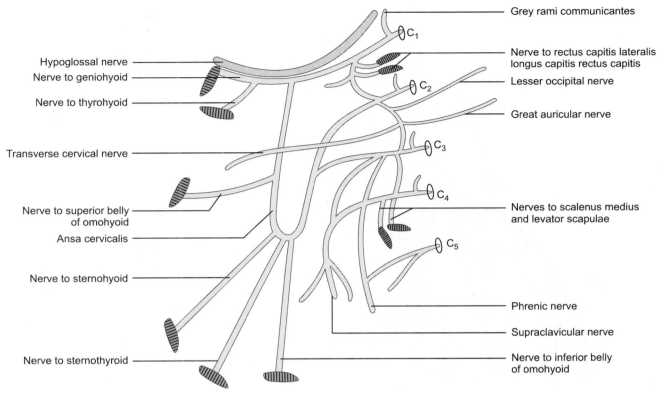

Fig. 9.2: Cervical plexus

cantes from the superior cervical ganglion of sympathetic trunk.

Phrenic Nerve

It arises from the ventral rami of $C_{3, 4, 5}$ spinal nerves, chiefly from C_4.

Distribution

a. Provides the sole motor supply to the diaphragm which is the main muscle of respiration.
b. Provides sensory innervation to the diaphragmatic pleura, pericardium and subdiaphragmatic pleura.

BRACHIAL PLEXUS

Brachial plexus is formed by the interconnection of **ventral primary rami of C_5, C_6, C_7, C_8 and T_1 spinal nerves.** It supplies the upper limb. It is made up of roots, trunks and cords which are divided into cervical, supraclavicular and infraclavicular parts respectively (Fig. 9.3) .

Prefix: when C_4 root is also involved in formation of brachial plexus is known as prefix.

Postfix: when T_2 root is involved in formation of brachial plexus is known as postfix.

Trunks of Brachial Plexus

The five spinal nerves form three trunks namely
1. **Upper Trunk:** It is formed by ventral rami of C_5 and C_6 nerves.
2. **Middle Trunk:** It is formed by ventral ramus of C_7 nerve.
3. **Lower Trunk:** It is formed by ventral rami of C_8 and T_1 nerves.

Divisions of Brachial Plexus

Each trunk divides into an anterior and a posterior division.

Cords of Brachial Plexus

Three Cords are formed by the different divisions of trunks. These cords are named according to their position with respect to 2nd part of axillary artery.
1. **Lateral cord:** Formed by joining of anterior divisions of upper and middle trunks.
2. **Medial cord:** Formed by continuation of anterior division of lower trunk.
3. **Posterior cord:** Formed by union of posterior division of all three trunks.

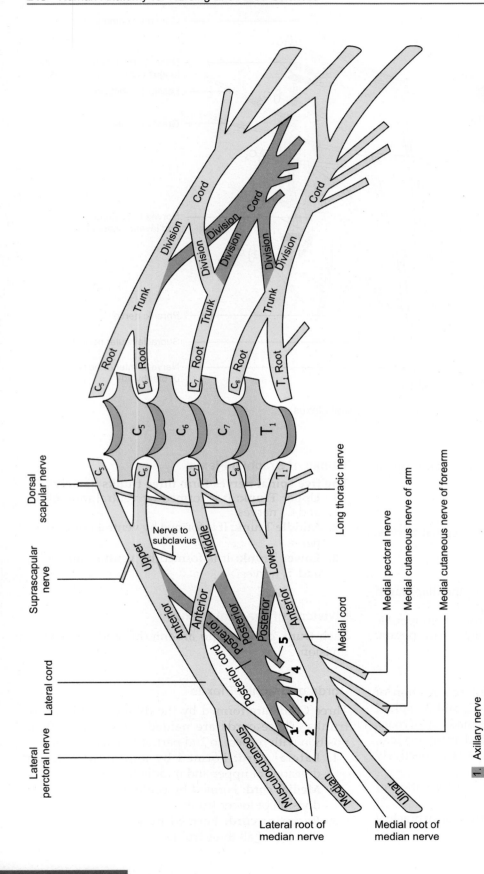

Fig. 9.3: Brachial plexus—diagrammatic representation

1. Axillary nerve
2. Radial nerve
3. Lower subscapular nerve
4. Thoraco dorsal nerve
5. Upper subscapular nerve

Branches of Brachial Plexus

Branches from the Roots
1. Dorsal scapular nerve (C_5)
2. Long thoracic nerve (C_5,C_6,C_7) **Nerve of Bell**
3. Branches to join phrenic nerve (C_5)
4. Branches to longus colli and scleneus muscles

Branches from Upper Trunk
1. Nerve to subclavius (C_5,C_6)
2. Suprascapular nerve (C_5,C_6)

Branches from Lateral Cord
1. Lateral pectoral nerve (C_5, C_6, C_7)
2. Musculo-cutaneous nerve (C_5, C_6, C_7)
3. Lateral root of median nerve (C_5, C_6, C_7)

Branches from Medial Cord
1. Medial pectoral nerve (C_8, T_1)
2. Medial cutaneous nerve of forearm (C_8, T_1)
3. Medial cutaneous nerve of arm (T_1, T_2)
4. Medial root of median nerve (C_8, T_1)
5. Ulnar nerve (C_7, C_8, T_1)

Branches from Posterior Cord
1. Upper (superior) subscapular nerves (C_5, C_6)
2. Lower (inferior) subscapular nerve (C_5, C_6)
3. Thoraco-dorsal nerve (C_6, C_7, C_8)
4. Axillary nerve (C_5, C_6)
5. Radial nerve (C_5, C_6, C_7, C_8, T_1)

LUMBAR PLEXUS (FIG. 9.4)

It is the plexus of nerves formed in the substance of psoas major muscle. It supplies lower limb and anterior abdominal wall. It is formed by ventral rami of L_1, L_2, L_3 supplemented by L_4 and subcostal spinal nerves. Ventral rami divide into ventral and dorsal divisions. These divisions reunite to give rise to lumbar plexus and its branches.

Prefix: If L_3 participates in lumbosacral trunk then it is called prefix.

Postfix: If L_5 participates in lumbosacral trunk and connects sacral plexus to lumbar plexus instead of L_4, it is post fix.

Branches of Lumbar Plexus

Nerve	Root value
1. Iliohypogastric	L_1
2. Ilioinguinal	L_1
3. Genitofemoral	L_1 L_2
4. Lateral femoral cutaneous nerve	L_2 L_3 (Dorsal division)
5. Accessory obturator nerve	L_3 L_4 (Dorsal division)
6. Femoral nerve	L_2 L_3 L_4 (Dorsal division)
7. Obturator nerve	L_2 L_3 L_4 (Ventral division)
8. Lumbo-sacral trunk	L_4 L_5
9. Muscular branches	
a. Quadratus lumborum	T_{12} to L_4
b. Psoas major	L_2 L_3 L_4
c. Psoas minor	L_1

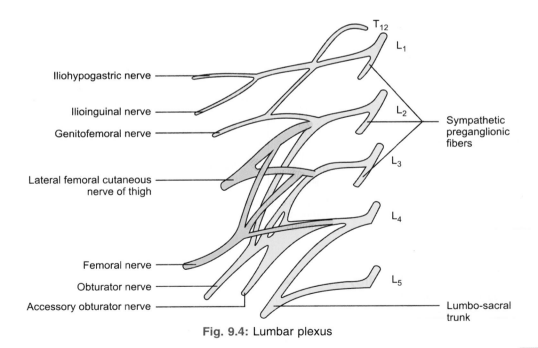

Fig. 9.4: Lumbar plexus

(Figs 9.6 to 9.13).

cutaneous nerve of arm.

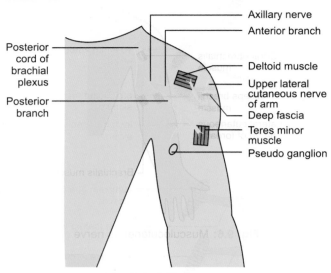

Fig. 9.8: Axillary nerve

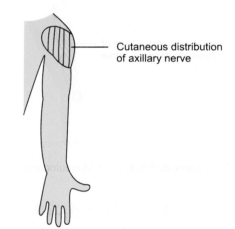

Fig. 9.9: Cutaneous distribution of Axillary nerve

3. **Articular branches:** To shoulder joint.
4. **Vascular branches** supply posterior circumflex humeral artery.

ULNAR NERVE (MUSICIANS NERVE)

Ulnar nerve is the direct continuation of medial cord of brachial plexus in axilla (Fig. 9.10).
Root value: Ventral rami of C_7 C_8 T_1 spinal nerves. It often receives contribution from C_7, these fibres supply flexor carpi ulnaris.

Branches
1. **Muscular branches**
   In forearm
   a. Flexor carpi ulnaris
   b. Medial half of flexor digitorum profundus
   In hand
   a. Palmaris brevis
   b. Abductor digiti minimi
   c. Flexor digiti minimi

d. Opponens digiti minimi
e. 3rd and 4th lumbricals
f. 4 palmar interossei
g. 4 dorsal interossei
h. Adductor pollicis
i. Flexor pollicis brevis
2. **Cutaneous branches**
   a. Dorsal cutaneous branch to dorsum of hand: It is given out 5 cm above wrist.
   b. Palmar cutaneous branch to palmar aspect of hand: It passes superficial to flexor retinaculum and supplies medial 1/3rd of palm and medial 1½ digits upto the dorsal aspect of the corresponding 1½ distal phalanx.

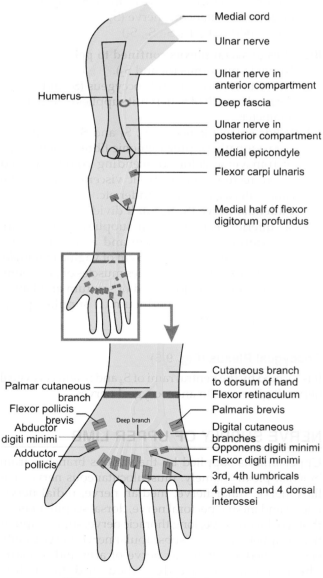

Fig. 9.10: Distribution of ulnar nerve

3. **Articular branches**
   a. Elbow joint
   b. Intercarpal joints
   c. Carpometacarpal joints
4. **Vascular branches** supply axillary, brachial, ulnar and deep palmar arteries.

MEDIAN NERVE (LABOURER'S NERVE)

It is formed in axilla by medial and lateral roots. Medial root comes from medial cord and lateral root comes from lateral cord of brachial plexus (Fig. 9.11).

Root value: Ventral rami of C_5, C_6, C_7, C_8, T_1 spinal nerves

Branches

1. **Muscular branches**
   In arm
   a. Nerve to pronator teres muscle.
   In the forearm
   a. Pronator teres muscle
   b. Flexor carpi radialis muscle
   c. Palmaris longus muscle
   d. Flexor digitorum superficialis muscle

   e. **Anterior interosseous nerve which supplies**
   — Flexor pollicis longus muscle
   — Pronator quadratus muscle
   — Lateral half of flexor digitorum profundus muscle
   In palm
   a. Abductor pollicis brevis muscle
   b. Flexor pollicis brevis muscle
   c. Opponens pollicis muscle
   d. 1st and 2nd lumbricals muscle
2. **Cutaneous branches**
   In forearm: Palmar cutaneous branch given just above the flexor retinaculum supplies central part of palm and adjacent part of thenar eminence
   In hand: Palmar digital nerves supply lateral three and half of the digits on palmar aspect and distal phalanges on the dorsal aspect
3. **Articular branches**
   a. Elbow joint
   b. Superior radioulnar joint
   c. Wrist joint
4. **Vascular branches** supply axillary and brachial arteries and their branches.

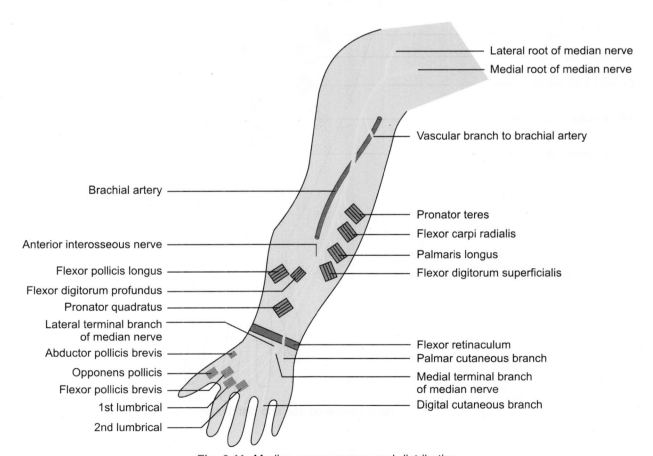

Fig. 9.11: Median nerve, course and distribution

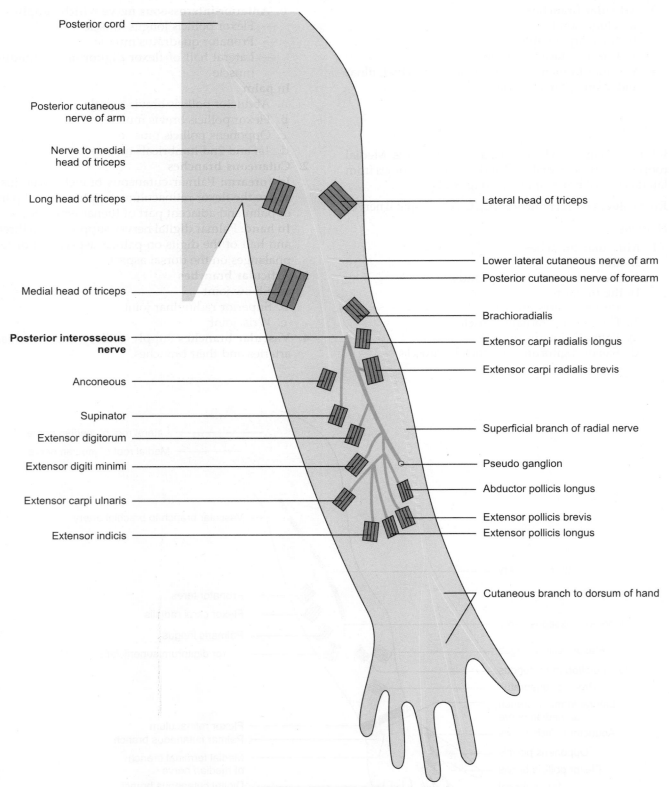

Posterior cord

Posterior cutaneous nerve of arm

Nerve to medial head of triceps

Long head of triceps

Medial head of triceps

Posterior interosseous nerve

Anconeous

Supinator

Extensor digitorum

Extensor digiti minimi

Extensor carpi ulnaris

Extensor indicis

Lateral head of triceps

Lower lateral cutaneous nerve of arm

Posterior cutaneous nerve of forearm

Brachioradialis

Extensor carpi radialis longus

Extensor carpi radialis brevis

Superficial branch of radial nerve

Pseudo ganglion

Abductor pollicis longus

Extensor pollicis brevis

Extensor pollicis longus

Cutaneous branch to dorsum of hand

Fig. 9.12: Radial nerve-course and distribution

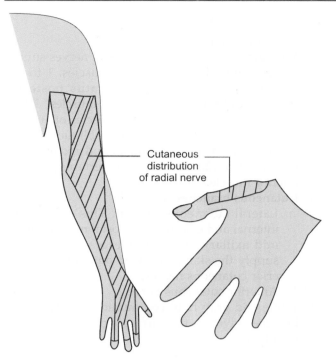

Fig. 9.13: Cutaneous distribution of radial nerve

RADIAL NERVE

It is the continuation of posterior cord of brachial plexus in axilla. It is the largest branch of brachial plexus. It terminates infront of the lateral epicondyle of humerus by dividing into a superficial terminal branch and the posterior interosseous nerve (Figs 9.12 and 9.13).

Root value: Dorsal branches of ventral rami of C_5, C_6, C_7, C_8, T_1

Branches

1. **Muscular branches**
   In axilla
   a. Long head of triceps
   b. Medial head of triceps
   In spiral groove
   a. Lateral head of triceps
   b. Medial head of triceps
   c. Anconeus
   Lower part of arm
   a. Brachioradialis
   b. Extensor carpi radialis longus
   c. Lateral part of brachialis
   Forearm: The muscles of forearm supplied by the **posterior interosseous nerve** which is the deep terminal branch of radial nerve. These are:
   a. Supinator
   b. Extensor carpi radialis brevis
   c. Extensor digitorum
   d. Extensor digiti minimi

   e. Extensor carpi ulnaris
   f. Abductor pollicis longus
   g. Extensor pollicis brevis
   h. Extensor pollicis longus
   i. Extensor indicis
   Posterior interosseous nerve also gives sensory branches to the radius, ulna and interosseous membrane.
2. **Cutaneous branches**
   In axilla
   a. Posterior cutaneous nerve of the arm supplies skin on the dorsal surface of arm upto olecranon process.
   In arm
   a. Posterior cutaneous nerve of forearm supplies skin of dorsal surface of forearm up to wrist.
   b. Lower lateral cutaneous nerve of arm supplies skin of lateral side of lower half of the arm.
   In forearm: Superficial terminal branch innervates lateral 2/3rd of dorsum of hand and dorsal aspect of lateral 31/2 digits except distal phalynx.
3. **Articular branches**
   a. Elbow joint
   b. Wrist joint
   c. Inferior radio ulnar joint
   d. Intercarpal joints
4. **Vascular branches:** To radial artery and part of deep palmar arch.

SYMPATHETIC INNERVATION OF UPPER LIMB

Preganglionic sympathetic fibres emerge from T_2 to T_6 spinal segments. Post ganglionic fibres arise from stellate ganglion and pass through grey rami communicants to the nerve roots forming brachial plexus. These postganglionic sympathetic fibres supply blood vessels of upper limb and sweat glands, arrector pilorus muscle of skin of upper limb. These fibres are vasomotor, secretomotor and pilomotor.

NERVE SUPPLY OF THORAX

The skin and muscles of thoracic wall are supplied by intercostal nerves. The various nerves supplying thoracic viscera are described along with the respective system.

INTERCOSTAL NERVES (FIG. 9.14)

- One intercostal nerve is present in each intercostal space on each side of thoracic cage. The 12th nerve is called subcostal nerve as it lies below the last rib. They arise as the ventral ramus of the corresponding thoracic spinal nerve.
- 3rd to 6th intercostal nerves are named typical intercostal nerves as they are confined to thorax.

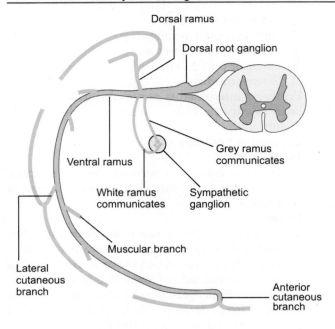

Fig. 9.14: Typical thoracic spinal nerve

Branches of an Intercostal Nerve

1. Collateral branch
2. **Muscular branches:** All intercostal nerves supply the corresponding intercostal muscles. 1 to 6th intercostal nerves supply serratus posterior superior and transversus thoracis muscles. 7th to 12th intercostal nerves supply muscles of anterior abdominal wall namely external oblique, internal oblique, transversis abdominis and rectus abdominis. 10th to 12th nerves supply serratus posterior inferior muscle.
3. **Cutaneous branches:** These are
   a. Lateral cutaneous branch: This pierces the internal and external intercostal muscles at the mid axillary line and emerges externally to supply the skin along with anterior and posterior cutaneous nerves.
   b. Anterior cutaneous nerve
4. White and gray rami communicantes: These are branches given to the corresponding sympathetic ganglion.

NERVE SUPPLY OF ABDOMEN AND PELVIS

The nerve supply to abdominal wall is described in chapter no. 10 (see page nos 302 to 304).

The nerve supply of various viscera of abdomen and pelvis is described along with the various systems.

NERVE SUPPLY OF LOWER LIMB

Lower limb is supplied by branches of lumbar plexus namely femoral nerve and obturator nerve and branches of sacral plexus namely sciatic nerve, tibial nerve, common peroneal nerve, superficial peroneal nerve, deep peroneal nerve and medial and lateral plantar nerves. The cutaneous nerve supply is derived from lumbar and sacral plexus (see page nos 304 to 306)

FEMORAL NERVE

It is a branch from the lumbar plexus and supplies muscles of the anterior compartment of the thigh as well as the skin of front of thigh, medial aspect of leg and foot (Fig. 9.15).

Root value: Dorsal branches of ventral primary rami of L_2, L_3, L_4 spinal nerves.

Branches

1. **From trunk:** They are three in number
   a. Nerve to iliacus muscle (few twigs to psoas major muscle)
   b. Nerve to pectineus muscle
   c. Vascular branches

- 1st intercostal nerve contributes to the lower trunk of brachial plexus and is distributed to the upper limb.
- 2nd intercostal nerve forms the intercostobrachial nerve which supplies the skin of upper arm.
- 7th to 11th intercostal nerves supply the skin over abdominal region in the anterior part beside giving few branches in the thorax. 12th thoracic nerve supplies anterolateral region of lower abdominal wall upto the upper part of gluteal region.

Course of a Typical Intercostal Nerve

- Each nerve arises from the corresponding intervertebral foramina lying medial to the superior costo- transverse ligament.
- It runs along with the vascular bundle in between the costal pleura and posterior intercostal membrane.
- Then it lies in the costal groove. The neurovascular bundle consists of the vein superiorly and nerve inferiorly with the artery in between.
- It further passes in front of internal thoracic artery and pierces successively the internal intercostal muscle, anterior intercostal membrane which is covered by pectoralis major and ends superfically as the anterior cutaneous nerve just lateral to the sternum.

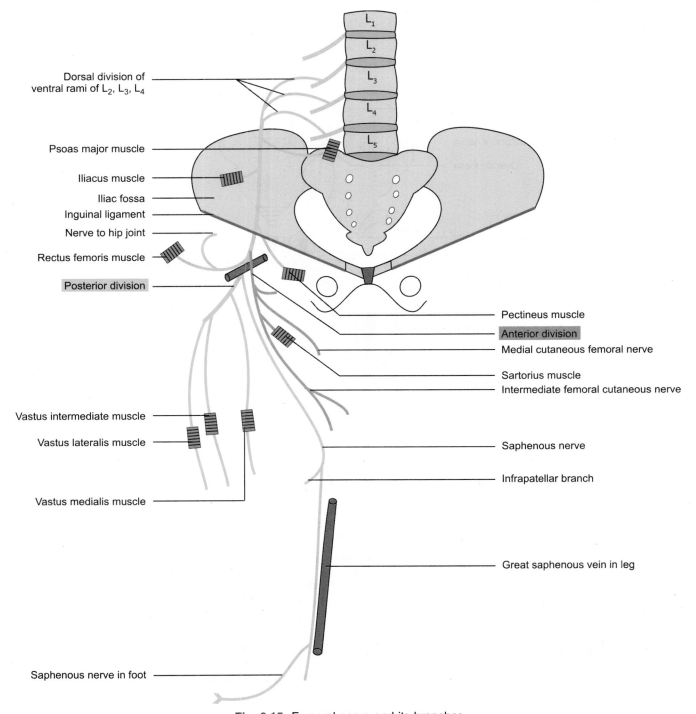

Fig. 9.15: Femoral nerve and its branches

2. **From anterior division:** They are three in number
   a. Intermediate femoral cutaneous nerve
   b. Medial femoral cutaneous nerve
   c. Nerve to sartorius muscle
3. **From posterior division:** It give rise to 5 branches
   a. Saphenous nerve (cutaneous)

b. Nerve to rectus femoris muscle, also supplies hip joint

c. Nerve to vastus medialis muscle

d. Nerve to vastus lateralis muscle

e. Nerve to vastus intermediate muscle

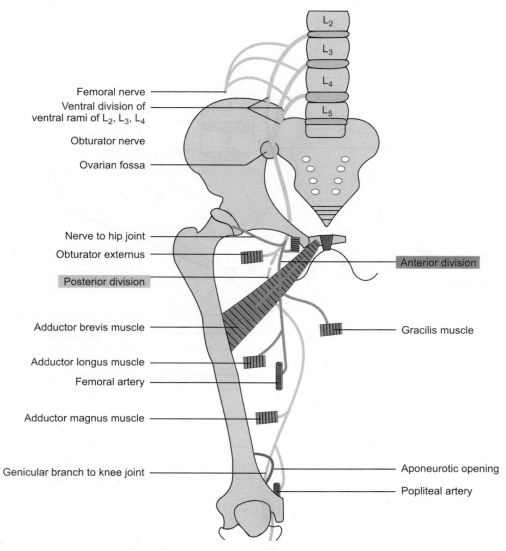

Fig. 9.16: Obturator nerve and its distribution

OBTURATOR NERVE

It is a branch of lumbar plexus. It supplies the medial compartment of thigh (Fig. 9.16).

Root value: Ventral branches of the ventral primary rami of L_2, L_3 and L_4 spinal nerves.

Branches

Anterior Division
1. **Muscular branches** to the following muscles
   a. Adductor longus
   b. Gracilis
   c. Pectineus
   d. Adductor brevis
2. **Articular branches** to hip joint.
3. **Cutaneous supply** to subsartorial plexus.
4. **Vascular branches** to femoral artery.

Posterior Division
1. **Muscular branches**
   a. Adductor Magnus—adductor part
   b. Obturator externus
   c. Adductor brevis
2. **Articular branches** to knee joint.
3. **Vascular branches** to popliteal artery.

SCIATIC NERVE

It is a nerve from the sacral plexus. It supplies the muscles of the back of thigh and divides into terminal branches namely tibial and common peroneal nerves. It is the thickest nerve of the body. In fact it is made up of two separate nerves enclosed in a common sheath (Figs 9.5, 9.17).

It terminates at the lower 1/3rd and upper 2/3rd of posterior aspect of thigh by dividing into tibial and common peroneal nerves.

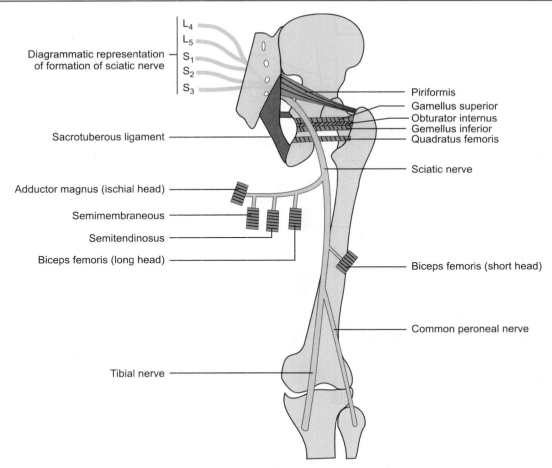

Diagrammatic representation of formation of sciatic nerve

L₄
L₅
S₁
S₂
S₃

Piriformis
Gamellus superior
Obturator internus
Gemellus inferior
Quadratus femoris

Sacrotuberous ligament

Sciatic nerve

Adductor magnus (ischial head)

Semimembraneous

Semitendinosus

Biceps femoris (long head)

Biceps femoris (short head)

Common peroneal nerve

Tibial nerve

Fig. 9.17: Sciatic nerve

Root Value: Ventral primary rami of L_4, L_5, S_1, S_2,S_3, spinal nerves.

Components: It has following two components

1. **Tibial:** It is the ventral division of ventral primary rami of L_4, L_5, S_1, S_2 and S_3.

2. **Common peroneal:** It is dorsal division of ventral primary rami of L_4, L_5, S_1 and S_2.

Branches

1. **Muscular branches**
   Branches containing tibial component supply the following muscles
   a. Semimembranous
   b. Semitendinosus
   c. Long head of biceps femoris
   d. Ischial head of adductor magnus
   Branch containing common peroneal component supplies:
   e. Short head of biceps femoris
2. **Articular branches to hip joint**

3. **Two terminal branches**
   a. Tibial nerve
   b. Common peroneal nerve

TIBIAL NERVE

It is the larger terminal division of sciatic nerve given at the apex of popliteal fossa or at the junction of upper 2/3rd and lower 1/3rd of thigh. It terminates deep to the flexor retinaculum by dividing into medial and lateral plantar nerves (Fig. 9.18).
Root value: Ventral division of ventral primary rami of L_4 L_5, S_1, S_2, S_3 spinal nerves.

Branches

1. **Muscular branches in popliteal fossa to the following muscles**
   a. Popliteus
   b. Soleus (from superficial surface)
   c. Two heads of gastrocnemius
   d. Plantaris

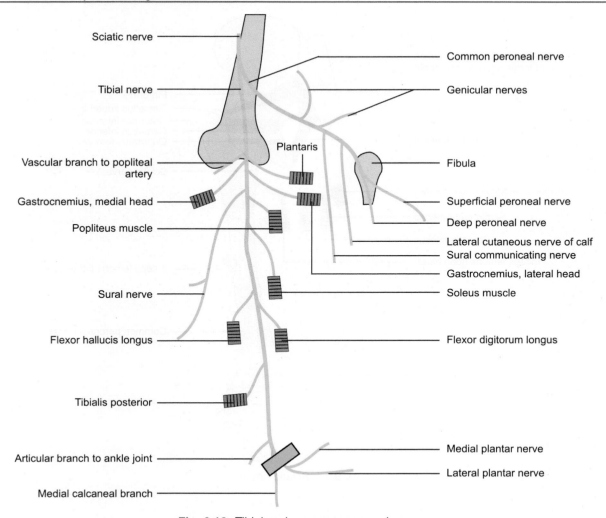

Fig. 9.18: Tibial and common peroneal nerves

2. **Muscular branches in leg to the following muscles**
   a. Soleus muscle (from deep surface)
   b. Tibialis posterior muscle
   c. Flexor digitorum longus muscle
   d. Flexor hallucis longus muscle
3. **Articular branches**
   a. Knee joint
   b. Ankle joint
4. **Cutaneous branches**
   a. **Sural nerve:** It supplies lateral and posterior part of lower one third of leg. Lateral side of foot and little toe is also supplied by sural nerve.
   b. **Medial calcanean branch:** Heel and medial side of sole and foot is supplied by medial calcanean branch.
5. **Vascular branches** supply popliteal artery and posterior tibial artery.

COMMON PERONEAL NERVE

It is the smaller terminal branch of sciatic nerve. It divides into deep and superficial peroneal branches at the neck of fibula (Fig. 9.18).

Root value: Ventral rami of L_4, L_5, S_1 and S_2 spinal nerves.

Branches

1. **Cutaneous branches**
   a. Sural communicating nerve.
   b. Lateral cutaneous nerve of calf.
2. **Articular branches:** To knee joint.
3. **Terminal branches**
   a. Deep peroneal nerve
   b. Superficial peroneal nerve

DEEP PERONEAL NERVE

It is the nerve of the anterior compartment of leg also known as **anterior tibial nerve**. It is a branch of common peroneal nerve (Fig. 9.19). It is given out on the lateral side of neck of fibula deep to peroneus longus muscle. It terminates by dividing into lateral and medial branches at the dorsum of foot.

Branches given in Leg

1. **Muscular branches to**
   a. Tibialis anterior muscle
   b. Extensor digitorum longus muscle
   c. Extensor hallucis longus muscle
   d. Peroneus tertius muscle
2. **Articular branches to ankle joint**

Branches given in Dorsum of Foot

1. **Medial branch gives rise to following branches**
   a. Two dorsal digital branches for cutaneous supply to cleft between the great toe and second digit.
   b. One communicating branch to medial branch of superficial peroneal nerve.
   c. One interosseous branch to 1st dorsal interosseous muscle.

2. **Lateral branch which gives rise to following branches**
   a. Articular branches to 2nd, 3rd and 4th toe.
   b. Second dorsal interosseous muscle.
   This lateral branch presents a **pseudoganglion** through which it supplies extensor digitorum brevis.

SUPERFICIAL PERONEAL NERVE

It is the terminal branch of common peroneal nerve (Fig. 9.20). It arises from common peroneal nerve on the lateral side of neck of fibula under cover of peroneus longus. It terminates as medial and lateral branches at the dorsum of the foot.

Branches
1. **Muscular branches:** It supplies following muscles
   a. Peroneus longus
   b. Peroneus brevis
2. **Cutaneous branches:** It supplies most of the dorsum of the foot.

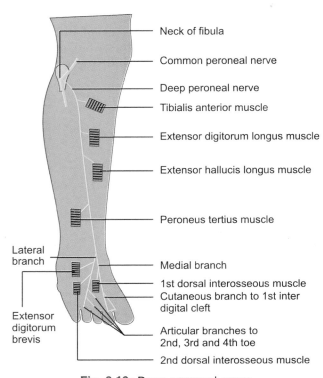

Fig. 9.19: Deep peroneal nerve

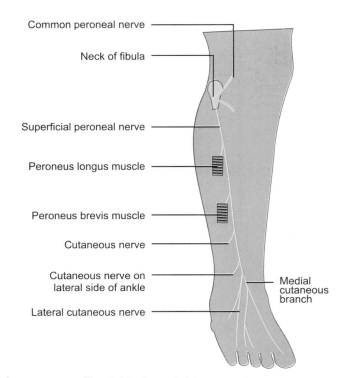

Fig. 9.20: Superficial peroneal nerve

NERVES OF THE FOOT

The foot is supplied by medial and lateral plantar nerves, branches of tibial nerve.

Medial Plantar Nerve

It is the larger terminal branch of **tibial nerve** (Fig. 9.21). It arises beneath flexor retinaculum and ends in the interval between abductor hallucis and flexor digitorum brevis.

Branches
1. **From trunk:** Two muscles are supplied by trunk of medial plantar nerve
   a. Abductor hallucis.
   b. Flexor digitorum brevis.
2. **Proper digital nerve to the hallux**
   a. Gives cutaneous branches to the medial side of great toe.
   b. Supplies flexor hallucis brevis muscle.
3. **Three common plantar digital nerves:** These supply

   a. Skin over lateral half of great toe and 2nd, 3rd and medial half of 4th toe including nail bed on dorsal surface
   b. The first common plantar digital nerve gives a branch to 1st lumbrical muscle.
4. **Articular branches**
   a. Tarsometatarsal joints
   b. Intertarsal joints
   c. Interphalangeal joints

Lateral Plantar Nerve

It is a terminal branch of tibial nerve (Fig. 9.22). It arises beneath flexor retinaculum. It ends by dividing into superficial and deep branches in the second layer of the sole.

Branches
1. **From Trunk**
   a. Branch to flexor digitorum accessorius muscle.
   b. Branch to abductor digiti minimi muscle.
   c. Cutaneous branch to lateral margin of sole.
2. **Superficial branch:** It gives rise to following branches:
   a. Skin of lateral 1½ digits including nail beds.
   b. Branches to flexor digiti minimi brevis muscle.
   c. Two interossei of 4th intermetatarsal space.
3. **Deep branch:** It give rise to following branches:
   a. Branch to adductor hallucis muscle.
   b. Branches to 2, 3, 4 lumbricals.
   c. All interossei except interossei of 4th space.
4. **Articular branches** to intertarsal tarsometatarsal and metatarsophalangeal and interphalangeal joints.

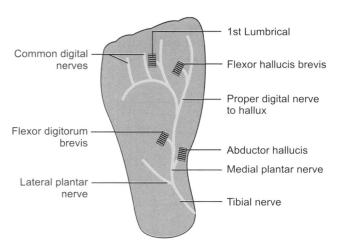

Fig. 9.21: Medial plantar nerve

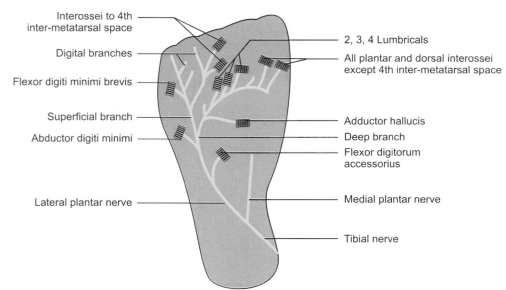

Fig. 9.22: Lateral plantar nerve

CRANIAL NERVES

There are twelve pairs of cranial nerves that carry information to and fro from head and neck region of body and various viscera (vagus nerve) to brain.

1. Olfactory nerve
2. Optic nerve
3. Oculomotor nerve
4. Trochlear nerve
5. Trigeminal nerve
6. Abducent nerve
7. Facial nerve
8. Vestibulo—cochlear nerve
9. Glossiogaryngeal nerve
10. Vagus nerve
11. Accessory Nerve
12. Hypoglossal nerve

There are seven functional components of the cranial nerves based on their position and the embryological origin of tissues which they supply. These are tabulated below:

Functional component	Tissue supplied	Basis of classification
Somatic efferent	Striated muscle of limbs and body wall, extrinsic muscles of the eye ball and muscles of tongue	These tissues are derived from somites and mesoderm of body wall.
General visceral efferent	Smooth muscles, glands, heart muscles	They form viscera of the body.
Special visceral efferent	Muscles of face, mastication, larynx and pharynx	These are muscles derived from the branchial arches.
General somatic afferent	Skin, tendon, muscle joints	Convey sense of touch, pain and temperature from skin and sense of proprioception from the joints.
Special somatic afferent	Eye (retina), ear and nose	Ectodermal origin of sense organs of vision, hearing and olfaction.
General visceral afferent	Viscera	Transmits pain from viscera.
Special visceral afferent	Tongue (Taste buds)	Endodermal in origin, an organ of special sense.

OLFACTORY NERVE

It is the nerve for sensation of smell (Fig. 9.23).

Functional Component

1. **Special somatic afferent :** For sense of smell.

Origin: The fibres arise from the central processes of bipolar neurons in the olfactory epithelium present in the upper part of nasal cavity, over superior nasal conchae and the upper part of nasal septum.

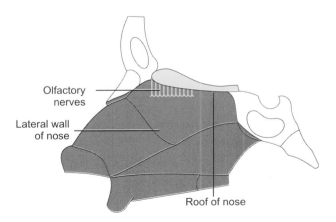

Olfactory nerves

Lateral wall of nose

Roof of nose

Fig. 9.23: Olfactory nerve

Course

- The fibres run upwards and unite to form about 20 small nerve bundles or filaments which are collectively known as olfactory nerves. Each nerve bundle is enclosed by the three meninges.
- The olfactory nerves pierce the cribriform plate of ethmoid to enter the cranial cavity and end in the olfactory bulb of the frontal lobe of brain lying immediately above the cribrifrom plate.

OPTIC NERVE

This is the nerve of sight (Fig. 9.24).

Functional Component

1. Special somatic afferent: For sense of vision
2. Afferent for visual reflex

Origin: The nerve fibers are made up of axons of ganglion cells of the retina. It is made up of about 1 million myelinated fibres.

Course

The nerve runs backwards and medially in the orbit and enters the cranial cavity through the optic canal. In the canal it is enclosed in three meninges i.e. dura, arachnoid and pia. It continues as the optic pathway.

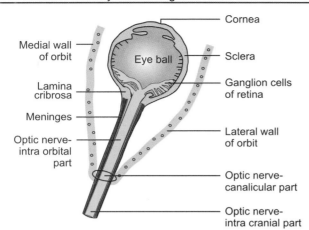

Fig. 9.24: Optic nerve

Parts of Optic Nerve
1. Intraorbital: 2.5 cm long.
2. Intra-canalicular: 0.6 cm long.
3. Intra-cranial: 1.0 cm long.

Visual Pathway

Retina is the photoreceptive layer of the eye. Impulses are generated in rods and cones of retina and are transmitted along the axons of ganglion cells of retina which converge to the optic disc and exit the eyeball as optic nerve (Fig. 9.25).

- The impulses course successively through optic nerve, optic chiasma and optic tract to relay in lateral geniculate body of corresponding side.

- The fibres originating from nasal halves of the retina cross to opposite side at the chiasma. Hence each optic tract consists of fibres from temporal region of retina of ipsilateral side (same side) and nasal region of retina of contra-lateral side (opposite side).
- The fibres from nuclei of lateral geniculate body extend to the visual cortex in the medial aspect of occipital lobe via the optic radiation.

OCULOMOTOR NERVE

Oculomotor is the third cranial nerve (Fig. 9.26).

Functional Components
1. **General visceral efferent:** Conveys preganglionic parasympathetic fibres for constriction of pupil and accommodation.
2. **General somatic efferent:** Motor to extraocular muscles of the eyeball.
3. **General somatic afferent:** Receives proprioceptive impulses from the muscles of the eyeball.

Nuclear Origin: Fibres arise from the oculomotor nuclear complex (motor nucleus and Edinger Westphal nucleus) situated in the periaqueductal grey matter of upper part of the midbrain at the level of superior colliculus.

Course
- The nerve emerges as a single trunk from the oculomotor sulcus of midbrain.
- It enters lateral wall of cavernous sinus in middle cranial fossa.

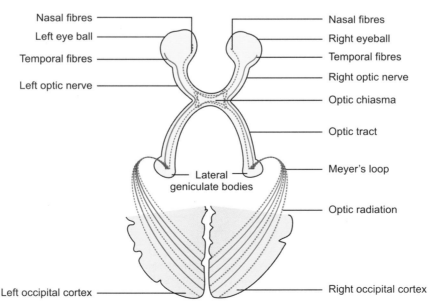

Fig. 9.25: Visual pathway

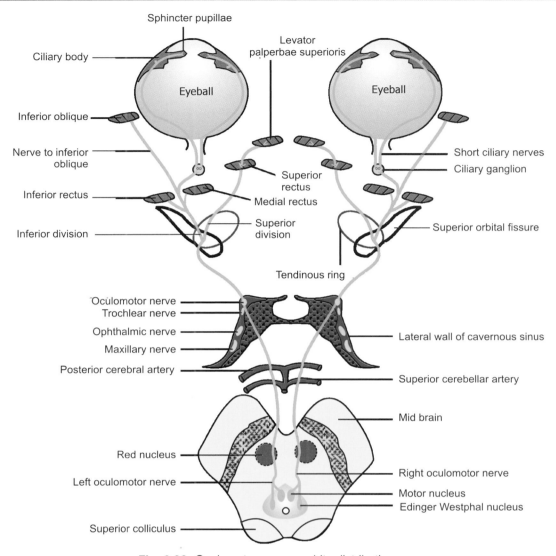

Fig. 9.26: Oculomotor nerve and its distribution

- It divides into superior and inferior rami and enters superior orbital fissure in the orbit.

Distribution

Superior ramus supplies:
  a. Levator palpebrae superioris muscle
  b. Superior rectus muscle
Inferior ramus supplies:
  a. Inferior rectus muscle
  b. Medial rectus muscle
  c. Inferior oblique muscle
  d. Branch to ciliary ganglion: It supplies cilliary muscle and iris.

CILIARY GANGLION

It is a peripheral parasympathetic ganglion, tophographically connnected with the nasociliary nerve, branch of ophthalmic division of trigeminal nerve.

However, functionally it is connected to the oculomotor nerve. It lies near the apex of the orbit, between the optic nerve and lateral rectus muscle (Figs 9.26 and 9.28).

Roots

1. **Motor (parasympathetic) root:** It is derived from the nerve to inferior oblique and consists of preganglionic parasympathetic fibres from Edinger-Westphal nucleus. These fibres relay in the ganglion. The postganglionic parasympathetic fibres arise from the cells of the ganglion and pass through short ciliary nerves to supply the ciliary muscle and sphincter pupillae.
2. **Sensory root:** It is derived from the nasociliary nerve. It consists of sensory fibres for pain, touch and temperature from the eyeball which pass through the ciliary ganglion without relaying in it.

3. **Sympathetic root:** It is derived from the sympathetic plexus around internal carotid artery. It consists of postganglionic sympathetic fibres from the superior cervical sympathetic ganglion. These fibres pass through the ganglion without relay, into the short ciliary nerves to supply the dilator pupillae and blood vessels of the eyeball.

Branches of Ciliary Ganglion

1. **Short ciliary nerves (8 to 10 in number):** They contain fibres from all the three roots. The nerves run above and below the optic nerve towards the eyeball. On reaching the eyeball they pierce the sclera around the attachment of optic nerve and pass forward in the space between the sclera and choroid to reach the target organs.

TROCHLEAR NERVE

Trochlear is the fourth cranial nerve. It is the most slender of all the cranial nerves and the only one which arises from the dorsal aspect of the brain (Fig. 9.27).

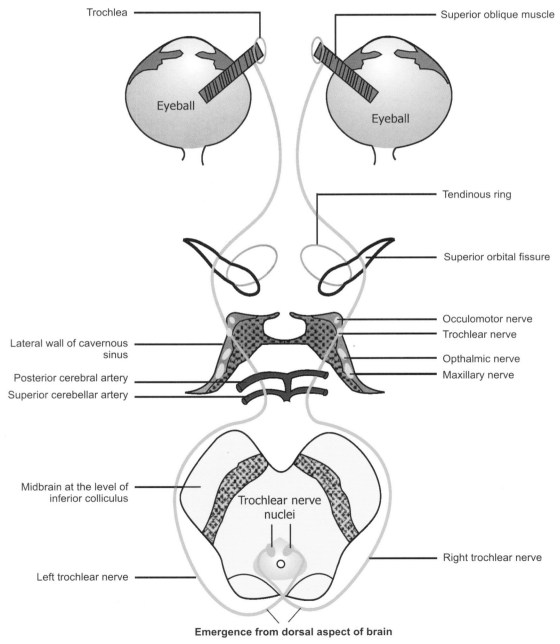

Fig. 9.27: Trochlear nerve and its distribution

Functional Components
1. **Somatic efferent:** Motor to superior oblique muscle.
2. **General somatic afferent:** Receives proprioceptive impulses from the superior oblique muscle.

Nuclear Origin: Fibres arise from the **trochlear nucleus** situated in the lower part of the midbrain at the level of inferior colliculus.

Course

- The two trochlear nerves arise from the dorsal surface of brain stem, one on each site of the frenulum veli. Fibres of both sides decussate with each other.
- It enters lateral wall of cavernous sinus in middle cranial fossa.
- It enters orbit through lateral part of superior orbital fissure.

Distribution of Trochlear Nerve

It supplies the superior oblique muscle.

TRIGEMINAL NERVE

The trigeminal nerve is the fifth cranial nerve. It is called trigeminal because it consists of three divisions (Fig. 9.28). These are
1. Ophthalmic nerve
2. Maxillary nerve
3. Mandibular nerve

These three nerves arise from a large semilunar trigeminal ganglion which lies in the trigeminal fossa. The fossa is present on the anterior surface of the petrous temporal bone near its apex. It is covered by a double fold of duramater which forms the trigeminal cave.

Functional Components
1. **General somatic afferent:** Receives exteroceptive sensations from the skin of face and mucosal surfaces and proprioceptive impulses from muscles of mastication.
2. **Special visceral efferent:** Motor to muscles of 1st branchial arch.

Nuclear Origin
1. **The sensory nuclei:** Sensory fibres arise from the trigeminal ganglion and enter the lateral aspect of the pons as the sensory root. The nuclei are arranged in three groups and their connections are as follows
   a. **Chief (principal) sensory nucleus of trigeminal:** It lies in the lateral part of pons, deep to the rhomboid fossa.
   b. **Spinal nucleus of trigeminal nerve:** It extends from the lower part of pons into medulla down

upto the 1st and sometimes the 2nd cervical segment of spinal cord.
   c. **Mesencephalic nucleus:** It lies in mid brain.
2. **The motor nucleus:** This lies in the pons close to the medial side of the chief sensory nucleus.

Course

- The trigeminal nerve arises from the ventral aspect of the pons by two roots, a large sensory and a small motor root.
- The motor root lies venteromedial to the sensory root.
- They pass forward in the posterior cranial fossa towards the apex of the petrous temporal bone.
- The two roots invaginate the dura of the posterior cranial fossa below the superior petrosal sinus forming the trigeminal cave.
- In this cave the sensory root joins the trigeminal ganglion.
- The motor root lies deep to the ganglion and does not join it. Instead, it passes out to join the mandibular nerve just at its emergence from the cranial cavity in the foramen ovale.

Distribution of Trigeminal Nerve

Three large nerves emerge from the convex antero-medial border of the trigeminal ganglion. These divisions of the trigeminal nerve are
1. Ophthalmic nerve
2. Maxillary nerve
3. Mandibular nerve

Ophthalmic Nerve

It is the smallest of the three divisions of trigeminal nerve. It is purely sensory and is given off in the beginning (Fig. 9.28).

It enters the orbit through the superior orbital fissure and divides into three branches namely lacrimal, frontal and nasociliary.

Branches of Ophthalmic Nerve

1. **Lacrimal nerve:** The lacrimal nerve supplies **lacrimal gland** and **conjunctiva** and finally pierces the orbital septum to also supply the **lateral part of upper eyelid.**
2. **Frontal nerve:** In the middle of orbit it divides into two branches namely
   a. **Supraorbital nerve:** It supplies the conjuctiva, upper eyelids and scalp as far back as the lambdoid suture.
   b. **Supratrochlear nerve:** It supplies the conjuctiva, upper lid and finally the skin of the lower part of forehead.

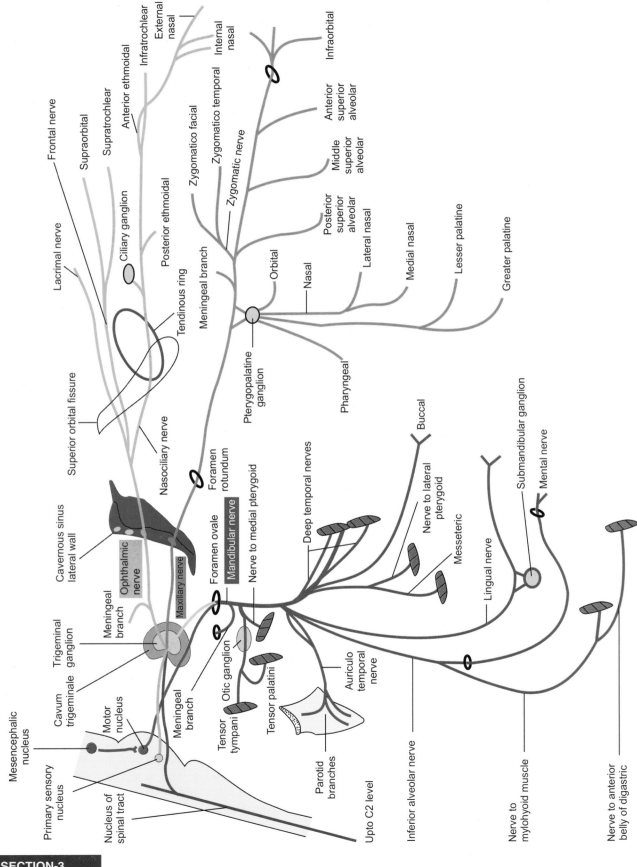

Fig. 9.28: Trigeminal nerve and its distribution (diagrammatic representation)

3. **Nasociliary nerve:** It enters orbit within the tendinous ring of superior orbital fissure and runs forwards and medially, crossing above the optic nerve from lateral to medial side along with the ophthalmic artery. On reaching the medial wall of the orbit it ends by dividing into anterior ethmoidal and infratrochlear nerves.

Branches of Nasociliary Nerve:
a. Sensory communicating branch to the ciliary ganglion is given just before crossing the optic nerve.
b. **Long ciliary nerves:** 2 or 3 in number. These arise from the nasociliary nerve as it crosses the optic nerve. They pass forward to enter the eyeball and supply sensory fibres to the **ciliary body, iris** and **cornea.**The long ciliary nerves also carry postganglionic sympathetic fibres to the dilator pupillae.
c. **Posterior ethmoidal nerve:** This enters the posterior ethmoidal foramen and supplies the ethmoidal and sphenoidal air sinuses.
d. **Anterior ethmoidal nerve:** It enters the anterior ethmoidal foramen and then passes through anterior ethmoidal canal to reach the anterior cranial fossa. Now it runs forwards over the cribriform plate of ethmoid and enters the nasal cavity by passing through a slit at the side of crista galli. In the nasal cavity the nerve lies in a groove on the posterior surface of the nasal bone and gives of internal nasal branches to the nasal septum and lateral wall of the nose. At the lower border of the nasal bone, the nerve leaves the nasal cavity and appears on the dorsum of nose as the **external nasal nerve.**
e. **Infratrochlear nerve:** This runs forwards on the medial wall of the orbit and ends by supplying the skin of both eyelids and adjoining part of the nose.

Maxillary Nerve

Maxillary nerve is the second division of trigeminal nerve. It is also purely sensory (Fig. 9.28).

Origin and Course
• It arises from the convex anterior border of the trigeminal ganglion and pierces the trigeminal cave of duramater to reach the lower part of the lateral wall of the cavernous sinus.
• The nerve leaves the middle cranial fossa through foramen rotundum and reaches the pterygopalatine fossa.
• It traverses in a straight line in the upper part of the fossa and enters orbit through the inferior orbital fissure where it is called as the infraorbital nerve.

• The infraorbital nerve (in fact a continuation of maxillary nerve) runs forwards along the floor of the orbit in the infraorbital groove and canal and appears on the face through the infraorbital foramen.
• Therefore, in its course the maxillary nerve traverses in succession, the middle cranial fossa, the pterygopalatine fossa and the orbit.

Branches

The maxillary nerve gives off the following branches.

In the Middle Cranial Fossa
1. **Meningeal branch:** Supplies the duramater of the middle cranial fossa.

In the Pterygopalatine Fossa
2. **Ganglionic (communicating) branches:** Are 2 in number. They suspend the pterygopalatine ganglion from the lower border of maxillary nerve in the pterygo-palatine fossa.
3. **Zygomatic nerve:** Enters the orbit through inferior orbital fissure and divides on the lateral wall of the orbit into two
   a. **Zygomatico-temporal:** This passes through a foramen in the zygomatic bone to supply the skin of the temple.
   b. **Zygomatico-facial:** It passes through a foramen in the zygomatic bone to supply the skin of the face on the prominence of cheek.
4. **Posterior superior alveolar nerve:** Enters the foramen on the posterior surface of the body of maxilla and supplies the mucous membrane of the maxillary air sinus. Then it breaks up to form the superior dental plexus which supplies the upper molar teeth and adjoining part of the gum.

In the Orbit (Infra Orbital Canal)
5. **Middle superior alveolar nerve:** Passes downwards and forwards along the lateral wall of the maxillary sinus to join the superior dental plexus and supplies the upper premolar teeth.
6. **Anterior superior alveolar nerve:** Runs in the anterior wall of the maxillary sinus through a bony canal called canalis sinusus and divides into two branches
   a. The dental branches which join the dental plexus and supply the canine and incisor teeth of upper jaw.
   b. The nasal branches which appear in the lateral wall of the inferior meatus and supply the mucous membrane of the lateral wall and the floor of the nasal cavity.

On the Face

7. **Palpebral branches:** These turns upwards and supply the skin of the lower eyelid.
8. **Nasal branches:** Supply the skin of the side of nose and the mobile part of the nasal septum.
9. **Superior labial branches:** Supply the skin and mucous membrane of the upper lip.

PTERYGOPALATINE GANGLION (SPHENOPALATINE GANGLION)

Pterygopalatine ganglion is the largest peripheral ganglion of the parasympathetic system. It serves as a relay station for the secretomotor fibres of the lacrimal glands and mucous glands of the nose, palate, pharynx and paranasal sinuses. Topographically, it is related to the maxillary nerve, but functionally, it is connected to the facial nerve through greater petrosal nerve (Fig. 9.28).
Location: It lies in the deep part of the pterygo-palatine fossa, suspended from the maxillary nerve by 2 roots.
Size: Head of a small tack

Roots or Connections

1. **Motor or parasympathetic root:** It is derived from the nerve of pterygoid canal which carries preganglionic parasympathetic fibres from superior salivatory nucleus located in the lower part of the pons. These fibres pass via the geniculate ganglion and greater petrosal nerve to relay in this ganglion. The post ganglionic fibres arise from the cells in the ganglion and provide secretomotor fibres to the lacrimal gland and mucous glands of the nose, palate, nasopharynx and paranasal sinuses. They pass via the maxillary nerve and its branches to the lacrimal nerve.
2. **Sympathetic root:** It is derived from the sympathetic plexus around the internal carotid artery which contains postganglionic fibres from the superior cervical sympathetic ganglion. These fibres pass through the ganglion without relay and form the deep petrosal nerve. This further joins with greater petrosal nerve and provides vasomotor supply to the mucus membrane of nose, paranasal sinuses, palate and pharynx.
3. **Sensory root:** It is derived from the maxillary nerve and passes through the ganglion without interruption to be distributed through the branches of the ganglion.

Branches and Distribution

These are virtually derived from the ganglionic branches of the maxillary nerve which passes through the ganglion without relay.
The ganglion provides four sets of branches namely

1. Orbital
2. Palatine
3. Nasal
4. Pharyngeal

Each branch carries parasympathetic, sympathetic and sensory fibres.

1. **Orbital branches:** They enter the orbit through inferior orbital fissure and supply the periosteum of orbit, orbitalis muscle and sphenoidal air sinuses.
2. **Palatine branches**
   a. **Greater (anterior) palatine nerve:** It descends through the greater palatine canal to emerge underneath the hard palate through the greater palatine foramen. From here it passes forwards along the lateral side of hard palate upto the incisive fossa. It supplies the mucus membrane of the hard palate and the adjoining gum. While in the bony canal it gives off posterior inferior nasal branches to supply the postero-inferior quadrant of the lateral nasal wall.
   b. **Lesser (middle and posterior) palatine nerves:** These run downwards through the greater palatine canal and then through the lesser palatine canals to emerge through lesser palatine foramina. They supply the soft palate and the palatine tonsil.
3. **Nasal branches:** These enter the nasal cavity through the sphenopalatine foramen and divide into two postero-superior branches namely,
   a. **Posterosuperior lateral nasal branches:** They are about 6 in number and supply the postero-superior quadrant of the lateral nasal wall.
   b. **Posterosuperior medial nasal branches:** They are 2 or 3 in number. These cross the roof of the nasal cavity and supply the nasal septum. One of these nerves which is the longest is called naso-palatine (spheno-palatine). It passes downwards and forwards along the nasal septum and reaches the under surface of the anterior part of hard palate through the lateral incisive foramen.
4. **Pharyngeal branch:** It passes backwards and supplies the mucus membrane of nasopharynx behind the auditory tube.

Mandibular Nerve

This is largest of the three divisions of the trigeminal nerve and is the nerve of the first branchial arch. It consists of both sensory and motor fibres (Fig. 9.28).
Origin: It is formed by two roots.
   a. **Larger sensory root:** Arises from the convex aspect of the trigeminal ganglion.
   b. **Small motor root:** Arises from the ventral aspect of pons and passes below the trigeminal ganglion.

Course: Both roots pass through the foramen ovale and join to form the main trunk which lies in the infratemporal fossa. After a short course the main trunk divides into a small anterior and a large posterior division.

Branches

From Main Trunk
1. **Nervous spinosus (meningeal branch):** Supplies the duramater of middle cranial fossa. It enters the middle cranial fossa along with middle meningeal artery through foramen spinosum.
2. **Nerve to medial pterygoid:** It supplies three muscles namely medial pterygoid, tensor palati and tensor tympani.
   It also forms the motor root of the otic ganglion.

From anterior division: It give rise to three motor and one sensory branches.
3. **Deep temporal nerves:** Two in number. They supply the temporalis muscle from its deep surface.
4. **Nerve to lateral pterygoid:** Supplies lateral pterygoid muscle.
5. **Masseteric nerve:** Supplies masseter muscle.
6. **Buccal nerve:** Supplies skin and mucus membrane of the cheek.

From posterior division: It gives rise to three sensory nerves namely
7. Auriculo-temporal nerve
8. Inferior alveolar nerve
9. Lingual nerve

Auriculo-temporal Nerve

It characteristically arises by two roots which unite to form a single trunk after encircling the middle meningeal artery.

Branches: It has mainly sensory supply
   a. **Auricular branches:** Supplies the pinna, external acoustic meatus and adjoining tympanic membrane.
   b. **Articular branches:** To temporo-mandibular joint.
   c. **Superficial temporal branches:** These supply the area of skin over the temple.
   d. **Communicating branches:** It receives postganglionic secretomotor fibres from otic ganglion to supply the parotid gland.

Inferior Alveolar Nerve

It is the larger terminal branch of mandibular nerve and it is a mixed nerve. It has most of the motor fibres of the trigeminal nerve.
Branches:
   a. **Inferior dental plexus:** Few nerve fibres in mandibular canal break away to form this plexus

which supplies the molar and premolar teeth and the adjoining gum of lower jaw.
   b. **Incisive nerve:** Supplies the canine and incisor teeth with the adjoining gum of lower jaw.
   c. **Mental nerve:** Supplies skin of chin and lower lip
   d. **Nerve to mylohyoid:** It supplies mylohyoid and anterior belly of digastric. It is given before the inferior alveolar nerve enters the mandibular foramen
   e. Communicating branch to the lingual nerve.

Lingual Nerve

It is the smaller terminal branch of mandibular nerve given off in front of the inferior alveolar nerve. About 2 cm. below the base of skull, in the infratemporal fossa, the chorda tympani nerve joins it posteriorly at an acute angle. It comes in direct contact with the mandible medial to the last molar tooth. Here it is covered by mucus membrane of gum only.

Branches
1. Sensory branches to mucus membrane of anterior 2/3rd of tongue, floor of mouth and adjoining area of gum.
2. Communicating branches
   a. **With chorda tympani:** The lingual nerve receives secretomotor fibres for submandibular and sublingual glands. It also conveys fibres for taste sensation from anterior 2/3rd of tongue to the chorda tympani.
   b. **With hypoglossal nerve:** Lingual nerve transmits proprioceptive sensations from the lingular muscles via its communicating branches to the hypoglossal nerve.

SUBMANDIBULAR GANGLION

It is the parasympathetic ganglion which provides a relay station for the secretomotor fibres that supply the submandibular and sublingual salivary glands. Topographically it is connected to lingual nerve but functionally it is connected to facial nerve through the chorda tympani branch (Fig. 9.28).

Size   : Pin-head
Shape   : Fusiform
Location : Submandibular region, on the outer surface of hyoglossus muscle. It is suspended from the lingual nerve by two roots or filaments.

Roots or Communications

1. **Parasympathetic root:** It lies posteriorly and is derived from the fibres of chorda tympani nerve communicating with lingual nerve. Preganglionic parasympathetic fibres arise from the superior

salivatory nucleus and pass successively through the facial nerve, chorda tympani nerve and lingual nerve to relay in the submandibular ganglion.

2. **Sympathetic root:** It is derived from the sympathetic plexus around facial artery. It conveys postganglionic fibres from the superior cervical ganglion of sympathetic trunk.They pass the ganglion without relay.

Branches

1. **Postganglionic parasympathetic fibres:** These arise as 5 to 6 branches which directly supply the submandibular gland. The fibres supplying sublingual and anterior lingual glands are conveyed via the lingual nerve through the anterior root of ganglion.
2. **Postganglionic sympathetic fibres:** These fibres are vasomotor to the submandibular and sublingual glands.

OTIC GANGLION

It is a parasympathetic ganglion connected to the mandibular division of trigeminal nerve which provides a relay station to the secretomotor parasympathetic fibres of the parotid gland. Topographically, it is connected to mandibular nerve but functionally, it is asociated with glossopharyngeal nerve (Fig. 9.28).

Size : Pin-head, 2 to 3 cm.

Shape : Oval

Location : Infratemporal fossa, just below foramen ovale.

Roots or Connections

1. **Parasympathetic root:** It is obtained from the lesser petrosal nerve. The preganglionic fibres arise in the inferior salivatory nucleus and pass via the tympanic branch of glossopharyngeal nerve followed by tympanic plexus to the lesser petrosal nerve. They relay in the otic ganglion
2. **Sympathetic root:** It is derived from the sympathetic plexus around middle meningeal artery and conveys postganglionic fibres from the superior cervical ganglion. These fibres do not relay in the ganglion.
3. **Somatic motor root:** It receives 1 to 2 fillaments from nerve to medial pterygoid. They pass through the ganglion without relay.

Branches and Distribution

1. Communicating branches to auriculotemporal nerve: These convey postganglionic parasympathetic secretomotor and sympathetic vasomotor fibres to the parotid gland.
2. Communicating branches to chorda tympani.

ABDUCENT NERVE

It is the 6th cranial nerve (Fig. 9.29).

Functional Components
1. **Somatic efferent:** Responsible for lateral movement of the eyeball. (Motor to lateral rectus)
2. **General somatic afferent:** Receives proprioceptive impulses from the lateral rectus muscle.

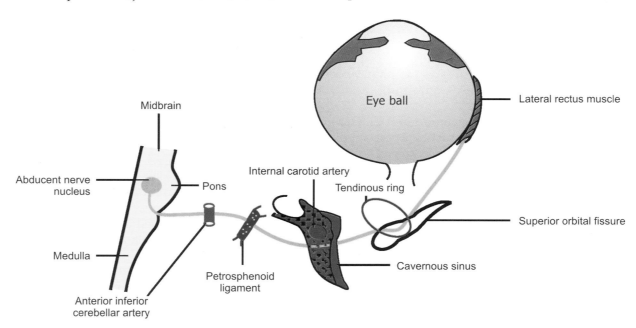

Fig. 9.29: Abducent nerve and its distribution

Nuclear origin: Fibres arise from the **abducent nucleus** located in the lower part of pons beneath the floor of 4th ventricle.

Course

- The abducent nerve arises from the ventral aspect of the brain stem, at the junction of lower border of pons and the upper end of pyramid of the medulla.
- **It takes a long intracranial course.** First it runs forwards, upwards and laterally in the cisterna pontis usually dorsal to the anterior inferior cerebellar artery.
- It pierces dura mater lateral to the dorsum sellae of the sphenoid and bends sharply forwards across the sharp upper border of the petrous temporal bone below the petrosphenoid ligament to enter the cavernous sinus.
- The nerve traverses the cavernous sinus lying at first lateral and then inferolateral to the internal carotid artery.
- Finally, it enters the orbit by passing through the superior orbital fissure within the common tendinous ring inferolateral to the occulomotor and nasociliary nerve.
- The nerve supplies lateral rectus muscle from its ocular surface.

Distribution

It supplies the lateral rectus muscle

FACIAL NERVE

Facial nerve is the seventh cranial nerve. It is a mixed nerve containing both sensory and motor fibres (Fig. 9.30).

Functional Components

1. **Special visceral efferent** is motor to muscles derived from 2nd branchial arch viz. muscles of facial expression.
2. **General visceral efferent:** Provides secretomotor fibres to
   a. Submandibular and sublingual salivary gland.
   b. Lacrimal gland.
   c. Mucous glands of the nose, palate and pharynx.
3. **Special visceral afferent:** Carries taste sensations from anterior 2/3rd of the tongue and palate.
4. **General somatic afferent:** For proprioceptive impulses from the muscles of facial expressions (muscles derived from 2nd branchial arch) and sensation from external auditory meatus.

Nuclear Origin: The facial nerve fibres are connected to the following four cranial nuclei.

1. **Motor nucleus of facial nerve:** This lies in the lower part of pons below and in front of the abducent nerve nucleus. The fibres supplying muscles of 2nd branchial arch originate here.
2. **Superior salivatory nucleus:** It also lies in the pons, lateral to the motor nucleus. It provides the preganglionic parasympathetic secretomotor fibres.
3. **Nucleus of tractus solitarius:** It receives those fibres of facial nerve which are responsible for taste sensation.
4. **Spinal nucleus of trigeminal nerve:** It lies in the medulla and receives fibres for pain and temperature sensations from the external auditory meatus.

Intracranial Course

- The facial nerve arises from the brain stem by two roots
  1. **Motor root:** It is larger and arises from the lower border of pons between the olive and inferior cerebellar peduncle.
  2. **Sensory root:** It arises from the lateral part of the groove between pons and medulla. The sensory root is attached between the motor root medially and the vestibulo-cochlear nerve laterally. Hence, it is also known as **'nervous intermedius'.**
- After arising from the brain stem the two roots of the facial nerve pass forwards and laterally along with the vestibulo-cochlear nerve and enter the internal acoustic meatus located on the posterior surface of the petrous temporal bone.
- They run through the meatus laterally and combine at its lower end to form a single trunk.
- The nerve then enters the facial canal in the petrous temporal bone and runs for a short distance laterally above the vestibule of internal ear.
- As it reaches the medial wall in the epitympanic part of the middle ear, it turns sharply backwards making an acute bend called the genu or knee of facial nerve. The nerve presents with a ganglion on this bend called the geniculate ganglion.
- The nerve now runs horizontally backwards in a bony canal above the promontory producing a bulge in the medial wall of the middle ear.
- On reaching the junction between the medial and posterior walls of the middle ear the nerve turns downwards and continues vertically in the facial canal located along the junction of the medial and posterior walls of the middle ear. It finally emerges out of the skull through the stylomastoid foramen.

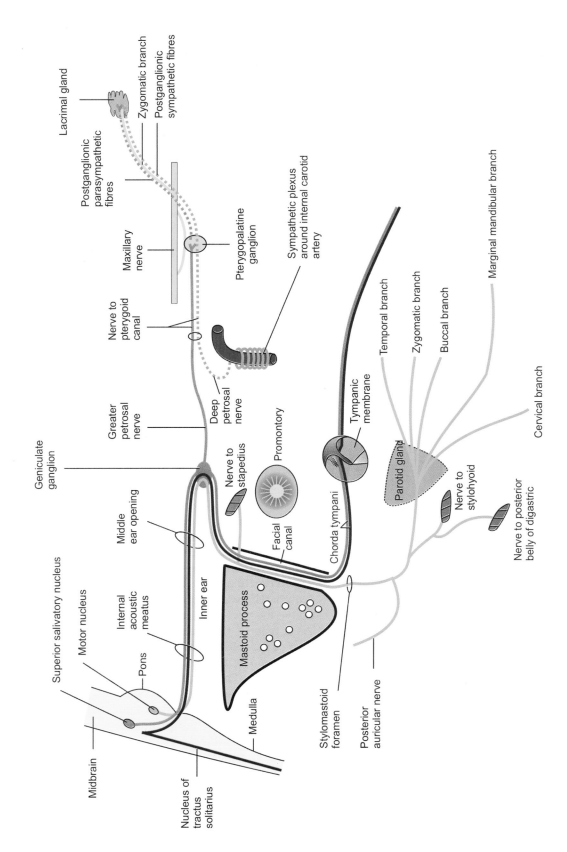

Fig. 9.30: Facial nerve and its distribution

Extracranial Course

On emerging from the stylomastoid foramen, the facial nerve curves forwards around the lateral aspect of the styloid process and enters the posteromedial aspect of the parotid gland. In the parotid gland it divides into its terminal branches.

Branches of the Facial Nerve

1. **Greater petrosal nerve:** It joins with the deep petrosal nerve to form nerve to pterygoid canal. This nerve conveys preganglionic secretomotor fibres to the lacrimal gland and nasal mucosa. They relay in the pterygopalatine ganglion.
2. A twig from geniculate ganglion joins the lesser petrosal nerve
3. **Nerve to stapedius:** It supplies stapedius muscle.
4. **Chorda tympani nerve:** It arises in the facial canal about 6 mm above the stylomastoid foramen and enters the middle ear. It passes forward across the inner surface of the tympanic membrane internal to the handle of malleus and then leaves the middle ear by passing through the petrotympanic fissure to appear at the base of skull. Here it runs downwards and forwards in the infratemporal fossa and joins the lingual nerve at an acute angle.
   The chorda tympani nerve carries
   a. Taste fibres from anterior 2/3rd of the tongue, except from vallate papillae.
   b. Secretomotor fibres to the submandibular and sublingual salivary glands.
5. **Posterior auricular nerve:** It arises just below the styloid foramen. It further divides into two branches
   a. Auricular branch, which supplies the muscles of auricle.
   b. Occipital branch, which supplies the occipital belly of the occipito-frontalis.
6. **Nerve to posterior belly of digastric:** It arises near the origin of posterior auricular nerve and supplies the posterior belly of digastric. It also gives a branch to the stylohyoid muscle.
7. **Terminal branches:** They are 5 in number and arise within the parotid gland. From above downwards they are
   a. Temporal branch
   b. Zygomatic branch
   c. Buccal branches
   d. Marginal mandibular branch
   e. Cervical branch
8. **Communicating branches:** It communicates with the branches of 5th, 8th, 9th, 10th cranial nerves and the sympathetic plexus around middle meningeal artery.

VESTIBULO-COCHLEAR NERVE

The vestibulo-cochlear is the 8th cranial nerve. It is a sensory nerve consisting of two components (Fig. 9.31).
1. **The cochlear nerve,** the nerve of hearing.
2. **The vestibular nerve,** the nerve of balance (equilibrium).

Functional Components
1. **Special somatic afferent:** Conveys the sensation of hearing from hair cells organ of Corti.
2. **Special visceral afferent:** For maintaining static and kinetic equilibrium.

Nuclear Origin: It arises from the following nuclei:
1. **Dorsal and ventral cochlear nuclei:** They are present in pons and give origin to the cochlear nerve.
2. **Vestibular nuclei:** They give origin to the vestibular nerve and are also present in the pons. They are four in number namely superior, inferior, medial and lateral

Intracranial Course

- The vestibular and cochlear components of the 8th cranial nerve arise from the brain stem at the junction of pons and medulla, in the region of cerebello-pontine angle. They lie lateral and posterior to the facial nerve at this point.
- The two components then pass forwards and laterally to enter the internal auditory meatus along with the facial nerve and run in the petrous temporal bone to the inner ear.

Connections and Distribution

1. The cochlear nerve consists of afferent fibres and is formed primarily by the central processes of **bipolar**

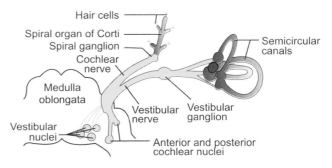

Fig. 9.31: Vestibulo-cochlear nerve

neurons which have their cell bodies in the spiral ganglion located in the petrous temporal bone at the modiolus. The peripheral processes of these cells end in relation to the inner and outer hair cells of the spiral organ of Corti. They are responsible for perception of sound waves.

2. The vestibular nerve also consists of afferent fibres which are formed by the central processes of bipolar neurons of the vestibular ganglion situated at the bottom of the internal acoustic meatus. The peripheral processes of these cells end in the macula of the saccule and utricle which are responsible for the static balance or equilibrium of the body and the ampullary cristae of semicircular canals which maintain the kinetic balance of the body.

GLOSSOPHARYNGEAL NERVE

It is the 9th cranial nerve. It is a mixed nerve containing both motor and sensory fibres. It is the nerve of the 3rd branchial arch (Fig. 9.32).

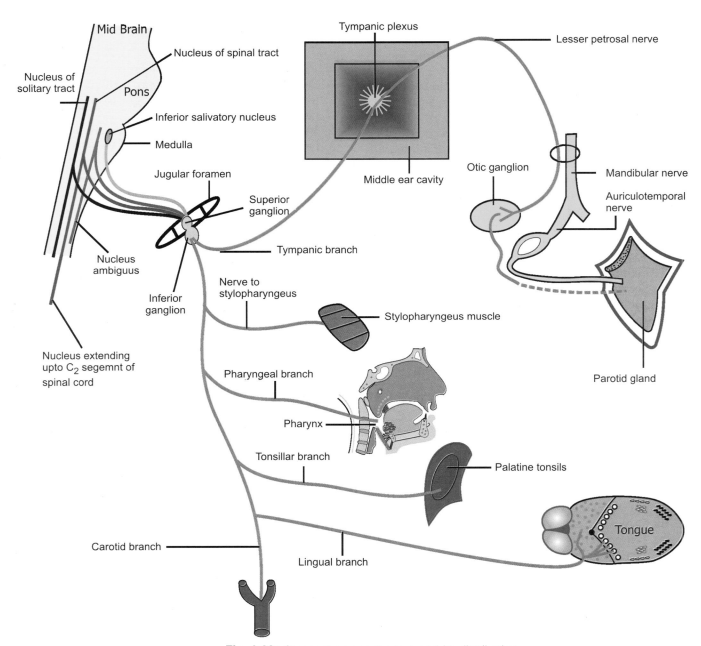

Fig. 9.32: Glossopharyngeal nerve and its distribution

Functional Components

1. **Special visceral efferent (SVE):** Motor to stylopharyngeus muscle
2. **General visceral efferent (GVE):** Secretomotor to parotid gland
3. **Special visceral afferent (SVA):** For taste sensations from posterior 1/3rd of the tongue including vallate papillae
4. **General visceral afferent (GVA):** Sensory to mucous membrane of the soft palate posterior 1/3rd of the tongue
5. **General somatic afferent (GSA):** For proprioceptive impulses from stylopharyngeus and skin of the auricle.

Nuclear Origin: The fibres of glossopharyngeal nerve are connected to the following four nuclei in the medulla oblongata.

1. **Nucleus ambiguus:** The special visceral efferent fibres originate from this nucleus
2. **Nucleus of tractus solitarius:** It receives afferent fibres of.
   a. Taste sensation from posterior 1/3rd of tongue
   b. General visceral sensations from the pharynx, tonsils and tongue
3. **Inferior salivatory nucleus:** It gives rise to preganglionic secretomotor fibres for the parotid gland
4. **Nucleus of spinal tract of trigeminal nerve:** The afferent fibres from stylopharyngeus and skin of the auricle terminate in this nucleus.

Intracranial Course

- The nerve arises from the upper lateral part of the medulla in the form of 3 to 4 rootlets.
- These unite to form a single trunk that runs forwards and laterally towards the jugular foramen.
- The nerve is associated with two ganglia in this region.
  1. **Superior ganglion:** This is smaller and lies at the upper end of jugular foramen
  2. **Inferior ganglion:** It is the larger of the two and is present just below the jugular foramen.

Extracranial Course

- The glossopharyngeal nerve emerges out of the jugular foramen at the base of the skull along with the 10th and 11th cranial nerves.
- It lies between the internal carotid artery and internal jugular vein at this point, in front of the vagus nerve
- Then, it passes forwards and downwards between the internal and external carotid arteries to reach the medial aspect of the styloid process

- It runs along with the stylopharyngeus, lying superficial to it and enters the triangular gap between the superior and middle constrictors of the pharynx
- Now it curves upwards around the lower aspect of stylopharyngeus to emerge deep to the stylohyoid ligament and posterior edge of hyoglossus muscle
- Here, it finally breaks up into its terminal lingual and tonsillar branches

Branches

1. **Communicating branches**
   - A twig to the ganglion of vagus nerve.
   - A twig to auricular branch of vagus nerve.
2. **Tympanic branch:** It conveys the secretomotor fibres from the inferior ganglion and enters the middle ear. It joins with fibres of the sympathetic plexus around internal carotid artery to form the tympanic plexus over the promontary. Branches from the tympanic plexus are
   a. **Lesser petrosal nerve:** The secretomotor fibres pass through lesser petrosal nerve to relay in the otic ganglion.
   b. **Twigs to tympanic cavity, auditory tube and mastoid air cells.**
3. **Carotid nerve:** It supplies the carotid sinus.
4. **Pharyngeal branch:** It joins the pharyngeal branches of the vagus and the cervical sympathetic chain to form the pharyngeal plexus on the middle constrictor of the pharynx.
5. **Branch to stylopharyngeus,** arises as the nerve winds round the stylopharyngeus muscle.
6. **Tonsillar branches,** supply the tonsil.
7. **Lingual branches:** Convey taste and common sensations from the posterior 1/3rd of the tongue and vallate papillae.

VAGUS NERVE

The vagus nerve is the 10th cranial nerve. It is a mixed nerve. Because of its extensive course and distribution it is named as vagus or wandering nerve. Its field of supply extends beyond the head and neck to the thorax and abdomen. It conveys most of the efferent fibres of the cranial part of the parasympathetic outflow. The fibres of cranial part of the accessory nerve also distribute through it (Fig. 9.33) .

Functional Components

1. **Special visceral efferent (SVE):** Motor to the muscles of palate, pharynx and larynx
2. **General visceral efferent (GVE):** For parasympathetic innervation of the heart, bronchial tree and most of the GIT.

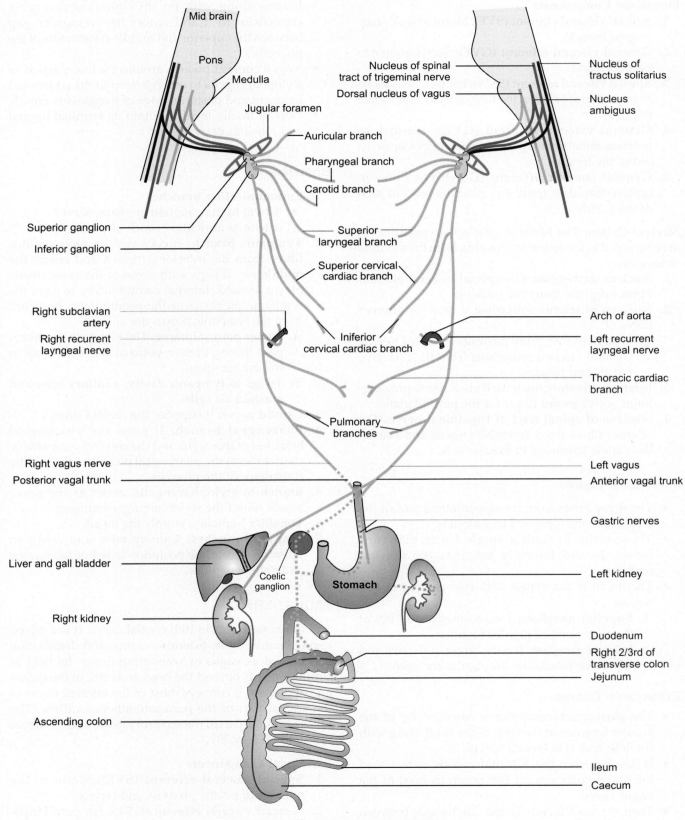

Fig. 9.33: Vagus nerve and its distribution

3. **Special visceral afferent (SVA):** Carries taste sensations from the posterior most part of the tongue and epiglottis.
4. **General visceral afferent (GVA):** For sensory innervation of the mucous membrane of pharynx, larynx, trachea, oesophagus and thoracic and abdominal viscera.
5. **General somatic afferent (GSA):** Carries general sensations from skin of the auricle and external acoustic meatus.

Nuclear Origin: Fibres of the vagus nerve arise from the following four nuclei in the medulla oblongata

1. **Nucleus ambiguus:** It gives rise to fibres for the special visceral efferent component or the branchio-motor fibres of vagus nerve.
2. **Dorsal nucleus of vagus:** This gives origin to the parasympathetic motor and secreto-motor fibres for heart, lungs, tracheobranchial tree and GIT. The viscero-sensory fibres from these organs also terminate in the dorsal nucleus.
3. **Nucleus of tractus solitarius:** This receives fibres of taste sensations i.e., the special visceral afferent component of vagus nerve.
4. **Nucleus of spinal tract of trigeminal nerve:** It is the nucleus for general somatic afferent fibres of vagus nerve. The auricular branch transmits sensations of pain and temperature from the auricle, external acoustic meatus and tympanic membrane.

Intracranial Course

- Vagus nerve arises from the lateral aspect of medulla between the olive and the inferior cerebellar peduncle in the form of about 10 rootlets which lie below the glossopharyngeal nerve.
- These nerve rootlets unite to form a single nerve trunk which runs laterally, crosses the jugular tubercle and then traverses the middle part of the jugular foramen along with the 9th and 11th cranial nerves to pass out of the cranial cavity. Here, the nerve is enclosed within the same dural sheath as the 11th the nerve. The 9th nerve however lies within a separate dural sheath.

Extracranial Course

- After coming out of the cranial cavity the nerve runs vertically downwards within the carotid sheath between the internal jugular vein laterally and the internal carotid artery medially, (common carotid artery in lower part upto the root of neck).
- **At the root of the neck**
  — The right vagus nerve enters the thorax by crossing in front of the right subclavian artery
  — Left vagus nerve enters the thorax by passing between the left common carotid and left subclavian arteries.

Vagus nerve in thorax

Right vagus nerve	Left vagus nerve
• It passes downward posteromedial to brachiocephalic vein and superior vena cava	• It passes downward between left common carotid and left subclavian arteries
• It passes behind root of right lung	• It is crossed superficially by phrenic nerve just above aortic arch
• It enters abdomen through esophageal opening in diaphragm	• It passes behind root of left lung through esophageal
• It enters abdomen opening in diaphragm	

Vagus nerve in abdomen

- Right and left vagus nerves enter abdomen through esophageal opening of diaphragm.
- Right and left vagus nerves form anterior and posterior vagal trunks.

Ganglia Associated with the Vagal Trunk

The upper part of the vagal trunk is associated with two ganglia.

1. **Jugular or superior ganglion:** It lies within the jugular foramen and is small in size.
2. **Inferior ganglion:** It is larger and lies just below the jugular foramen.It is also known as ganglion nodosum. Both the ganglia contain cell bodies of the sensory fibres of vagus nerve.

Branches of Vagus Nerve

In Head and Neck

1. **Meningeal branch:** It supplies the duramater of posterior cranial fossa.
2. **Auricular branch of the vagus:** It supplies the skin on the back of the meatus and the adjoining auricle. It then enters the meatus between its bony and cartilaginous parts to supply the floor of the meatus and the tympanic membrane.
3. **Pharyngeal branch:** It takes part in the formation of pharyngeal plexus. It supplies the following muscles
   a. All the muscles of the pharynx except stylo-pharyngeus which is supplied by the glossopharyngeal nerve.
   b. All muscles of the soft palate except tensor palati which is supplied by the mandibular nerve, through nerve to medial pterygoid.
4. **Branches to carotid body and carotid sinus.**
5. **6 (nerve of 4th arch):** It further divides into
   a. **External laryngeal nerve:** It runs downwards along with the superior thyroid vessels and supplies the cricothyroid muscle. It also gives

twigs to the inferior constrictor and pharyngeal plexus.

b. **Internal laryngeal nerve:** It passes downwards and forwards, towards the gap between the middle and inferior constrictors. It pierces the thyrohyoid membrane of the larynx and supplies:
  i. Mucous membrane of larynx above the vocal cords
  ii. Mucous membrane of the pharynx, epiglottis, vallecula and the posterior most part of the tongue.

6. **Recurrent laryngeal nerve (nerve of 6th arch)**
   - **On the right side,** it arises at root of the neck from the right vagus nerve as it crosses in front of the subclavian artery. Then it ascends up (in a recurrent direction) behind the subclavian and the common carotid arteries in the tracheo-oesophageal groove.
   - **On the left side,** it arises from the vagus nerve as it crosses the arch of aorta on its lateral aspect. Hence, the left recurrent laryngeal nerve originates in thorax. It hooks below the arch of aorta on the left side of the ligamentum arteriosum and passes up behind the arch on its way to the tracheo-oesophageal groove of left side.
   - In the neck each nerve ascends upwards in the respective tracheo-eosophageal grooves.
   - Each nerve passes in close relation to the respective inferior thyroid artery at the inferior pole of the thyroid gland and ascends up on the medial surface of the gland.
   - Then each passes deep to the inferior constrictor of pharynx.
   - Finally, each nerve enters the larynx behind the crico-thyroid joint.

   Branches of recurrent laryngeal nerve
   a. **Sensory supply:** To the mucus membrane of the larynx below the vocal cords.
   b. **Motor supply:** To all the intrinsic muscles of larynx except, cricothyroid which is supplied by the external laryngeal nerve.

7. **Cardiac branches:** They are two in number, superior and inferior cardiac branch. The branches from both sides form the cardiac plexus and supply the heart.
8. Branches to the trachea and oesophagus, supply the muscus glands and mucus membrane
9. Communicating branch to inferior cervical ganglion.
10. **Articular branches:** To cricothyroid and cricoarytenoid joints.
11. Twig to inferior constrictor muscle of pharynx.

In Thorax

1. Left recurrent laryngeal nerve
2. Pulmonary branches to form pulmonary plexus along with sympathetic fibres
3. Cardiac branches to form deep cardiac plexus
4. Esophageal branches

In Abdomen

Distribution of anterior vagal trunk

Branch	Distribution
1. Hepatic branches	• Liver • Biliary apparatus • Prepyloric stomach • Pyloric sphincter and duodenum
2. Gastric branches	• Anterior superior surface of stomach
3. Renal branches	

Distribution of Posterior Vagal Trunk

Branches	Distribution
1. Gastric branches (Nerve of Latajel)	They supply postero-inferior postero-inferior surface of stomach
2. Coeliac branches	Duodenum, jejunum, ileum, ascending colon, right 2/3rd of transverse colon
3. Renal branches	

ACCESSORY NERVE

It is the 11th cranial nerve. It is purely motor and consists of two roots (Fig. 9.34).

a. **Cranial root:** The fibres of this root are distributed through vagus and hence it is termed as being accessory to vagus
b. **Spinal root:** It has an independent course and is sometimes regarded as the true accessory nerve.

Functional Components
1. **Special visceral efferent:** Motor to muscles of soft palate, pharynx and larynx.
2. **General somatic efferent:** Motor to sternocleidomastoid and trapezius.

Nuclear Origin: It arises from two sites:
1. **Cranial root:** It arises from the lower part of nucleus ambiguus and dorsal nucleus of vagus in the medulla.
2. **Spinal root:** These fibres arise from an elongated motor nucleus extending from C_1 to C_5 spinal segments which lies in the lateral part of anterior grey column.

Intracranial Course of Cranial Root

- The cranial root arises by 4 or 5 rootlets from the posterolateral sulcus of the medulla, between the olive and inferior cerebellar peduncle. The rootlets are attached in line with rootlets of the vagus nerve above.
- These rootlets unite together to form a single trunk which runs laterally along with 9th and 10th cranial nerves to reach the jugular foramen where it is joined by the spinal root.

Extracranial Course

- The combined trunk comes out of the cranial cavity through the jugular foramen enclosed in a dural sheath along with the vagus nerve.
- Immediately after coming out of the cranial cavity the two roots again separate. The cranial root joins the vagus nerve just below its inferior ganglion. Its fibres are distributed through the branches of the vagus nerve to the muscles of the palate, pharynx and larynx.

- The spinal root of accessory nerve descends vertically downwards between the internal jugular vein and the internal carotid artery.
- The nerve pierces the sternocleidomastoid muscle at the junction of its upper 1/4th with the lower 3/4th and supplies it.
- It passes through the muscle and emerges through its posterior border a little above its middle to enter the posterior triangle of the neck. Here, it is related to the superficial cervical lymph nodes.
- It runs downwards and backwards underneath the fascial roof of the posterior triangle, parallel to the fibres of levator scapulae.
- It leaves the posterior triangle by passing along with C_2, C_3 and C_4 spinal nerves under the anterior border of trapezius, 5cm above the clavicle.
- The C_2 and C_3 spinal nerves supply proprioceptive fibres to the sternocleidomastoid, while C_3 and C_4 supply proprioceptive fibres to the trapezius muscle.

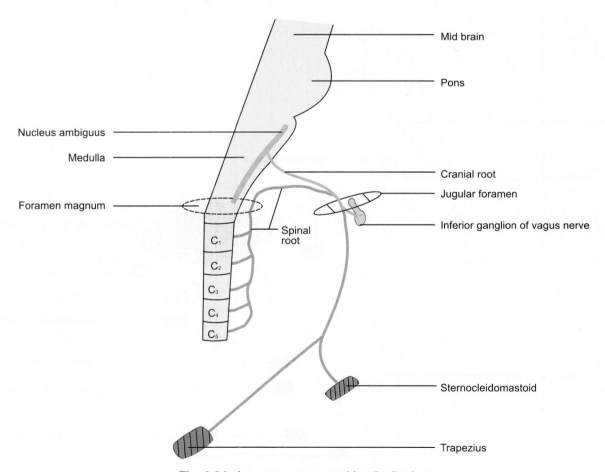

Fig. 9.34: Accessory nerve and its distribution

Course of Spinal Root

- The spinal root arises by a number of rootlets from the lateral aspect of spinal cord along a vertical line between the ventral and dorsal roots of the spinal nerves.
- These rootlets unite to form a single trunk which ascend up in the vertebral canal and enters the cranial cavity through foramen magnum.
- The spinal root leaves the skull through the jugular foramen where it fuses with the cranial root.

Branches of Accessory Nerve

1. **Muscular branches**
   a. To sternocleidomastoid along with C_2 and C_3 nerves.
   b. Supplies trapezius along with C_3 and C_4 nerves.
2. **Communicating branches:** It communicates with the following cervical spinal nerves.
   a. C_2, deep to sternocleidomastoid.
   b. C_2,C_3, in the posterior triangle.
   c. C_3 and C_4, deep to trapezius.

HYPOGLOSSAL NERVE

It is the 12th cranial nerve. It is purely motor (nerve of the occipital myotomes) (Fig. 9.35).

Functional Component

1. **General somatic efferent:** Motor to the muscles of the tongue, both extrinsic and intrinsic which are derived from occipital myotomes.

Nuclear origin: The hypoglossal nerve arises from the hypoglossal nucleus present in the posterior part of medulla oblongata. The fibres run forward through the substance of the medulla, lateral to the medial lemniscus to emerge on the ventral aspect of the medulla oblongata.

Intracranial Course

- The hypoglossal nerve arises in the form of 10 to 15 rootlets from the ventral aspect of medulla in the anterolateral sulcus between the pyramid and the olive.
- The rootlets of the hypoglossal nerve run laterally and pass behind the vertebral artery where they merge to form 2 bundles of nerve fibres.

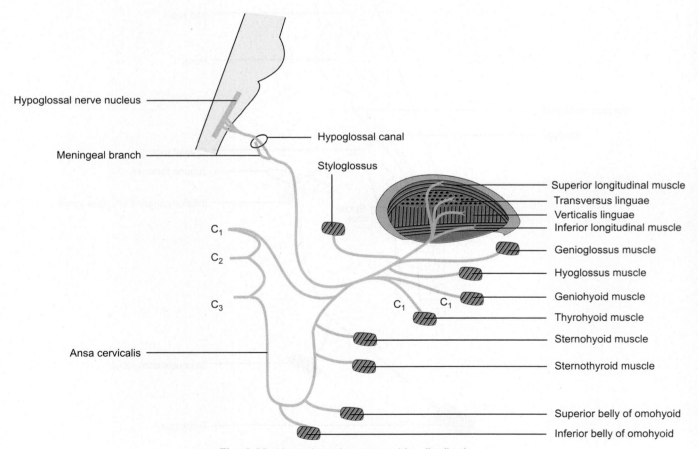

Fig. 9.35: Hypoglossal nerve and its distribution

- The two roots pierce the dura mater and pass through the anterior condylar canal (hypoglossal canal) in the occipital bone to come out of the cranial cavity. In the canal, the two roots unite to form a single trunk.

Extracranial Course

- After coming out of the cranial cavity the nerve lies deep to the internal carotid artery and the 9th, 10th and 11th cranial nerves.
- It then passes downwards and laterally over the accessory nerve and the vagus nerve to reach the interval between the internal carotid artery and internal jugular vein.
- At the level of angle of mandible, the nerve curves downwards and forwards crossing over the internal and external carotid arteries and over the 1st part of lingual artery to reach the posterior margin of hyoglossus muscle.
- It passes over the hyoglossus and reaches the digastric triangle, lying deep to the tendon of posterior belly of digastric and stylohyoid .
- Then, it runs upwards and forwards lying below the submandibular ganglion, submandibular gland and its duct along with the lingual nerve.
- At the anterior margin of hyoglossus it crosses over the 3rd part of lingual artery and pierces the genioglossus to reach the tip of tongue.
- Finally, it ends by dividing into its terminal branches.

Branches of Hypoglossal Nerve

1. **Muscular branches:** They supply all the muscles of the tongue except palatoglossus which is supplied by the cranial root of accessory nerve via the pharyngeal plexus.
2. **Branches of the hypoglossal nerve containing C_1 fibres**
   a. Meningeal branch: It supplies the duramater of posterior cranial fossa.
   b. Descendens hypoglossi or upper root of ansa cervicalis: It arises from the nerve as it crosses the internal carotid artery. It runs downwards to join the inferior root of ansa cervicalis at the level of cricoid cartilage.
   c. Nerve to thyrohyoid muscle
   d. Nerve to geniohyoid muscle
3. **Communicating branches:** The hypoglossal nerve communicates with the following
   a. Superior cervical ganglion of sympathetic trunk.
   b. Inferior ganglion of vagus nerve.
   c. Loop of fibres of C_1 and C_2 spinal nerves
   d. Pharyngeal plexus.
   e. Lingual nerve

The anatomy and functions of autonomic nervous system.

CLINICAL AND APPLIED ASPECT

NERVES OF UPPER LIMB

Brachial Plexus

- **Erb's point (Fig. 9.36):** This corresponds to a point in the upper trunk where the following six nerves meet
  1. Root of C_5
  2. Root of C_6
  3. Suprascapular nerve

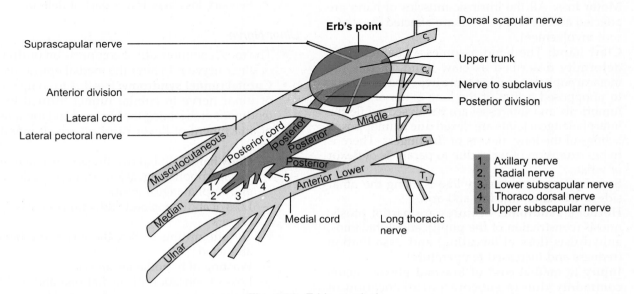

Fig. 9.36: Erb's paralysis

4. Nerve to subclavius
5. Anterior division of upper trunk
6. Posterior division of upper trunk
- **Erb's Duchenne palsy (Fig. 9.36)** is due to injury to the upper trunk of brachial plexus at the Erb's point. It usually occurs following undue separation of head from shoulder. This is usually seen following difficult deliveries, especially in breech delivery. It can also occur due to prolonged abnormal posture during surgery under anaesthesia.
  The following clinical signs are usually observed.
  — **Motor Loss:** The following muscles are paralysed
    1. Supraspinatus
    2. Infraspinatus
    3. Biceps brachii
    4. Coracobrachialis
    5. Deltoid
    6. Teres minor
    7. Subclavius
  — **Sensory loss:** Occurs on lateral side of forearm
  — **Position of upper limb**
    1. Upper limb is by the side of the body and adducted, due to paralysis of deltoid, coracobrachialis and subclavius.
    2. It is medially rotated, due to loss of function of teres minor and infraspinatus muscles.
    3. Fore arm is pronated because of paralysis of biceps brachii muscle.
    4. This is also known as waiter's tip hand.
- **Klumpke's paralysis:** It results due to lesions involving the lower trunk of brachial plexus (C_8 and T_1 nerve roots). It can be caused by forceful upward traction of the arm. The area of distribution of T_1 is mainly involved. The following clinical signs are observed.
  Motor loss: All the intrinsic muscles of hand are affected and flexors of wrist are affected due to C_8 root involvement.
  Claw hand: The hand assumes a characteristic deformity described as claw hand. In this the metacarpophalangeal joints are hyperextended due to unopposed action of the long extensors as the lumbricals and interossei are paralysed while the interphalangeal joints are flexed due to unopposed actions of the long flexors of the fingers. There is hyper extension of wrist due to paralysis of flexor of wrist.
  Sensory loss: The sensory loss is along the ulnar side of the hand, forearm and arm.
  Horner's syndrome: Features are partial ptosis, miosis (constriction of the pupil), enophthalamos, anhydrosis (loss of sweating) and vasodilation (redness and increased temperature).
- **Injury to medial cord of brachial plexus** occurs commonly due to subcoracoid dislocation of humerus. This presents as follows:

— Claw hand, due to involvement of ulnar nerve and medial root of median nerve.
— Sensory loss on the ulnar side of forearm and hand, due to involvement of medial cutaneous nerve of forearm and ulnar nerve.
- **Lateral cord of brachial plexus** can be injured in dislocation of shoulder joint. It presents as follows
  — Mid prone forearm with sensory loss on the radial side of forearm.
  — Loss of flexion at elbow joint, due to involvement of musculo-cutaneous nerve
  — Loss of flexion of wrist, due to involvement of lateral root of median nerve.
- Injury to nerve of Bell can occur as a result of carrying heavy load on the shoulder and sudden pressure on the shoulder from above. It leads to paralysis of serratus anterior muscle. The patient present with protrusion of medial border of scapula which is known as winging of scapula.

Musculocutaneous Nerve

Isolated lesion of musculocutaneous nerve is rare. It may be involved in injury to upper arm and fracture of humerus. It presents as weakness of flexion of elbow and loss of sensation at the extensor aspect of forearm

Axillary Nerve

- Axillary nerve usually gets injured due to
  a. Fracture of surgical neck of humerus.
  b. Dislocation of shoulder joint.
  Clinical presentation
  a. Loss of abduction of arm due to paralysis of deltoid.
  b. Loss of rounded contour of shoulder due to flattening of deltoid.
  c. Sensory loss over lower part of deltoid.

Ulnar Nerve

- The most common site of compression or division of ulnar nerve is behind the medial epicondyle.
- **Cubital tunnel syndrome:** It is due to compression of ulnar nerve in cubial tunnel formed by the tendinous arch joining the humeral and ulnar heads of attachment of flexor carpi ulnaris. It manifests as:
  — **Claw hand:** Medial two fingers are extended at metacarpophalangeal joints and partially flexed at interphalangeal joints
  — Loss of abduction and adduction of medial four fingers
  — On attempting to flex the wrist, the hand is abducted
  — Wasting of hypothenar muscles
  — Loss of sensation of medial one and a half of digits and adjoining medial side of the hand.

- **Ulnar paradox:** An injury to the ulnar nerve at the elbow appears to produce lesser degree of claw hand than when it gets injured at the wrist.
- Test for ulnar nerve palsy
  — Patient is unable to hold a sheet of paper between index and middle finger.
  — Patient cannot abduct or adduct the medial four digits while placing the flat hand on the table.
- Ulnar nerve can be felt behind the medial epicondyle. It is easily felt when thickened in patient with leprosy. Other nerves felt in patient with leprosy are:
  — Common peroneal nerve, above the neck of fibula.
  — Upper branches of facial nerve, those branches which lie during their course on zygoma.
  — Radial nerve, in the radial groove.
  — Median nerve, just proximal to wrist joint.
  — Posterior tibial nerve, at the ankle joint.

Median Nerve

- Median nerve is most likely to be damaged above elbow in supracondylar fracture.
  — There is loss of
    1. Flexion of second phalanges of all digits.
    2. Flexion of terminal phalanges of index and middlefinger.
    3. Abduction of thumb.
    4. Cutaneous sensation on palmar aspect of 3½ digits and dorsal surface of same digits over distal phalanx.
  — There is wasting of muscles of thenar eminence.
  —. It presents as **Ape-like hand.**

- **Carpal tunnel syndrome:** It occurs due to compression of median nerve in the carpal tunnel which is formed by the concavity of carpal bones bridged by flexor retinaculum. Any decrease in volume of carpal tunnel leads to compression of median nerve.

  Common causes of carpal tunnel syndrome are:
  — Acromegaly
  — Rhematoid arthritis
  — Pregnancy
  — Myxoedema

  Presentation: It is more common in females. There is pain and burning sensation in lateral 3½ digits.

  On examination
  — **Motor loss:** Paralysis of abductor pollicis brevis, opponens pollicis, flexor pollicis, 1st and 2nd lumbricals.
  — **Sensory loss:** Palmar surface of lateral 3 ½ digits and distal phalanges of the same digits on the dorsal aspect.

  — **Trophic changes:** These changes are due to loss of vasomotor regulation by sympathetic innervation.

  Treatment: A cut is given through the flexor retinaculum to release the pressure.

- Injury to median nerve in the middle of the forearm leads to Pointing index finger.

Radial Nerve

- **Saturday night palsy or honey moon palsy:** It is the compression of radial nerve in radial groove due to placing the out stretched arm on an arm chair. Its a reversible condition and usually occurs during weekends due to abnormal posture after excessive alcohol consumption.

  Presentation:
  — **Wrist drop**—flexed, flaccid hand with fingers flexed at proximal phalanges and extended at middle and distal interphalangeal joint.
  — Extended forearm.
  — Loss of cutaneous sensation on the dorsum of hand.

- **Features of injury to radial nerve at or below elbow:** There is no wrist drop due to sparing of brachioradialis and extensor carpi radialis longus because they receive their nerve supply proximal to elbow joint.

- Crutch paralysis occurs due to the damage of radial nerve in the axilla from constant pressure of crutches used by disabled persons. The second most common nerve involved in crutch paralysis is Ulnar nerve

- When radial nerve is injured in radial groove, long head of triceps muscle is spared.

NERVES OF THORAX

Intercostal Nerves

Intercostal neuralgia is most commonly a result of herpes zoster infection. The virus lies dormant in the dorsal root ganglion of a intercostal nerve. In the event of any stress, e.g., fever there is flaring up of inflammation. This leads to pain along the distribution of the nerve and is called intercostal neuralgia. The skin of the dermatome supplied by the nerve shows erythematous vesicular rash with intense burning. The rash does not cross the midline.

NERVES OF LOWER LIMB

Obturator Nerve

- The pain in disease of hip joint may be referred to the medial side of thigh or knee joint along the obturator nerve since obturator nerve supplies both the joints.

- In inflammation of ovary, localized peritonitis affecting the ovarian fossa eventually leads to irritation of obturator nerve. Pain may be referred in such a condition to the hip, knee or inner side of thigh.
- Appendicitis involving the appendix in the pelvic position irritates the obturator nerve, hence leads to spasm of the muscles of the medial compartment of the thigh.

Sciatic Nerve

- **Sciatica:** It is a lay man's term. It is not a disease but a symptom due to the compression of one or more roots forming sciatic nerve.
  Cause: Disc prolapse, osteoarthritis
  Presentation: Radiating pain along the cutaneous distribution of sciatic nerve at the following sites:
  a. Gluteal region
  b. Back of thigh
  c. Lateral side of leg
  d. Dorsum of foot
- Root value of posterior femoral cutaneous nerve is $S_{1,2,3}$. Parasympathetic supply to pelvic viscera also comes from $S_{2,3,4}$. Hence, pain may be referred from the pelvic viscera along the distribution of posterior femoral cutaneous nerve i.e. back of thigh and calf. It needs to be differentiated from sciatica.
- After sitting for a long time there may be compression of the sciatic nerve against femur. This leads to numbness of the lower limb, and is known as sleeping foot.
- Sciatic nerve can be injured due to
  — Dislocation of hip
  — Fracture pelvis
  — Intramuscular injection

Effects of sciatic nerve injury: Injury to the sciatic nerve leads to the condition known as **foot drop.** This foot drop is passive in which the foot hangs downward by its own weight due to the paralysis of following muscles:
  a. Hamstring muscles.
  b. All the muscles of leg and foot.
There will be a loss of sensation on back of thigh and entire leg except the area innervated by saphenous nerve.

- In case of paralysis of common peroneal nerve or deep peroneal nerve the muscles of the posterior compartment of the leg are not affected and this causes active plantar flexion of the foot. This is known as active foot drop.

Tibial Nerve

Injury of tibial nerve leads to
- The patient will come walking on heel. The foot is dorsiflexed, everted and person cannot stand on toes.
- There is paralysis of gastrocnemius, soleus, popliteus, tibialis posterior, flexor digitorum longus, flexor hallucis longus and all intrinsic muscles of the foot except extensor digitorum brevis.
- There is loss of sensation on the entire sole of foot and terminal phalanges on the dorsal aspect.
- It can also lead to local autonomic changes leading to trophic ulcers on the leg.

Common Peroneal Nerve

The common peroneal nerve is commonly injured due to fracture at the neck of fibula. Characteristic features are:
- There will be foot drop of the active type.
- The foot will be fully plantar flexed, inverted and adducted. Dorsiflexion of middle and terminal phalanges of lateral four toes is retained due to the contraction of interossei and lumbrical muscles.
- The following muscles will be paralysed in injury of common peroneal nerve:
  — Tibialis anterior
  — Extensor hallucis longus
  — Extensor digitorum longus
  — Peroneus tertius
  — Peroneus longus
  — Peroneus brevis
  — Extensor digitorum brevis
- **Sensory loss:** There will be a loss of sensation on most of the dorsum of the foot and outer surface of lower third of the front of the leg.

Deep Peroneal Nerve

Injury to deep peroneal nerve leads to:
- Patient will walk on toes due to overaction of plantar flexors as dorsiflexors are paralysed due to injury of deep peroneal nerve.
- Patient will complain of loss of sensation in the 1st interdigital cleft on the dorsum of the foot.

Superficial Peroneal Nerve

Injury to superficial peroneal nerve leads to:
- The patient will walk on lateral border of foot due to overaction of invertors as evertors are paralysed.
- There will be loss of sensation in the most part of the dorsum of the foot.

CRANIAL NERVES

Olfactory Nerves

Lesion of olfactory nerves results in the loss of sense of smell called anosmia. The sense of smell also plays an important role in the finer appreciation of taste.

Optic Nerve and Visual Pathway

Lesions of visual pathway at following sites leads to different presentations. These are (Fig. 9.37):
1. Optic nerve lesion causes total blindness of corresponding eye.
2. Lesions of optic chiasma causes bitemporal hemianopia.
3. Lesion of optic tract causes contralateral homonymous hemianopia.
4. Partial lesion of visual cortex causes upper or lower quadrantic homonymous hemianopia.

Oculomotor Nerve

Complete involvement of the oculomotor nerve will result in the following signs and symptoms:
- Ptosis (drooping of upper eyelid), due to paralysis of levator palpebrae superioris
- Lateral squint, due to unopposed action of lateral rectus.
- Dilatation of pupil, due to unopposed action of dilator pupillae
- Loss of accomodation, convergence and light reflex, due to, paralysis of ciliary muscle, medial rectus and constrictor pupillae.

- Diplopia (double vision), where the false image is higher than the true image.

Trochlear Nerve

Complete lesion of trochlear nerve results in inability to turn the eye downwards and laterally due to paralysis of superior oblique muscle.

Abducent Nerve

The abducent nerve is commonly involved in cases of increased intracranial pressure due to the following reasons:
- The nerve is very slender and takes a long intracranial course from the pontomedullary junction to the orbit.
- At the upper border of the petrous temporal bone, the nerve makes a sharp bend.
- Downward shift of the brainstem through foramen magnum results in stretching of the nerve.

Abducent nerve palsy results in medial or convergent squint and diplopia due to paralysis of lateral rectus.

Facial Nerve

Facial palsy: It is the paralysis of the facial nerve. It is of two types
1. Upper motor neuron type
2. Lower motor neuron type

Upper motor neuron facial palsy (Fig. 9.38): It is due to involvement of the cortico-nuclear fibres i.e. the upper motor neurons. These fibres arise in the cerebral cortex,

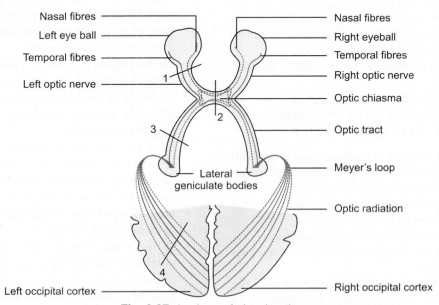

Nasal fibres
Left eye ball
Temporal fibres
Left optic nerve
1
3
2
Lateral geniculate bodies
4
Left occipital cortex

Nasal fibres
Right eyeball
Temporal fibres
Right optic nerve
Optic chiasma
Optic tract
Meyer's loop
Optic radiation
Right occipital cortex

Fig. 9.37: Lesions of visual pathway

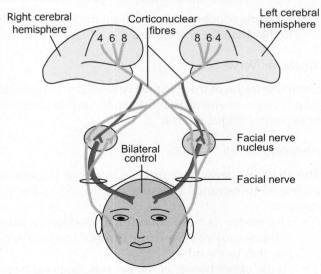

Right cerebral hemisphere

Corticonuclear fibres

Left cerebral hemisphere

4 6 8

8 6 4

Bilateral control

Facial nerve nucleus

Facial nerve

Fig. 9.38: Central connections of facial nerves

pass through internal capsule and end in the motor nucleus of the facial nerve. These are most commonly involved in patients with cerebral haemorrhage which is always associated with hemiplegia. Since the lesion is above the nucleus, it is also called as supranuclear type of facial palsy.

It leads to paralysis of the contralateral lower part of face below the palpebral fissure. The upper part of the face is spared because the part of facial nucleus which supplies it, is innervated by corticonuclear fibres from both the cerebral hemispheres.

Lower motor neuron facial palsy: It is further of 2 types

a. Nuclear paralysis: It is due to involvement of the nucleus of facial nerve. This can occur due to poliomyelitis or lesions of the pons. The motor nucleus of facial nerve is close to the abducent nerve which is also usually affected.

Effect: Paralysis of muscles of the entire face on ipsilateral side.

b. Infranuclear paralysis: This occurs due to involvement of the facial nerve. Clinical effects vary according to the site of injury of the nerve.

Facial nerve can get injured at various sites (Fig. 9.39)
Site 1: Injury proximal to the geniculate ganglion produces the following sign and symptoms

- Diminished lacrimation, due to involvement of secretomotor fibres to lacrimal gland
- Hyperacusis, due to paralysis of stapedius
- Loss of facial expression, due to paralysis of muscles of facial expression
- Loss of salivation and taste sensations in the anterior 2/3rd of tongue, due to involvement of chorda tympani.

Site 2: Injury in the middle ear segment of the nerve. All effects as at site 1 occur except that there will be no loss of lacrimation.

Site 3: Lesion in the vertical course of the facial nerve within the mastoid bone. All effects as seen in lesion of site 1 occur except that there will be no hyperacusis and no loss of lacrimation.

Site 4:
- Injury at or distal to the stylomastoid foramen – It is the common site of involvement especially in young children. In a child the mastoid process is absent and the stylomastoid foramen with facial nerve are superficial. Thus the nerve is easily injured by any incisions given around the ear. It leads to
  — Paralysis of muscles of facial expression
  — No loss of lacrimation
  — No hyperacusis
  — No loss of taste sensations
  — No loss of salivation.

Bell's palsy: It is a lower motor neuron type of facial nerve involvement. It has a varied etiology e.g. exposure to sudden cold, middle ear infections. Mostly it is idiopathic, believed to be a viral infection. It leads to paralysis of muscles of facial expression. There may be associated symptoms according to the site of lesion. It requires only supportive therapy and physiotherapy. In majority it recovers completely with in 2 to 8 weeks. Facial muscles of the same side are paralysed and this leads to the following features :

- **Facial asymmetry:** due to unopposed action of muscles of the normal side. There is deviation of angle of mouth to the opposite side.
- **Loss of wrinkles on forehead:** due to paralysis of fronto-occipitalis muscle
- **Widening of palpebral fissure and inability to close the eye:** due to paralysis of orbicularis oculi.
- **Inability of angle of mouth to move upwards and laterally during laughing:** due to paralysis of zygomaticus major.
- **Loss of naso-labial furrow:** due to paralysis of levator labii superioris alaeque nasi.
- **Accumulation of food into the vestibule of mouth:** due to paralysis of buccinator muscle.
- **Dribbling of saliva from the angle of mouth:** due to paralysis of orbicularis oris.
- **When one presses the cheek with inflated vestibule, the air leaks out between the lips:** due to paralysis of orbicularis oris.
- **Loss of resistance while blowing out air in mouth:** due to paralysis of buccinator.

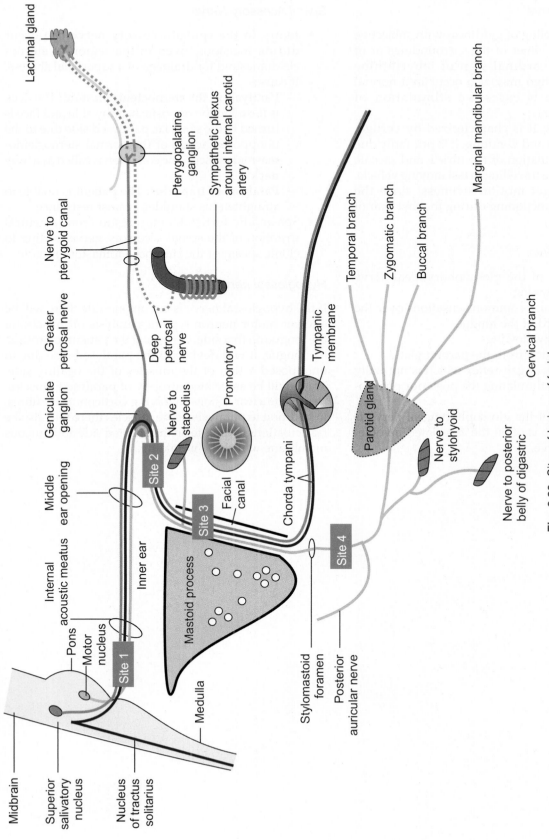

Lacrimal gland

Pterygopalatine ganglion

Sympathetic plexus around internal carotid artery

Nerve to pterygoid canal

Greater petrosal nerve

Deep petrosal nerve

Geniculate ganglion

Nerve to stapedius

Promontory

Tympanic membrane

Temporal branch

Zygomatic branch

Buccal branch

Marginal mandibular branch

Site 2

Middle ear opening

Facial canal

Chorda tympani

Parotid gland

Cervical branch

Internal acoustic meatus

Inner ear

Site 3

Nerve to stylohyoid

Pons

Motor nucleus

Mastoid process

Site 4

Nerve to posterior belly of digastric

Midbrain

Superior salivatory nucleus

Nucleus of tractus solitarius

Site 1

Medulla

Stylomastoid foramen

Posterior auricular nerve

Fig. 9.39: Sites of lesions of facial nerve

Vestibulo-cochlear Nerve

- **Vertigo:** Is the feeling of giddiness with subjective sense of rotation either of the surroundings or of oneself. It is a cardinal sign of labyrinthine dysfunction. Vertigo may also occur in a normal person if there is excessive stimulation of semicircular ducts.
- **Motion sickness:** It is characterized by vertigo, headache, nausea and vomiting. It is primarily due to excessive stimulation of the utricle and saccule during motion like travelling in fast moving vehicle. Infants do not get motion sickness, since the labyrinth is not functioning during the first year of life.

Glossopharyngeal Nerve

- Complete lesion of the glossopharyngeal nerve results in the following
  - Loss of taste and common sensations over the posterior 1/3rd of the tongue.
  - Difficulty in swallowing.
  - Loss of salivation from the parotid gland.
  - Unilateral loss of gag-reflex which is normally produced by stimulating the posterior pharyngeal wall.

Complete lesion of the glossopharyngeal nerve is rare in isolation. There is often the associated involvement of the vagus nerve.

Spinal Acessory Nerve

- Injury to the spinal accessory nerve can occur during incisions given in the region of sternocleidomastoid for drainage of a superficial abscess. It causes
  - **Paralysis of the sternocleidomastoid:** The neck is flexed to the opposite healthy side and face is turned to the same i.e. paralysed side due to the unopposed action of the normal sternocleidomastoid muscle. The condition is called as a 'wry neck'.
  - **Paralysis of trapezius:** The patient is unable to straighten his shoulder against resistance.
- Spasmodic torticollis may result from a central irritation of the spinal accessory nerve leading to clonic spasm of the sternocleidomastoid muscle.

Hypoglossal nerve

If the hypoglossal nerve is cut on one side there will be a lower motor neuron type of paralysis of muscles of the tongue on that side. On asking the patient to protude his tongue, it will deviate to the paralysed side due to unopposed action of the muscles of the healthy side. There will be associated atrophy of paralysed muscles. In supranuclear lesions involving corticonuclear fibres, in addition to paralysis of the muscles there will also be fasciculations in tongue on the affected side and mucous membrane will show wrinkling.

Chapter 10

Somatosensory, Somatomotor and Autonomic Nervous System

SOMATOSENSORY SYSTEM

This system is responsible for receiving and transmitting various impulses from the external environment to the higher centers or brain in the body. These impulses are interpreted and appropriate response is elicited for benefit of the body for survival and existence. It consists of the following parts:

1. Sense organ/receptors
2. Sensory pathways
3. Higher centres: Integration primarily occurs in thalamus and cerebral cortex.

SENSE ORGANS

The central nervous system (CNS) receives impulses from internal and external environment of body by means of stimulation of sensory receptors. Sensory receptors are mostly modified nerve endings. They also be consist of specialized cells supplied by nerve endings. These receptors respond to a specific stimulus and generate action potentials in neurons which are transmitted to CNS.

The sensory receptors along with the surrounding non-neuronal cells form a sense organ. Each receptor is specialized to respond to one type of stimulus or energy form, either mechanical, chemical, thermal etc and converts it to electrical impulses in the afferent neuron.

Various types of receptors are:

1. **Special sense receptors:** Located close to CNS and innervated by cranial nerves. Examples, vision, hearing, smell, taste, acceleration etc.
2. **Cutaneous or skin receptors:** Present in the skin and respond to touch, pressure, pain and temperature. Sensations are carried by cutaneous branches of spinal nerves.
3. **Deep sense receptors:** Present in joints and muscles. They generate impulses of position sense via spinal or cranial nerves, e.g. golgi tendon organ.
4. **Visceral sense organs:** Present in various viscera, glands and tissues. They are innervated with autonomic nerves. Examples are visceral pain receptors, baroreceptors, chemoreceptors etc.

Receptors can be classified according to the type of stimulus that they respond to:

1. **Chemoreceptors:** e.g., receptors for taste and smell, receptors for change in osmolality (osmoreceptors in hypothalamus) etc.

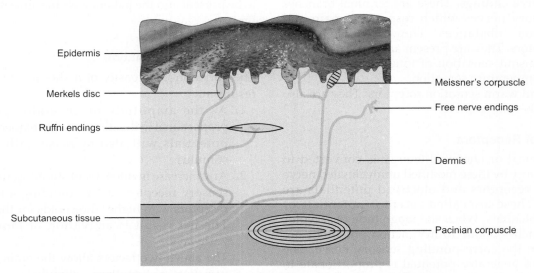

Fig. 10.1: Sensory receptors in skin and subcutaneous tissue

2. **Mechanoreceptors:** Touch and pain receptors.
3. **Thermoreceptors:** Receptors which respond to hot and cold temperatures.
4. **Nociceptors:** Receptors which respond to painful stimuli (free nerve endings in skin).
5. **Photoreceptors:** Rods and cones of retina which respond to light.

The receptors are also named according to their function:

1. **Telereceptors:** Receptors which are concerned with perceiving sensations from a distance eg. hearing and vision.
2. **Exteroceptors:** Receptors that receive stimuli from the immediate external environment eg. touch, temperature receptors.
3. **Interoceptors:** Receptors that are stimulated by changes in internal environment of the body eg. osmoreceptors, baroreceptors etc.
4. **Proprioceptors:** Receptors that are concerned with sensing position of body at a given time and space, e.g., golgi tendon organ, muscle spindles, proprioceptive receptors at joints.

Cutaneous receptors (Fig. 10.1): Skin is the largest sensory organ. Cutaneous receptors are made of modifications of unmyelinated nerve endings. They are of the following types:

a. **Merkel's discs:** These are expanded nerve tips, responsible for sensation of touch.
b. **Meissner's corpuscles:** These are encapsulated nerve endings, responsible for sensation of touch.
c. **Pacinian corpuscles:** These are encapsulated nerve endings responsible for sensation of pressure.
d. **Ruffini's endings:** These are encapsulated expanded nerve terminals. They are slow adapting touch receptors.
e. **Krause's end-bulbs:** These are spherical receptors placed in dermis and respond to pressure.
f. **Free nerve endings:** These are terminal branches of sensory nerves which respond to pain and injurious substances. They are also called nociceptors. They are present around hair follicles and transmit sensation of touch. They may also carry temperature sensation.
g. **Cold and warm** sensation receptors. They are also called thermoreceptors.

Excitation of Receptors

The mechanical or chemical energy is converted to electrical energy by these modified unmyelinated nerve endings or receptors and electrical potentials are generated. These are called receptor potentials or generator potentials. When the magnitude of receptor potential reaches about 10 mV, action potentials are generated in the corresponding sensory nerve. The magnitude of generator potential is proportionate to intensity of stimulus.

Adaptation

Continuous application of a stimulus of same intensity results in desensitization of the receptor. The lack of change in stimulus intensity results in decline of action potentials in sensory nerves. There are two types of adaptation receptors:

1. **Phasic receptors:** These adapt rapidly, examples Pacinian and Meissner's corpuscles. Thus sensation of wearing clothes is not felt unless they are removed or worn.
2. **Tonic receptors:** These adapt very slowly and incompletely. Various examples are baroreceptors, lung inflation receptors, cold and pain receptors, muscle spindle receptors. These are essential as they regulate internal homeostasis.

Doctorine of Specific Nerve Energies

The impulses produced by a sensation is carried from the receptor via sensory nerves to a specific part of the brain. Hence, if the nerve pathway in between the two is stimulated at any point in between, without actual stimulus on receptor, the sensation felt is same as the one produced by the corresponding receptor.

Law of Projection

In continuation with the above fact, stimulation of the sensory pathway arising from any of the receptors evokes a response in the brain that is felt at the site of receptor. This explains 'phantom limb'. In patients with an amputated limb, the nerve endings are cut and on regeneration they may be stimulated by small stimuli of pressure and temperature. The sensation is felt as though coming from the site where the receptors used to be present and the patient feels the amputated part of limb.

Intensity Discrimination

The variation in intensity of a stimulus on a receptor results in:

1. As the amplitude of generator potential is proportional to the stimulus, the frequency of action potentials will also increase with increasing stimulus.
2. Any increase in intensity of stimulus, recruits more sensory receptors in surrounding area and also receptors with higher thresholds for that stimulus. The net result is activation of more afferent pathways.

The above two factors allow the brain to perceive variation in strength of a stimulus.

SENSORY PATHWAYS

Characteristic features of sensory pathways

- The sensory pathways are also called **ascending pathways** as they ascend from periphery to the brain.
- These pathways are also known as three neuronal pathways (except spinocerebellar pathway). This means that conscious integration of sensory input involves three sets of neurons.
- The primary afferent neurons that receive impulses from receptors have their cell bodies in the dorsal root ganglia of spinal nerve root or corresponding cranial nerve nuclei in brain. These are called first order neurons.
- **All modalities of sensation reach spinal cord by way of dorsal root of spinal nerve except special senses.**
- Dorsal root ganglia have unipolar neurons with a peripheral process that ends on various peripheral receptors and a central process that passes via the dorsal root of spinal nerve to the spinal cord.
- The 1st order neurons of most sensations (except dorsal column tracts which relay in medulla) relay in spinal cord with the neurons situated in the posterior grey column of spinal cord. Neurons of the posterior grey column of spinal cord receive medial and lateral divisions of the dorsal root of spinal nerves. The axons of the second order neurons of a particular sensation are grouped together to form a tract.
  - Ascending tracts to thalamus: Spinothalamic tracts.
  - Ascending tracts to the brain stem nuclei (Medulla): Fasciculus gracilis and cuneatus.
  - Ascending tracts to the cerebellum: Spinocerebellar tracts.
- Axons of 2nd order neurons ascend to the thalamus and relay in the ventero-postero-lateral nucleus of thalamus.
- Axons of principal sensory nucleus, nucleus of spinal tract, trigeminal nerve and relay in ventro-postero-medial nucleus of thalamus.
- 3rd order neurons arising from thalamus finally end in the somatosensory cortex of brain.
- All sensations pass through thalamus except sense of olfaction (smell).

Spinothalamic Pathway (Fig. 10.2)

There are two spinothalamic pathways. These tracts are situated in the anterior and lateral funiculus of the white matter.
  a. Lateral spinothalamic tract
  b. Anterior spinothalamic tract

Lateral Spinothalamic Tract (Fig. 10.2)

Origin: Laminae I to IV of spinal grey matter.
Termination: Area 3, 1, 2 of cerebral cortex.

Crossing over: Fibres cross in the corresponding spinal segment anterior to the central canal of spinal cord.

Course

- 1st order neurons lie in the dorsal root ganglion.
- 2nd order neurons lie in the posterior grey column of spinal cord. Axons of the 2nd order neurons ascend in the contralateral lateral funiculus of spinal cord in the lateral spinothalamic tract.
- This tract ascends through the medulla, pons and midbrain as the **spinal lemniscus.**
- The 2nd order neurons finally relay in the VPL nucleus of the thalamus.
- 3rd order neurons lie in the ventro-postero-lateral nucleus of thalamus and axons of these neurons ascend through the internal capsule and then the thalamic radiations to area no. 3, 1, 2 of the cerebral cortex.
  Somatotropic arrangement: Fibres from sacral region are most superficial while the cervical fibres lie deepest with the rest, in between.
Sensations carried: Pain and temperature

Anterior Spinothalamic Tract (Fig. 10.2)

Origin: Laminae I to IV of spinal grey matter.
Termination: Joins with the medial lemniscus in medulla.
Crossing over: Fibres cross 2 to 3 segments above the spinal segment from the entry of the 1st order neurons.
Course

- 1st order neurons lie in the dorsal root ganglion
- 2nd order neurons are present in the spinal cord and axons of these neurons ascend through the contralateral anterior funiculus of spinal cord as the anterior spinothalamic tract.
- This tract joins the medial lemniscus in medulla and ascends further to terminate in VPL nucleus of thalamus.
- 3rd order neurons from VPL nucleus of thalamus ascend to terminate in the same cortical area of 3, 1 and 2.
Sensations carried: Non-discriminatory touch and pressure.

Dorsal White Column or Fasciculus Gracilis and Cuneatus (Fig. 10.3)

These are situated in the posterior funiculus of white matter.
Origin: 1st order neurons lie in the dorsal root ganglion (proprioceptive and exteroceptive).
Crossing over: In the middle part of medulla.
Termination: Area 3, 1, 2 of cerebral cortex.
Course

- The medial division of the dorsal root of spinal nerve is made up of central processes of the dorsal root ganglion neurons (1st order neuron). Their axons ascend upto the medulla oblongata as fasciculus gracilis and cuneatus.

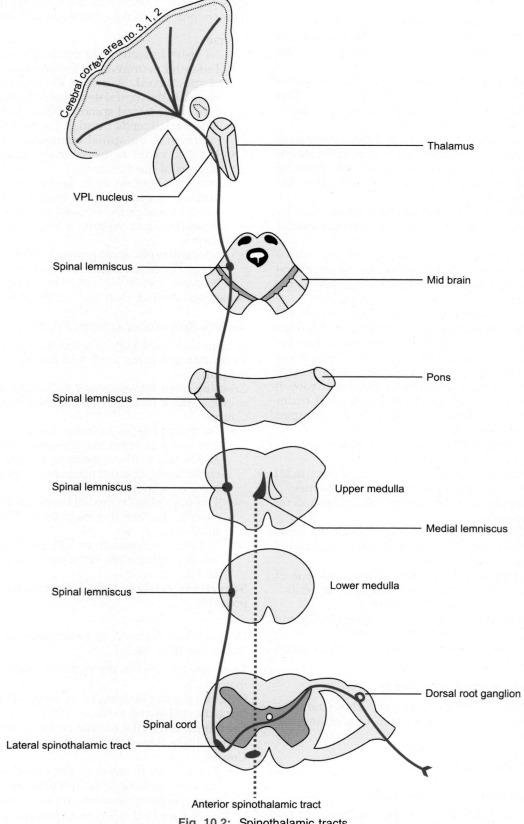

Fig. 10.2: Spinothalamic tracts

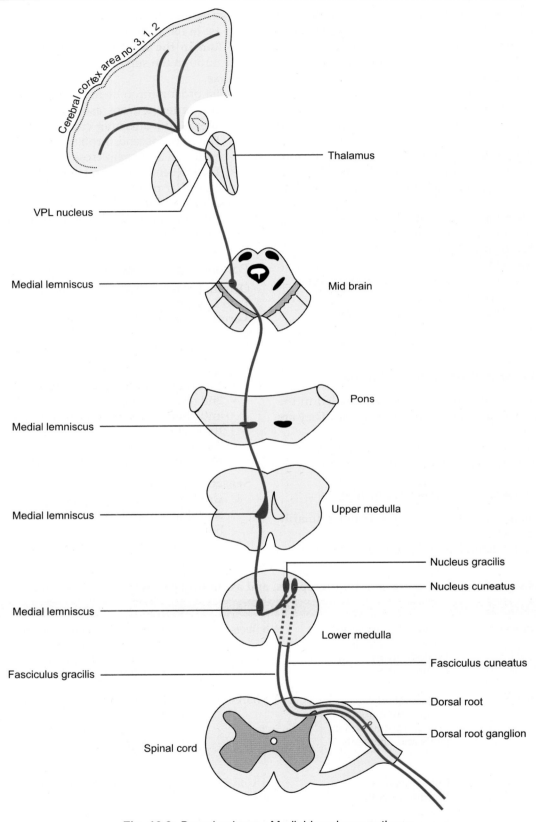

Fig. 10.3: Dorsal column—Medial lemniscus pathway

- 2nd order neurons lie in nucleus gracilis and nucleus cuneatus in the medulla. The axons of 2nd order neurons crosses over and decussate at medulla (sensory decussation)and form the medial lemniscus on each side of midline dorsal to the pyramids.
- Medial leminiscus ascends up through pons, midbrain and relays in the VPL nucleus of thalamus.
- 3rd order neurons lie in thalamus and their axons pass through the internal capsule and thalamic radiations to finally reach area no. 3, 1, 2 of cerebral cortex.
  Somatotopic arrangement: Medial most fibres are from sacral region and the lateral most fibres are from the cervical region.

Sensations carried
1. Movement, kinetic conscious proprioception
2. Discriminatory touch
3. Position, static conscious proprioception
4. Pressure
5. Vibration.

Spinocerebellar Pathway (Tract) (Fig. 10.4)

It is a two neuronal pathway which is situated in the posterior and lateral funiculus of white matter. They are two in number:
a. Anterior (ventral) spinocerebellar pathway.
b. Posterior (dorsal) spinocerebellar pathway.

Anterior Spinocerebellar Pathway (Fig. 10.4)

Origin: Laminae V to VII of spinal grey matter, primarily in T_1 to L_2 segments.
Termination: Ipsilateral anterior cerebellar vermis.

Crossing over: Fibres cross over twice
1. 1st in the same spinal segment.
2. **2nd in the midbrain:** The recrossed fibres pass through the superior cerebellar peduncle.

Course
- 1st order neuron lie in dorsal root ganglion
- 2nd order neurons ascend through the opposite lateral funiculus after crossing over
- The fibres ascend through the medulla, pons and midbrain and again cross over to the same side
- The tract enters the cerebellum through the superior cerebellar peduncle

Sensation carried
a. Unconscious proprioception from lower limb
b. Exteroceptor information from lower limb

Posterior Spinocerebellar Pathway (Fig. 10.4)

Origin: Lamina VII of spinal grey matter, primarily in T_1 to L_2 segments.
Termination: Rostral and caudal part of cerebellar vermis.
Crossing over: There is no crossing over

Course
- 1st order neurons lie in dorsal root ganglion
- 2nd order are present in laminae VII of spinal cord and their axons ascend in the ipsilateral lateral funiculus
- The tract passes through medulla and pons and reaches ipsilateral cerebellar cortex

Sensation carried
1. Unconcious proprioceptive touch and pressure sensations from lower limb and lower half of the body.
2. Conscious proprioception from lower limb.

The various sensations, their corresponding receptors, and ascending pathways in spinal cord:

Sensation	Receptors involved	Afferent fibers	Ascending spinal tract
Touch and pressure	Meissner's corpuscles Pacinian corpuscles Merkel's disks Ruffini endings	A b fibers	Anterior spinothalamic tract (carries crude touch sensation) Dorsal column (carries fine touch sensation and tactile discrimination)
Proprioception	Muscle spindle, Golgi tendon organ, Pacinian corpuscles in joints and ligaments	A a fibres	Dorsal column (responsible for concious proprioception) Posterior and anterior spinocerebellar tracts (responsible for unconcious proprioception)
Temperature	Cold receptors Warmth receptors	A d, C fibers C fibers	Lateral spinothalamic tract
Pain	Free nerve endings (Nociceptors)	A d, C fibers	Lateral spinothalamic tract

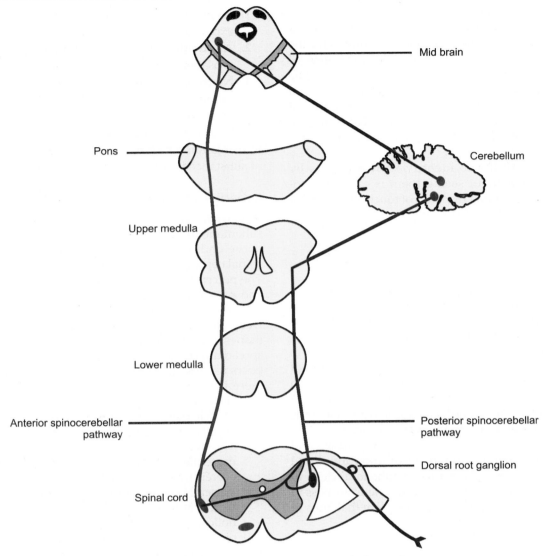

Fig. 10.4: Anterior land Posterior spinocerebellar pathways

Rostral Spinocerebellar Tract

Equivalent to anterior spinocerebellar tract. It carries similar sensations from upper limb.

HIGHER CENTERS OF SOMATOSENSORY INPUT

The higher centers for receiving and intergrating various sensory inputs are the thalamus and the cerebral cortex.

Thalamus

It is the major relay station for various sensations of the body. 3rd order neurons arise from thalamus and ascend to cerebral cortex. The functions of thalamus are described in detail on page no. 220.

Cerebral Cortex

The location of primary and secondary somasthetic (sensory) areas has been described on page no. ....

- **Somatic sensory area I:** It is located in the post central gyrus, area 3, 1, 2 and receives inputs from thalamus.
- **Somatic sensory area II:** It lies below somatic sensory area I. It receives inputs from area no. 3, 1, 2 also besides the thalamus.

The sensory area of cerebral cortex of one side receives afferents from opposite side of the body. The cortical representation of each area of the body depends on its sensory innervation. Hence fingers, lips, toes are represented by large areas as compared to the trunk and back.

Two point discrimination: It is the minimal distance at which one can recognize 2 similar stimuli as separate. This depends on intactness of touch receptors and the cortical (parietal lobe) component. This sense of discrimination varies normaly in different parts of the body. In fingers two touch points separated by 3 mm are felt separate while in the back two points are felt separated only at a distance of 65 mm. The ability of two point discrimination is tested in an individual with eyes closed.

Stereognosis: Ability to identify known objects by handling them without seeing them is called stereognosis. It is an integrated response of touch and pressure pathways and cerebral cortex.

SENSORY PATHWAY FROM FACE AND ORAL CAVITY

General sensations of pain, temperature, touch and pressure from skin of face and part of scalp, external ear and anterior part of oral cavity are carried by the various divisions of trigeminal nerve.

1st order neurons lie in the trigeminal ganglion in sensory nucleus of trigeminal nerve and nucleus of spinal tract of trigeminal nerve. 2nd order neurons from these nuclei relay in the thalamus in ventro-postero-medial nucleus and 3rd order neurons from thalamus form thalamic radiations to the cerebral cortex.

Sensations of proprioception from eye muscle and muscles of facial expression and masdication are carried by the 1st order neurons of mesencephalic nucleus of trigeminal nerve in midbrain. 1st order neurons pass to thalamus and then 2nd order neurons from thalamus to the cerebral cortex.

PAIN SENSATION

Receptors for pain sensation consist of naked nerve endings present in all parts of body.

Pain has two components which are:
1. Fast pain which is transmitted by A fibers to spinal cord.
2. Slow pain which is transmitted by C fibers to dorsal root ganglion.

Neurotransmitter for fast pain transmission is glutamate and for slow pain is substance P. There is some element of presynaptic inhibition of pain transmission at dorsal root ganglion by collaterals from other neurons, e.g., touch neurons or interneurons.

Post Traumatic Nerve Pain

After injury to an area, during healing, pain persists which can be described as:

1. **Hyperalgesia:** In this a minor stimulus produces excess pain.
2. **Allodynia:** It is the perception of pain when other sensations like touch are stimulated.
3. **Neuropathic pain:** It is a form of severe pain that radiates along the nerve distributions.

The occurrence of such pain is due to increase sensitivity of peripheral pain receptors, increased synaptic transmission which may be due to increase production of substance P or lack of presynaptic inhibition.

Superficial Versus Deep Pain

Superficial pain: It is the pain sensation from skin and subcutaneous tissue. The skin is richly supplied with nerve endings. The pain pathway extends from the spinal nerves, spinal cord, thalamus upto cerebral cortex. The perception of pain is subcortical but discrimination and meaningful interpretation of the painful stimulus is by the cerebral cortex.

Deep pain: It is the pain sensation arising from deeper tissues, muscles and viscera. The receptors are few and spread apart, and the pain is poorly localized. Afferent fibers usually travel along the autonomic nerves and so there is an associated response of sweating, increase heart rate and fall in BP seen with such pain.

- Muscle pain occurs as a result of decrease in blood supply. It is due to the release of Lewis P factor. The accumulation of P factor increases during muscular activity and hence pain is aggravated by exercise, e.g., as seen in pain of angina.
- Visceral pain is another example of deep pain and is poorly localized. It occurs due to distension of hollow viscera, excessive contractions above level of obstruction in intestines, inflammation of capsule of a viscus, ischemia and accumulation of noxious metabolites or spasm of smooth muscles. The deep pain usually causes reflex spasm of surrounding skeletal muscles. Example, Inflammation of abdominal viscera causes reflex spasm of anterior abdominal wall muscles associated in that area. This is felt as '**guarding**' during examination.

Experience of Pain

Pain fibers from spinal cord have multiple connections in the reticular formation, hypothalamus and limbic system, finally ending in thalamus which connects to cerebral cortex. Hence, painful stimuli result in emotional responses like anxiety and fear, stress responses, withdrawal responses and memory responses.

Itching and Tickling Sensation

Itching and tickling sensations are carried by free nerve ending of C fibers and pass along pain fibers to lateral spinothalamic tract of spinal cord. Scratching activates the fast conducting afferent neurons that inhibit transmission of itch sensation. These sensations are primarily due to mild stimulations of skin or mucus membranes. Endogenous chemicals like histamine and kinins released during inflammatory response can stimulate itching.

CUTANEOUS NERVE SUPPLY OF THE BODY

Skin is the largest sense organ of the body. It has numerous receptors for sensation of touch, pressure, temperature and pain and provides somatic afferent input to the central nervous system. The knowledge of cutaneous nerve supply has important clinical significance for clinching diagnosis in certain conditions.

CUTANEOUS NERVE SUPPLY OF SCALP

Each half of the scalp is supplied by eight sensory nerves (Fig. 10.5).

In front of the ear: These are four in number and all are branches of the trigeminal nerve
1. Supratrochlear nerve
2. Supraorbital nerve
3. Zygomaticotemporal nerve
4. Auriculotemporal nerve

Behind the ear: These are also four in number and arise from the cervical plexus
5. Great auricular nerve ($C_{2,3}$)
6. Lesser occipital nerve (C_2)
7. Greater occipital nerve (C_2)
8. Third occipital nerve (C_3)

CUTANEOUS NERVE SUPPLY OF FACE (FIGs 10.5 and 10.6)

The face receives its sensory innervation from following two sources:
1. **Trigeminal nerve:** The three divisions of trigeminal nerve supply almost the entire skin of face except an area over the angle of mandible.
   a. Branches from ophthalmic division
      i. Lacrimal nerve
      ii. Supraorbital nerve
      iii. Supratrochlear nerve
      iv. Infratrochlear nerve
      v. External nasal nerve
   b. Branches from maxillary division
      i. Infraorbital nerve
      ii. Zygomatico-facial nerve
      iii. Zygomatico-temporal nerve
   c. Branches from mandibular division
      i. Mental branch
      ii. Buccal branch
      iii. Auriculotemporal nerve

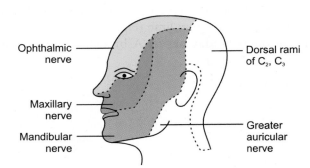

Fig. 10.6: Sensory distribution of face and scalp

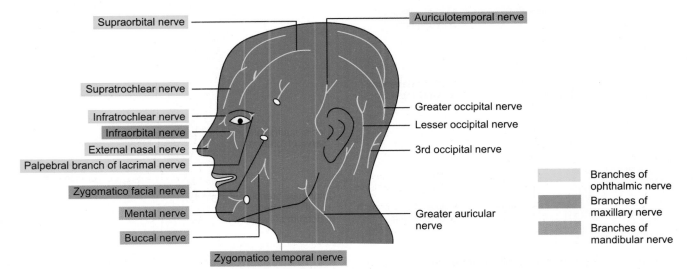

Fig. 10.5:   Sensory supply to face and scalp

CHAPTER-10

2. **Great auricular nerve (C₂):** This branch of cervical plexus supplies the area of skin over the angle of mandible.

CUTANEOUS NERVE SUPPLY OF NECK

It is derived from the following branches of cervical plexus (Figs 10.5, 10.13 and 10.14):

1. Lesser occipital nerve, C_2
2. Great auricular nerve, $C_{2,3}$
3. Transverse cutaneous nerve of neck, $C_{2,3}$
4. Supraclavicular neves, $C_{3,4}$
5. Medial branches of dorsal rami of $C_{3,4,5}$ spinal nerves

Lesser occipital nerve, greater auricular nerve and medial branches of dorsal rami of $C_{3,4,5}$ supply the posterior aspect of neck while the transverse cutaneous and supraclavicular nerves supply the anterior and lateral surfaces of neck.

CUTANEOUS NERVE SUPPLY OF UPPER LIMB

Following cutaneous nerves are present in the superficial fascia and supply upper limb (Figs 10.7 and 10.8).

1. **Supraclavicular nerve:** A branch from cervical plexus (C_3, C_4).

2. **Intercostobrachial nerve (T₂):** It is the lateral cutaneous branch of T_2 spinal nerve.
3. **Upper lateral cutaneous nerve of arm:** A branch from axillary nerve (C_5, C_6)
4. **Posterior cutaneous nerve of arm:** A branch of radial nerve.
5. **Lower lateral cutaneous nerve of arm:** A branch from radial nerve (C_5, C_6).
6. **Medial cutaneous nerve of arm:** A branch from medial cord of brachial plexus (T_1, T_2).
7. **Lateral cutaneous nerve of forearm:** A branch from musculo cutaneous nerve (C_5, C_6).
8. **Posterior cutaneous nerve of forearm (C_6, C_7, C_8):** A branch of radial nerve.
9. **Medial cutaneous nerve of forearm:** A branch from medial cord of brachial plexus (C_8, T_1).
10. **Palmar cutaneous branch of ulnar nerve:** A branch from ulnar nerve (C_8).
11. **Palmar cutaneous branch of median nerve:** A branch from median nerve (C_6, C_7).
12. **Superficial branch of radial nerve:** A branch from radial nerve (C_6, C_7).
13. **Dorsal cutaneous branch of ulnar nerve:** A branch from ulnar nerve (C_8).

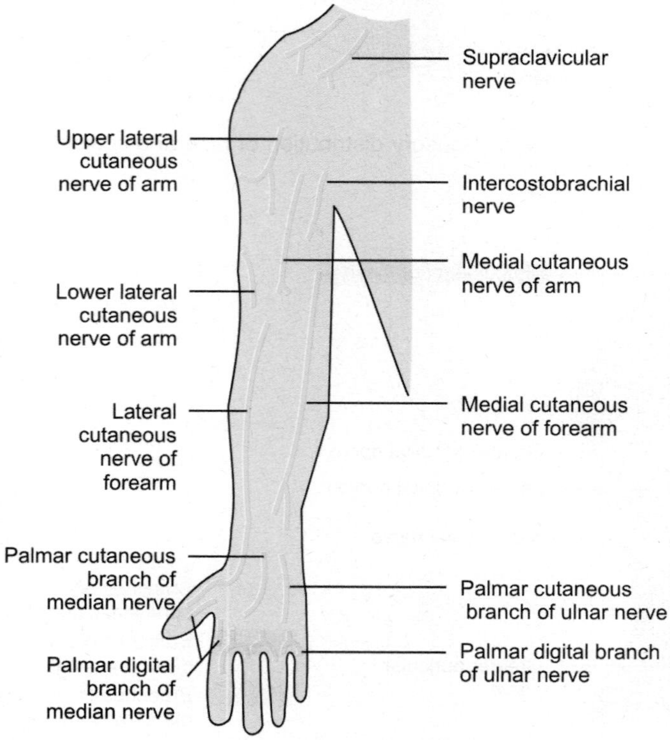

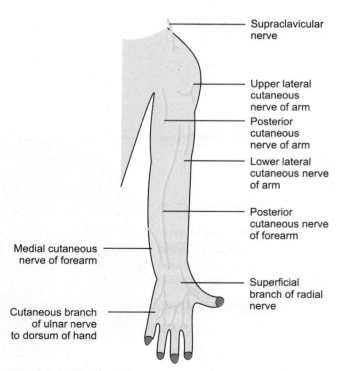

Fig. 10.7: Cutaneous nerve supply of upper limb, ventral or anterior surface

Fig. 10.8: Cutaneous nerve supply of upper limb, dorsal or posterior surface

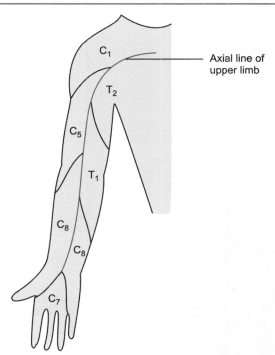

Fig. 10.9: Segmental innervation of upper limb (ventral aspect)

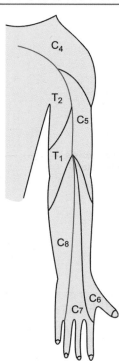

Fig. 10.10: Segmental innervation of upper limb (dorsal aspect)

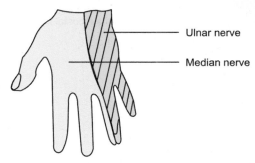

Fig. 10.11: Cutaneous nerve supply of palmar aspect of hand

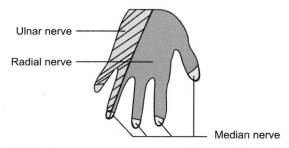

Fig. 10.12: Cutaneous nerve supply of dorsal aspect of hand

Dermatomes of Upper Limb (Figs 10.9 and 10.10)

- **Dermatome is defined as the area of skin supplied by a single spinal segment.**
- The upper limb is supplied by ventral rami of C_5 C_6 C_7 C_8 and T_1.
- Dermatome along preaxial border or radial border of the arm is supplied by C_5 and forearm is supplied by C_6. It includes thumb also.
- Dermatome along the postaxial border of arm is supplied by T_1 and forearm is supplied by C_8 including little finger.
- Central part of the hand is supplied by C_7.

- The area over the deltoid is supplied by C_4 and axillary region is supplied by T_2.

Cutaneous distribution of palmar and dorsal aspects of hand (Figs 10.11 and 10.12)

1. **Palmar aspect:** Medial 1 1/2 digits and medial 1/3rd of palm is supplied by ulnar nerve. Lateral 3 ½ digits and lateral 2/3rd of palm is supplied by median nerve.
2. **Dorsal aspect:** Medial 1 1/2 digits and medial 1/3rd of dorsum of hand is supplied by ulnar nerve. Lateral 3 1/2 digits except distal phalanx and lateral 2/3rd dorsum of hand is supplied by radial nerve. Skin over distal phalanges of lateral 3 1/2 digits is supplied by median nerve.

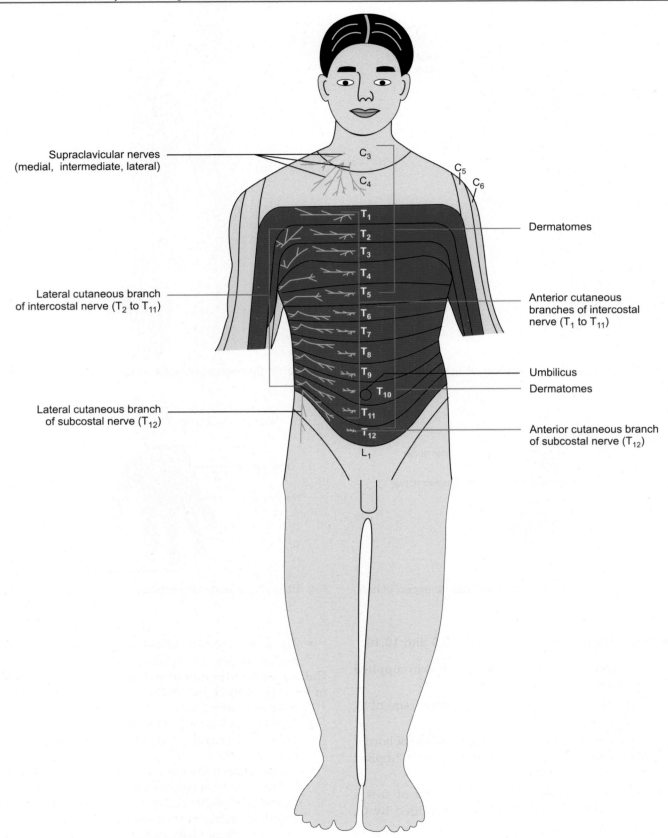

Supraclavicular nerves
(medial, intermediate, lateral)

C₃

C₄

C₅

C₆

Dermatomes

T₁
T₂
T₃
T₄
T₅

Anterior cutaneous
branches of intercostal
nerve (T₁ to T₁₁)

Lateral cutaneous branch
of intercostal nerve (T₂ to T₁₁)

T₆
T₇
T₈
T₉
T₁₀

Umbilicus
Dermatomes

T₁₁

Lateral cutaneous branch
of subcostal nerve (T₁₂)

T₁₂

Anterior cutaneous branch
of subcostal nerve (T₁₂)

L₁

Fig. 10.13: Cutaneous nerve supply of front of thorax and abdomen

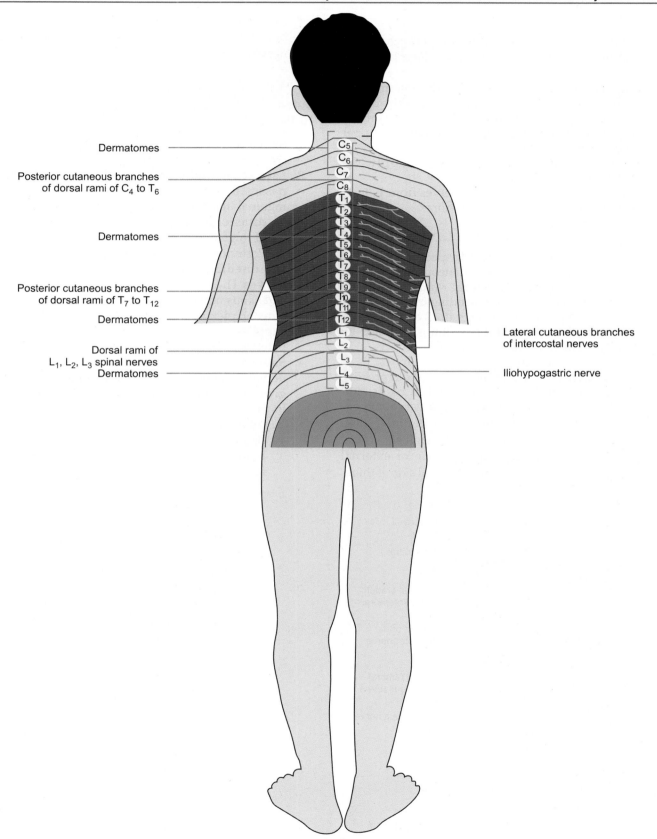

Dermatomes

Posterior cutaneous branches of dorsal rami of C_4 to T_6

Dermatomes

Posterior cutaneous branches of dorsal rami of T_7 to T_{12}

Dermatomes

Dorsal rami of L_1, L_2, L_3 spinal nerves
Dermatomes

C_5
C_6
C_7
C_8
T_1
T_2
T_3
T_4
T_5
T_6
T_7
T_8
T_9
T_{10}
T_{11}
T_{12}
L_1
L_2
L_3
L_4
L_5

Lateral cutaneous branches of intercostal nerves

Iliohypogastric nerve

Fig. 10.14: Cutaneous nerve supply of back of thorax and abdomen

CUTANEOUS NERVE SUPPLY OF THORAX

Skin of thorax is supplied by following branches from cervical plexus and intercostal nerves (Figs 10.13 and 10.14).

1. **Supraclavicular nerves (C_3, C_4):** The intermediate supraclavicular nerves supply the skin below clavicle upto the second rib while the lateral supraclavicular nerves supply the skin over upper and posterior part of shoulder.
2. T_1 to T_6 intercostal nerves: The supply the anterolateral of thorax.
3. Dorsal rami of thoracic spinal nerves from T_1 to T_6 supply the posterior aspect of thorax.

CUTANEOUS NERVE SUPPLY OF ABDOMINAL WALL

- Skin of the anterior and lateral aspect of abdominal wall is supplied by lateral cutaneous and anterior cutaneous branches of ventral rami of lower six thoracic nerves (T_7 to T_{12}) extending from xiphisternum to symphysis pubis (Figs 10.13 and 10.14)
  1. **At the level of umbilicus** skin is supplied by T_{10} segment of the spinal cord.
  2. **Above umbilicus** skin is supplied by T_9, T_8, T_7 spinal nerves. T_7 supplies near xiphoid process.
  3. **Below umbilicus** skin is supplied by T_{11} and T_{12} and L_1 nerves. Iliohypogastric nerve emerges 2.5 cm above the superficial inguinal ring. Ilioinguinal nerve emerges through superficial inguinal ring and supplies skin of external genitalia and upper part of medial side of thigh.

- The posterior aspect of abdomen is supplied by branches of dorsal rami of lower six thoracic spinal nerves.

CUTANEOUS NERVE SUPPLY OF LOWER LIMB

Cutaneous Nerve Supply of Front of Thigh (Figs 10.15, 10.16)

1. **Subcostal nerve (T_{12}):** It supplies at the level of iliac crest and anterior superior iliac spine.
2. **Lateral femoral cutaneous nerve (L_2 and L_3):** It passes behind and through the substance of inguinal ligament. It divides into two branches.
   a. Anterior branch, supplies anterolateral surface of thigh and forms patellar plexus.
   b. Posterior branch, supplies gluteal region.
3. **Intermediate and medial femoral cutaneous nerves (L_2, L_3 and L_4):** Intermediate femoral cutaneous nerve supplies front of thigh and forms patellar plexus. Medial femoral cutaneous nerve supplies medial lower 1/3rd of thigh and forms patellar plexus.
4. **Saphenous nerve (L_3 and L_4):** Longest cutaneous nerve of the body. It is a branch of femoral nerve given in the thigh but does not supply the thigh. Its branches are
   a. Infra patellar branch
   b. Branches to supply medial side of ankle
   c. Branches to supply medial side of dorsum of foot upto first metatarsophalangeal joint

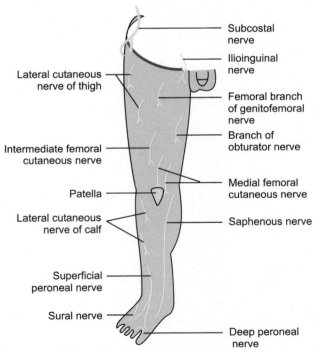

Fig. 10.15: Cutaneous innervation of lower limb—anterior aspect

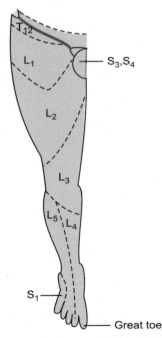

Fig. 10.16: Segmental supply of lower limb anterior aspect

5. **A branch from anterior division of obturator nerve (L_2, L_3 and L_4):** It supplies upper 1/3rd of medial side of thigh.
6. **Ilioinguinal nerve (L_1):** Supplies area below the pubic tubercle.
7. **Femoral branch of genitofemoral nerve (L_1):** It supplies below the middle 1/3rd of inguinal ligament.

Cutaneous Nerve Supply of Front of the Leg and Dorsum of the Foot (Figs 10.15 to 10.17)

1. **Saphenous nerve (L_3 L_4):** It supplies upper 2/3rd of medial side of the leg and the medial border of the dorsum of the foot.
2. **Lateral cutaneous nerve of calf:** It supplies upper 2/3rd of the leg laterally.
3. **Superficial peroneal nerve:** It supplies lower 1/3rd of the leg laterally. It also supplies most of the dorsum of foot except following areas.
   a. **Sural nerve:** It supplies lateral margin of the foot.
   b. **Saphenous nerve:** It supplies medial margin of the foot.
   c. **Deep peroneal nerve:** It is sensory to 1st interdigital cleft.
   d. **Medial and lateral plantar nerves:** They supply terminal phalanges on the dorsum of the foot.

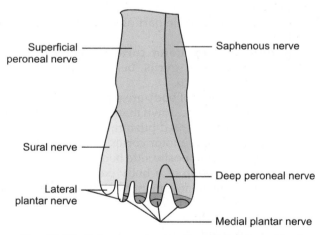

Fig. 10.17: Cutaneous innervation of dorsum of foot

Cutaneous Nerve Supply of Gluteal Region and Back of Thigh (Figs 10.18 to 10.20)

Cutaneous nerves converge towards the centre of gluteal region. They are 45 in number.
From above (lateral to medial side)
1. Lateral cutaneous branch of subcostal nerve (T_{12}).
2. Lateral cutaneous branch of iliohypogastric nerve (L_1).
3. Lateral branches of dorsal rami from L_1, L_2, L_3 spinal nerves.

From below (medial to lateral side)
4. Recurrent gluteal branches of posterior femoral cutaneous nerve (S_1, S_2, S_3).
5. Perforating branches of S_2, S_3 nerves which appear after piercing the sacrotuberous ligament.
From front
6. Posterior branch of lateral femoral cutaneous nerve (L_2).
From behind
7. Lateral branches of dorsal rami of S_1, S_2, S_3 spinal nerves.
Following nerves supply skin of back of thigh
1. Posterior femoral cutaneous nerve of thigh: It supplies major part of back of thigh
2. Branch from lateral femoral cutaneous nerve of thigh
3. Branch from medial cutaneous nerve of thigh
4. Branch from obturator nerve

Cutaneous Nerve Supply of Posterior Surface of Leg (Figs 10.18 to 10.20)

1. **Posterior femoral cutaneous nerve:** It supplies upper part of back of leg.
2. **Sural nerve:** It supplies the lower part of skin of half and accompanies the short saphenous vein.
3. **Lateral cutaneous branch:** It supplies the upper and lateral part of calf.

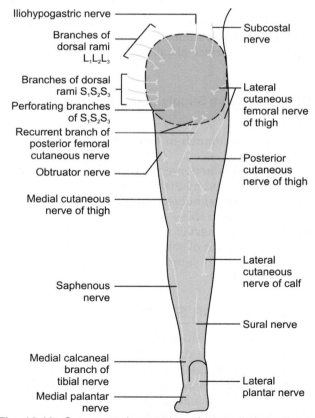

Fig. 10.18: Cutaneous innervation of lower limb—posterior aspect

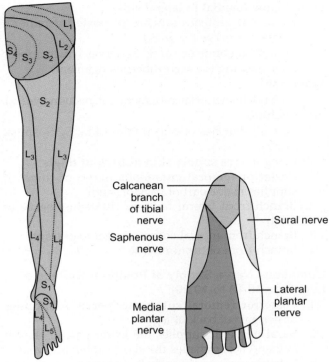

Fig. 10.19: Segmental supply of lower limb—posterior aspect

Fig. 10.20: Cutaneous nerve supply of sole

4. **Saphenous nerve:** It supplies the medial side of calf.
5. **Calcanean branch of tibial nerve:** It supplies posterior surface of calcaneus and weight bearing area of heel.

Cutaneous Nerve Supply of the Sole (Figs 10.18 to 10.20)

1. **Calcanean branch of tibial nerve:** It supplies the heel.
2. **Medial plantar nerve:** It supplies the medial aspect of the sole and medial 3½ toes.
3. **Lateral plantar nerve:** It supplies lateral part of sole and lateral 1½ toes.
4. **Saphenous nerve:** It supplies middle 1/3rd of medial margin of sole.
5. **Sural nerve:** It supplies posterior 2/3rd of lateral margin of sole.

SOMATOMOTOR SYSTEM

This system deals with initiation of command, planning, integration and finally the execution of voluntary movements of the body in a coordinated manner. The motor pathway is responsible for integration of inputs from various lavels and brings about:
1. Voluntary muscular activity.
2. Adjustments of body posture.

3. Coordination between various muscle groups for smooth and precise motor activity (fine skillful movements).

This enables the survival and existance of the body, e.g., movements for work, movements to obtain and ingest food, etc. The somatomotor system consists of the following parts:
1. Higher center: Cerebral cortex, basal ganglia, brain stem and cerebellum.
2. Motor pathways: The actvity in higher centers is transmitted to the motor neurons of spinal cord and motor neurons of cranial nerves.
   a. The fibers from motor cortex of cerebrum to cranial nerve nuclei and their distribution form **corticobulbar tract.**
   b. The fibers descending from the motor cortex to the spinal cord are named **corticospinal tract.**
3. Spinal nerves and cranial nerves.
4. Effector organ.

HIGHER CENTERS OF SOMATOMOTOR SYSTEM

Cerebrum

The various motor areas of cortex have been discussed on page nos 214 to 216.
1. **Motor cortex (area no. 4):** It is located in the precentral gyrus.
2. **Premotor cortex (area no. 6 and 8):** It is located in posterior and middle part of superior and middle frontal gyrus.
3. **Supplementory motor cortex:** It is located just above cingulated gyrus, behind medial frontal gyrus, below area 6.
   — Various parts of body are represented on motor cortex in upside down manner (Fig. 8.16). Facial area is represented bilaterally while for rest of body one side motor cortex controls the motor function of opposite side body.
   — Representation of a body part is proportional to the skill of movement of that part for example hand movements and area of speech has large representation.
   — Supplementary motor cortex helps in programming of motor sequences.
   — Premotor cortex has connections with motor cortex, brain stem and corticospinal fibers and probably helps in posture control.

Basal Ganglia

The anatomical and functional organization of basal ganglia is given on page no. 219.
• Basal ganglia receive connections from all parts of cerebral cortex and from thalamus.

- The various parts of basal ganglia are inter-connected .
- Efferents from globus pallidus pass to the thalamus and further to the prefrontal and motor cortex of cerebral hemispheres.
- Basal ganglia are connected to the substantia nigra.
- The basal ganglia are involved in planning and programming of various movements. It helps in regulating muscle tone through its connections with substantia nigra, thalamus and cerebral cortex.

Brain Stem

The anatomical and functional organization of medulla, pons and midbrain is given on page nos 226 to 234.
- Brain stem provides passage to the various ascending and descending pathways.
- The reticular formation of brain stem has multiple connections with higher centers and the motor neurons of spinal cord. It controls the activity of γ-motor neurons.
- Vestibular nuclei of brain stem are connected to the cerebellum and are responsible in control of posture and equilibrium of body.
- The brain stem also has the vital centers of the body namely, respiratory and cardiovascular centers. These have to and fro connections with higher centers and affect the motor activity of the organs.

Cerebellum

The anatomical and functional organization of cerebellum is given on page nos 234 to 237.
- Afferents to cerebellum (mossy fibres and climbing fibres) provide input from
  1. Inferior olivary nucleus via dorsal and ventral spinocerebellar tracts, responsible for proprioceptive impulses from body.
  2. Vestibular nuclei of brain stem provide vestibular impulses from the labyrinths of the ear.
  3. Cerebral cortex via pontocerebellar tract provide input from cerebral cortex.
  4. Inferior and superior colliculi via tectocerebellar tract provide auditory and visual inputs.
- Efferent fibres from cerebellar cortex.
  1. The axons of neurons of cortex (Purkinje cells and granule cells) end on the deep nuclei of cerebellum while axons of basket cells and golgi cells and on Purkinje cells and the molecular layer of cerebellar cortex.
  2. Efferents from deep nuclei pass to the brain stem and thalamus.
- These fine interconnections of cerebellum are responsible for its functions which are control of

muscle tone and stretch reflexes, coordination of voluntary and involuntary movements and control of posture and equilibrium of the body.

MOTOR PATHWAYS

The fibers descending from the motor cortex to the spinal cord are divided into two pathways:
1. **Pyramidal tract:** It consists of fibers from motor cortex of cerebrum that pass down via medullary pyramids to spinal cord.
   — 80% of fibres cross to opposite side at the medualla and form lateral corticospinal tract and the rest pass down as anterior corticospinal tract.
   — The fibers end on the ventral horn cells of spinal cord. These are called **upper motor neuron fibers.**
   — Axons of motor neurons (A α and γ neurons) from ventral horn of spinal cord then supply the muscles of the body. These are called **lower motor neuron fibers.**
   — Corticospinal tracts are described below.
   — Functions of corticospinal and corticobulbar tracts are primarily, initiation of skilled voluntary movements of body. They are also involved in posture regulation and coordination of action of various muscle groups of the body.
2. **Extra pyramidal tract:** It consists of rest of the fibers descending from the brain which do not pass via medullary pyramids. These fibers have multiple synapses with basal ganglia, hypothalmus and the reticular formation. Descending pathways that contribute to the extrapyramidal system:
   — Rubrospinal tract
   — Tectospinal and tectobulbar tract
   — Reticulospinal tract
   — Vestibulospinal tract
   — Medial longitudinal fasciculus (or bundle)

   Functions of extrapyramidal tracts:
   1. Corticobulbar (corticonuclear) fibers control the movement of the eye balls.
   2. They are responsible for control of tone, posture and equilibrium.
   3. They control complex movements of the body and limb such as coordinated movements of arms and legs during walking.
   4. They exert tonic inhibitory control over the lower centres.
   5. If the pyramidal tracts are damaged, they can carry out voluntary movement to some extent.

The pyramidal and extrapyramidal tracts control the motor neurons of the opposite side of the spinal cord.

CHAPTER-10

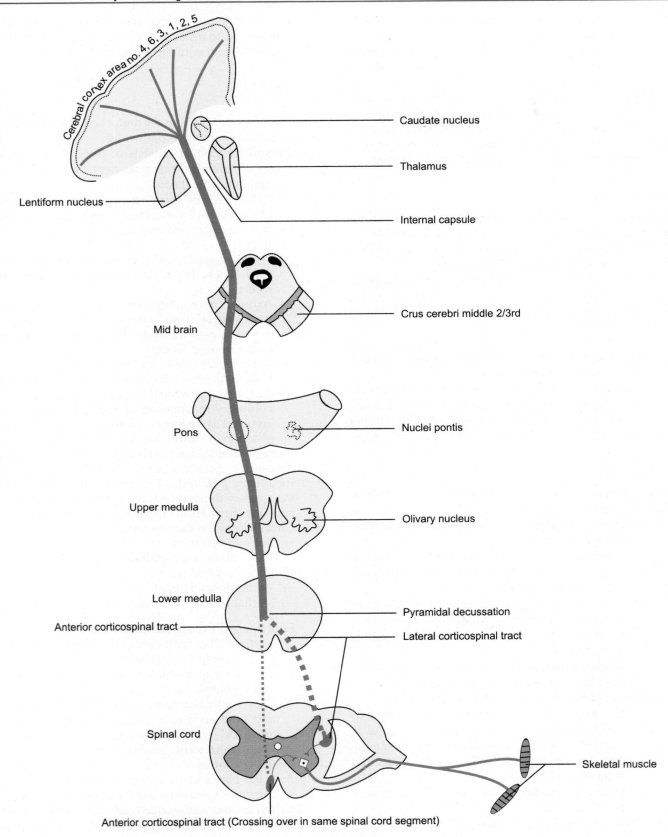

Fig. 10.21: Corticospinal tracts

Corticospinal Tract

It is also known as the pyramidal tract. It is made up of axons of pyramidal cells of cerebral cortex (Fig. 10.21).

Origin: The fibres arise from functional area no. 4, 6, 3, 1, 2, 5 of cerebral cortex. 1/3rd fibres arise from area 4, 1/3rd from area 6, and rest 1/3rd from area 3, 1 and 2, 5

Termination: The fibres of corticospinal tract terminate on neurons of lamina IV to VII (posterior and lateral grey colums) of spinal grey matter. It is connected to alpha and gamma neurons of lamina IX through interneurons.

Course: Fibres of corticospinal tract passes successively through
- The corona radiata
- Posterior limb of internal capsule
- Middle 2/3rd of cerebral peduncle of mid brain
- Ventral part of pons
- Pyramid of medulla
- In the lower part of medulla, 75 to 90% fibres cross to the opposite side and form lateral cortico-spinal tract in the spinal cord
- 25 to 10% fibres remain uncrossed and form anterior corticospinal tract of the cord.

Lateral Corticospinal Tract

It extends up to the S_4 segment of spinal cord and lies in the lateral funiculus of the spinal cord. It may also contain some uncrossed fibres.

Somatotopic arrangement of lateral corticospinal tract fibres
Cervical fibres are deeper and lower limb fibres are most superficial.

Anterior Corticospinal Tract

It extends up to the mid thoracic region and lies in the anterior funiculus of spinal cord. It crosses to the opposite side in the spinal segment where it would terminate.

Functions of Corticospinal Tract

It is stimulatory to the flexor muscles and inhibitory to the extensor muscles. It is concerned with skillful voluntary movements of the non-postural type.

SPINAL NERVES AND CRANIAL NERVES

These are the peripheral extentions from spinal cord motor nuclei and cranial nerve nuclei that carry the motor fibres to the effector organs. The course and distribution of various spinal nerves and cranial nerves has been discribed in chapter no. 9.

EFFECTOR ORGAN

Skeletal musculature of the body forms the effector organ of the somatomotor system. The motor fibres end on extrafusal skeletal muscle fibres and result in contraction of muscles.

Final common pathway: The motor neurons that supply extrafusal fibers of skeletal muscles are stimulated by various reflex arcs and are also responsible for voluntary movements in the body. Thus the stimulation of α-motor neurons is the final common pathway that causes contraction of muscles. It responds by integrating inputs from reflex arc, pyramidal tracts from cerebral cortex, reticular formation, cerebellum and vestibular nuclei.

REFLEXES

Reflex is a motor response to a stimulus which is independant of voluntary control which means it is

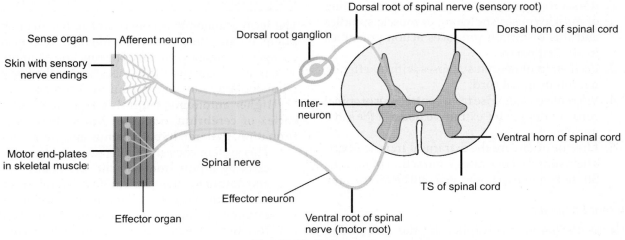

Fig. 10.22: Reflex arc

brought about without the involvement of cerebral cortex. The basic unit of a reflex is the **reflex arc** which consists of the following parts (Fig. 10.22):

1. Sense organ
2. Afferent neuron, usually from dorsal root ganglia of spinal cord or cranial nerve ganglia.
3. Synapses, single or multiple that set up excitatory post synaptic potentials (EPSP) or inhibitory post synaptic potentials (PSP).
4. Efferent neuron
5. Effector organ

Monosynaptic Reflexes

These have a simple reflex arc and consist of a single synapse between the afferent and efferent neurons.

Stretch Reflex

- It is a monosynaptic reflex.
- When skeletal muscle is stretched, it contracts. This is stretch reflex.
- Clinical examples are; knee reflex, in which tapping on tendon of quadriceps femoris muscle leads to knee jerk; triceps reflex, by tapping on tendon of triceps brachii there is reflex extension of elbow.
- Reflex arc of stretch reflex:
  1. **Sense organ:** It is the skeletal muscle spindle. It is made up of specialized muscle fibers enclosed in connective tissue. This forms intrafusal fibers. Extrafusal fibers are the contractile units of muscle. Intrafusal fibers are of two types:
     a. **Nuclear bag fibers:** Supplied by annulospiral endings of group I a sensory nerve fibers.
     b. **Nuclear chain fibers:** Supplied by flower spray endings of group II sensory nerve fibers.
     Muscle spindle fibers have their own motor supply derived from A γ-efferents.
  2. The afferent neurons are from the corresponding dorsal root ganglion of spinal cord. Stretching of muscle causes stretching of muscle spindles and this distortion produces action potentials in afferent nerves.
  3. Each afferent neuron synapses with an efferent neuron in spinal cord.
  4. Efferent neurons arise from ventral root of spinal cord and supply the extrafusal fibers of the same muscle.
  5. Effector organ are the extrafusal muscle fibers. Their stimulation causes contraction of muscle. Stronger the stretch, stronger will be contraction.

γ-efferent Stimulation

γ-efferent discharge is controlled by the descending motor tracts from various parts of the brain. Stimulation of γ-efferents leads to contraction of muscle spindle fibers which further stretches the nuclear bag fibers. Thus they indirectly stimulate reflex contraction of muscle via stretch reflex.

Golgi Tendon Organ

It is a net like collection of nerve endings present among the fascicles of muscle fibers at the tendinous ends. Stimulation of this organ sets up impulses in afferent neurons which end on inhibitory interneurons and inhibit the efferent neurons supplying the muscle. These nerve endings are stimulated by contraction of muscle fibers and lead to a reflex relaxation response. They are also stimulated when the muscle is excessively stretched and cause relaxation instead of contraction. Hence, they are responsible for inverse stretch reflex.

The muscle spindles and golgi tendon organs thus regulate the extent and force of muscle contraction. They also act as protective reflexes.

Polysynaptic Reflex

The reflex arc of a polysynaptic reflex has a number of inter neurons intersposed between the afferent and efferent neurons.

Withdrawl Reflex

- It is a typical example of polysynaptic reflex.
- When a painful stimulus is applied to the skin, subcutaneous tissue or muscle it leads to withdrawl of stimulated area away from stimulus. This generally occurs due to stimulation of flexor muscles and inhibition of extensor muscles.
- Multiple interneurons which may vary from 2 to 100 are present between afferent and efferent neurons.

AUTONOMIC NERVOUS SYSTEM (ANS)

The term autonomic is convenient rather than appropriate, because this system is intimately responsive to changes in somatic activities. The function of autonomic system is to maintain the homeostasis of the body and regulates body functions for survival and existence.

Higher autonomic control is from the prefrontal cortex of cerebrum, nuclei of brain stem, reticular formation, thalami, hypothalamus and limbic lobe.

- This system consists of afferent and efferent fibres carrying inputs from somatic and cranial sources and output to innervate various visceral structures. Autonomic nervous system is responsible for the involuntary activities of the body and controls function of heart, lungs, smooth muscles and various glands.

- ANS consists of a sensory (afferent) pathway and a motor (efferent) pathway.
- Neurons of afferent pathway arise from various visceral receptors and pass through dorsal root of spinal nerves or corresponding cranial nerves.
- Efferent pathway consists of pre-ganglionic and post-ganglionic neurons:
  a. **Pre-ganglionic fibers:**
     - These arise from neruons present in the intermediolateral gray column of spinal cord or corresponding cranial nerve nuclei and relay in the autonomic ganglia situated outside the CNS (Examples are otic and pterygo palatine ganglion of parasympathetic pathway and various sympathetic ganglia of the sympathetic chain).
     - Axons of pre-ganglionic fibers are mostly myelinated, B-fibers.
     - The neurotransmitter secreted at the endings of preganglionic fibers is acetylcholine.
  b. **Post-ganglionic fibers:**
     - These arise from the neuronal cells in various autonomic ganglia and pass to the corresponding effector organs.
     - Axons of post-ganglionic fibers are mostly unmyelinated, C fibers.
     - The neurotransmitter secreted at the endings of post-ganglionic parasympathetic fibers is acetylcholine while of post-ganglionic sympathetic fibers is nor-adrenaline.
- Postganglionic fibres are more numerous. This helps in diffusion of activity.
- The ratio of postganglinic : preganglionic fibres is more in the sympathetic than in parasympathetic nervous system.

   Autonomic nervous system can be studied in two parts:
   1. Sympathetic nervous system
   2. Parasympathetic nervous system

SYMPATHETIC NERVOUS SYSTEM

It is the larger component of autonomic nervous system. It is made up of two ganglionated trunks and their branches, plexuses and subsidiary ganglia (Fig. 10.23). It innervates the following structures:
   1. All sweat glands
   2. Arrector pilorum muscle
   3. Muscular wall of arteries
   4. Abdomino-pelvic viscera
   5. Esophagus, lung, heart
   6. Non striated muscles of the urogenital system
   7. Iris
   8. Eye lids

Efferent pathway of sympathetic nervous system forms the lateral grey column of T_1 to L_2 spinal segments hence it is also known as thoraco-lumbar outflow. It arises from the intermedio-medial and intemedio-lateral neural group of spinal grey column. It consists of a total of 14 nerves. It has been suggested (Mitchell, 1953) that neurons like those of lateral grey column exist at other levels also. Nervi terminalis may be a rostral extension of sympathetic system containing efferent postganglionic fibres distributed to vessels and glands of nasal cavity.

Parts of Sympathetic Nervous System

It consists of the following parts (Fig. 10.23)
   1. **Sympathetic trunks with sympathetic ganglia (lateral ganglia):** There are two sympathetic trunks, one lying on each side of vertebral column. Each trunk extends from the base of skull to the coccyx. At the level of 1st coccygeal vertebra the two trunks unite to form a single ganglion called gaglion impar. Each trunk presents with 22 to 23 ganglia. These are:
      a. **Three cervical ganglia:** Superior cervical ganglion, middle cervical ganglion and Inferior cervical ganglion.
         Stellate ganglion: Sometimes inferior cervical ganglion fuses with 1st thoracic ganglion to form the stellate or cervicothoracic ganglion.
      b. 10 to 12 thoracic ganglia
      c. 4 lumbar ganglia
      d. 4 to 5 sacral ganglia
   2. **Subsidiary ganglia:** These consist of the following:
      Intermediate or collateral ganglia
      a. Coeliac ganglia
      b. Superior mesenteric ganglia
      c. Inferior mesenteric ganglia
      d. Aortico renal ganglia
      e. Neurons in the superior hypogastric plexus
      Terminal ganglia: It is formed by the suprarenal medulla and consists of chromaffin cells.
   3. **Preganglionic neurons and fibres**
      - The preganglionic neurons are located in the lateral horn or intermediomedial and intermediolateral groups of neuronal cells of the spinal grey column. They extend from the 1st thoracic to 2nd or 3rd lumbar segments of the spinal cord.
      - Preganglionic fibres are known as the white rami communicantes and they emerge from T1 to L_2 spinal segments through the ventral root and trunk of the spinal nerves to reach the corresponding ganglion of the sympathetic chain.
      - These fibres are thinly myelinated.

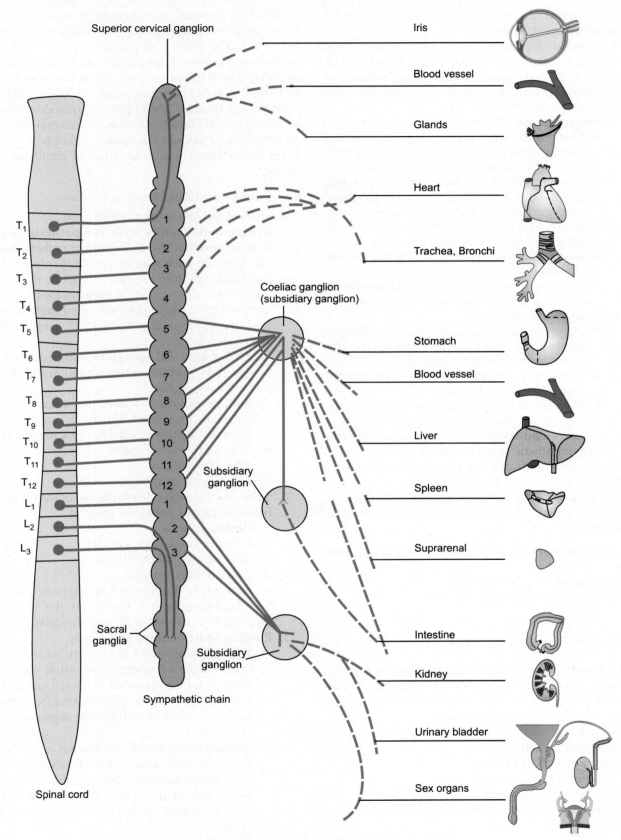

Fig. 10.23: Sympathetic innervation

- **Mode of termination of preganglionic fibres.** It can occur in following ways
  a. Relay into the corresponding ganglion. directly or through interneurons
  b. Some fibres either ascend or descend in the sympathetic chain and relay in the upper or lower ganglia of the sympathetic chain.
  c. A few fibres pass the corresponding ganglion without relay to end in the collateral ganglia, e.g. splanchnic nerves of thorax and lumbar regions.
  d. Some fibres pass without relay and terminate in the terminal ganglion (suprarenal medulla).

4. **Postganglionic neuron and fibres**
   - Postganglionic neurons lie either in the ganglia of sympathetic chain or in the collateral or subsidiary ganglia.
   - Postganglionic fibres arise from these ganglia.
   - They are nonmyelinated.
   - **Mode of termination of post ganglionic fibres** can be in any one of the following ways
     a. Some postganglionic fibres pass back to the corresponding spinal nerve via the grey rami communicantes.
     b. Postganglionic fibres also pass through medial branches of the ganglia and supply the viscera.
     c. A few fibres either ascend or descend in the sympathetic chain and pass as grey rami to the other spinal nerves or as their medial branches.
     d. Postganglionic fibres arising from collateral ganglia reach the target organs via plexuses around corresponding arteries (periarterial sympathetic plexuses).

Components of Sympathetic System

1. **Sensory component:** It conveys the visceral sensation of pain. The cell bodies of these nerves lie in the dorsal root ganglia of the thoracic and upper two lumbar spinal nerves.
2. **Motor component:** The cell bodies of preganglionic neurons lie in the thoracic and upper two lumbar segments of spinal cord in the lateral horn of spinal cord while the postganglionic neurons lie in the sympathetic chain ganglia and the collateral ganglia. The postganglionic fibres primarily supply the heart, smooth muscles and glandular cells. They secret non-adrenaline on the surface of effector cells. Hence the sympathetic nervous system is also called the adrenergic system.

The sympathetic nervous system is divided into the following five parts

1. **Cranial part:** Preganglionic fibres arise from the first thoracic (T_1) spinal segment. Postganglionic fibres arise from the superior cervical ganglion and ascend along the internal carotid artery. The plexus around internal carotid artery continues further around the anterior cerebral, middle cerebral and anterior communicating arteries.
2. **Cervical part:** It includes the superior, middle and inferior cervical ganglia.
   a. **Superior cervical ganglion:** It lies at the level of C_2 and C_3 vertebra. Preganglionic fibres come from 1st and 2nd thoracic spinal segments. Postganglionic fibres leave the superior cervical ganglion as the lateral, medial, anterior and ascending branches. Their distribution is as follows. The ascending branches form plexus around internal carotid artery and continues with plexus around its branches.
   Branches
   i. Inferior vagal ganglion
   ii. Hypoglossal nerve
   iii. Superior vagal ganglion
   iv. Inferior ganglion of glossopharyngeal nerve
   v. Superior bulb of internal jugular
   vi. Grey rami communication to upper four cervical nerves
   vii. Carotid body
   viii. Pharyngeal plexus
   ix. Cardiac branches
   x. Communicate with vagus
   xi. Form plexus around the facial artery and supply the submandibular gland
   xii. Form plexus around the middle meningeal artery and supply otic gaglion
   xiii. Supply facial sweat glands via trigeminal branches
   b. **Middle cervical ganglion:** It lies at the level of C_6 vertebra. Preganglionic fibres arise from T_1 to T_3 spinal cord segments. Distribution of postganglionic fibres
   i. Grey rami are given to C_5 and C_6 spinal nerves.
   ii. Supplies thyroid and parathyroid glands.
   iii. Cardiac branches to deep cardiac plexus.
   iv. Communicating branches to external laryngeal and recurrent laryngeal nerves.
   c. **Stellate ganglion:** It is formed by the fusion of C_7, C_8 and T_1 ganglia of the sympathetic chain. It lies at the level of base of transverse process of C_7 and neck of 1st rib. Preganglionic fibres are derived from T_1 to T_3 spinal segments. Postganglionic fibres are distributed as
   i. Grey rami communicantes to C_7, C_8, T_1, spinal nerves
   ii. Cardiac branches to deep cardiac plexus
   iii. Branches to subclavian artery.
   iv. Branches to vertebral artery.

v. Form periarterial plexus around inferior thyroid artery which supplies the thyroid gland.
3. **Thoracic part:** It is made up of 11 sympathetic ganglia ie, forms 70% of the population. T_2 to T_9 ganglia lie against the heads of corresponding ribs while T_{10}, T_{11}, T_{12} ganglia lie in front of the corresponding vertebral bodies. Preganglionic fibres are derived from T_1 to T_{11}. Postganglionic fibres are distributed as follows:
   a. Grey rami communicantes to all thoracic spinal nerves.
   b. Medial branches of thoracic ganglia give rise to
      i. Greater splanchnic nerve, from T_5 to T_9: Joins the coeliac plexus.
      ii. Lesser splanchnic nerve, from T_9 to T_{11}: Ends in the aortico-renal ganglia.
      iii. Least splanchnic nerve, from T_{11} to T_{12}: Ends in the renal ganglia.
   c. Small branches to esophagus and trachea.
   d. Pulmonary plexus (T_2 to T_5).
   e. Deep cardiac plexus (T_2 to T_5).
4. **Lumbar part:** This consists of 4 intercommunicating ganglia which lie extra peritoneally. Preganglionic fibres are derived from L_1 and L_2 spinal segments. Postganglionic fibres are distributed as follows:
   a. Grey rami communicantes to L_1, L_2, L_3 spinal nerves. These further form plexuses around femoral and obturator arteries.
   b. L_2 ganglion gives rises to a special branch which joins the inferior part of aortic plexus.
   c. L_3 and L_4 join the inferior hypogastric plexus, as far as the proximal part of the femoral artery
5. **Pelvic part:** It is made up of 4 to 5 sympathetic ganglia. They lie over the sacrum medial to the anterior sacral foramina. Preganglionic fibres arise from T_{10} to L_2 spinal segments. Postganglionic fibres are distributed as follows:
   a. Medial branch to inferior hypogastric plexus, from S_1, S_2 ganglia.
   b. Grey rami communicantes to S_3, S_4, S_5 sacral ganglia.

Functions of Sympathetic System
1. **Fibres which return to spinal nerve are:**
   a. Vasoconstrictor to blood vessels
   b. Accompanying motor nerves are vasodilatory to muscles
   c. Secretomotor to sweat gland
   d. Motor to arrector pilorus
2. **Those reaching viscera cause:**
   a. Vasoconstriction
   b. Bronchial, bronchiolar dilatation
   c. Modification of secretion
   d. Pupillary dilatation
   e. Alimentary contraction.

PARASYMPATHETIC NERVOUS SYSTEM
It is also known as the **cranio-sacral outflow (Fig. 10.24).** This system regulates the internal environment of the body in resting condition.

Parts of Parasympathetic Nervous System
It is made up of the following parts (Fig. 10.24):
1. **Cranial part:** It includes four parasympathetic ganglia related to head and neck. These are:
   a. Ciliary ganglion
   b. Pterygopalatine ganglion (spheno palatine)
   c. Submandibular ganglion
   d. Otic ganglion
   Preganglionic fibres are carried by II, VII, IX, X cranial nerves. **Parasympathetic nuclei present in the brain:**
   1. Edinger-Westphal nucleus
   2. Superior salivatory nucleus
   3. Inferior salivatory nucleus
   4. Dorsal nucleus of vagus
2. **Sacral part:** Preganglionic fibres arise from lateral horn cells of S_2 S_3 and S_4 spinal segments. These fibres form the pelvic splanchnic neves, also known as **nervi erigentes.** Pelvic splanchnic nerves relay into terminal ganglia which lie close to the pelvic viscera. The postganglionic fibres supply the following organs
   a. Left 1/3 of transverse colon
   b. Descending colon
   c. Sigmoid colon
   d. Rectum
   e. Anal canal
   f. Urinary bladder
   g. Testes or ovaries
   h. Penis or clitoris
   i. Uterine tubes and uterus in females
   j. Prostate

Components of Parasympathetic System
1. **Sensory component:** Sensory fibres of parasympathetic system convey following sensations:
   a. Hunger
   b. Nausea
   c. Visceral reflexes like carotid sinus reflex, Hering Breuer's reflex, reflex act of micturition and visceral pain sensations from visceral organs
2. **Motor component:** It consists of preganglionic neurons which lie in various brain stem nuclei and S_2, S_3 and S_4 spinal cord segments (cranio-sacral outflow). Postganglionic neuronal cell bodies lie in the four parasympathetic ganglia mentioned above and the various terminal ganglia.

Functions of Parasympathetic System
Parasympathetic system is responsible for regulating the homeostasis in normal conditions. Hence, it predominates during normal, usual functioning of the human being. Sympathetic system on the other hand predominates in emergency conditions.

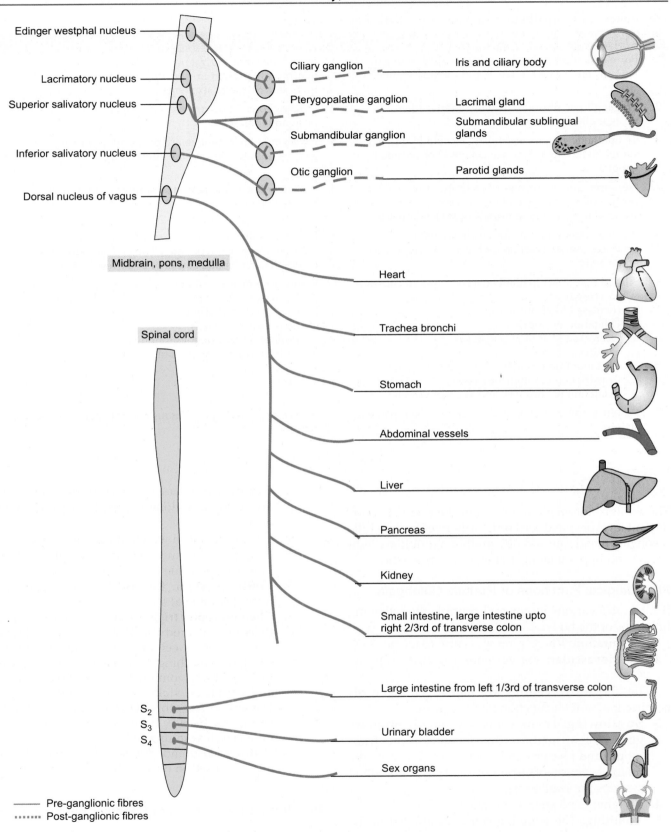

Fig. 10.24: Cranio-sacral out flow of parasympathetic system

Differences in sympathetic and parasympathetic nervous system

Sympathetic nervous system	Parasympathetic nervous system
1. Forms the thoraco-lumbar outflow. Preganglionic neurons are located in the T_1 to L_2 spinal segments.	1. Forms the cranio-sacral outflow. Preganglionic neurons are present in various brain stem nuclei and S_1, S_2 and S_3 sacral segments.
2. Preganglionic fibres are usually shorter than postganglionic fibres.	2. Preganglionic fibres are usually longer than postganglionic fibres.
3. Sympathetic ganglia are mostly located in the sympathetic trunk. Few are collateral or terminal ganglia.	3. Parasympathetic ganglia are primarily terminal ganglia, located close to the effector organs.
4. Noradrenaline is the neurotransmitter produced at postganglionic nerve endings (except in region of sweat gland and blood vessels of skeletal muscles).	4. Acetylcholine is the neurotransmitter produced at the postganglionic ends.
5. It is the system for reaction to an emergency. Produces a mass reaction mobilising all resources of the body.	5. It is an essential system to maintain the resting internal homeostasis of body. Thus it has a basal tone related to actions that conserve body resources.
6. Stimulation of sympathetic nervous system causes a. Increase heart rate b. Increase blood pressure c. Dilatation of pupils d. Decreased intestinal peristalsis e. Closure of sphincters — Inhibition of micturition and defecation f. Constriction of cutaneous vessels g. Dilatation of coronary and skeletal vessels	6. Stimulation of parasympathetic nervous system causes a. Decrease in heart rate b. Constriction of pupils c. Increased peristalsis d. Promotes glandular secretion e. Aids in evacuation of bladder and bowel
7. Posterior part of hypothalamus controls sympathetic activity.	7. Anterior part of hypothalamus controls parasympathetic activity.

CENTRAL REGULATION OF VISCERAL FUNCTION

The various automatic functions of the body at controlled at level of spinal cord (micturition reflex), medulla oblongata (heart rate and BP), midbrain (pupillary light reflex) and hypothalamus (temperature regulation).

Physiological Functions of Medulla Oblongata

It integrates various inputs and controls the following functions of the body:
1. **Respiration:** Via respiratory centre (page no. 386)
2. **Cardiovascular:** Via vasomotor centre (page no. 444)

The above two centres are named vital centres because loss of their function leads to death.

3. **Swallowing:** Is controlled by central program generator of medulla that receives input from mouth and pharynx and cerebrum to integrate the motor responses of respiratory and gastro-intestinal systems for swallowing.
4. Coughing and sneezing (page no. 387)
5. **Vomiting:** The vomiting centre is situated in the reticular formation of medulla and receives impulses from:

a. Irritant receptors in gastrointestinal tract, afferents pass along sympathetic and vagus nerves.
b. Vestibular nuclei which in turn are stimulated by impulses from vestibular apparatus of ear. This is responsible for motion sickness.
c. **Limbic system:** Responsible for vomiting during emotional stresses.
d. **Chemoreceptor trigger zone:** It is a zone in area prostima of medulla itself which contains chemoreceptor cells that respond to various substances reaching them. They are responsible for stimulating vomiting in diseases like uremia and radiation sickness, and emetic drugs. Dopamine receptors (D_2 type) and serotonin receptors (5-HT_3 type) are believed to be involved in vomiting reflex. Hence are of anti-D_2 drugs like domperidone and anti-5HT_3 drugs like ondansetron effectively controls vomiting.

Physiological Functions of Reticular Formation

It forms an important component of the somatic and visceral pathways of the body. It is essential for life. The neurons of reticular formation are grouped in medulla forming centres for respiration, cardiovascular function etc.

Important Functions of Sympathetic Nervous System

1. Vasoconstriction.
2. Increase heart rate, stroke volume and contractility of heart.
3. Relaxation of bronchial muscles and decrease secretion of bronchial glands.
4. Dilatation of pupil of eye.
5. Increase secretion of salivary glands.
6. Relaxation of intestinal muscles and constriction of sphincters with inhibition of secretion of intestinal glands.
7. Relaxation of detrusor muscle and constriction of urinary spincter.
8. Secretomotor to sweat glands.
9. Endocrine function—stimulates glycogenolysis in liver, inhibit insulin and glucagon secretion and increases breakdown of fat.

Important Functions of Parasympathetic Nervous System

1. Vasodilatation.
2. Decrease heart rate, stroke volume and contractility of heart.
3. Contraction of bronchial muscles and increase secretion of bronchial glands.
4. Constriction of pupil of eye.
5. Decrease secretion of salivary glands.
6. Contraction of intestinal muscles and relaxation of sphincters with stimulation of secretion of intestinal glands.
7. Contraction of detrusor muscle and relaxation of urinary spincter.
8. Endocrine function: stimulates glycogen synthesis in liver, stimulates insulin and glucagon secretion and decreases breakdown of fat.

CLINICAL AND APPLIED ASPECT

CUTANEOUS NERVE SUPPLY

- In a case of spinal cord injury, neurological evaluation is done by examining the presence or absence of various sensations like touch, pain and temperature in various dermatomes. This can help to identify the spinal cord segment at which it has been damaged.
- Knowledge of the dermatomal nerve supply helps to localise area of referred pain.

PAIN SENSATION

Referred pain: Deep pain usually from the viscera is perceived at a somatic point away from the viscera. This is called referred pain. This occurs because the dermatomal supply of the two parts is by the same spinal segment. Visceral pain is poorly localized and brain is conditioned over a period of time to receiving somatic impulses. Thus, a stimulus from a viscera is perceived as arising from the somatic part of the body supplied by the nerve of same dermatome (Fig. 53.3). Examples are:
- Cardiac pain: It is referred to inner aspect of left upper arm. Spinal segment T_2 is involved.
- Irritation of right side of diaphragmatic peritoneum by an underlying inflamed gall bladder leads to perception of shoulder tip pain. Spinal segment C_3 is involved.
- Pain due to appendicitis is felt at the umbilicus. Spinal segment T_{10} is involved.

Analgesia: Analgesia is inhibition of pain. Analgesia can be brought about by:
- **Counter irritants:** Stimulation of touch receptors (acupressure and acupuncture therapy) is seen to reduce pain. These act by stimulating neurons that give collaterals which result in presynaptic inhibition of transmission of pain impulses at level of dorsal root ganglion. Other examples are use of TENS (transcutaneous electric nerve stimulation) and cutaneous gels or sprays which also acts as irritants.
- **Central inhibition:** Acute stress is known to reduce pain.
- **Opioid analgesia:** Opioids receptors are present in the brain and spinal cord (dorsal root ganglion). The stimulation of these receptors in the brain, leads to activation of inhibitory pathway that descends from brain to spinal cord. In the dorsal root ganglion stimulation of opioid receptors may cause presynaptic inhibition of release of substance P. This leads to reduced sensation of pain. Exogenous opioids like morphine act in brain and spinal cord and cause analgesia. Endogenous opioids or endorphins are produced at site of injury and also may be responsible for reduced sensation of pain due to stress, acupuncture.

CHAPTER-10

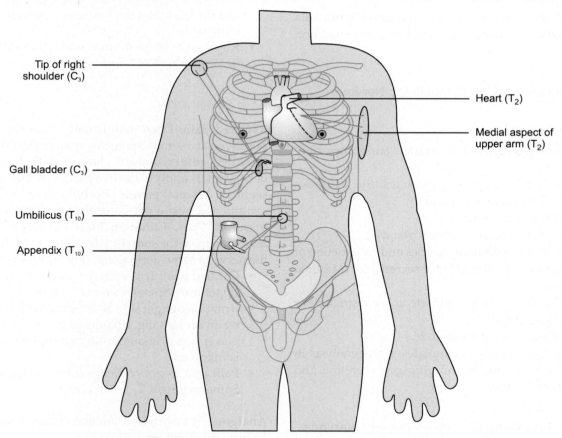

Fig. 10.25: Diagrammatic representation of common sites of referred pain

SOMATOMOTOR SYSTEM

Pyramidal tract: There are 1 million fibres in each pyramidal tract. Alpha and gamma motor neurons are activated simultaneously by stimulation of the corticospinal tract. Myelination of corticospinal tract starts at 3 years of age and completes by puberty. Lesion of corticospinal tract leads to an upper motor neuron type of paralysis. It is characterized by

    a. Spastic paralysis
    b. Hyperreflexia: Exaggerated tendon reflexes
    c. Hypertonia: Increased muscle tone
    d. Babinski extensor response is positive.

Generally it is associated with a lesion in the extrapyramidal tracts also. Rarely, there is an isolated lesion of corticospinal tract.

If the corticospinal tract is involved above the pyramidal decussation in medulla then contralateral side will be affected. Below pyramidal decussation, same side of the body will be affected as the side of lesion.

Initial manifestations in a patient with corticospinal tract lesion

- Flaccid paralysis
- Absence of deep tendon reflexes

Manifestation after few days and weeks

- Loss of voluntary movement or impairment of voluntary movement of the affected side there can be **Hemiplegia** – Paralysis of upper and lower limbs of the same side, **Monoplegia** – When one limb is affected, **Paraplegia** – When both lower limbs are affected
- Exaggerated deep tendon reflexes
- Hypertonia of the affected side
- Clasp knife rigidity
- Loss or diminution of superficial reflexes
- Positive Babinski sign
- Partial atrophy of muscles due to disease

Babinski's sign: When the lateral aspect of the sole of a patient is scratched, there occurs dorsiflexion of great toe and fanning out of other toes. Babinski sign is positive in the following conditions:

- Lesions of pyramindal tract
- Infants
- Poisoning

In normal individuals scratching of sole leads to dorsiflexion of all toes.

Lesions of pyramidal tract can be divided functionally into upper motor neuron lesions and lower motor neuron lesions. Damage to upper motor neuron fibers is associated with hypertonic or spastic paralysis of the involved muscles, hyperactive stretch reflexes and positive Babinski sign. Damage to lower motor neuron fibers is associated with flaccid or hypotonic paralysis of the affected muscle, loss of stretch reflexes and atrophy of the muscle. Babinski sign is negative.

AUTONOMIC NERVOUS SYSTEM

Horner's syndrome: It is a clinical condition occuring usually due to lesion of ascending cervical sympathetic chain.

Characteristic Features

- **Partial ptosis:** Due to involvement of Muller's muscle (smooth part of the levator palpebrae superioris).
- **Miosis (constriction of the pupil):** Due to involvement of dilator pupillae (unopposed action of constrictor pupillae).
- **Enophthalamos:** Due to involvement of orbitalis muscle (muscle of Muller) which helps to maintain the normal position of the eye ball.
- **Anhydrosis (loss of sweating):** Due to involvement of sympathetic innervation of sweat glands
- **Vasodilatation (redness and increased temperature):** Due to involvement of the sympathetic innervation of blood vessels in the head and face.

CHAPTER-10

Chapter 11

Special Senses

VISION

Sense of vision includes image formation, transmission of image to brain and recognition and interpretation of image. The various structures involved in this function are eyeball and its surrounding structures, visual pathway, reflex pathways associated with visual pathway and occipital cortex (visual area of cerebral hemisphere).

EYELIDS

Eyelids are the movable curtains present in front of the eyeball. They protect the eye from injury, foreign bodies and bright light and help to keep the cornea moist and clean. They are two in number on each side, one upper and one lower. The upper and lower eyelids are separated at their free margins by a palpebral fissure. The lateral 5/6th of the lid margin presents with an outer and an inner lip. The outer lip has two or more layers of eyelashes or cilia and associated openings of sweat glands and sebaceous glands. Medial end of the margin does not have any cilia. It presents with a lacrimal papilla which has the lacrimal punctum at its summit. This punctum leads to the lacrimal canaliculus medially, which drains the lacrimal fluid (tears). Margins of the upper and lower eyelids meet at an angle at their lateral and medial ends respectively.

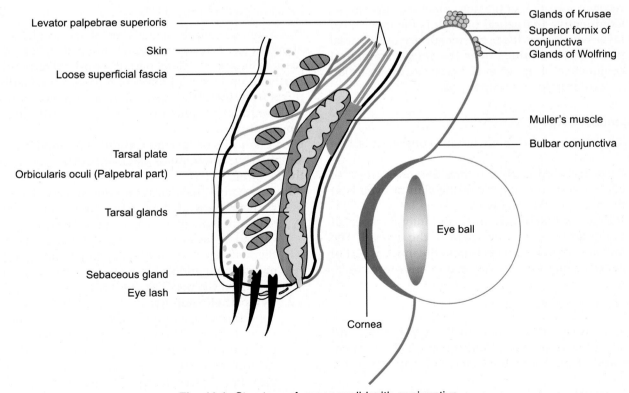

Fig. 11.1: Structure of upper eyelid with conjunctiva

Structure of the Eyelid (Fig. 11.1)

Each eyelid made up of five layers. From without inwards these are:

1. **Skin:** It is thin and continues with the conjunctiva at the margin of the eyelid. It consists of
   a. Large sebaceous glands (**Zies glands**) which open at the lid margin closely associated with cilia.
   b. Modified sweat glands (**Moll'glands**) which lie along the lid margin closely associated with Zies glands.
   c. Skin of upper eyelid receives the insertion of levator pelpebral superioris.
2. **Superficial fascia:** It is devoid of fat and contains the palpebral part of orbicularis oculi muscle.
3. **Palpebral fascia (orbital septum):** It is a sheet of fascia which connects the anterior surface of the tarsal plate with the bony orbital margin.
4. **Tarsal plate:** It is a sheet of dense fibrous tissue present adjacent to the palpebral margins. It provides stiffness to the lids. The tarsal glands (**meibomian glands**) are embedded in the posterior surface of the tarsal plate. These channels open in a row behind the cilia along the inner lip of margin of eyelid.

   The upper and lower tarsal plates fuse medially and laterally to form the medial and lateral palpebral ligaments respectively. Upper tarsal plate also receives insertion of levator palpebrae superioris.
5. **Conjunctiva (palpebral part):** It is the inner most layer which lines the posterior surface of the tarsal plate and continues over the sclera. Palpebral conjunctiva of upper eyelid receives the insertion of levator palpebrae superioris.

Conjunctiva (Fig. 11.1)

It is a transparent mucus membrane consisting of two parts:

1. **Palpebral conjunctiva:** It lines the inner aspect of eyelids and continues with the skin of eyelids at the margins. It is highly vascular.
2. **Bulbar conjunctiva:** It covers the anterior aspect of the outer most coat or sclera of the eyeball. The bulbar conjunctiva reflects onto the inner aspect of eyelids along the superior and inferior fornices.

LACRIMAL APPARATUS

The structures concerned with the production and drainage of lacrimal (tear) fluid constitute the lacrimal apparatus. Components of lacrimal apparatus are (Fig. 11.2)

1. Lacrimal gland and its ducts.

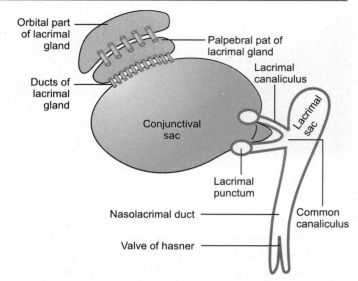

Fig. 11.2: Right Lacrimal apparatus

2. Accessory lacrimal glands.
3. Conjunctival sac.
4. Lacrimal puncta and canaliculi, common canaliculus.
5. Lacrimal sac.
6. Nasolacrimal duct.

Lacrimal Gland (Fig. 11.2)

It is a lobular, tubulo-acinar type of serous gland. It is about the size of an almond and is situated in the lacrimal fossa of the antero-lateral part of the orbital roof (orbital part) and upper eyelid (palpebral part). About a dozen ducts from the gland open into the superior fornix of the conjunctiva and pour lacrimal fluid into the conjunctival sac.

Nerve supply to lacrimal gland: Lacrimal gland is supplied by secretomotor parasympathetic and sympathetic fibres.

1. **Parasympathetic secretomotor supply:** Parasympathetic pre ganglionic fibres arise from superior salivatory nucleus in the pons. These fibres are carried by facial nerve. Pre-ganglionic parasympathetic fibres relay in the pterygopalatine ganglion and post ganglionic fibres are carried by zygomatic branch of the maxillary nerve.
2. **Sympathetic supply:** Post ganglionic fibres from superior cervical ganglion are carried along internal carotid artery. These fibres give rise to the deep petrosal nerve which joins greater petrosal nerve to form nerve to pterygoid canal. Sympathetic fibres pass through the pterygopalatine ganglion without relay and supply the gland.

Accessory Lacrimal Glands

These are glands of Krusae and Wolfring which are present in the superior fornix. They also secrete lacrimal fluid.

Conjunctival Sac

It is a potential space present between the palpebral conjunctiva and bulbar conjunctiva. The periodic blinking of eyelids helps in spreading the lacrimal fluid over the eye that keeps the cornea moist and prevents it from drying. Most of the fluid evaporates and the remaining fluid is drained by the lacrimal canaliculi.

Lacrimal Puncta and Canaliculi

Each lacrimal canaliculus begins from a lacrimal punctum present at the summit of the lacrimal papilla located at the medial end of the free margin of eyelid. Each is 10 mm long. The superior canaliculus of upper eyelid, first runs upwards and then downwards and medially while the lower canaliculus, in lower eyelid first runs downwards and then horizontally and medially. The two canaliculi join to form the common canaliculus. The common canaliculus drains into the Lacrimal sac. These canaliculi drain the lacrimal fluid from the conjunctival sac to the lacrimal sac.

Lacrimal Sac

It is a membranous sac, 12 mm long and 8 mm wide, located in the lacrimal groove on the medial wall of the orbit, behind the medial palpebral ligament. The lacrimal sac continues inferiorly with the nasolacrimal duct.

Nasolacrimal Duct

It is a membranous duct, 18 mm long which runs downwards, backwards and laterally from the lacrimal sac and opens in the inferior meatus of the nose. It is lodged in the nasolacrimal canal formed by the articulation of maxilla, lacrimal bone and inferior nasal concha. It drains the lacrimal fluid from lacrimal sac to the nose. Its opening in the nose is guarded by a fold of mucous membrane called lacrimal fold or valve of Hasner. This prevents retrograde entry of air and nasal secretions into the eye when one blows his nose.

BONY ORBIT (FIGs 11.3 and 11.4)

The orbits are a pair of bony cavities, situated one on either side of the root of the nose in the skull. Each orbit is a four sided pyramid with its apex directed behind, at the optic canal and base in front, represented by the orbital margin. The medial walls of the two orbital cavities are parallel to each other but the lateral walls are set at right angles to each other.

Boundaries of the Orbit

1. **Medial wall:** It is the thinnest. It is formed by four bones. They are, from before backwards.
    a. Frontal process of maxilla
    b. Lacrimal bone
    c. Orbital plate of ethmoid
    d. Body of sphenoid.
2. **Lateral wall:** It is the strongest and is formed by two bones.
    a. Zygomatic bone, in front
    b. Orbital surface of greater wing of sphenoid, behind.
3. **Floor:** It is formed by three bones.
    a. Orbital surface of the body of maxilla
    b. Zygomatic bone, anterolaterally

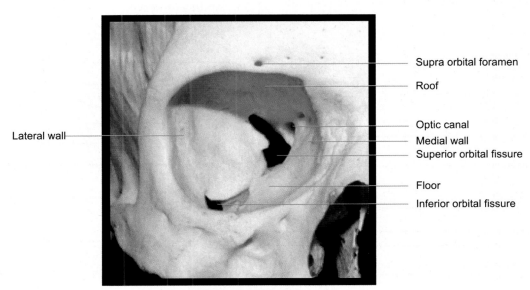

Lateral wall

Supra orbital foramen

Roof

Optic canal

Medial wall

Superior orbital fissure

Floor

Inferior orbital fissure

Fig. 11.3: Right bony orbit

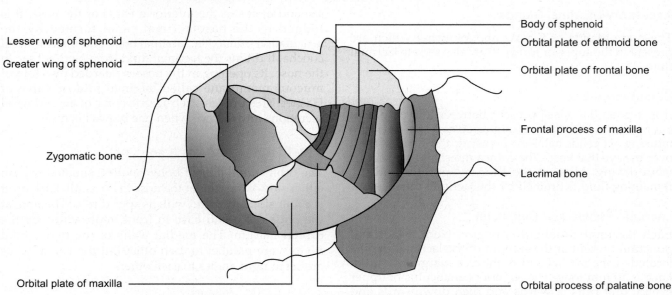

Fig. 11.4: Right bony orbit-diagrammatic representation

c. Orbital process of palatine bone, postero-medially.
4. **Roof:** It is formed by two bones.
   a. Orbital plate of frontal bone, in front
   b. Lesser wing of sphenoid, behind.

Apex of the orbit: Is formed by the centre of the bony bridge between optic canal and superior orbital fissure.
Base of the orbit: Is open and quadrangular in shape. Its boundaries form the orbital margins.

Superior Orbital Fissure (Fig. 11.5)

It is a retort shaped gap between the posterior part of lateral wall and roof of the bony orbit. It connects the orbit to middle cranial fossa. The fissure is divided into

three parts by a tendinous ring attached in a circular manner. The ring provides a common origin for the four extraocular muscles of the eyeball.

Structures Passing Through Superior Orbital Fissure

In superolateral compartment
1. Lacrimal nerve.
2. Trochlear nerve.
3. Frontal nerve.
4. Superior ophthalmic vein.
5. Recurrent meningeal branch of lacrimal artery.

In intermediate/central compartment
1. Upper and lower divisions of oculomotor nerve
2. Nasociliary nerve
3. Abducent nerve

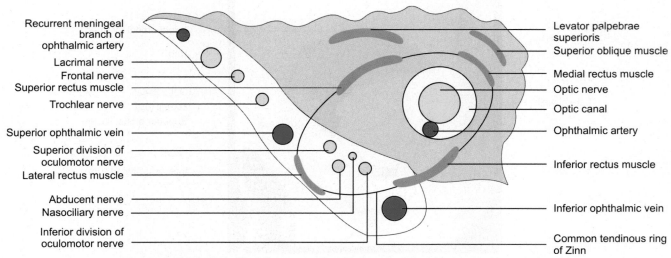

Fig. 11.5: Superior orbital fissure, optic canal and origin of extra ocular muscles

In inferomedial compartment

Inferior ophthalmic vein

Inferior Orbital Fissure

It is a gap present between the posterior part of lateral surface and floor of bony orbit. It connects orbit to the infratemporal and pterygo-palatine fossae.

Structures Passing Through Inferior Orbital Fissure

1. Infraorbital vessels.
2. Infraorbital nerve.
3. Zygomatic nerve.
4. Orbital branch of pterygopalatine ganglion.
5. Communicating vessels between inferior ophthalmic veins and pterygoid venous plexus.

Contents of the Orbit (Fig. 11.6)

1. Eyeball
2. Muscles of orbit
3. Fascia bulbi
4. Nerves
   a. Optic nerve
   b. 3rd, 4th and 6th cranial nerves
   c. Ophthalmic nerve
5. Ophthalmic artery
6. Superior and inferior ophthalmic veins
7. Lacrimal gland
8. Orbital fat

MUSCLES OF THE ORBIT

There are seven voluntary and three involuntary muscles in the orbit.

Extraocular Muscles of the Eyeball (Figs 11.5, 11.6)

Six muscles move the eyeball and one muscle moves the upper eyelid. These consist of
1. **Four recti muscles**
   a. Superior rectus.
   b. Inferior rectus.
   c. Medial rectus.
   d. Lateral rectus.
2. **Two oblique muscles**
   a. Superior oblique.
   b. Inferior oblique.
3. **Levator palpebrae superioris muscle**

Nerve supply of extra-ocular muscles

1. **Medial rectus:** Oculomotor nerve, inferior division.
2. **Lateral rectus:** Abducent nerve.
3. **Superior rectus:** Oculomotor nerve, superior division.
4. **Inferior rectus:** Oculomotor nerve, inferior division.
5. **Superior oblique:** Trochlear nerve.
6. **Inferior oblique:** Oculomotor, inferior division.

Movements of the Eyeball

Movements of eyeball are considered in relation to three axes. These are vertical, transverse and anteroposterior.

Associated movements of the two eyeballs

1. **Conjugate movements:** When both the eyes move in same direction with their visual axes being parallel to each other.
2. **Disconjugate movements:** When the axes of both eyes converge or diverge in one movement.

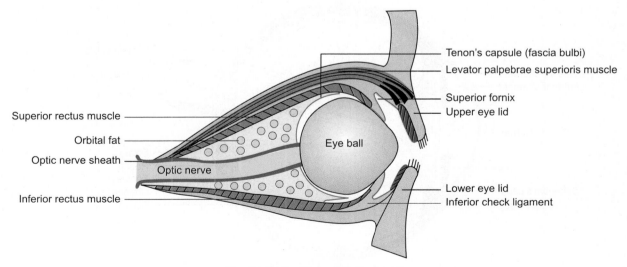

Fig. 11.6: Sagittal section of orbit

Movement of eyeball	Muscle responsible	Axis of movement
1. **Elevation**	1. Superior rectus 2. Inferior oblique	Transverse axis through equator
2. **Depression**	1. Inferior rectus 2. Superior oblique	Transverse axis through equator
3. **Adduction**	1. Medial rectus 2. Inferior rectus 3. Superior rectus	Vertical axis through equator
4. **Abduction**	1. Lateral rectus 2. Inferior oblique 3. Superior oblique	Vertical axis through equator
5. **Rotatory movements**		Anteroposterior axis from anterior to posterior pole of eyeball
a. Intorsion	1. Superior rectus 2. Superior oblique	Medial rotation of the 12'o clock position of cornea
b. Extorsion	1. Inferior rectus 2. Inferior oblique	Lateral rotation of the 12'o clock position of cornea

Levator Palpebrae Superioris Muscle

Origin: It arises from the undersurface of the lesser wing of sphenoid above the optic canal by a narrow tendon.

Insertion: It inserts in the form of three lamellae into the skin of upper eyelid, upper margin of the superior tarsus, superior fornix of the conjunctiva.

Nerve supply: Upper ramus of oculomotor nerve.

Actions: Elevation of upper eyelid.

Involuntary Extra Ocular Muscles

These are minor muscles related to the eyelid.
  1. Superior tarsal muscle
  2. Inferior tarsal muscle
  3. Orbitalis muscles (Muller's muscle)

Nerve supply: They receive postganglionic sympathetic fibres from superior cervical ganglion.

EYE BALL (BULBUS OCULI)

Eyeball is the organ of sight. It functions like a camera and has a lens system for focussing images (Fig. 11.7).

Location: The eyeball occupies anterior half of the orbital cavity. Optic nerve emerges from it, a little medial to its posterior pole.

Shape and Size: It is almost spherical in shape and has a diameter of about 24 mm.

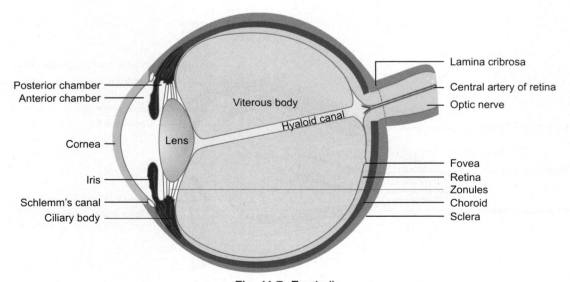

Fig. 11.7: Eye ball

Fascial Sheath of Eyeball or Fascia Bulbi (Fig. 11.6)

The fascia bulbi **(Tenon's capsule)** is a membranous envelope of the eyeball. It extends from the optic nerve behind to the sclero-corneal junction in front. It is separated from the sclera by the episcleral space and forms a socket for the eyeball to facilitate free ocular movements. The fascia bulbi is pierced by
1. Tendons of 4 recti and 2 oblique muscles of the eyeball.
2. Ciliary nerves and vessels around the entrance of optic nerve.

Tunics of the Eyeball

The eyeball consists of three concentric coats:
1. An outer fibrous coat consisting of sclera and cornea.
2. A middle vascular coat consisting of choroid and ciliary body.
3. An inner nervous coat consisting of the retina and iris.

Sclera

Sclera forms the posterior five-sixths of the outer coat. It is opaque and consists of dens fibrous tissue A small portion of it is visible as the 'white of the eye' in the palpebral fissure It is continuous anteriorly with the cornea.
Functions:
1. Helps to maintain the shape of the eyeball.
2. Protects internal structures.
3. Provides attachment to muscles that move the eyeball.

Cornea

The cornea forms the anterior one-sixths of the outer coat. It is transparent and more convex than the sclera. It is avascular and is nourished primarily by permeation from the periphery. It not only permits the light to enter the eye but also refracts the entering light. It is highly sensitive to touch and is supplied by the ophthalmic division of trigeminal nerve.

Middle Coat of the Eyeball

The middle coat is often called as the vascular coat because it contains most of the blood vessels of the eyeball. This coat also contains a large number of melanin containing cells. It is divided into three parts, from behind forwards these are, choroid, cillary body and iris. These three parts together form the **uvea** or **uveal tract.**

Choroid

Choroid is the larger posterior part of the vascular coat of eyeball. It is a brown, thin and highly vascular membrane lining the inner surface of the sclera. Anteriorly, it is connected to iris by the ciliary body and posteriorly, it is pierced by the optic nerve.
Functions: The inner surface of choroid is firmly attached to the retina and nourishes the rods and cones of the retina by diffusion.

Ciliary Body (Fig. 11.8)

Ciliary body is present in the form of a circular thickening in the vascular tunic. It extends from the choroid posteriorly at the level of ora-serrata of retina to the iris anteriorly, at the level of corneo-scleral junction. The iris is attached along its lateral margin. The ciliary body suspends the lens via suspensory ligaments or zonules. Its outer surface lines the inner aspect of the sclera

Structure of ciliary body: It is made up of:
1. Stroma of collagen fibres with vessels and nerves.
2. Ciliary muscles: These consist of smooth muscle fibres which are arranged in an outer radial and an inner circular fashion.
   Action: The ciliary muscle acts as a sphincter. When the radial and circular fibres contract, the choroid is pulled towards the lens reducing the tension on the suspensory ligaments. This allows the lens to assume a more spherical form because of its own elastic nature and results in an increase in the refraction.This process is called accommodation. This allows a person to adjust for near vision.
3. Bilaminar ciliary epithelium linning the inner surface of the ciliary body.

Functions of Ciliary Body
1. It helps in the suspensation of lens.
2. It is responsible for accomodation of eye.

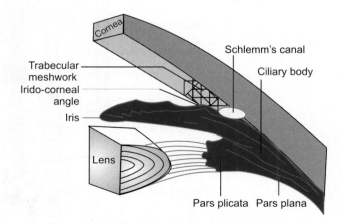

Fig. 11.8: Irido-corneal angle (sagittal section)

3. The vessels in ciliary body secrete the aqueous humor of the eye.

Iris

Iris is a pigmented contractile diaphragm present between the cornea and the lens. It is attached along periphery to the choroid by the ciliary body. In the centre it presents with an opening called the pupil which regulates the entry of light into the eye.

Structure of iris: The iris consists of four layers. From anteroposterior these are
1. Anterior mesothelial lining
2. Connective tissue stroma containing pigment cells and blood vessels.
3. Layer of smooth muscle which consists of two parts, namely:
   a. **Constrictor pupillae:** It is an annular band of muscle fibres encircling the pupil. It constricts the pupil in response to parasympathetic stimulation.
   b. **Dilator pupillae:** It constsits of radially arranged fibres from circumferance of the pupil. It dilates the pupil in response to sympathetic stimulation.
4. Posterior layer of pigmented cells which is continuous with the ciliary part of retina.

Retina—The Inner Nervous Coat of Eyeball

Retina is the innermost coat of the eyeball. Retina lies between the choroid externally and the hyaloid membrane of the vitreous internally. Its thickness decreases gradually from behind forwards.It is insensitive to light and is made up of pigmented cuboidal epithelium

Structure of retina: It is primarily made up of two layers namely, outer retinal pigment epithelium and inner neuro sensory layer. The inner sensory layer of retina is sensitive to light and is made up photoreceptor cells called rods and cones as well as numerous relay neurons viz. bipolar neurons and ganglion cells. This layer ends at a crenated margin anteriorly, called the ora serrata. Retina is divided into ten layers for the purpose of description. These layers are (Fig. 11.9):

1. **Retinal pigment epithelium:** It is insensitive to light and is made up of pigmented cuboidal epithelium. This is the outer most layer lying next to choroid. It prevents scattering of light and provide nutrition to rods and cones.
2. **Layer of rods and cones:** They are photoreceptors.
3. **Outer limiting membrane:** It is made up of processes of Muller's cells which are connective tissue cells of retina.
4. **Outer nuclear layer:** It is form by the nuclei of rods and cones.

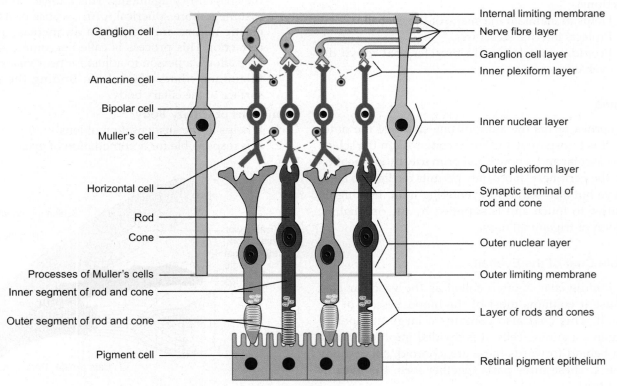

Fig. 11.9: Layers of retina

Labels (left): Ganglion cell, Amacrine cell, Bipolar cell, Muller's cell, Horizontal cell, Rod, Cone, Processes of Muller's cells, Inner segment of rod and cone, Outer segment of rod and cone, Pigment cell

Labels (right): Internal limiting membrane, Nerve fibre layer, Ganglion cell layer, Inner plexiform layer, Inner nuclear layer, Outer plexiform layer, Synaptic terminal of rod and cone, Outer nuclear layer, Outer limiting membrane, Layer of rods and cones, Retinal pigment epithelium

5. **Outer plexiform layer:** It is formed by the connections of rods and cones with bipolar cells and horizontal cells.
6. **Inner nuclear layer:** It is form by nuclei of bipolar cells.
7. **Inner plexiform layer:** It is form by connections of bipolar cells with the ganglion cell and amacrine cells.
8. **Ganglion cell layer:** It is form by ganglion cells.
9. **Nerve fibre layer:** It is form by axons of ganglion cells which form optic nerve.
10. **Internal limiting membrane:** It is form by process of Muller's cells.

Blood Supply of the Retina

1. The deeper part of the retina, i.e., up to the bipolar neurons is supplied by the central artery of the retina, a branch of ophthalmic artery.
2. The superficial part of the retina upto the rods and cones is nourished by diffusion from the capillaries of the choroid.

Venous Drainage of Retina

It is by the central vein of retina which drains into the cavernous sinus.

Compartments of Eye Ball

The interior of the eyeball is divided by the lens into two compartments namely, anterior and posterior compartment.

Anterior Compartment

It is further divided into two chambers by the iris.
1. **The anterior chamber:** It lies between the iris and cornea.
2. **The posterior chamber:** It lies between iris and lens.
   The two chambers are filled with aqueous humor which helps in maintaining the intraocular pressure.

Aqueous Humor

It is an aqueous fluid secreted by the non-pigmented epithelium of ciliary body. It helps to maintain the intraocular pressure. The aqueous humor is rich in ascorbic acid, glucose and aminoacids. It nourishes the cornea and the lens which are otherwise avascular.

Circulation of aqueous humor: The aqueous humor is secreted in the posterior chamber by the vessels in the ciliary processes. From here it passes into the anterior chamber through the pupil. Then it passes through the spaces in the irido-corneal angle, located between the fibres of ligamentum pectinatum, to enter the canal of Schlemm, a venous ring. Finally, it drains into the anterior ciliary veins.

Posterior Compartment

- It lies behind the lens and is much larger than the anterior compartment.
- It constitutes posterior 4/5th of the inner part of eyeball.
- It is surrounded almost completely by the retina and is filled with a colourless, transparent jelly like substance called vitreous humour/vitreous body. The vitreous humour is enclosed in a delicate hyaloid membrane.
- The vitreous humor also helps in maintaining the intraocular pressure and the shape of the eyeball. Further it holds the lens and the retina in place.

LENS

The lens is an unusual biological structure. It is also known as the crystalline lens. It is transparent and biconvex shaped body which is placed between the anterior and posterior compartments of the eyeball and is suspended from the ciliary body by zonular fibres.

External features: It presents with an anterior surface and a posterior surface. It has anterior and posterior poles. These are the centre points of the respective surfaces. The line connecting anterior and posterior poles forms the axis of the lens. The equator of lens constitutes the circumference of the lens.

Structure of Lens (Fig 11.10): It is an avascular structure and does not have any nerve fibres. Lens consists of the following parts:
1. Lens capsule: It encloses the entire lens and receives the zonular fibres. It is thickest anteriorly.
2. Anterior epithelium of cuboidal epithelium.
3. Lens fibres: These form the bulk of the lens. Center of lens contains oldest fibres and is hard. This is

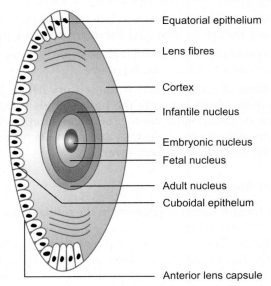

Fig. 11.10: Structure of lens

called nucleous. Peripheral part is made up of recently formed fibres.

Suspensory Ligaments of the Lens (Zonules of Zinn)

The lens is suspended between the anterior and posterior compartments of the eye by the suspensory ligaments.These ligaments extend from the ciliary body to the lens capsule and are present mostly in front of the equator.

PHYSIOLOGY OF EYE

Functions of the Eye

As mentioned before the eye functions much like a camera. The iris allows light to enter the eye through its aperture called pupil. The light rays are focussed by the lens (also by cornea and humours) on the photosensitive retina. The light striking the retina is converted into action potentials that are relayed through optic pathways to the visual cortex of the brain where an image is perceived.

Mechanism of Optics of the Eye

The light rays entering the eye are focussed on the retina to form an image. The focussing power or refractive power of human eye is 60 diopters.

Function of cornea: It provides the clear path for entry of light rays and acts as a refractive surface.

Function of lens: It acts as a biconvex lens which focusses the light rays on retina. The curvature of lens changes to see near objects (accomodation).

Function of aqueous humor: It maintains the intraocular pressure of eye and acts as a refractive surface.

Function of iris: It acts to regulate the amount of light entering the eye by changing the aperture of the pupil.

Function of vitreous humor: It gives shape to the eyeball and acts as a refractive media of eye.

Functions of retina: Retina is the sensory neural layer of eyeball which converts the light signals to action potentials in the optic nerve. The pigment epithelium of retina absorbs the light rays and prevents reflection into the inner neurosensory layer.

Visual Receptors

Receptors for vision are present in the retina of the eye. They are of two types:
1. **Rods:** They contain photosensitive pigment, rhodopsin and are extremely sensitive to light. They are responsible for vision in dim light, i.e., scotopic vision or night vision.

2. **Cones:** They contain photosensitive pigment, iodopsin and are sensitive to bright light and colors. They are responsible for vision in day light, i.e., photopic vision.

Each receptor is made up of an outer segment consisting of saccules and disks containing the photosensitive pigment and an inner segment containing the cell body with nucleus and the synaptic terminal.

Neuronal Cells of Retina

There are four types of neuronal cells in retina namely:
1. Bipolar cells
2. Ganglion cells
3. Horizontal cells
4. Amacrine cells

The synaptic zone of rods and cones synapses with dendrites of bipolar cells which further synapse with ganglion cells. **The axons of ganglion cells form the optic nerve.** Horizontal cells inter-connect the receptors while amacrine cells inter-connect ganglion cells. There is significant convergence at the synaptic level. This means one bipolar cells makes synapses with a number of receptor cells and one ganglion cell makes synapses with a number of bipolar cells.

Mechanism of Generation of Visual Impulses

- The light waves are transmitted, refracted and converged on the retina by the optical system of eye consisting of cornea, aqueous humor, pupil, lens, and vitrous humor anteroposteriorly.
- The total refractive power of eye is 60 diopters.
- The eye responds to light of wavelengths between 397 to 723 nm. Ultra violet light rays <397 are absorbed by choroid while infrared rays >723 nm are absorbed by cornea.
- The stimulation by light causes changes in the photosensitive molecules present in rods and cones which results in changes in Na^+ efflux and setting up of action potentials that are transmitted via optic nerve to the brain.

Photosensitive Compounds of Rods and Cones

- Photosensitive pigments are made up of compexes of opsin and $retinene_1$. Opsin is a protein molecule while $retinene_1$ is a derivative of vitamin A.
- Exposure to light changes the configuration of retinine from cis-configuration to trans configuration.
- Normally Na^+ channels of the rods and cones are open and current flows from the inner to outer segments of these cells. A change in configuration

of retinene₁ results in change of configuration of opsin. This initiates cellular changes that lead to closure of Na⁺ channels. There is hyperpolarisation of receptor cells which results in initiation of impulses in neuronal cells.

- Transformed retinene₁ seperates from opsin. This is called bleaching. It is reduced to vitamin A which again combines with opsin to form rhodopsin.

Visual Pathway (Optic Pathway)

The retina is the photoreceptive layer of the eye and impulses generated in rods and cones of retina are finally transmitted along the axons of ganglion cells of retina which converge to the optic disc and exit the eyeball as optic nerve (Fig. 11.11).

- The impulses course through optic nerve, optic chiasma and optic tract to relay in lateral geniculate body of corresponding side.
- The fibres originating from nasal halves of the retina cross to opposite side at the chiasma. Hence each optic tract consists of fibres from temporal region of retina of ipsilateral side and nasal region of retina of contra-lateral side.
- The fibres from nuclei of lateral geniculate body extend to the visual cortex (area no. 17, 18 and 19) in the medial aspect of occipital lobe via the optic radiation.

Dark Adaptation

When a person enters a dark room, with dim lighting from a bright area, it takes some time for the eyes to see clearly that is it takes time for the eyes to get adjusted to lower threshold of light. This is called dark adaptation. There are two components to this adaptation namely:

1. **Rapid response:** It is of small magnitude due to adaptation of cones. It takes 5 minutes.
2. **Slow response:** It is due to adaptation of rods and take upto 20 minutes for complete response.

It is associated with dilatation of pupil.

Light Adaptation

As a person moves from a dark room to bright light, the light is uncomfortable but in 5 minutes the eyes adapt to increase the threshold. Also pupil contracts (light reflex) to restrict light entry.

Visual Acuity

- It is defined as the minimum distance between two lines that allow them to be perceived as two and not single.
- It is different from visual threshold which is minimum amount of light that gives a sensation of light.

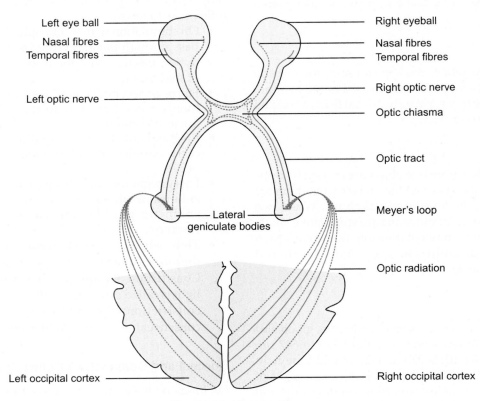

Fig. 11.11: Visual pathway

Left eye ball
Nasal fibres
Temporal fibres
Left optic nerve
Lateral geniculate bodies
Left occipital cortex

Right eyeball
Nasal fibres
Temporal fibres
Right optic nerve
Optic chiasma
Optic tract
Meyer's loop
Optic radiation
Right occipital cortex

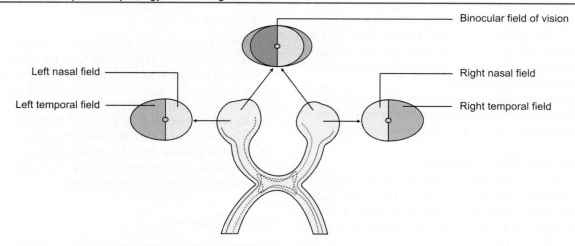

Fig. 11.12: Diagrammatic representation of visual fields and binocular vision

- Hence, it is the degree to which one can see clearly the details and contours of an object.
- Visual acuity is tested with the help of **Snellen charts.** The patient is seated comfortably and the chart is kept at a distance of 6 meters (relaxed vision) with adequate illumination.
- Visual acuity is altered in various eye conditions that interfere with light transmission. Examples corneal opacity, lens opacity (cataract), refractive errors, diseases of retina especially macular edema etc.

Visual Fields

It is the extent to which the eye can seen the outside world. The field of vision of each eye is limited by more medially and eyebrow superiorly. Visual fields are tested by the perimeter (Fig. 11.12).

Binocular Vision

The visual impulses from one object are carried by optic pathway of both the eyes and the images from them are fused into one at the level of visual cortex. When two corresponding points of the retina are stimulated, single image is seen. This is binocular vision. Binocular vision provides us with ability to appreciate depth and proportion of an object.

Colour Vision

There are three primary colours namely, red, green and blue. The red light has a wavelength of 723 to 647 nm green light wavelength is 575 to 492 nm and blue light wavelength is 492 to 450 nm. Mixing of wavelengths of these colours in variable proportion produces the full spectrum of colours. Colour vision is the function of cones of retina. There are three types of cones namely, red sensitive, green sensitive and blue sensitive and the sensations are integrated by the ganglion cells of retina, lateral geniculate bodies and visual cortex (area no. 19).

Pupillary Light Reflex Pathway

Pupillary light reflex is defined as contraction of the pupil of the eye when it is exposed to bright illumination (Fig. 11.13). The path of nerve impulses causing this reflex is as follows:

- On stimulation with bright light the nerve impulses pass through ganglion cells of retina, optic nerve, optic chiasma and optic tract to pretectal nucleus of mid brain.
- Fibres of secondary neurons from pretectal nuclei then convey impulses to the Edinger-Westphal nuclei bilaterally.
- Preganglionic fibres from Edinger-Wesphal nuclei carry impulses to ciliary ganglia via oculomotor nerve.
- Past ganglionic fibres from ciliary ganglion on each side travel along short ciliary nerves to supply sphincter pupillae muscle which contracts in response.
- Thus, when one eye is exposed to a beam of light, the pupil of both eyes contract together and equally. Constriction of pupil which is exposed to beam of light is called direct light reflex while simultaneous constriction of pupil of opposite eye is called consensual or indirect light reflex.

Corneal and Conjunctival Reflex Pathway

On touching the cornea or conjunctiva there is blinking of eyes. This is a protective reflex.

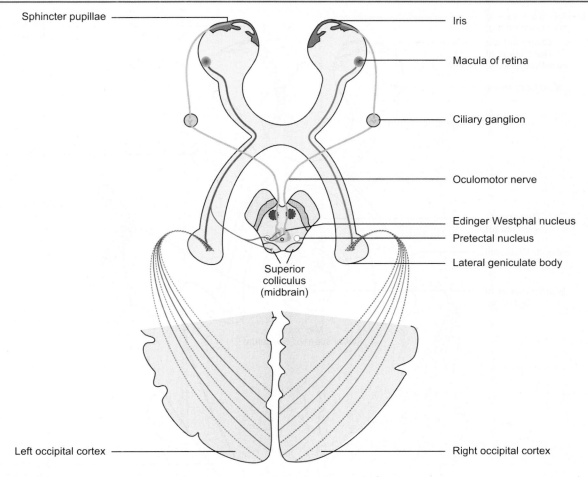

Fig. 11.13: Patyhway of light reflex

- Afferent impluses are transmitted by ophthalmic division of trigeminal nerve to ventral posterior medial nucleus of thalamus and relay in post central gyrus of cortex.
- Efferent impluses travel down from motor cortex to facial nerve nucleus, along facial nerve and via its branches to the orbicularis occuli muscles causing its contraction and blinking of eye lids.

Near Vision Reflex Pathway (Fig. 11.14)

In order to view near objects the eyes respond by:
1. Convergence of eyes.
2. Contraction of ciliary muscles leading to change in shape of anterior surface of lens, **accommodation reflex**.
3. Constriction of pupils to increase depth of focus.
   - Afferent path is along optic nerves, optic chiasma, optic tracts, lateral geniculate bodies,

optic radiation to the visual areas in cerebral cortex. Then impulses are transmitted to pretectal region and Edinger-Westphal and motor nuclei of oculomotor nerve via superior longitudinal fasciculus, frontal eye field and internal capsule.
- Efferent path consisting parasympathetic fibres arises from Edinger-Westphal nucleus and travel along oculomotor nerve to relay in ciliary ganglion. Post ganglionic fibres supply ciliary muscle and sphincter pupillae via short ciliary nerves.
- Efferent fibres from oculomotor nerve supply medial rectus muscle of eyeball.

Eye Movements

Movements of eye ball are well coordinated in order to maintain binocular vision. The extraocular muscles and the various eye movements are described above.

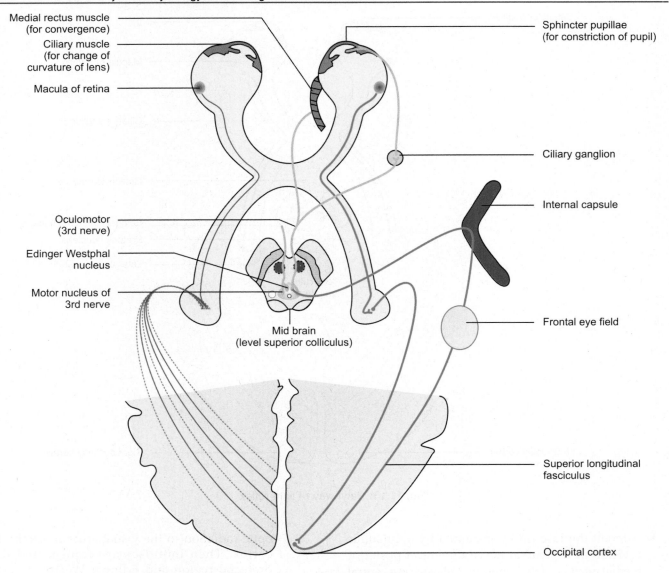

Fig. 11.14: Near vision reflex pathway

HEARING AND EQUILIBRIUM

Ear is the organ of hearing. It is also concerned with maintaining the balance of the body. It consists of three parts:
1. External ear
2. Middle ear
3. Internal ear

EXTERNAL EAR (FIG. 11.15)

It consists of two parts namely
1. Pinna
2. External auditory meatus

Pinna or Auricle

- It is a shell like projection present one on each side of the head.

- It consists of a single crumpled plate of elastic fibro-cartilage closely lined by the skin.
- The lowest part is however, soft and consists of fibrofatty tissue only. This is called lobule.
- The skin of pinna is adherant to the underlying cartilage. Sebaceous glands are present in the region of concha. Coarse hairs may be present in some elderly males along the tragus, antitragus and intertragic notch. **(It is a Y-linked genetic expression.)**

Anatomical Features

Lateral surface: It presents with a number of elevations and depressions.
1. **Concha:** A large central depression that leads into the external auditory meatus.

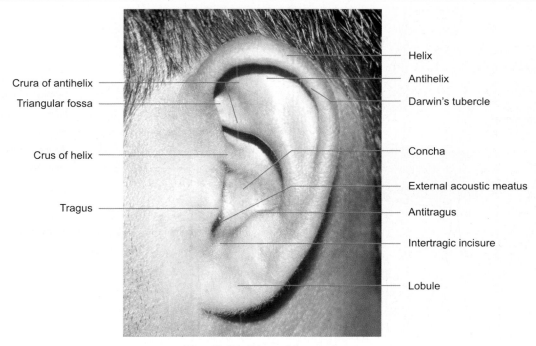

Crura of antihelix

Triangular fossa

Crus of helix

Tragus

Helix

Antihelix

Darwin's tubercle

Concha

External acoustic meatus

Antitragus

Intertragic incisure

Lobule

Fig. 11.15: Parts of external ear

2. **Helix:** The outer prominent rim of pinna.
3. **Antihelix:** The prominent margin lying in front of and parallel to the helix. It encircles the concha in a C-shaped manner except in the anterior part.
4. **Scaphoid fossa:** Area between helix and antihelix.
5. **Cymba concha:** Small part of concha present above the crus of helix. It corresponds internally to the suprameatal triangle on skull.
6. **Tragus:** A triangular flap of cartilage present in front of depression of concha. It guards the entry into the external auditory meatus.
7. **Antitragus:** An elevation on the lower end of antihelix lying just opposite the tragus.
8. **Lobule of pinna:** Skin covered flap of fibro fatty tissue that hangs below the anti-tragus.

Medial surface (Cranial surface): It presents with elevations corresponding to the depressions of the lateral surface.
1. **Eminentia conchae:** Lies opposite the concha.
2. **Eminentia triangularis:** Lies opposite the triangular fossa.

Muscles of Pinna

The muscles are auricularis anterior, auricularis posterior, auricularis superior, helicis major and minor, tragicus and antitragicus etc. They serve minimal or no significant function in human beings. They are supplied by facial nerve.

Blood Supply of Pinna

1. Posterior auricular branch of external carotid artery.
2. Anterior auricular branches of superficial temporal artery.
3. Branches of occipital artery.

The veins follow arteries and drain into external jugular and superficial temporal veins

Lymphatic Drainage of Pinna

1. Parotid lymph nodes: In front of tragus
2. Mastoid lymph nodes: Behind the auricle
3. Upper group of deep cervical lymph nodes

Nerve Supply of Pinna

1. Great auricular nerve
2. Lesser occipital nerve
3. Auriculo-temporal nerve
4. Auricular branch of vagus nerve

External Auditory/Acoustic Meatus

It is a 24 mm long canal which extends from the bottom of the concha to the tympanic membrane (Fig. 11.16). It consists of two parts:
1. **Cartilaginous part:** It forms the lateral or outer 1/3rd of the meatus.
2. **Bony part:** Medial or inner 2/3rd of the meatus is bony. It is formed by

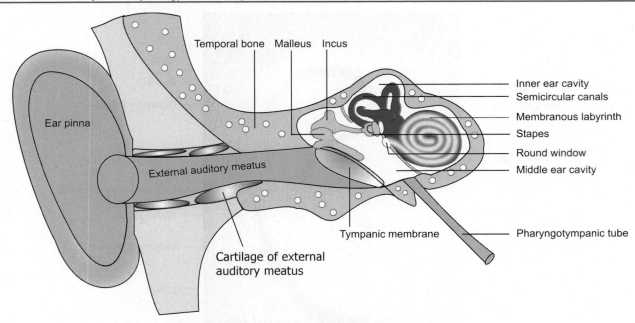

Fig. 11.16: Different parts of the ear (coronal section)

a. **Tympanic plate of temporal bone:** Anteriorly and inferiorly
b. **Squamous part of temporal bone:** Superiorly and posteriorly

At the medial end of the bony canal a tympanic sulcus is present that lodges the tympanic membrane. which is obliquely placed.

Direction of meatus: The external auditory meatus has a peculiar S-shaped course. From lateral to medial side it curves as follows :
a. Medially, upwards and forwards.
b. Medially, upwards and backwards.
c. Medially, forward and downwards.

The meatus is lined by skin which is adherant to the perichondrium and periosteum of the meatus. The cartilaginous part has ceruminous glands which are modified sweat glands. These produce ear wax or cerumen. The wax prevents maceration of the lining epithelium by water and also aids in opposing entry of insects into the ear.

Blood Supply of External Auditory Meatus

1. Posterior auricular branch of external carotid.
2. Deep auricular branch of maxillary artery.
3. Anterior auricular branches of superficial temporal artery.

The veins run along with arteries and drain into external jugular and maxillary veins.

Nerve Supply of External Auditory Meatus

1. **Auriculo-temporal nerve:** It supplies the roof and anterior wall of meatus.

2. **Auricular branch of vagus nerve** (The only cutaneous branch of vagus nerve): It supplies the floor and posterior wall of meatus.

TYMPANIC MEMBRANE (EAR DRUM)

It is a thin translucent membrane attached to the sulcus in the tympanic plate of temporal bone and it separates the external auditory meatus from the middle ear. It is oval in outline, a little less than ½ inch (12 mm) in its greatest (vertical) diameter (Fig. 11.17).

Anatomical Features

- The tympanic membrane is directed laterally, forward and downwards. It makes an angle of 55° with the floor of the external auditory meatus.
- Two folds, the anterior and posterior malleolar folds extend downwards from the two ends of the upper circumferance and converge at the level of lateral process of malleus.
- The tympanic membrane is divided into two parts namely **Pars tensa,** the greater part of membrane

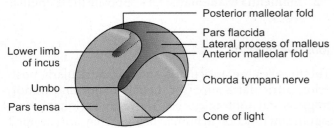

Fig. 11.17: Right tympanic membrane

which is taut and **Pars flacida,** It is the part of membrane which is thin and lax present in a small triangular area above the lateral process of malleus between the two malleolar folds.

- The ear drum has two surfaces
  — **Lateral surface:** Is concave and directed downwards, forwards and laterally.
  — **Medial surface:** It is convex and is attached to the handle of malleus. The point of attachment is maximally convex and is called the umbo.

Structure of Tympanic Membrane

The tympanic membrane is composed of following three layers
  a. **Outer cutaneous layer:** Which is continuous with the skin of the external auditory meatus.
  b. **Middle fibrous layer:** In the pars flacida there is loose connective tissue instead of fibrous tissue.
  c. **Inner mucous layer:** Which is continuous with mucous lining of the middle ear.

Blood Supply of Tympanic Membrane

1. Deep auricular branch of maxillary artery.
2. Stylomastoid branch of posterior auricular artery.
3. Anterior tympanic branch of maxillary artery.

The veins runs along with arteries. From the lateral surface they drain into the external jugular vein while from the medial surface they drain into the pterygoid venous plexus.

Nerve Supply of Tympanic Membrane

1. Auriculotemporal nerve
2. Auricular branch of vagus nerve
3. Glossopharyngeal nerve

MIDDLE EAR (SYN. TYMPANIC CAVITY)

The middle ear is a narrow, slit-like, air filled space in the petrous part of the temporal bone between the external ear and the inner ear (Fig. 11.18).

Shape and size: It is like a cube compressed from side to side. In coronal section the cavity of middle ear appears biconcave. The medial and lateral walls are close to each other in the centre.

Measurements

Vertical diameter : 15 mm
Anteroposterior : 15 mm
Transverse diameter : At roof it is 6 mm, in the center it is 2mm and at floor it is 4 mm.

Communications

1. Anteriorly, with nasopharynx, through pharyngo-tympanic tube,
2. Posteriorly, with mastoid (tympanic) antrum and mastoid air cells through aditus to antrum.

Contents of the Middle Ear

1. Three small bones (ear ossicles): malleus, incus and stapes.
2. Two muscles: tensor tympani and stapedius.
3. Two nerves: chorda tympani and tympanic plexus.
4. Vessels supplying and draining the middle ear.

   The mucous membrane lining the middle ear forms folds which project into the cavity, giving it a honey-combed appearance.

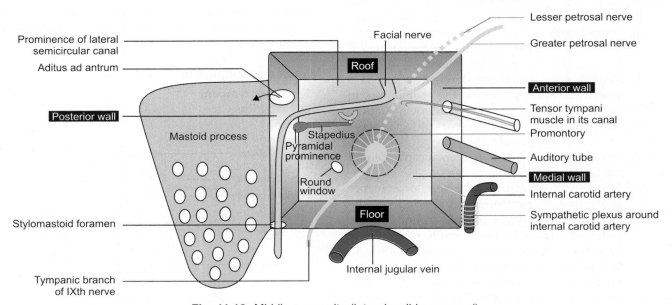

Fig. 11.18: Middle ear cavity (lateral wall is removed)

Boundaries of Middle Ear (Fig. 11.18)

1. **Roof:** It is wider than the floor and is formed by a thin sheet of bone called tegmen tympani. It separates the tympanic cavity from the middle cranial fossa and the temporal lobe of brain.

2. **Floor:** It is formed by a thin bony plate of petrous temporal which lodges the superior bulb of internal jugular vein inferiorly.

3. **Anterior wall:** It presents with the following features from above downwards:
   a. Semicanal for tensor tympani muscle
   b. Canal for bony part of pharyngotympanic tube which is directed forwards, downwards and medially.
   c. The lowest part is formed by the posterior wall of the bony carotid canal. This separates the cavity from the internal carotid artery and the sympathetic plexus of nerves around it.

4. **Posterior wall:** It presents with the following features:
   a. An opening in the upper part which communicates with mastoid antrum. It lies above the level of tympanic membrane.
   b. Vertical part of bony canal for facial nerve in lower part.
   c. A pyramidal prominence which contains the stapedius muscle. It is present in front of the upper part of facial canal.

5. **Medial wall:** It separates the tympanic cavity from the internal ear. It presents with following features
   a. **Promontory:** It is a large rounded elevation formed by the first (basal) turn of the cochlea. It is covered by the tympanic plexus.
   b. **Fenestra vestibuli (oval window):** It is a fenestration present behind the promontory in upper part that is closed by the base of stapes.
   c. Prominence of the oblique part of facial nerve canal, above the oval window.
   d. Prominence of lateral semicircular canal, behind the facial canal.
   e. Processus trochleariformis, a bony prominence above and in front of the oval window. The tendon of tensor tympani hooks around it before inserting into the handle of malleus.
   f. Fenestra cochleae (round window), below and behind the promontory. It is closed by the mucous membrane of middle ear also called secondary tympanic membrane.

6. **Lateral wall:** It is mainly formed by the tympanic membrane. The portion situated above the tympanic membrane is called as epitympanic recess. It is formed by the squamous part of temporal bone and opens posteriorly into aditus ad antrum.

Ear Ossicles (Fig. 11.19)

Malleus

It consists of the following parts:
1. **Head,** lies in the epitympanic part and articualtes with the incus.
2. **Neck**
3. **Three processes**
   • Handle, which is directed downwards and embedded in the medial surface of the tympanic membrane.
   • Anterior process
   • Lateral process

Incus

It consists of the following parts:
1. **Body:** Articulates with malleus
2. **Short process**
3. **Long process:** Articulates with stapes

Stapes

It resembles a stirrup and presents with the following parts:
1. **Head:** articulates with incus
2. **Neck**
3. **Anterior and posterior limbs:** These arise from neck and diverge to attach to the base.
4. **Base:** Also called foot plate. It is reniform in shape and is connected to the fenestra vestibuli by an annular ligament.

Muscles of Middle Ear

1. Tensor tympani
2. Stapedius

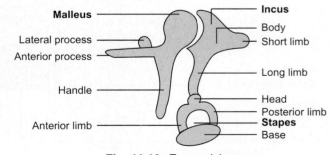

Fig. 11.19: Ear ossicles

Action of muscles: The tensor tympani makes the tympanic membrane taut while the stapedius draws the stapes laterally. This exerts a dampening effect on sound vibrations which is particularly useful in presence of a loud noise to prevent damage to the internal ear.

Arterial Supply of Middle Ear

1. Stylomastoid artery.
2. Anterior tympanic artery.
3. Petrosal branch of middle meningeal artery.
4. Superior tympanic branch of middle meningeal artery.
5. Branches from ascending pharyngeal artery and internal carotid artery.

Nerve Supply of Middle Ear

1. Superior and inferior carotico-tympanic nerves, from sympathetic plexus around internal carotid artery.
2. Tympanic branch of glossopharyngeal nerve.

INTERNAL EAR

The internal ear is located within the petrous part of the temporal bone.

Structure

- It consists of a complex series of fluid filled spaces called the membranous labyrinth.
- This membranous labyrinth is loged within similarily arranged bony cavities forming the 'bony labyrinth'.
- The membranous labyrinth is filled with endolymph and bony labyrinth with perilymph.

Bony Labyrinth

The bony labyrinth consists of a complex series of bony canals in the petrous part of temporal bone. It is made up of the following three parts which communicate with each other (Fig. 11.20).

Vestibule

- The vestibule is the middle part of the bony labyrinth and is located immediately medial to the tympanic cavity.

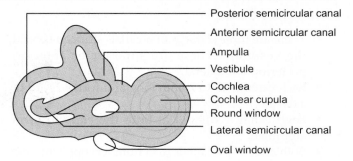

Fig. 11.20: Bony labyrinth

Posterior semicircular canal
Anterior semicircular canal
Ampulla
Vestibule
Cochlea
Cochlear cupula
Round window
Lateral semicircular canal
Oval window

- It lodges the utricle and saccule of the membranous labyrinth.
- Its lateral wall opens into the tympanic cavity by an oval aperture called fenestra vestibuli which is closed by the foot-plate of the stapes.
- Posteriorly, it receives the opening of three semicircular canals.
- Anteriorly, it is continuous with the cochlea.

Cochlea

- The cochlea is a helical tube of about 2½ turns. It is named cochlea due to its resemblance to the shell of a snail.
- It forms the anterior part of the bony labyrinth.
- Its basal coil forms the promontory of the middle ear and opens into the vestibuli posteriorly.
- The cochlea possesses a bony core or central bony pillar called modiolus which contains the spiral ganglion and transmits the cochlear nerve.
- A spiral ridge of the bone projects from the modiolus which partly divides the cochlear canal into two parts:
  a. Scala vestibuli, above
  b. Scala tympani, below
- The partition between scala vestibuli and scala tympani is completed by the basilar membrane which extends from the tip of spiral lamina to lateral wall of cochlea.
- The scala vestibuli communicates with the scala tympani at the apex of the cochlea by a small opening called helicotrema.
- Both scala have perilymph.
- The scala tympani is closed by a bony lamina at the end of the basal turn while the scala vestibuli opens into the anterior wall of vestibule.

Semicircular Canals

- There are three semicircular canals situated behind the vestibule. These are superior or anterior, posterior, and lateral.
- Each canal is 15 to 20mm long and forms 2/3rd of a circle.
- Each canal is dilated at both the ends to form ampullae.
- Both ends of the canals (6 in number) open into the vestibule by five openings.
- The three canals are set at a right angle to each other.

POINT TO REMEMBER

The lateral semicircular canals of both ears lie in the same plane. The anterior semicircular canal of one side is parallel to the plane of the posterior semicircular canal of the other side.

Membranous Labyrinth (Figs 11.21 and 11.22)

- The membranous labyrinth, as mentioned earlier, consists of closed membranous sacs and ducts intercommunicating with each other.
- It lies within the bony labyrinth.
- The membranous labyrinth consists of 3 parts
- **Cochlear duct,** within the bony cochlea. It is a spiral-shaped duct consisting of 2 and 3/4th turns. It lies in the bony cochlear canal between the scala vestibuli and scala tympani. The cochlear duct contains the spiral organ of Corti.

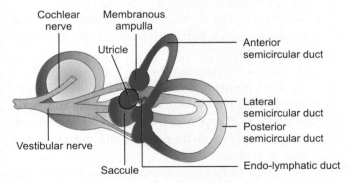

Fig. 11.21: Membranous labyrinth

Spiral Organ of Corti (Fig. 11.22)

- **It is the peripheral organ of hearing** present in the cochlear duct. It rests on the basilar membrane.
- **Structure:** It consists of
  — Inner and outer rod cells

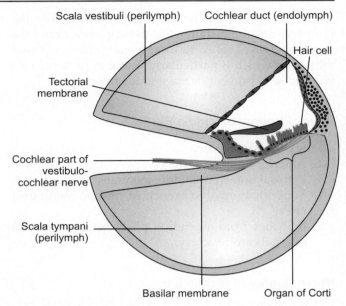

Fig. 11.22: Vertical section of Cochlea showing organ of Corti, hair cells, tectorial membrane, scala vestibuli, scala tympani and Cochlear duct

  — Inner and outer hair cells: These respond to vibrations induced in the endolymph by the sound waves.
  — Supporting cells (Deiter's and Hensen's cells)
  — Tunnel of Corti
  — Membrana tectoria: It is made up of a gelatinous substance and covers the hair cells.
- The organ of Corti is innervated by the peripheral processes of bipolar neurones located in the spiral ganglion which is located in the spiral canal.
  — The spiral canal is located within the modiolus at the base of the spiral lamina.
  — The central process of these ganglion cells forms the cochlear nerve.
- **Saccule and utricle,** within the vestibule. The inner aspect of medial wall of saccule and anterior wall of utricle possess the sensory end organs called maculae. They contain hair cells, supporting cells and a covering gelatinous mass impregnated with calcium salts called the otolithic membrane. The maculae are also called the static balance receptors and give infromation about the position of head. They respond to movement of fluid when there is linear acceleration of head. They are supplied by the peripheral processes of the neurons of vestibular nerve.
- **Three semicircular canals,** within the respective semicircular canals. Three semicircular ducts are present within the corresponding bony semicircular canals along their outer walls. Each duct is dilated at both its ends forming an ampulla lodged in the corresponding bony ampulla. The three ducts open into the utricle at both their ends by five openings. The inner aspect of the medial wall of the ampulla

of each duct possesses sensory end organs called crista ampullaris or ampullary crests. Crista ampullaris consists of hair cells, supporting cells and a gelatinous mass called cupula covering the sterocilia and kinocilia of hair cells. The semicircular ducts are responsible for sensing the rotatory movements of the head and help to maintain the kinetic balance of the body.

Arterial Supply of Internal Ear

1. Labyrinthine artery, branch of basilar artery.
2. The organ of Corti has no blood vessels but receives oxygen via the cortilymph.

Nerve Supply of Internal Ear

1. The utricle, saccule and semicircular ducts receive fibres from vestibular nerve.
2. The cochlear duct (organ of Corti) receives fibres from cochlear nerve.

PHYSIOLOGY OF HEARING

The external ear and middle ear are primarily concerned with transmission of soundwaves to the cochlea (inner ear) which houses the sense organ of hearing.

Functions of external ear: It captures the sound waves and transmits them inside. The wax produced by ceruminous glands keeps the epithelium of external ear moist preventing dryness and also prevents maceration of epithelium due to water.

Function of tympanic membrane: The tympanic membrane vibrates in response to sound wavesand transmits them to the middle ear ossicles.

Transmission of Sound Waves

- The sound waves are captured by the pinna and passed to tympanic membrane via the external auditory canal.
- This sets up vibrations in tympanic membrane which are transmitted to the ossicles of middle ear.
- The movements are passed successfully from malleus, incus to the foot of stapes that sets up vibrations in the cochlea fluid in scala vestibule.
- The pressure of sound waves is increased 22 times as it passes from the tympanic membrane to foot of stapes.
- The movement of fluid in inner ear sets up pressure changes on inner hair cells which initiates action potentials in them and hence in auditory nerves.
- Loudness of sound is proportional to amplitude of sound waves while pitch of sound is proportional to frequency of sound waves striking the ear.
- Intensity of sound is measured on decibel scale. The human ear can hear sound waves with frequencies ranging from 20 to 20,000 Hertz (Hz) only.

The primary receptor cells of hearing are inner hair cells in organ of Corti which initiate action potentials in the auditory nerve fibers.

Auditory Pathway

The organ of Corti is the peripheral receptor of auditory pathway. Hair cells of organ of Corti are the receptor cells which are innervated by the dedrites of bipolar cells located in spiral ganglion of modiolus (Fig. 11.23).

- Afferents impulses are transmitted via axons of the bipolar cells which form the cochlear division of vestibulocochlear nerve (8th cranial nerve).
- These relay in the dorsal and ventral cochlear nuclei located at the upper part of medulla and lower part of pons.
- The fibres from ventral cochlear nuclei decussate to opposite side forming trapezoid body at basilar part of pons.
- Fibres from ipsilateral dorsal cochlear nucleus and contra-lateral ventral cochlear nucleus pass through superior olivary nucleus (some fibres relay here) and ascend up as lateral lemniscus successively through inferior colliculus of midbrain, medial geniculate body, auditory radiation to the auditory cortex on superior temporal gyrus.

Masking: Masking is the phenomenon in which presence of one sound decreases the ability to hear another sound. Example, we cannot hear clearly human voice if loud music is playing.

Localization of direction of sound depends upon the differences in the time of sound waves reaching the two ears and the variation in the intensity of sound waves reaching the two ears. This is integrated at level of auditory cortex and any diseases of the cortex can affect sound localization.

Vestibular Pathway

Peripheral receptors for vestibular pathway are the cristae ampularis of the semicircular canals and the macular located in saccule and utricle of vestibule. They are innervated by the distal processess of bipolar cells of vestibular ganglion situated in the lateral part of internal acoustic meatus.

- The afferent impulses are transmitted from the receptors to the proximal processes of bipolar cells which formed the vestibular division of vestibulo-cochlear nerve.
- The fibres relay in vestibular nuclei located in upper part of medulla and lower part of pons. Further transmission is complex and fibres go along various pathways.

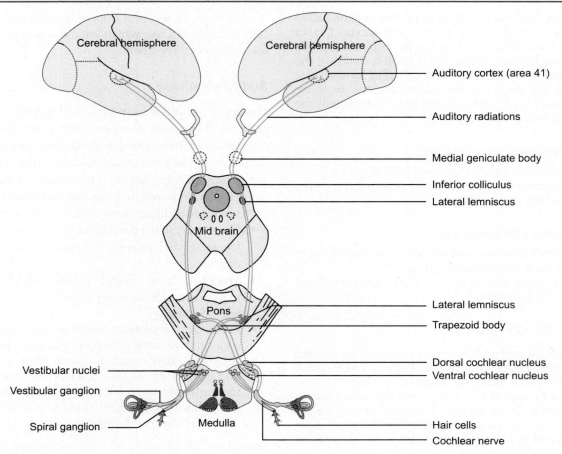

Fig. 11.23: Auditory pathway

— Ascend to cerebellum via inferior cerebellar peduncle.
— Descend in spinal cord as the vestibulospinal tract.
— Cross to vestibular nuclei of opposite side.
— Have to and fro connection with reticular formation.
— Ascend to cerebral cortex of temporal lobe.
— Have connection with nuclei of 3rd 4th and 6th cranial nerve via medial longitudnal bundle.

Function of vestibular pathway: This pathway intergrates multiple inputs and helps to co-ordinates movements of head, neck and body to maintanance of balance and provides subjective awareness of motion.

SMELL

Sense of smell or olfaction is not very well developed in human beings as compared to animals like dogs. Sense of smell is a function of the olfactory epithelium of nose and the olfactory pathway.

OLFACTORY EPITHELIUM

Olfactory epithelium is a specialised thickened epithelium present on the roof of nose (Fig. 11.24), superior concha, upper most part of middle concha and the adjoining nasal septum. It is made up of olfactory receptor neurons, sustentacular cells and basal cells. The olfactory neurons are bipolar neurons with numerous dendrites and a single axon. An unbranched dendrite

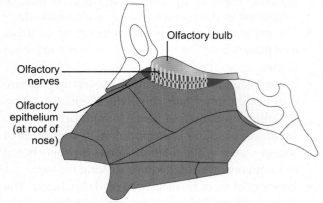

Fig. 11.24: Olfactory epithelium and nerves

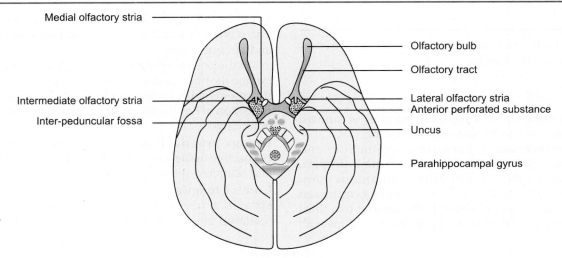

Fig. 11.25: Olfactory pathway

from the neuron extends on to epithelial surface as an expanded ending. This dendritic ending has numerous cilia which radiate from its surface and are bathed in the mucus secretions of the nasal epithelium. The expanded ends are called olfactory rods and are the receptors for sensation of smell. The axons of many such bipolar neurons join to form rootlets of olfactory nerve which pass out from the roof of nose through the cribriform plate of ethmoid bone to end in olfactory bulb.

OLFACTORY PATHWAY (FIGs 11.24 and 11.25)

Olfactory pathway is made up of the following:
1. Olfactory nerve
2. Olfactory bulb: The olfactory nerves relay on the mitral and the tuft cells of olfactory bulb. Axons of these cells form the olfactory tracts.
3. Anterior olfactory nucleus: It is an accesory nucleus of the olfactory pathway connected to the olfactory bulb and cerebral cortex.
4. Olfactory tract: Each tract divide into medial and lateral olfactory stria which pass on the anterior perforated substance to reach the cerebral cortex.
6. Olfactory cortex: The olfactor stria and in the piriform cortex of cerbrum which consists of:
   a. Pre-piriform cortex: It includes lateral olfactory gyrus and gyrus ambiens.
   b. Para-amygdaloid region in temporal lobe.
   c. Entorhinal area: Area no. 28.

The pririform cortex has connections with orbitofrontal cortex, thalamus, hypothalamus and limbic system.

PHYSIOLOGY OF SMELL

- The receptors of sense of smell as already mentioned are the olfactory neurons which have expanded dendritic ends called **olfactory rods.** These olfactory rods contain cilia which project into the nasal mucus.
- Mucus is produced by gland cells of the nasal (respiratory) epithelium situated below olfactory mucus membrane.
- Odor producing molecules enter nose along with air and dissolve into the nasal mucus which presents them to the olfactory receptors.
- Chemical stimulation of the neuron receptors leads to setting up of action potential in the axons of receptors which form the olfactory nerves. These nerves in turn form complex synapses called olfactory glomeruli with mitral cells and tufted cells in olfactory bulb.
- The axons of cells from olfactory bulb pass to olfactory cortex of brain (area no. 28).
- About 10,000 smells can be identified by human nose.
- Differentiation of intensity of odor is less, about 30% change of odor intensity is required to detect it as a change.
- Molecules with high water and lipid solubility give stronger odors.
- When there is a continuous exposure to a strong smell, adaptation of the receptors for that smell occurs and gradually perception of the smell is lost during that time.

Irritant Receptors in Nose

- Free nerve endings, from trigeminal nerve are interspersed in olfactory mucus membrane. These are stimulated by irritant odors like that of formalin, peppermint and onion fumes and macromolecules like pepper powder.
- They respond by stimulating the reflex of sneezing, lacrimation and excess mucus production.

TASTE

Organ of taste sensation are the taste buds present primarily over the tongue.

TONGUE (FIGs 11.26 and 11.27)

Tongue is made up of interlacing bundles of striated muscle fibres coverd by mucous membrane.

Mucous membrane: It consists of epithelium and underlying connective tissue called lamina propria. Epithelium is mostly striatified squamous non-keratinized type and at places is thinly keratinized stratified squamous epithelium. In the anterior two-third of dorsal surface of the tongue, epithelium presents with a number of upward projections known as papillae. Three types of papillae are present: Filiform, fungiform and circumvallate.

In the posterior one-third of the dorsal surface of the tongue the mucosa does not have any papillae. However, it presents with surface projections due to underlying collection of lymphoid follicles (lingual tonsil) below the epithelium.

Lamina propria: It is thin and is made up of dense connective tissue with elastic fibres, blood vessels, nerves and scattered lymphatic cells.

Core of tongue: It consists of interlacing bundles of striated muscle fibres with connective tissue and scattered mucous and serous lingual glands.

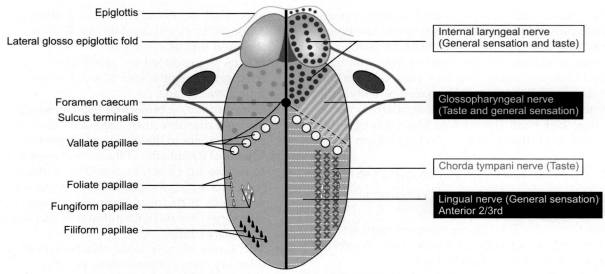

Fig. 11.26: Sensory supply of tongue

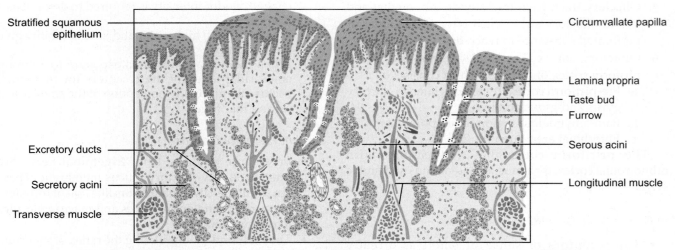

Fig. 11.27: Transverse section of tongue: stain—hematoxylin-eosin under high magnification

Taste Buds (Fig. 11.29)

- Taste buds are barrel shaped structures, narrower at the ends and broader in the middle which are distributed within the epithelium of oral cavity. They open to the surface of lingual epithelium by a taste pore.
- Taste buds are made up of cluster of modified epithelial cells which are of two types:
  a. Gustatory cells: These are slender rod shaped cells with a central nucleus. Free surface of these cells present with short hairs projecting into lumen of pit surrounding the taste buds.
  b. Supporting or sustentacular cells: These are spindle shaped.
- The base of each bud is penetrated by the afferent gustatory fibres.
- All papillae except filiform papillae contain taste buds.
- **Taste buds are present at the following sites**
  — Anterior 2/3rd of dorsum of tongue
  — Inferior surface of soft palate
  — Palatoglossal arches
  — Posterior surface of epiglottis
  — Posterior wall of oropharynx

Physiology of Taste (Figs 11.28 and 11.29)

- The sense organs for taste are taste buds which are present in between the epithelial cells of tongue.

Microvilli extend from gustatory cells to the pores which sense the changes in chemical in the saliva.
- Each taste bud is innervated by about 50 nerve endings and each nerve fiber receives input from upto 5 taste buds.
- Taste buds are present over fungiform and vallate papillae of the tongue (no taste buds are present on filiform papillae) and are distributed in the mucosa of epiglottis, palate and oropharynx.
- The ingested substances responsible for taste sensations are dissolved in saliva and presented to the microvilli of gustatory receptor cells. This leads to opening up of H^+ or Na^+ channels in the chemoreceptors leading to alteration in polarization of cell membrane and setting up of action potentials in the nerve endings.
- Sensory fibers from taste buds on anterior 2/3rd of tongue except circumvallate papillae travel in chorda tympanic nerve while from circumvallate papillae travel in glossopharyngeal nerve. The sensations from palate, pharynx and epiglottis are carried by internal laryngeal nerve a branch of vagus nerve.
- These fibers project on the nucleus of tractus solitarius in medulla oblongata. Second order neurons from here cross to other side and ascend in the dorsomedial part of medial lemniscus and terminate in the venteroposterolateral nucleus of

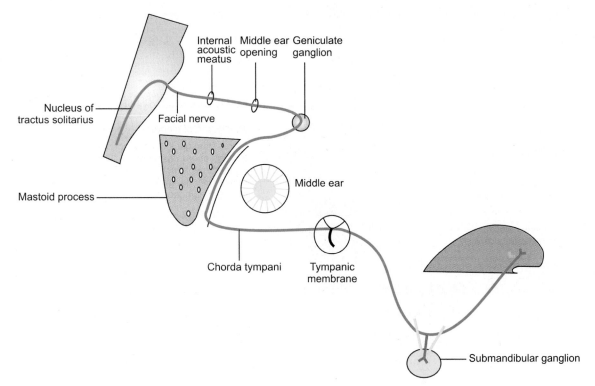

Fig. 11.28: Nerve supply to taste buds of anterior 2/3rd of tongue except circumvallate papillae

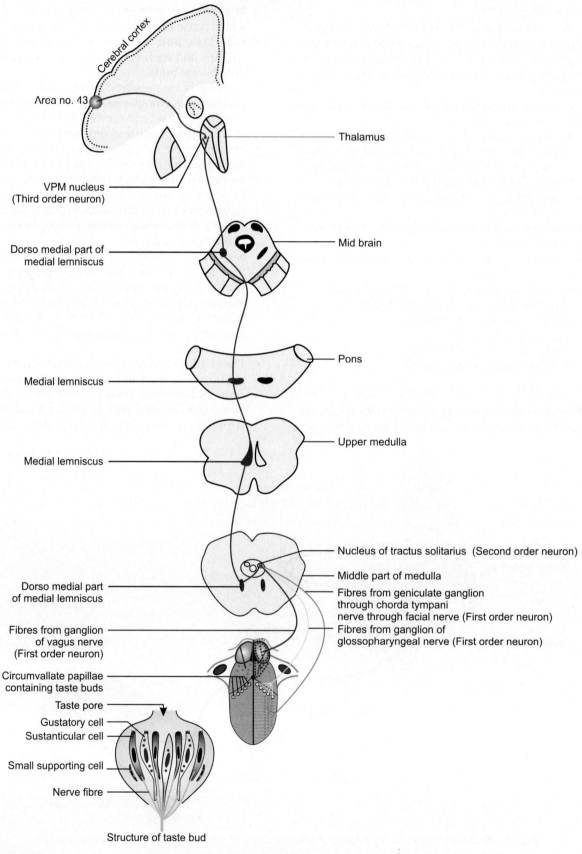

Cerebral cortex

Area no. 43

Thalamus

VPM nucleus
(Third order neuron)

Dorso medial part of
medial lemniscus

Mid brain

Medial lemniscus

Pons

Medial lemniscus

Upper medulla

Nucleus of tractus solitarius (Second order neuron)

Middle part of medulla

Dorso medial part
of medial lemniscus

Fibres from geniculate ganglion
through chorda tympani
nerve through facial nerve (First order neuron)

Fibres from ganglion
of vagus nerve
(First order neuron)

Fibres from ganglion of
glossopharyngeal nerve (First order neuron)

Circumvallate papillae
containing taste buds

Taste pore

Gustatory cell

Sustanticular cell

Small supporting cell

Nerve fibre

Structure of taste bud

Fig. 11.29: Structure of taste bud and taste pathway

thalamus. Axons of 3rd order neurons pass to the taste projection area in the post-central gyrus of cerebral cortex (area no. 43). Fibres from thalamus have connection with hypothalamus which further connects to limbic system. This explains the emotional factors involved in taste sensation.

- There are four basic taste modalities appreciated by humans, these are; **sweet, sour, bitter and salt.** The threshold for bitter substances is the lowest while it is highest for sweet (except saccharin) substances.
- The concentration of a substance needs to be changed by more than 30% for the change in intensity of taste to be appreciated at the cortical level.
- Adaptation to taste of a substance occurs when it is placed continuously in one part of mouth.

CLINICAL AND APPLIED ASPECT
EYELID AND LACRIMAL APPARATUS

- **Stye** is an acute suppurative inflammation of a Zies gland. The pus points near the base of the cilia. Epilation of the eyelash helps to drain the pus.
- **Chalazion (internal stye):** It is the inflammation of a tarsal (meibomian) gland. The swelling points on the inner aspect of the eyelid.
- Inflammation of lacrimal sac is called **dacryo-cystitis.** It hampers the drainage of lacrimal fluid into the nose. This causes overflow of the lacrimal fluid from the conjunctival sac on to the face, a condition called epiphora.
- **Ptosis:** Paralysis of levator palpebrae superioris leads to ptosis, i.e., drooping of upper eyelid. This can occur either due to damage of oculomotor nerve or due to damage to the cervical sympathetic chain (as in Horner's syndrome).

ORBIT

Squint: Unilateral paralysis of an extraocular muscle (usually due to damage of the corresponding nerve). This produces strabismus or squint. It may result in **diplopia** or double vision. Diplopia occurs because light from an object is not focussed on identical areas of both retinae. The real image falls on the macula of the unaffected eye while the false image falls on some peripheral part of the retina in the paralysed eye leading to diplopia.

CORNEA

- Due to ageing there is fatty degeneration along the periphery of the cornea. This becomes visible as a white ring in old people and is known as **arcus senilus.**

- Transparency of cornea is essential for adequate vision. It can be affected by following conditions.
  - **Injuries:** This is the most common cause of corneal opacities as any injury heals by fibrosis.
  - **Inappropriate use of contact lenses:** Semisoft lenses should not be worn for long periods as they are impermeable to gases. The central part of cornea receives oxygen from air by diffusion and this gets cut off by such lenses. Soft lenses are relatively more permeable to gases and can be used for longer hours.
  - **Vitamin A deficiency** in childhood leads to destruction of cornea which is known as keratomalacia. Healing is by fibrosis which results in opacification of cornea.
- **Astigmatism:** Loss of normal curvature of cornea is known as astigmatism. In this case the cornea is more curved in one meridian than the other. It leads to eye strain due to irregular refraction of light.

RETINA

- The following features are observed on the retina as seen through the ophtahalmoscope (Fig. 11.30).
  a. **Macula lutea** is a pale yellowish area seen near the posterior pole. It is approximately 5 mm in diameter. A small pit in its center is called the fovea centralis. This is the point where light is normally focussed. Fovea is that portion of retina which has the maximum concentration of cones. Hence, it is the site of greatest visual acuity, i.e., the ability to see fine images.
  b. **Optic disc:** It is a white spot seen about 3 mm medial to the macula. It has a depressed area in the center called the 'physiological cup'. Nerve

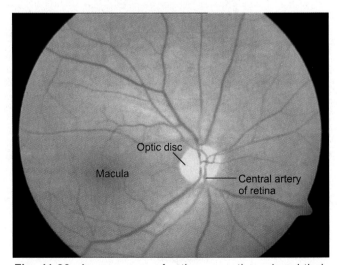

Fig. 11.30: Appearance of retina seen through ophthal-moscope

fibres from retina meet and pass through this region of the eyeball and form the optic nerve. The blood vessels of retina also pass through this spot. There are no photoreceptor cells in the optic disc. Hence, it does not respond to light. Therefore, the optic disc is also called as the 'blind spot'.

c. **Central artery of the retina:** It enters the eye through center of the optic disc. It divides into superior and inferior branches, each of which then divides into temporal and nasal branches. The retinal veins follow the arteries. The branches of the central artery of retina are seen radiating over the edges of the optic disc. They are smaller and paler than veins. At points where they cross the veins, the wall of the veins can be seen through them. In patients with high blood pressure the arteries may appear narrowed. Haemorrhages may be seen around the arteries.

• **Papilloedema:** Normal optic disc as seen on ophthalmoscopy appears as a cup shaped area, paler than the surrounding area i.e., the fundus. The edges of the cup are sharp and well defined. In patients with raised intracranial pressure the optic disc is congested. The cup gets obscured and the disc margin is blurred. This is known as papilloedema. Intracranial pressure gets transmitted to the disc via the meningeal coverings which continue over the optic nerve. The raised pressure also compresses the central retinal artery which lies in the subarachnoid space around the optic nerve.

• In retinal detachment there is separation of the two layers of retina. Retinal pigment epithelium separates from the neurosensory layer of retina.

• **Night blindness:** As retinene$_1$ is derived from vitamin A, any deficiency of this vitamin will lead to visual abnormalities. The deficiency initialy affects the function of rods and hence there is difficulty in seeing in dim light or darkness. This is called nyctalopia or night blindness. Prolonged deficiency subsequently hampers the function of cones also. It also leads to epithelial changes in the form of thickening of conjunctiva and dryness due to loss of tear film which damages cornea.

OPTICS OF EYE

• **Emmetrotia:** It is the normal focussing eye in which parallel rays of light from infinity are focussed on the retina, when accomodation is at rest.

• **Refractive error (Ametropia) (Fig. 11.31):** This is a clinical condition characterised by defect in the image forming mechanism of the eye in which the rays coming from an object are not focussed on the retina. It can be classified into the following types:

a. **Myopia or near sightedness:** This occurs when the axial length of eye ball is increased or the refractive power of lens is increased. The light rays from a distant object are focused in front of the retina and hence the image appears blurred. It can be treated by using appropriate concave lenses.

b. **Hypermetropia or far sightedness:** This occurs when the axial length of eye ball is decreased or the refractive power of lens is decreased. The

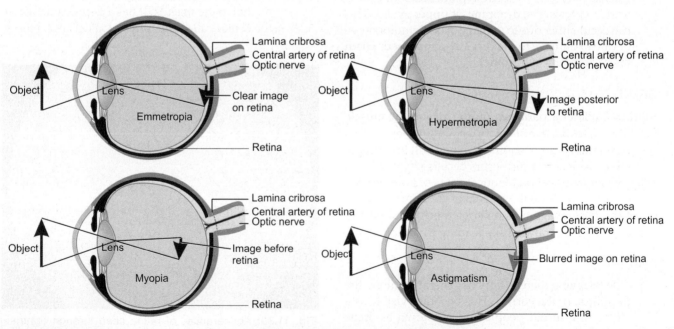

Fig. 11.31: Emmetropia and refractive errors of eye

light rays from a near object are focused behind the retina and hence the appears blurred. It can be treated by using appropriate convex lenses.

   c. **Astigmatism:** In this there is defective focusing of an image on the retina due to alteration in the horizontal and vertical curvatures of the cornea. It is treated by using cylindrical lenses.

- **Presbyopia:** It is the inability to clearly see the near objects. This occurs in old age due to gradual loss of power of accomodation of eye and increase in opacification of the lens. The primary complaint is difficulty in reading. It is treated by using appropriate convex lenses.

- **Accommodation:** Change in focal length of the lens of the eye when it focuses on a nearby object is called accommodation. This occurs by the contraction of ciliary muscles and enables us to see both the far and near objects with the same lens.

LENS AND AQUEOUS HUMOR

- **Glaucoma:** It is an abnormal increase in the intraocular pressure of eye. Glaucoma usually occurs due to a block in the circulation and drainage of the aqueous humor. In acute conditions there is severe pain due to pressure on the highly sensitive cornea. Chronic glaucoma results in gradual pressure necrosis of the retina with decreasing vision and eventually blindness.

- **Opacification of the lens is known as cataract:** The most common cause is senile cataract, i.e., cataract of old age. The lens absorbs much of the ultraviolet rays and increasingly becomes yellow with ageing. It also becomes hard and ultimately opaque so that light cannot pass through. This results in blindness which is easily cured by surgery.

EXTERNAL EAR

- We know that external auditory meatus is S shaped. Hence, in order to examine the canal and view the tympanic membrane the auricle is pulled upwards, backwards and laterally to straighten the external meatus before inserting the ear speculum. In newborn babies and young children the bony part of meatus is poorly developed and is in the form of a bony rim. Hence, the ear speculum should be inserted minimally and carefully as otherwise the tympanic membrane can be easily damaged.

- **Ceruminosis** is the excessive collection of wax in the meatus. This causes blocked ear and decrease in hearing. The wax can be washed out by syringing with a warm jet of water. However, this can lead to stimulation of auricular branch of vagus nerve which results in coughing and vomiting during the procedure and rarely, can even cause sudden cardiac inhibition. There is also a high chance of injury to the tympanic membrane. Thus, wax now a days is removed by gentle suction in the meatus. It is not advisable to use earbuds to clean wax as they push the wax further inside which gets stuck.

- An infection of the lining of meatus is very painful because the lining of skin is intimately adherent to the underlying cartilage and bone.

TYMPANIC MEMBRANE

- Since the tympanic membrane is transluscent, on examination with otoscope, one can see the underlying handle and lateral process of malleus and the long process of incus. The greater part of membrane (pars tensa) is taut. Above the lateral process of malleus, a small triangular area of the membrane is seen which is thin and lax (pars flacida). This triangular area is seen to be bounded by two distinct folds, anterior and posterior malleolar folds which reach down to the lateral process of the malleus.

  The point of greatest concavity on the external surface of the membrane is known as **umbo**. This marks the attachment of the handle of the malleus to the membrane. On illumination, the normal tympanic membrane appears pearly grey in colour and reflects a 'cone of light' in its antero-inferior quadrant with the apex at umbo. This picture is due to its angulated alignment in the external auditory canal.

- **Myringotomy** means incision in tympanic membrane. It is usually given to drain pus collected in middle ear in acute ear infection. The best site of incision is in the postero-inferior quadrant where the bulge is usually most prominent. The risk of injury to chorda tympani nerve is also minimal in such an incision because it runs on the inner aspect of tympanic membrane downwards and forwards lateral to the long process of incus.

MIDDLE EAR

- **Otitis media:** This is the term given for infections of middle ear cavity. Acute infections commonly lead to radness tympanic membrane and pain. They may result in pus formation and rupture of the membrane with discharge of pus from ear. In severe cases infection can spread to mastoid antrum and mastoid air cells through aditus-ad-antrum. Since the mastoid antrum is intimately related posteriorly to the sigmoid sinus and cerebellum, both these structures may also be involved.

- In children upper respiratory tract infections are fairly common. The infection spreads easily from nasopharynx to the middle ear via the eustachian tube because the tube is short and more horizontal in position.
- The pharyngo-tympanic tube connects nasopharynx to the middle ear cavity and helps to equalize the pressure on either side of tympanic membrane. The tubal opening in nasopharynx is slit like and normally remains closed except while yawning or swallowing. When it opens, the air in middle ear escapes and equalizes with atmosphere pressure. The pressure of air at higher altitudes is less. Hence when ascending up a mountain in a vehicle or travelling by air plane, the pressure changes can lead to ear ache. This is because on ascent the middle ear pressure (internal) will exceed the pressure in external ear (external). The tympanic membrane as a consequence is pushed outwards leading to pain. This is relieved normally by constant swallowing. However, in people suffering from common cold the tubal opening may be blocked due to swelling and the pain cannot be relieved as the escape of air is prevented. During descent, the pressure changes are reversed and air is sucked into the middle ear cavity via the tube. **Pain during descent is more** because the slit like tubal opening allows easy escape of air during ascent while the sucking in of air during descent via the opening is more difficult.

INTERNAL EAR

- **Vertigo:** It is the sensation of rotational acceleration in the absence of actual rotation. In young patients it is generally a benign idiopathic condition. There is stimulation of crista ampullairs on its own in a particular head posture. It can also be a sign of labryintitis specially in elderly.
- **Motion sickness:** When exposed to constant acceleration and deceleration movements, e.g., while traveling in car or bus, some people experience nausea, vomiting hypotension, sweating and palpitations. This is associated with excessive vestibular stimulation and mediated by the connections of vestibular pathway with medulla oblongata and cerebellum.
- **Caloric stimulation:** When either hot or cold water is instilled into the external ear, the temperature difference results in setting up of convection currents in semicircular canals which stimulates vertigo, nausea and nystagmus.

PHYSIOLOGY OF HEARING

- **Deafness:** It is the loss of sense of hearing. Hearing loss can vary from impaired or decrease sensation of hearing to a complete loss of hearing or deafness. There are two types of hearing loss.
  1. Conductive type of hearing loss: It occurs due to impaired transmission of sound waves due to pathology of external ear, (e.g., presence of wax) or middle ear (otitis media)
  2. Sensorineural type of hearing loss: It occurs due to damage to inner ear, i.e., cochlea or the vestibulo-cochlear nerve.

SENSE OF SMELL

Anosmia: It is the complete loss of sensation of smell.
Hyposmia: It is the partial loss of sensation of smell.
Dysosmia: It is the altered or distorted sense of smell.

These conditions can arise due to changes in mucus membrane due to aging, exposure to infections especially sinusitis and in presence of nasal polyps.

SENSE OF TASTE

Ageusia: It is athe absence of sensation of taste.
Hypogeusia: It is the decrease in taste sensation.
Dysgeusia: It is the presence of altered taste sensation.
These can be caused by drugs like penicillamine, metronidazole etc.

Chapter 12

Respiratory System

INTRODUCTION

Respiratory system deals with absorption of O_2 from air and removal of CO_2 from the body via lungs.

Anatomy of Respiratory System

It can be studied in two parts (Fig. 12.1):

1. **Respiratory tract or air passage:** It consists of the following parts:
   Upper Respiratory Tract
   - Nose and paranasal sinuses
   - Pharynx
   - Larynx
   - Trachea with two principal bronchi

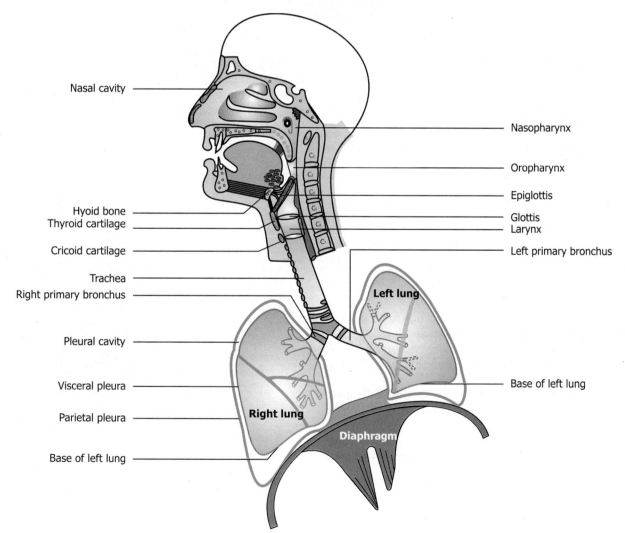

Nasal cavity

Hyoid bone
Thyroid cartilage
Cricoid cartilage
Trachea
Right primary bronchus
Pleural cavity
Visceral pleura
Parietal pleura
Base of left lung

Nasopharynx
Oropharynx
Epiglottis
Glottis
Larynx
Left primary bronchus

Left lung
Right lung
Base of left lung
Diaphragm

Fig. 12.1: Respiratory system

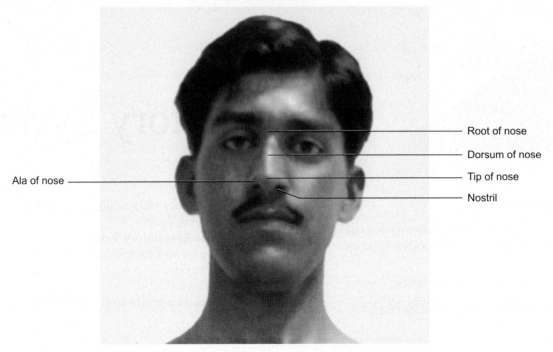

Fig. 12.2: Photograph showing various parts of external nose

Lower Respiratory Tract
- Bronchopulmonary tree on each side
- Two lungs enclosed in pleura
2. **Musculo-skeletal framework:** enclosing the lung and pleura. It is made up of
   - Thoracic cage
   - Intercostal muscles
   - Diaphragm

NOSE

Nose is the most proximal part of the upper respiratory system which is lined by respiratory and olfactory epithelium. It consists of external nose and nasal cavity.

External Nose (Fig. 12.2)

External nose forms a pyramidal projection in the middle of the face. It presents with the following features
   a. **Tip (or apex):** It is the lower free end of the nose
   b. **Root:** The upper narrow part attached to the forehead is the root of nose.
   c. **Dorsum of the nose:** Is formed by a rounded border between the tip and root of nose along with the adjoining area.
   d **Nostrils or anterior nares:** These are two piriform shaped apertures present at the broad lower part of the nose.

Structure of External Nose
It is made up of cartilaginous framework supported by bones and is covered with skin.

Skeleton of external nose: It is formed by the following bones and cartilages (Fig. 12.3).
   a. **The bony framework** comprises of the following
      1. Two nasal bones, forming the bridge of the nose.
      2. Frontal processes of maxillae.

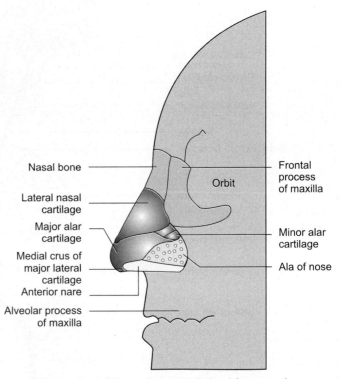

Fig. 12.3: External nose—skeletal framework

b. **The cartilaginous framework (Fig. 12.3)** comprises of 5 main cartilages and several additional tiny ones. The important cartilages are
   1. **Two lateral alar cartilages**, one upper and one lower.
   2. **A single median septal cartilage**
   3. **Two major alar cartilages:** Each major alar cartilage comprises of a medial and a lateral crus.

NASAL CAVITY

Nasal cavity extends from the nostrils (anterior nares) to the posterior nasal aperture (choanae). It is subdivided into two parts by a nasal septum. Each half is again called as the nasal cavity.

Each nasal cavity presents with the following boundaries.
   a. Roof
   b. Floor
   c. Mecdial wall or nasal septum
   d. Lateral wall

Roof of Nasal Cavity

It is very narrow and is mainly formed by the cribriform plate of the ethmoid bone. It is lined by the olfactory epithelium

Floor of Nasal Cavity

The floor is almost horizontal and is formed by the upper surface of hard palate which separates it from the oral cavity.

Medial Wall of Nasal Cavity or Nasal Septum

It is formed by various bones and cartilages (Fig. 12.4).
The bones are
   1. Perpendicular plate of ethmoid bone: Forms the anterosuperior part of septum.
   2. Vomer: Forms the posteroinferior part of the septum.
   3. Frontal crest of nasal bone lies in front of ethmoid
   4. Nasal spine of frontal bone.
   5. Sphenoidal crest lies behind the ethmoid
   6. Nasal crest lies in the lower most part. It is formed by fusion of the two palatine processes of maxilla and the two horizontal plates of palatine bone, in the lower most part.

The cartilages are
   1. Septal cartilage: Its forms the major anterior part of the septum
   2. Septal processes of major alar cartilages.
   3. **Jacobson's cartilage:** It lies between the vomer and septal cartilage.

Most of the septum on each side is lined by mucous membrane except at the lower mobile part which is lined by the skin.

The septum is generally slightly deviated to one side.

Arterial Supply of the Nasal Septum (Fig. 12.5)

The nasal septum is supplied by the following arteries:
   1. Septal branch of anterior ethmoidal artery, branch of ophthalmic artery.
   2. Septal branch of sphenopalatine artery, branch of maxillary artery.

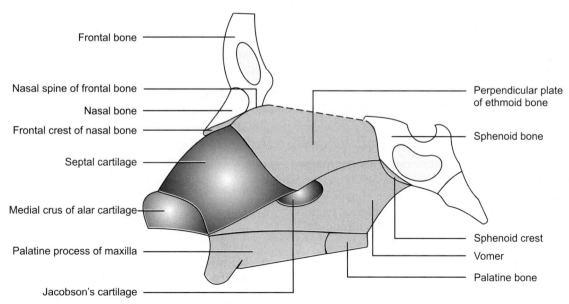

Fig. 12.4: Skeletal framework of nasal septum

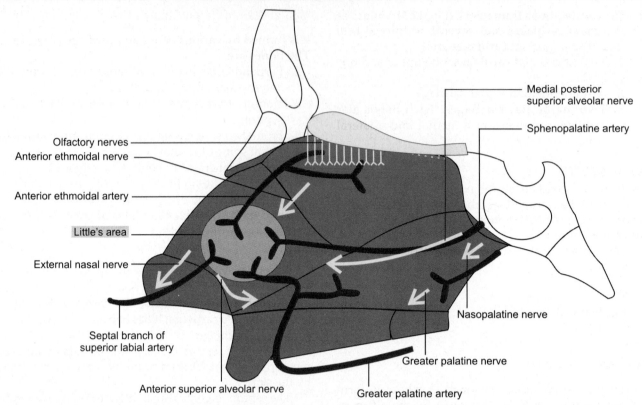

Fig. 12.5: Arterial and nerve supply of nasal septum

3. Septal branch of greater palatine artery, branch of maxillary artery
4. Septal branch of superior labial artery, branch of facial artery

Nerve Supply of the Nasal Septum (Fig. 12.5)

1. Olfactory nerves, about 15 to 20 in number supply the olfactory zone, present along the roof of nose. These nerves pierce the cribriform plate of ethmoid and enter the cranial cavity to end in the olfactory bulbs of the forebrain.
2. Inter nasal branch of anterior ethmoidal nerve, from nasociliary nerve supplies the anterosuperior part.
3. Medial posterior superior alveolar nerve, branch of pterygopalatine ganglion supplies the intermediate part.
4. Nasopalatine nerve supplies the posterior part.
5. Nasal branch of greater palatine nerve also supplies the posterior part
6. Anterior superior alveolar nerve, branch of maxillary nerve supplies the antero-inferior part.
7. External nasal nerve, branch of anterior ethmoidal nerve, supplies the lower mobile part.

Lateral Wall of the Nasal Cavity

It is also formed by bones and cartilages (Fig. 12.6). The bones are

Anteriorly
1. Nasal bone
2. Frontal process of maxilla
3. Lacrimal bone
4. Superior and middle conchae
5. Uncinate process of ethmoid, below the middle concha
6. Inferior concha

Posteriorly
7. Perpendicular plate of palatine
8. Medial pterygoid plate of sphenoid
   The bony part is lined by mucus membrane

The cartilages are
1. Lateral nasal cartilage (upper nasal cartilage)
2. Major alar cartilage (lower nasal cartilage)
3. 3 or 4 tiny alar cartilages
   This part is lined by skin

Subdivisions of the Lateral Wall

a. **Anterior part** presents a small depressed area called the vestibule. It is lined by skin which contains short, stiff and curved hairs called **vibrissae.**
b. **Middle part** is known as atrium of the middle meatus.
c. **Posterior part** presents the conchae and the spaces separating them which are called meatuses.

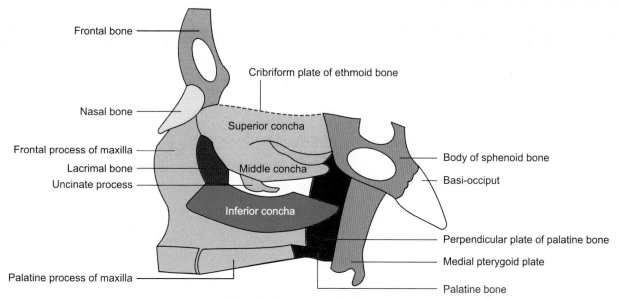

Fig. 12.6: Lateral wall of nose

Main Features of the Lateral Wall (Fig. 12.7)

1. **Conchae:** There are three curved bony projections directed downwards and medially from the lateral wall. They are
   a. **Superior concha:** It is the smallest concha.
   b. **Middle concha:** It covers the maximum number of openings. The superior and middle conchae are part of the ethmoidal labryrinth.
   c. **Inferior nasal concha:** Is the largest concha and is an independent bone.
   Sometimes a supreme nasal concha is also present.
2. **Meatuses:** These are the passages, present beneath the overhanging conchae.
   a. **Inferior meatus:** Is the largest and lies underneath the inferior nasal concha.
   b. **Middle meatus:** Lies underneath the middle concha.
   c. **Superior meatus:** Is the smallest meatus and lies below the superior concha.
3. **Spheno-ethmoidal recess:** It is a triangular depression, above and behind the superior concha.
4. **Atrium of middle meatus:** It is a shallow depression present in front of the middle meatus and above the vestibule of the nose. It is limited above by a faint ridge, the agger nasi. The curved muco-cutaneous junction between the atrium and the vestibule of nose is called as limen nasi.

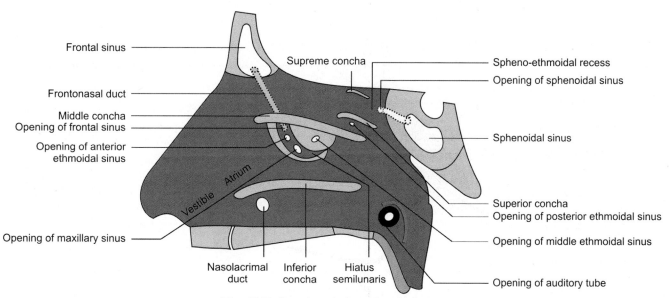

Fig. 12.7: Openings in lateral wall of nose

Openings in the Lateral Wall of the Nose (Fig. 12.7)

Site	Opening/Openings
Sphenoethmoidal recess	Opening of sphenoidal air sinus
Superior meatus	Openings of posterior ethmoidal air sinuses
Middle meatus	
• On bulla ethmoidalis	Openings of middle ethmoidal air sinuses
• In hiatus semilunaris	
— Anterior part	Opening of frontal air sinus
— Middle part	Opening of anterior ethmoidal air sinus
— Posterior part	Opening of maxillary air sinus
Inferior meatus	Opening of nasolacrimal duct (at the junction of anterior 1/3rd and posterior 2/3rd)

Arterial Supply of the Lateral Wall (Fig. 12.8)

1. Anterior ethmoidal artery. It supplies the antero-superior quadrant.
2. Branches of facial artery, supply the antero-inferior quadrant.
3. Sphenopalatine artery, supplies the postero-superior quadrant.
4. Greater palatine artery, supplies the postero-inferior quadrant, and its terminal branches supply the antero-inferior quadrant.

Nerve Supply of the Lateral Wall (Fig. 12.8)

1. Olfactory nerve, supply the upper part just below the cribriform plate upto the superior concha.
2. Anterior ethmoidal nerve, it supplies the antero-superior quadrant.
3. Anterior superior alveolar nerve, it supplies the antero-inferior quadrant.
4. Posterior lateral nasal branches of pterygo-palatine ganglion.

5. Anterior palatine branches of pterygo-palatine ganglion, from maxillary nerve.

Mucosal Lining of Nose

Nasal cavity is lined by skin at the entrance which contains hair follicles. Most of the nasal cavity is lined by respiratory epithelium consisting of pseudo-stratified, ciliated columnar epithelium with goblet cells which secrete mucus. A specialized epithelium, olfactory epithelium is present in the upper most part, i.e., roof of the nasal cavity.

Functions of Nose

1. The mucosa of nasal cavity is highly vascular and this helps in air conditioning (warming/cooling) and humidification of the inspired air.
2. Mucous secretions and hairs at the entrance of nasal cavity help in entrapement of foreign particles, preventing their entry into the respiratory tract.
3. Olfactory epithelium has receptors for sense of smell.

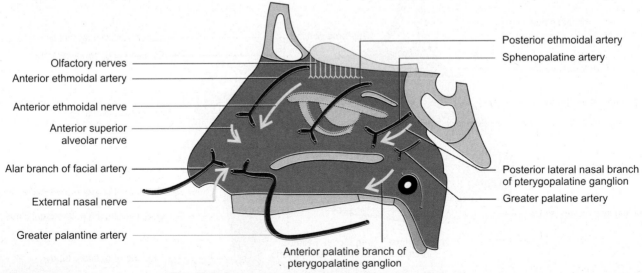

Fig. 12.8: Arterial and nerve supply of lateral wall of nose

PARANASAL AIR SINUSES

Paranasal air sinuses are air filled spaces within the bones around the nasal cavity. They are lined by mucous membrane consisting of ciliated columnar epithelium. All sinuses are related to the orbit and they communicate with the nasal cavity through various narrow channels (Figs 12.7, 12.9).

All paranasal sinuses are arranged in pairs except the ethmoidal sinuses which are arranged in three groups.

The paranasal sinuses are
1. **Frontal air sinuses:** The frontal air sinuses are contained in the frontal bone deep to supraciliary arches. They are related to the orbit inferiorly. Each sinus drains into the anterior part of the hiatus semilunaris of the middle meatus of nasal cavity through the frontonasal duct.
2. **Ethmoidal air sinuses:** The ethmoidal air sinuses are made up of a number of air cells present within the labyrinth of ethmoid bone. They are divided into following three groups
   a. Anterior group consisting of upto 11 cells
   b. Middle group consisting of 1 to 7 cells
   c. Posterior group also consisting of 1 to 7 cells
   Lateral wall of the sinuses is related to the orbit. The first two groups of air sinuses drain into middle meatus of nasal cavity while the posterior group opens into the posterior part of superior meatus.

3. **Maxillary air sinuses:** It is described below.
4. **Sphenoidal air sinuses:** The right and left sphenoidal sinuses lie within the body of sphenoid. They lie above and behind the nasal cavity and are separated from each other by a thin septum. The two sinuses are usually asymmetrical. Each sinus drains into spheno-ethmoidal recess of the nasal cavity.

Maxillary Air Sinus (Antrum of Highmore)

It is the largest paranasal-air sinus and is present in the body of maxilla, one on either side of the nasal cavity. It drains into the hiatus semilunaris of the middle meatus, in the posterior part.
Measurements

Vertical	:	3.5 cm
Transverse	:	2.5 cm
Antero-posterior	:	3.25 cm

Parts of Maxillary Sinus and Their Relations

Maxillary sinus is pyramidal in shape. It has the following parts
   a. **Roof,** formed by floor of the orbit
   b. **Floor** (is very small), formed by the alveolar process of the maxilla. It lies about 1.25 cm below the floor of the nasal cavity. This level corresponds to the level of ala of nose.

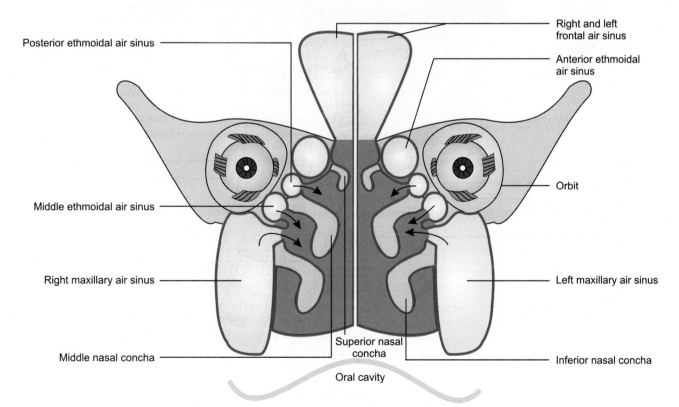

Fig. 12.9: Coronal section of head showing paranasal air sinuses (Diagrammatic representation)

c. **Base,** formed by the nasal surface of body of maxilla. It presents with the opening or ostium of the sinus in its upper part which communicates with the middle meatus.

d. **Apex,** extends into the zygomatic process of maxilla.

e. **Anterior wall** is related to infraorbital plexus of nerves. Within this wall runs the anterior superior alveolar nerve in a bony canal called the **canalis sinuosus.**

f. **Posterior wall** forms the anterior boundary of infratemporal fossa. It is pierced by the posterior superior alveolar nerves.

It is supplied by branches of anterior, middle and posterior superior alveolar arteries which are branches of maxillary artery. It is drained by tributaries of facial vein and pterygoid plexus of veins. Lymphatics from maxillary sinus drain into submandibular lymph nodes. Nerve supply of maxillary sinus is via.

• Anterior, middle and posterior superior alveolar nerves, branches of maxillary nerve.
• Infraorbital nerves.

Functions of Paranasal Sinuses

1. They help in air conditioning of the inhaled air.
2. The air filled spaces help to make the skull lighter.
3. They help to add resonance to the voice.

PHARYNX

Pharynx is a musculo-fascial tube extending from the base of skull to the oesophagus. It is situated behind the nose, mouth and larynx with which it communicates. It acts as a common channel for both deglutition and respiration (Fig. 12.10).

Measurements

Length : 12 to 14 cm
Width : Upper part 3.5 cm, Lower part 1.5 cm

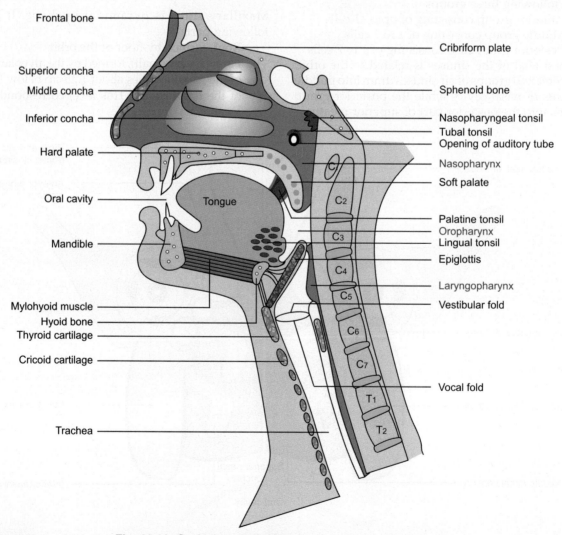

Fig. 12.10: Sagittal section of head and neck showing pharynx

Subdivisions of Pharynx

The pharynx is divided into three parts. From above downwards these are
1. Nasopharynx
2. Oropharynx
3. Laryngopharynx

Nasopharynx (Fig. 12.10)

- Nasopharynx is the part which lies above the soft palate.
- Superiorly, it is limited by the body of sphenoid and basi-occiput.
- It communicates anteriorly with the nasal cavities through posterior nasal apertures.
- Inferiorly, it communicates with the oropharynx at the pharyngeal (nasopharyngeal) isthmus. Pharyngeal isthmus, is an opening bounded anteriorly by the soft palate and posteriorly by the posterior wall of the pharynx.
- Two important structures lie in this part of pharynx. These are
  - **Nasopharyngeal (pharyngeal) tonsil:** It is a median collection of lymphoid tissue beneath the mucous membrane of the roof and the adjoining posterior wall of this region.
  - **Orifices of the pharyngotympanic tube or auditory tube** (Eustachian tube)
    - Each tubal opening lies 1.2 cm behind the level of inferior nasal concha, in the lateral wall of nasopharynx.
    - The upper and posterior margins of this opening are bounded by a tubal elevation which is produced by the collection of lymphoid tissue called the **tubal tonsil.**
  - Two mucous folds extend from this elevation, namely.
    - **Salpingopharyngeal fold:** This extends vertically downwards and fades on the side wall of the pharynx. It contains the salpingopharyngeus muscle
    - **Salpingopalatine fold:** This extends downwards and forwards to the soft palate. It contains the levator palati muscle.
    - There is a deep depression behind the tubal elevation which is known as the **pharyngeal recess or fossa of Rosenmuller.**

Oropharynx (Fig. 12.10)

- Oropharynx extends from the palate above to the tip of epiglottis below.
- It communicates anteriorly with the oral cavity through the oropharyngeal isthmus.

Boundaries of oropharyngeal isthmus

Above : Soft palate
Below : Dorsal surface of the posterior third of the tongue
Lateral, (on each side): Palatoglossal arch, containing the palatoglossus muscle.
The oropharyngeal isthmus is closed during deglutition to prevent regurgitation of food from pharynx into the mouth.
- Inferiorly, it continues with the laryngopharynx at the upper border of epiglottis.
- Posteriorly, oropharynx lies over the C_2 and C_3 vertebrae, separated from them by the retropharyngeal space and its contents.
- Lateral wall of oropharynx presents with the following features on each side.
  - **Tonsillar fossa:** A triangular fossa which lodges the palatine tonsil.
  - **Palato-glossal arch:** Fold of mucus membrane which forms the anterior wall of the fossa. It overlies the palatoglossus muscle
  - **Palato-pharyngeal arch:** Fold of mucus membrane which forms the posterior wall of the fossa. It overlies the palato-pharyngeus muscle. The two arches meet above at the soft palate.

Laryngopharynx (Fig. 12.10)

- Laryngopharynx extends from upper border of the epiglottis to the lower end of pharynx and continues as the oesophagus at the level of C_6 vertebra.
- Its communicates anteriorly in the upper part with the laryngeal cavity through the laryngeal inlet and inferiorly with the oesophagus at the pharyngo-oesophageal junction (the narrowest part of the GIT after appendix).
- Below the laryngeal inlet, its anterior wall is formed by the posterior surfaces of arytenoids and lamina of cricoid cartilages.
- Posteriorly, it overlies the bodies of C_4, C_5 and C_6 vertebra separated from them by the retropharyngeal space.
- **This part presents two important features**
  - **The laryngeal inlet:** Is the opening into the larynx. It is bounded antero-posteriorly by the epiglottis, aryepiglottic folds and inter-arytenoid fold. The laryngeal inlet closes during deglutition to prevent entry of food into the laryngeal cavity by the approximation of the two aryepiglottic folds in midline.
  - **Piriform fossa:** It is a deep recess seen in the inner aspect of the anterior part of lateral wall of laryngopharynx, on each side of the laryngeal inlet. These recesses are produced due to inward

bulging of the lamina of thyroid cartilage on each side of midline into this part of pharynx.

Boundaries of Piriform Fossa

Medial: Aryepiglottic fold.

Lateral: Mucous membrane covering the medial surface of the lamina of thyroid cartilage and thyrohyoid membrane.

Important Feature: The internal laryngeal nerve and superior laryngeal vessels pierce the thyrohyoid membrane and traverse underneath the mucous membrane of the floor of the piriform fossa to reach the medial wall of pharynx.

Structure of the Pharynx

The wall of the pharynx consists of following layers, from within outwards these are

1. Mucosa
2. Submucosa
3. Muscular coat
4. Loose areolar sheath or the buccopharyngeal fascia

Mucosa

The mucosa of pharynx is made up of stratified squamous epithelium except, in the region of nasopharynx where it is lined by ciliated pseudostratified columnar epithelium.

Submucosa

The submucosa is thick and fibrous. It is called the pharyngobasilar fascia.

Muscular Coat

The muscular coat consists of striated muscles which are arranged in an outer circular layer and an inner longitudinal layer. The circular layer comprises of three pairs of constrictors (Fig. 12.11)

1. Superior constrictor
2. Middle constrictor
3. Inferior constrictor

The longitudinal coat comprises of three pairs of longitudinal muscles

1. Stylopharyngeus
2. Palatopharyngeus
3. Salpingopharyngeus

Constrictor Muscles of the Pharynx (Figs 12.11, 12.12)

- Constrictor muscles form the main bulk of the muscular coat of pharyngeal wall.
- They arise from the posterior openings of the nose, mouth and larynx. The fibres pass backwards in a fan-shaped manner into the lateral and posterior walls of the pharynx and get inserted into the

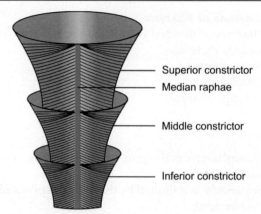

Fig. 12.11: Arrangement of constrictor muscles

median fibrous raphe on the posterior aspect of the pharynx. This raphae extends from the base of the skull (pharyngeal tubercle) to the oesophagus.

- The three constrictor muscles are arranged like flower pots placed one inside the other but are open in front for communication with the nasal, oral and laryngeal cavities. Thus, the inferior constrictor muscle overlaps the middle constrictor which in turn overlaps the superior constrictor muscle (Fig. 12.11).
- The muscles are supplied by pharyngeal branches of cranial root of accessory nerve carried by the vagus nerve. These fibres form a pharyngeal plexus along with branches from glossopharyngeal nerve and superior cervical sympathetic ganglion over the middle constrictor. The latter are sensory to the pharynx and are responsible for the swallowing reflex.
- The inferior constrictor is in addition supplied by the external laryngeal and recurrent laryngeal nerves.

Actions: They aid in deglutition by the coordinated contractions.

Longitudinal Muscles of the Pharynx: These muscles run longitudinally from above downwards to form the longitudinal muscle coat of pharynx (Fig. 12.12).

1. Stylopharyngeus
2. Palatopharyngeus
3. Salpingopharyngeus

Actions: They elevate the larynx and shorten the pharynx during swallowing. At the same time palatopharyngeus acts as a sphincter that closes the pharyngeal isthmus.

Passavant's ridge: Some fibres of palatopharyngeus, arising from the palatine aponeurosis sweep horizontally backwards forming a 'U'-shaped loop within the wall of pharynx underneath the mucosa. This is seen as a raised area called the Passavant's ridge. This U-shaped muscle loop acts as the palato-pharyngeal sphincter.

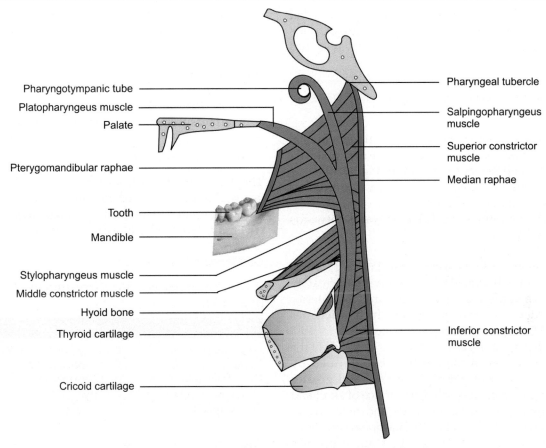

Fig. 12.12: Constrictor and longitudinal muscles of the pharynx

Labels:
- Pharyngotympanic tube
- Platopharyngeus muscle
- Palate
- Pterygomandibular raphae
- Tooth
- Mandible
- Stylopharyngeus muscle
- Middle constrictor muscle
- Hyoid bone
- Thyroid cartilage
- Cricoid cartilage
- Pharyngeal tubercle
- Salpingopharyngeus muscle
- Superior constrictor muscle
- Median raphae
- Inferior constrictor muscle

Loose Areolar Sheath of the Pharynx

A loose areolar membrane also called the 'buccopharyngeal fascia' covers the outer surface of the muscular coat of pharynx. It extends anteriorly across the pterygomandibular raphe to cover the outer surface of the buccinator also.

Nerve Supply of the Pharynx

a. **Motor supply:** All the pharyngeal muscles are supplied by the cranial root of accessory nerve (carried via pharyngeal branch of vagus and pharyngeal plexus) except the stylopharyngeus which is supplied by the glossopharyngeal nerve.

b. **Sensory supply**
   1. Nasopharynx is supplied by pharyngeal branch of the pterygo-palatine ganglion which carries fibres from maxillary division of trigeminal nerve
   2. Oropharynx is supplied by glossopharyngeal nerve
   3. Laryngopharynx is supplied by the internal laryngeal nerve.

Pharyngeal Plexus of Nerves

The pharyngeal plexus of nerves lies between the buccopharyngeal fascia and the muscular coat of middle constrictor.

It is formed by the following nerves
   1. Pharyngeal branch of vagus carrying fibres from cranial part of the accessory nerves.
   2. Pharyngeal branch of the glossopharyngeal nerve.
   3. Pharyngeal branch from superior cervical sympathetic ganglion.

Functions of Pharynx

- Nasopharynx and Oropharynx provide passage for air and helps to maintain the warmth and humidity of the air.
- Oropharynx and Laryngopharynx provide passage for food.
- Nasopharyngeal, tubal and palatine tonsils form a part of Waldeyer's ring (see page no. 472). They guard the respiratory and food passages.
- Pharynx acts as a resonating passage and aids in phonation.

CHAPTER-12

- The eustachian tube open into the nasopharynx and it helps to equalise air pressure in middle ear cavity. This helps in conduction of sound waves and facilitates hearing.

PHARYNGOTYMPANIC TUBE (AUDITORY TUBE) (FIG. 12.13)

- The auditory tube is an osseo-cartilaginous channel which connects the lateral wall of nasopharynx with the middle ear (tympanum) (Fig. 12.13).
- It maintains the equilibrium of air pressure on either side of tympanic membrane.
- It is 4 cm long and is directed downwards, forwards and medially.
- The tube comprises of two parts
  a. **Osseous or bony part:** Forms lateral 1/3rd of the tube. It extends from the tympanic cavity downwards and forwards towards the anterior border of petrous temporal which articulates with the greater wing of sphenoid.
  b. **Cartilaginous part:** Forms anterior 2/3rd of the tube. It lies in the sulcus tubae, formed by articulation of petrous temporal and greater wing of sphenoid on undersurface of skull and runs downwards, forwards and medially to open into the lateral wall of nasopharynx above the superior constrictor. It is made up of a triangular plate of elastic fibrocartilage bent in such a way so that it forms the superior and medial wall of the tube. The infero-lateral gap is filled by a fibrous membrane.

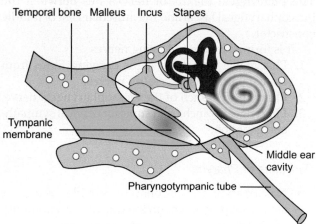

Fig. 12.13: Pharyngotympanic tube

LARYNX

It is situated in the neck and extends from upper border of the epiglottis, at the laryngeal inlet, to the lower border of the cricoid cartilage, at the level of C_6 vertebra. It acts as a watch dog for lower respiratory tract (Fig. 12.14).

It lies under the skin, fascia of neck and the strap muscles of anterior triangle of neck. Posteriorly it is related to laryngopharynx.

Measurement

Length	:	36 to 44 mm
Inner diameter	:	40 to 44 mm

The measurements are greater in males than females.

Structure of Larynx

The skeletal framework of larynx is made up of 9 cartilages which are connected to one another by ligaments and membranes. It is lined by mucus membrane and covered externally by muscles of larynx.

Cartilages of Larynx

It has three paired and three unpaired cartilages (Fig. 12.14).

Paired cartilages	Unpaired cartilages
They are small and comprise of	They are large and comprise of (from above downwards)
1. Arytenoid	1. Epiglottis
2. Corniculate	2. Thyroid
3. Cuneiform	3. Cricoid

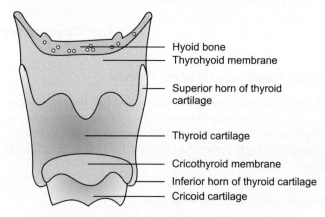

Fig. 12.14: Cartilages of larynx (anterior view)

Epiglottis (Figs 12.15 and 12.17)

- It is a leaf like structure that extends upwards behind the hyoid bone and the base of the tongue.
- The upper broad end is free while the narrow lower end is connected to the posterior surface of the thyroid angle by the thyroepiglottic ligament.
- The anterior surface of epiglottis is connected with the base of tongue by a median and two lateral glosso-epiglottic folds. The depression on each side of the median fold is called as **vallecula.**
- The anterior surface is also connected below to the hyoid bone by the hyo-epiglottic ligament.

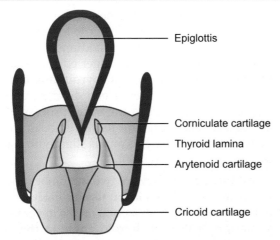

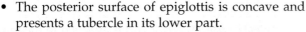

Fig. 12.15: Cartilages of larynx (posterior view)

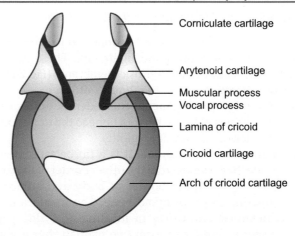

Fig. 12.16: Cartilages of larynx (anterior view)

- The posterior surface of epiglottis is concave and presents a tubercle in its lower part.
- Both the surfaces are covered with mucus membrane.
- The lower part of the lateral border provides attachment to aryepiglottic folds on each side.

Thyroid Cartilage (Figs 12.14 and 12.15)

- It consists of two quadrilateral laminae which are fused anteriorly at an angle called the thyroid angle. The angle measures 90° in males and 120° in females.
- The thyroid angle is more prominent in males and is responsible for a prominence on the front of neck called 'Adam's apple'.
- Upper border, from before backwards is convexoconcave and gives attachment to the thyrohyoid membrane.
- The lower border is straight anteriorly and curves, with concavity downwards, on each side in the posterior part.
- The outer surface can be felt under the skin. The inner surface of the thyroid cartilage is covered with mucus membrane. In the median plane it provides attachment to the following structures on each side of midline. From above downwards these are
  1. Thyroepiglottic ligament
  2. Vestibular ligaments
  3. Vocal ligaments.
- The posterior border of each lamina is free and extends above and below as the superior and inferior horns. It provides a conjoined insertion to following three muscles
  1. Stylopharyngeus
  2. Palatopharyngeus
  3. Salpingopharyngeus
  The lower horns articulate with cricoid cartilage.

Cricoid Cartilage (Figs 12.14 to 12.16)

- The cricoid cartilage is situated at the level of C_6 vertebra and completely encircles the lumen of the larynx. It is shaped like a **signet ring** with a narrow anterior arch and a broad posterior lamina.
- The outer surface of junction of the two parts on each side articulates with the corresponding inferior horn of thyroid cartilage. It can be felt below the thyroid cartilage separated by a groove.
- The inner surface of cartilage is lined by ciliated pseudostratified columnar epithelium.
- The lateral ends of the upper border of posterior lamina of the cartilage present with a convex articular shoulder that articulates with the base of arytenoid cartilages.

Arytenoid Cartilages (Figs 12.15 and 12.16)

- Each arytenoid cartilage is pyramidal in shape and presents, an apex, a base, 2 processes-**muscular** and **vocal** and 3 surfaces–anterolateral, medial and posterior.
- The apex is directed upwards while the base is directed below and is concave. The base articulates with the corresponding lateral end of upper border of lamina of cricoid cartilage.
- The medial surface is directed towards the cavity and lined by mucus membrane.

Corniculate Cartilages (Figs 12.15 to 12.18)

These are tiny cartilages lying in the posterior-inferior part of the aryepiglottic folds, above the apex of the arytenoid.

Cuneiform Cartilages (Figs 12.17 and 12.18)

These are tiny rods of cartilage situated in the aryepiglottic fold anterosuperior to the corniculate cartilages.

CHAPTER-12

Ligaments and Membranes of the Larynx

The cartilages of larynx are interconnected to each other by various membranes and ligaments. These can be divided into extrinsic and intrinsic membranes (Fig 12.17).

Extrinsic ligaments and membranes of larynx

1. **Hyoepiglottic ligament:** This extends from posterior aspect of body of hyoid bone to the upper part of anterior surface of epiglottis.
2. **Thyrohyoid membrane:** It is a fibroelastic membrane that extends from the upper border of thyroid cartilage to upper border of body and adjacent superior cornu of hyoid bone. The membrane is thickened anteriorly in midline and along its posterior border to form one median thyrohyoid ligament and lateral thyrohyoid ligaments on each side.
3. **Thyroepiglottic ligament:** It extends from the lower narrow end of epiglottis to the posterior surface of thyroid angle below thyroid notch and above the vestibular ligament.
4. **Crico-tracheal ligament:** It connects the lower border of anterior arch of cricoid cartilage with the first tracheal ring.

Intrinsic Ligaments and Membranes of Larynx

1. **Cricothyroid membrane/Crico-vocal membrane:** It is made up of yellow elastic tissue. It is attached to the upper border of anterior arch of cricoid cartilage and extends upwards. Anteriorly, the median part of the membrane is thickened and extends from upper border of cricoid cartilage to lower border of thyroid cartilage forming median cricothyroid ligament. Anterior end of upper edge is attached to the posterior surface of thyroid angle in the middle while the posterior end diverges on each side and is attached to the vocal process of the arytenoid cartilage. The upper edge is free in between the attachments and is slightly thickened to form the vocal ligament.

Vocal ligaments: They are two in number and are made up of yellow elastic tissue. Each extends anteroposteriorly from a point on the lower part of posterior surface of thyroid angle to the vocal process of arytenoid cartilage on each side.

2. **Quadrangular membrane:** It is a fibrous sheet extending from epiglottis to the thyroid cartilage. Upper border is free and forms aryepiglottic fold on each side. Anterior end is attached to the lower part of lateral margin of epiglottis and posterior end is illdefined and passes the the upper end of arytenoid cartilage. Its lower edge is also free. The lower edge is attached anteriorly to the inner aspect of thyroid angle above the cricothyroid membrane. Posteriorly, it attaches to the antero-lateral surface of arytenoid cartilage in front of muscular process. This lower edge is slightly thickened to form the vestibular ligament.

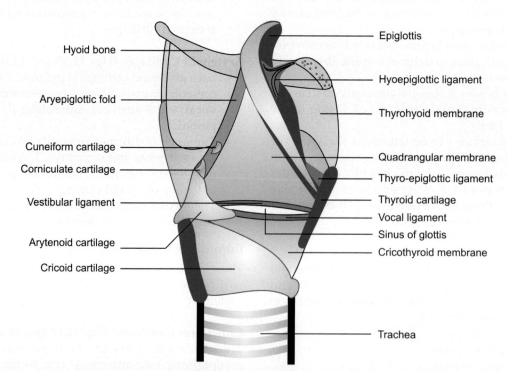

Fig. 12.17: Sagittal section of larynx showing cartilages, ligaments and membranes of larynx

Vestibular ligaments: Each is made up of fibrous tissue and extends anteroposteriorly from a point on posterior surface of the angle of thyroid to the lateral surface of the arytenoid cartilage on each side.

Cavity of the Larynx

It extends from the inlet of larynx to the lower border of cricoid cartilage. The anterior wall of laryngeal cavity is longer than the posterior wall (Fig. 12.18).

Laryngeal Inlet

The inlet to larynx is obliquely placed and slopes downwards and backwards. It opens into the laryngo-pharynx (Fig. 12.18).

Boundaries of Laryngeal Inlet

Anterior : Broad upper end of epiglottis

Posterior : Inter-arytenoid fold of mucous membrane

Lateral : Ary-epiglottic fold of mucous membrane on each side. It over lies the aryepiglottic muscle and has the corniculate and cuneiform cartilages at its posterior end.

Thus, the inlet consist of an anterior (2/3rd) membranous part and a posterior (1/3rd) cartilaginous part.

Inner Aspect of Laryngeal Cavity

The inner aspect of laryngeal cavity is lined by mucous membrane which extends from upper free border of aryepiglottic fold to the lower border of cricoid. Aryepiglottic fold overlies the upper border of quadrangular membrane and has the cuneiform and corniculate cartilages at its posterior end (Fig. 12.18). The lining membrane presents with two folds:

1. **Vestibular folds or false vocal cords:** These are folds of mucus membrane that are produced by the underlying vestibular ligaments. The space between the two vestibular fold is called as **rima vestibuli.** They prevent exit of air from the lungs. Hence, **they act as exit valves.** They are approximated when a person holds his breath after deep inspiration in order to increase the intra thoracic or abdominal pressure as in coughing or defecation.

2. **Vocal folds or true vocal cords:** These are folds of mucus membrane that are produced by the underlying vocal ligaments and lie below the false vocal cords. The space between the right and left vocal folds is called as **'rima glottidis'**

   Rima glottidis: It consists of two parts:
   - **Intermembranous part:** It lies between the two vocal cords, forms anterior 3/5th of rima glottidis.
   - **Intercartilaginous part:** It lies between inner aspect of the vocal process and medial surface

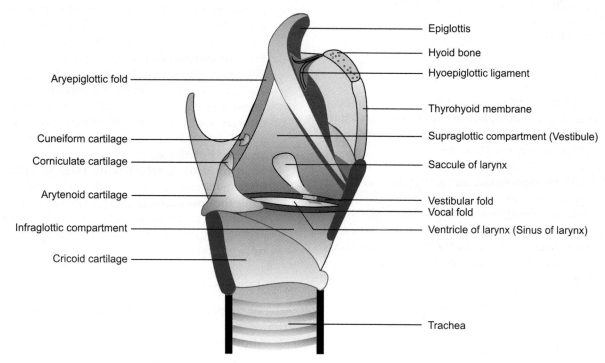

Fig. 12.18: Sagittal section of larynx showing interior aspect

Aryepiglottic fold

Cuneiform cartilage

Corniculate cartilage

Arytenoid cartilage

Infraglottic compartment

Cricoid cartilage

Epiglottis

Hyoid bone

Hyoepiglottic ligament

Thyrohyoid membrane

Supraglottic compartment (Vestibule)

Saccule of larynx

Vestibular fold
Vocal fold

Ventricle of larynx (Sinus of larynx)

Trachea

of arytenoid cartilage on each side, forms posterior 2/5th of rima glottidis.

Vocal cords act as entry valves. They prevent entry of all substances through rima glottis except air. Speech (phonation) is produced by vibrations of the vocal cords. The greater the amplitude of vibration, the louder is the sound. Pitch of sound is controlled by the frequency of the vibrations.

Since the males have longer vocal cords than females, they have louder but low pitched voices than females.

Subdivisions of Laryngeal Cavity

The laryngeal cavity is divided into the following three parts by vestibular and vocal folds:

1. **Vestibule or the supraglottic compartment:** It is the part present between laryngeal inlet and the vestibular folds.
2. **Sinus of larynx or the glottic compartment:** This lies between the vestibular and the vocal folds.
3. **Infraglottic compartment:** It is the area present below the vocal folds.

Epithelial Lining of Larynx

The mucus membrane of larynx primarily consists of ciliated pseudostratified columnar epithelium. The following areas are however, covered by stratified squamous non-keratinized epithelium:

1. Upper part of posterior surface of epiglottis
2. Aryepiglottic folds
3. Vocal folds

Muscles of Larynx

Muscles of larynx can be studied as:

1. Extrinsic muscles of larynx: These muscles attach from neighbouring structures of the neck to the cartilages of larynx. They are
   a. Infra-hyoid muscles of anterior triangle of neck namely, thyrohyoid, sternothyroid and sterno-hyoid muscles.
   b. Inferior constrictor muscle of pharynx.
   c. Stylopharyngeus and palatopharyngeus muscles. The extrinsic muscles move the larynx up and down during swallowing and speech.
2. Intrinsic muscles of larynx: These muscles are present within the larynx it self and act to open or close various parts of laryngeal cavity.

Intrinsic Muscles of the Larynx

The intrinsic muscles of larynx are arranged in the following groups according to their actions.

- **Muscles that open or close the laryngeal inlet**
  1. Oblique arytenoids: Close the inlet of larynx
  2. Aryepiglotticus: Close the inlet of larynx
  3. Thyroepiglotticus: Open the inlet of larynx
- **Muscles that open or close the glottis**
  1. Posterior cricoarytenoids: Open the glottis
  2. Lateral cricoarytenoids: Close the glottis
  3. Transverse arytenoids: Close the glottis
- **Muscles that increase or decrease the tension of vocal cords.**
  1. Cricothyroid: Tense the vocal cords
  2. Thyroarytenoid: Relax the vocal cords
  3. Vocalis: Tense the vocal cords.

All the intrinsic muscles of the larynx are supplied by the recurrent laryngeal nerve except cricothyroid which is supplied by external laryngeal nerve.

Various Positions of Rima-glottidis

The positions of membranous and cartilagenous parts of rima-glottidis varies with different functions. These are described below:

1. **Position during normal respiration (Fig. 12.19A):** The inter membranous part is triangular in shape while the inter cartilaginous part is rectangular. The vocal process of arytenoid cartilages are parallel to each other.
2. **Position during forced inspiration (Fig. 12.19B):** The rima-glottidis widens to form a diamond shaped cavity. The intermembranous and inter-cartilaginous parts appear triangular. The action of posterior cricoarytenoid muscles abducts and rotates the arytenoids laterally.
3. **Position during phonation or speech (Fig. 12.19C):** The intermembranous and intercartilaginous parts are adducted to reduced the rima-glottidis to a linear fissure. Action of lateral cricoarytenoid muscles and transverse arytenoid muscles bring about adduction and medial rotation of the arytenoid cartilages.
4. **Position during whispering (Fig. 12.19D):** The intermembranous part is adducted and narrow while the inter-cartilaginous part is widened. Action of lateral cricoarytenoid muscles rotates the arytenoid cartilages that closes the anterior part of rima-glottidis.

Blood Supply of Larynx

Arterial supply of larynx is derived from the following arteries:

1. **Above the vocal folds:** It is supplied by superior laryngeal artery, a branch of superior thyroid artery.
2. **Below the vocal folds:** Is is supplied by inferior laryngeal artery, a branch of inferior thyroid artery.

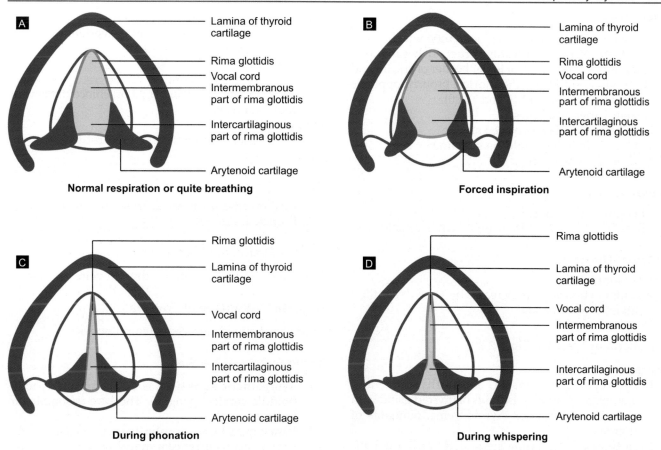

Fig. 12.19: Various positions of vocal cords and shapes of rima glottidis

The veins run along with the arteries. Superior laryngeal vein drains into superior thyroid vein and inferior laryngeal vein drains into inferior thyroid vein.

Lymphatic Drainage of Larynx

The lymphatics from larynx pass to the following lymph nodes:
1. **Above the vocal cords:** Lymphatics run along the superior thyroid vessels and drain into antero-superior group of deep cervical lymph nodes.
2. **Below the vocal cords:** It drains into postero-inferior group of cervical lymph nodes.

Nerve Supply of the Larynx

1. **Motor supply:** All the intrinsic muscles of the larynx are supplied by the recurrent laryngeal nerve except cricothyroid which is supplied by external laryngeal nerve.
2. **Sensory supply:** The mucous membrane of larynx is supplied by two nerves:

a. **Above the vocal folds:** It is supplied by the internal laryngeal nerve, a branch of superior laryngeal nerve.
b. **Below the vocal folds:** It is supplied by recurrent laryngeal nerve.

Functions of Larynx

- Larynx primarily functions as an air passage that allows only entry of air and prevents entry of food particles or any foreign body. Closure of laryngeal inlet is brought about by approximation of aryepiglottic folds overlapped by epiglottis. Closure of laryngeal cavity is brought about by approximation of vocal cords.
- **Vestibular cords act as exit valves.** The approximation of these cords helps to hold breath after deep inspiration that result in increase intra abdominal pressure. This is essential to complete the act of micturition, defeaction and parturition (child birth).
- **Function of phonation** is brought about by vibrations of vocal cords during expiration.

TRACHEA

It is a wide membrano-cartilaginous tube which forms part of the upper respiratory tract. It begins as a continuation of the larynx at lower border of cricoid and ends by dividing into right and left bronchi opposite the sternal angle (Figs 12.10 and 12.20).

Its extent varies as follows:
1. C_6 to T_4 in cadavers placed supine
2. C_6 to T_6 in living adults on standing
3. C_6 to T_3 in newborn

Measurements

Length	:	10 cm
Breadth	:	2 cm in male, 1.5 cm in female

Internal Diameter

- 12 mm in adult
- 3 mm in newborn. It increases by 1mm /year till it attains the adult size.

Relations of Trachea (Fig. 12.20)

Anterior
1. **In neck:** Skin, fascia, sternothyroid and sternohyoid muscles, isthmus of thyroid gland with superior and inferior thyroid veins, remnants of thymus
2. **In thorax:** Manubrium sterni, left brachiocephalic vein, proximal part of brachiocephalic and left common carotid arteries, deep cardiac plexus, arch of aorta at lower end.

Posterior
1. Esophagus, separates it from the vertebral column.
2. Left recurrent laryngeal nerve.

On Right Side
1. Right lung and pleura.
2. Superior vena cava and right brachiocephalic vein.
3. Right vagus nerve.

On Left Side
1. Arch of aorta and left common carotid artery.
2. Left lung.

Arterial Supply of Trachea

1. **Inferior thyroid arteries:** This is the main supply.
2. Bronchial arteries.

Venous Drainage of Trachea

Trachea is drained by inferior thyroid veins.

Lymphatic Drainage of Trachea

Pretracheal and paratracheal lymph nodes.

Nerve Supply of Trachea

1. **Sympathetic supply:** It is derived from T_1 to T_5 (middle cervical ganglia). They are vasomotor in function.
2. **Parasympathetic supply:** It is derived from the vagus and recurrent laryngeal nerves. The fibres are motor to tracheal muscles, secretomotor to glands and sensory to the mucus membrane of trachea.

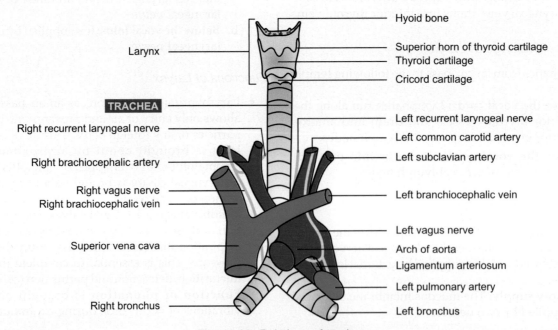

Larynx
TRACHEA
Right recurrent laryngeal nerve
Right brachiocephalic artery
Right vagus nerve
Right brachiocephalic vein
Superior vena cava
Right bronchus

Hyoid bone
Superior horn of thyroid cartilage
Thyroid cartilage
Cricord cartilage
Left recurrent laryngeal nerve
Left common carotid artery
Left subclavian artery
Left branchiocephalic vein
Left vagus nerve
Arch of aorta
Ligamentum arteriosum
Left pulmonary artery
Left bronchus

Fig. 12.20: Relations of trachea

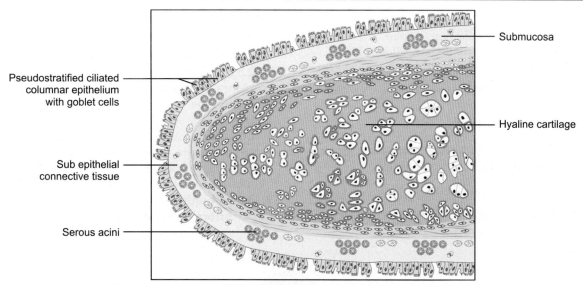

Fig. 12.21: Transverse section of trachea (Stain-hematoxylin-eosin under low magnification)

Structure of Trachea (Fig. 12.21)

- Trachea consists of 16 to 20 C-shaped cartilaginous rings with fibrous tissue, smooth muscle fibres and mucous membrane.
- The mucous membrane consists of pseudostratified ciliated columnar epithelium with goblet cells lying on a layer of connective tissue.
- Subepithelial connective tissue contains serous glands and elastic fibres. Numerous aggregations of lymphoid tissue are present in the subepithelial connective tissue.
- The outermost layer consists of C-shaped rings of hyaline cartilage bridged by fibrous tissue posteriorly to complete the circle.
- In between two rings the gap is filled by circularly arranged smooth muscle fibres.

BRONCHIAL TREE

Trachea ends by dividing into two principal bronchi (Primary pulmonary bronchi), right and left bronchi.

Each principal bronchus divides at the hilum of the corresponding lung giving rise to lobar bronchi (secondary pulmonary bronchi). Right bronchus gives rise to superior, middle and inferior lobar bronchi while left bronchus gives rise to superior and inferior lobar bronchi.

Each lobar bronchus gives rise to segmental or tertiary pulmonary bronchi. The tertiary bronchi divide further into successive generations of smaller bronchi and bronchioles within the parenchyma of lung.

Differences between right and left bronchus

Right Bronchus	Left Bronchus
1. It is wider and shorter	1. It is narrower and longer
2. Extra pulmonary part– it is 2.5 cm in length	2. Extra pulmonary part—it is 5 cm in length
3. It is more vertical and makes an angle of 25° with median plane	3. It is more oblique and makes an angle of 45° with median plane
4. It enters hilum at level of T_5 vertebra	4. It enters hilum at level of T_6 vertebra
5. Within the lung root, pulmonary artery is present anteriorly to the bronchus. Bronchus divides into an upper-eparterial branch and a lower hyparterial branch under the artery.	5. The bronchus passes behind and below the pulmonary artery without dividing
6. Intrapulmonary part: It divides into superior, middle and inferior lobar bronchi	6. Intrapulmonary part: It divides into superior and inferior lobar branches

Each principal bronchus gives rise to 23 generations of bronchi and bronchioles. The 16th generation bronchioles are known as terminal bronchioles which gives rise to respiratory bronchioles (17th to 22nd generation). The respiratory bronchioles gives rise to alveolar ducts and alveoli (alveolar sacs).

CHAPTER-12

LUNG

Lung is the organ of respiration. A pair of lungs are present in the thoracic cavity (Figs 12.22 and 12.23) .

Each lung is enveloped by double layer serous membrane known as pleura.

Anatomical Features of Lung

Color: Lungs are rosy pink in new born and dark gray in adults due to deposits of carbon particles.

Texture: They are elastic and spongy.

Shape: Each lung is conical in shape with one side flattened.

Presenting Parts

1. **Apex:** It is the rounded upper end of lung which extends above the anterior end of 1st rib to about 2.5 cm above the clavicle. It is covered by cervical pleura and further externally by the suprapleural membrane.
2. **Base:** It is semilunar in shape and is concave downwards as it rests on the dome of diaphragm. On right side, the right lobe of liver lies below the diaphragm and on the left side are present the left lobe of liver, fundus of stomach and spleen.
3. **Three borders**
   a. **Anterior border:** It is thin and lies in the costomediastinal recess of pleura. Below the 4th

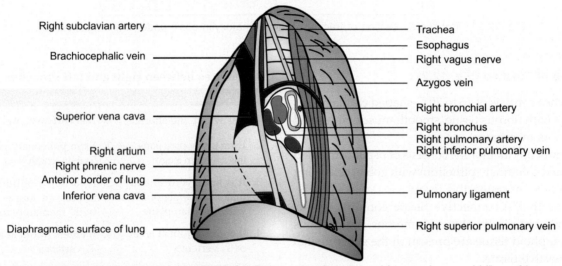

Fig. 12.22: Medial (mediastinal) surface of right lung showing visceral impressions and hilum of lung

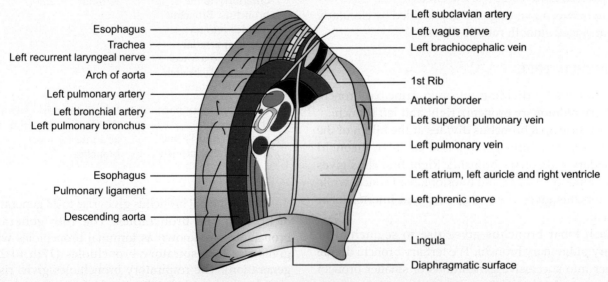

Fig. 12.23: Medial (mediastinal) surface of left lung showing visceral impressions and hilum of lung

costal cartilage on left side it presents with a cardiac notch to accommodate the heart.

   b. **Posterior border:** It is thick and rounded. It extends from above downwards along the anterior surfaces of the heads of 1st to 10th ribs. It is related to the sympathetic trunk with the splanchnic nerves posteriorly.

   c. **Inferior border:** It is the border external to the base which separates it from upper surface of lung.

4. **Two surfaces**

   a. **Costal surface:** It is the outer smooth and convex surface of the lung covered by the costal pleura. It is related to inner surfaces of the ribs and the costal cartilages with intervening intercostal spaces. The ribs form their impressions on the lung.

   b. **Medial surface:** It is divided into two parts

      i. **Anterior or mediastinal surface:** It is concave medially.

      ii. **Posterior or vertebral surface:** This lies behind the esophagus and is flat. It is related to the sides of vertebral bodies upto T_{10}, intervertebral discs, origin of posterior intercostal vessels and splanchnic nerves.

Mediastinal Surface of Lung

• The characteristic feature of mediastinal surface of lung is the hilum present in the posterior half. Hilum is a roughly triangular area that gives passage to the bronchi, pulmonary and bronchial vessels, nerves and lymphatics.

• The mediastinal pleura at the hilum forms a tubular sheath which connects the hilum to the mediastinum. This is called the root of lung.

Contents of Root of Lung

1. Bronchus
2. Pulmonary artery: Single
3. Pulmonary vein: Two are present
4. Bronchial arteries
5. Bronchial veins
6. Pulmonary plexus of nerves
7. Bronchopulmonary lymph nodes
8. Areolar tissue

Arrangement of structures with in the root or hilum of lung (Figs 12.22, 12.23). From before backwards

1. Superior pulmonary vein
2. Pulmonary artery
3. Bronchus with its vessels

Impressions and Relations of Mediastinal Surface

These occur due to various mediastinal structures which lie in relation to this surface of the lung. The pleura separates these structures from the lung (Figs 12.22, 12.23).

Right lung	Left lung
— Anterior surface of right auricle	— Left atrium and left auricle
— Right atrium	— Anterior surface of right ventricle
— Part of right ventricle	— Phrenic nerve
— Phrenic nerve	— Pulmonary trunk
— Superior vena cava	— Arch of aorta
— Origin of right brachiocephalic vein	— Subclavian artery
— Azygos vein-arches over the hilum	— Esophagus
— Origin of right subclavian artery	— Descending thoracic aorta
— Trachea	— Esophagus, inferiorly
— Esophagus	

Lobes of Lung

The right lung is divided into three lobes by an oblique and a horizontal fissure. The left lung is however divided into two lobes by a single oblique fissure.

Right Lung	Left Lung
1. Upper lobe	1. Upper lobe
2. Middle lobe	2. Lower lobe
3. Lower lobe	

Lingula of Left Lung

It is a tongue shaped projection of lung below the cardiac notch.

Arterial Supply of Lung

Lung is supplied by bronchial and pulmonary arteries.

1. **Bronchial arteries:** These arteries supply lung upto respiratory bronchioles and then anastomose with pulmonary arteries.

   a. Right bronchial artery: Is single and is a branch of the 3rd posterior intercostal artery or upper left bronchial artery.

   b. Left bronchial arteries: Are two in number and arise from the descending thoracic aorta.

2. **Pulmonary arteries:** These carry deoxygenated blood from the right side of heart to the alveoli for exchange of gases, i.e., oxygenation. Pulmonary trunk is the continuation of infundibulum of right ventricle and divides into right and left pulmonary arteries which enter the respective lungs at the hilum. The branches of pulmonary arteries supply alveoli and anastomose with bronchial arteries.

Venous Drainage of Lung

Lung is drained by bronchial and pulmonary veins

1. **Bronchial veins:** They have two parts

   a. **Superficial bronchial veins:** These drain the pleura and the extra pulmonary bronchi. On right side they end in the azygos vein and on left side they end in left superior intercostal vein or hemiazygos vein.

b. Deep bronchial veins drain rest of the bronchial tree and the lung parenchyma. They open into pulmonary veins.

2. **Pulmonary veins:** These are formed by confluence of pulmonary capillaries. Two pulmonary veins arise from each lung and drain into the left atrium of the heart.

Lymphatic Drainage of Lung

The lymph from both the lungs is drained into respective bronchopulmonary lymph nodes present at the hilum of lung.

Nerve Supply of Lung

1. **Parasympathetic supply:** It is derived from vagus nerve. The fibres are motor to bronchial muscles, and secretomotor to glands of bronchial tree. They also convey sensory fibres for stretch and cough reflex. Parasympathetic stimulation causes broncho constriction.

2. **Sympathetic supply:** Preganglionic fibres are derived from spinal segments of T_2 to T_5. Their action is opposite to the parasympathetic and causes broncho dilatation.

The parasympathetic and sympathetic fibres form anterior and posterior pulmonary plexus in front and behind the lung roots respectively on each side.

BRONCHO-PULMONARY SEGMENTS

Broncho-pulmonary segment is the independent functional unit of lung made up of a tertiary bronchus with its bronchial tree up to the alveoli accompanied by

an independent branch from pulmonary artery. The venous drainage is however intersegmental (Figs 12.24 to 12.26). **Each lung has ten broncho-pulmonary segments.**

Right lung segments	Left lung segments
1. **Upper lobe**	1. **Upper lobe**
— Apical	— Apical
— Posterior	— Posterior
— Anterior	— Anterior
	— Upper lingual
	— Lower lingual
2. **Middle lobe**	2. **Lower lobe**
— Medial	— Apical
— Lateral	— Medial basal
3. **Lower lobe**	— Anterior basal
— Apical	— Lateral basal
— Medial basal	— Posterior basal
— Anterior basal	
— Lateral basal	
— Posterior basal	

Structure of Lung

The lung parenchyma is made up of the broncho-pulmonary tree accompanied by branches of pulmonary artery and tributaries of pulmonary veins with associated lymphatics and nerves enclosed in a connective tissue framework.

Each lung is enclosed within a serous membrane, the visceral peritoneum. Underlying the serosal membrane is a layer of connective tissue. A number of trabeculae extend from the connective tissue layer into the substance of lung dividing it into lobules. These trabeculae carry the bronchioles and their vessels.

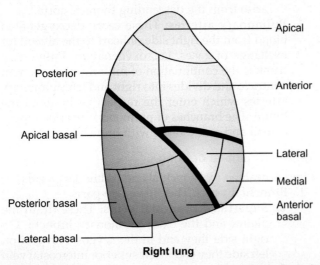

Right lung

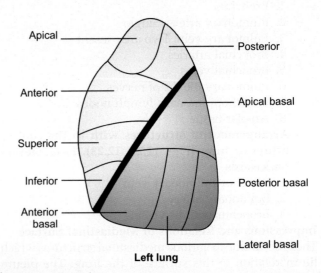

Left lung

Fig. 12.24: Broncho-pulmonary segments

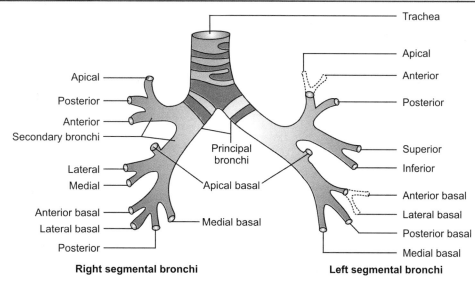

Trachea

Apical
Posterior
Anterior
Secondary bronchi

Principal
bronchi

Apical basal

Lateral
Medial

Anterior basal
Lateral basal
Medial basal
Posterior

Apical
Anterior
Posterior

Superior
Inferior

Anterior basal
Lateral basal
Posterior basal
Medial basal

Right segmental bronchi   **Left segmental bronchi**

Fig. 12.25: Segmental bronchi or tertiary bronchi

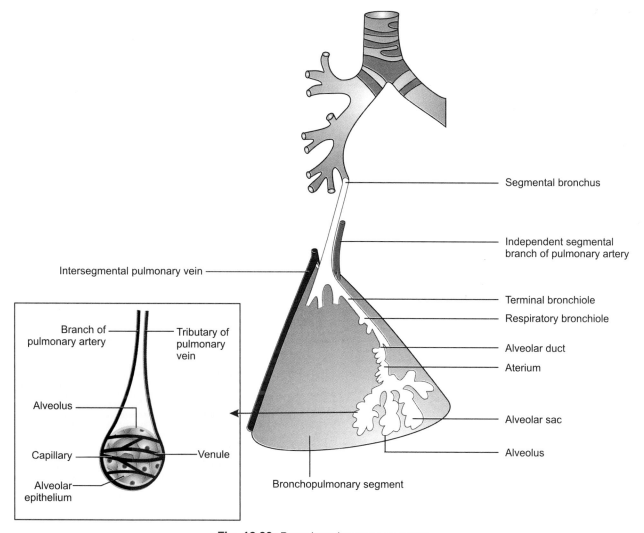

Segmental bronchus

Independent segmental
branch of pulmonary artery

Intersegmental pulmonary vein

Terminal bronchiole
Respiratory bronchiole
Alveolar duct
Aterium

Alveolar sac

Alveolus

Branch of
pulmonary artery

Tributary of
pulmonary
vein

Alveolus

Capillary

Venule

Alveolar
epithelium

Bronchopulmonary segment

Fig. 12.26: Bronchopulmonary segment

CHAPTER-12

Characteristic histological features of different parts of airway present in the lung (Fig. 12.27)

Feature	Intrapulmonary bronchus	Bronchiole	Terminal bronchiole	Respiratory bronchiole	Alveoli
1. Epithelium	Ciliated columnar pseudostratified with goblet cells	Simple columnar with goblet cells	Simple cuboidal, goblet cells are rare	Low cuboidal. No goblet cells	Simple squamous type with pneumocyte type I and type II cells
2. Subepithelial connective tissue	Present as a thick layer. Has mucus glands	Present but there are no glands	Decreased in thickness. No glands	Very thin No glands	Predominantly made of elastic fibres and capillaries
3. Cartilage	A complete ring of cartilage is present	No cartilage	No cartilage	No cartilage	No cartilage
4. Smooth muscle	Several layers of smooth muscle fibres are present	Smooth muscle content is relatively high	Gradual decrease in smooth muscle fibres	Not present or only few fibres are seen	No smooth muscle fibres present

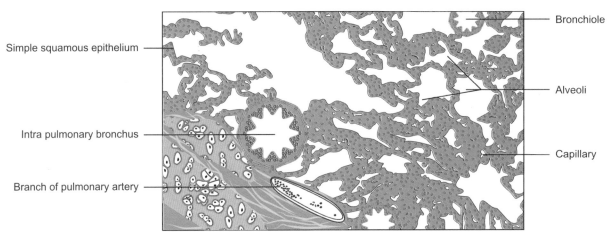

Simple squamous epithelium

Intra pulmonary bronchus

Branch of pulmonary artery

Bronchiole

Alveoli

Capillary

Fig. 12.27: Histology of lung (Stain—hematoxylin-eosin under low magnification)

On microscopy lung parenchyma is made up of clusters of alveolar sac and ducts. Interspersed between the alveoli are present respiratory bronchioles, terminal bronchioles, bronchioles and intrapulmonary bronchi. Branches of pulmonary arteries and veins are seen along the bronchi and bronchioles (Figs 12.25 and 12.26).

Alveolar sacs are surrounded by pulmonary capillaries. Exchange of gases occurs across the alveolo—capillary membrane made up of (Figs 12.26 to 12.28):

1. Epithelium of alveoli: It consists of flat, squamous, epithelium.
2. Basement membrane of epithelium.
3. Basement membrane of endothelium.
4. Endothelial cells of pulmonary capillary.

Structure of alveoli: Alveoli are lined by two types of cells:

1. **Pneumocyte-I:** These are the most common cells making the basic structure of alveoli. They are flattened squamous cells.

2. **Pneumocyte-II:** These are rounded cells present in between the squamous cell. They bear microvilli and secrete surfactant.

The connective tissue between alveoli has lymphocytes, macrophages, mast cells, plasma cells and fibroblasts.

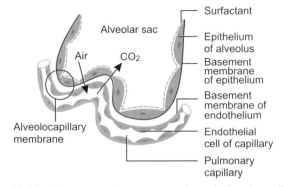

Alveolar sac

Air

CO$_2$

Alveolocapillary membrane

Surfactant

Epithelium of alveolus

Basement membrane of epithelium

Basement membrane of endothelium

Endothelial cell of capillary

Pulmonary capillary

Fig. 12.28: Diagrammatic representation of alveolocapillary membrane

Functions of Lung and Tracheo-bronchial Tree

- Lung is the organ of exchange of gases, i.e., oxygen and carbondioxide which provides for oxygenation of blood.
- Surfactant secreted by pneumocyte-II of alveoli prevents the collapse of alveoli. This maintains patency of alveoli and allows for exchange of gases to occur during inspiration and expiration.

Defence Mechanisms of Respiratory System

- Mucus secreted by goblet cells of upper respiratory tract helps to entrap foreign particles. The cilia of epithelium beat upwards and push the mucus towards the nose and exterior.
- Mucus also contains IgA antibodies that provide local immunity.
- Alveolar macrophages engulf foreign particles and destroy them by phagocytosis.
- Preventing reflexes like cough reflex, sneezing reflex and bronchoconstriction reflex help to clear the passage from inhaled foreign particles. The afferents of the reflex arise from irritant receptors present in the tracheo bronchial tree and travel in the vagus nerve.

Non-respiratory Functions of Lung

- Angiotensin converting enzyme is present in pulmonary capillary endothelium. This converts angiotensin-I to angiotensin-II which is responsible for maintenance of blood pressure.
- APUD cells or neuro-endocrine cells are present in the bronchiolar tree. They produce various vasoactive substances like VIP and substance P which may have a role in maintaining tone of bronchioles.
- Lung contains tissue type plasminogen activator which converts plasminogen to plasmin. Thus, it has a role in fibrinolytic mechanism of the body.

PLEURA

It is a closed serous sac which is invaginated from the medial side by two lungs. This invagination leads to formation of two layers of pleura over the lung namely, visceral pleura and parietal pleura with a potential space between these two layers. This space is known as pleural cavity.

Visceral Pleura

It is also known as the pulmonary pleura. It is attached with the connective tissue of lung and can not be separated from it. It invests the entire lung except at two areas (Fig. 12.29).

1. The hilum
2. Area of attachment of pulmonary ligament.

Parietal Pleura

The visceral pleura reflects over itself at the hilum to form an external layer covering the lung known as parietal pleura. For the purpose of description parietal pleura is divided into different parts according to the place where it is present.

1. **Cervical pleura (Figs 12.29 to 12.31):** This covers the apex of the lung. It continues as the mediastinal pleura medially and the costal pleura inferiorly. It is covered by Sibson's fascia or suprapleural membrane externally.
2. **Costal pleura (Figs 12.29 to 12.31):** It covers the major surfaces of lung. It is present inner to sternum, ribs with intercostal spaces and lateral sides of vertebral bodies.
   Vertical extent: It continues upwards as the cervical pleura. Inferiorly, it is reflected over the diaphragm at the base of lung along the line of costo-diaphragmatic reflection.
   Horizontal extent: In the median plane it continues as mediastinal pleura behind the sternum along the costo mediastinal reflection. Laterally, it passes along the curve of lungs, inner to the endothoracic fascia lining the ribs and intercostal spaces. Posteriorly at the side of vertebral column, it continues medially with the mediastinal pleura along the costo vertebral reflection.
3. **Mediastinal pleura:** It covers the medial side of lung and forms the lateral boundary of the mediastinum on either side. At the hilum, mediastinal pleura encloses various structures at the root of lung in a tubular fashion. It is reflected onto the lung as the visceral pleura at hilum of lung.
   Structures enclosed by the pleura at the hilum- From before backwards
   a. Pulmonary vein

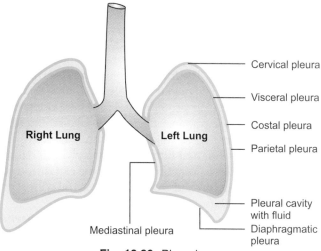

Fig. 12.29: Pleural sac

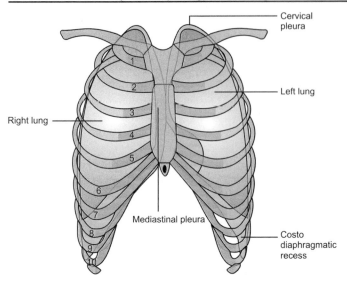

Fig. 12.30: Extent of pleura and lung in respect of ribs and costal cartilages (anterior aspect)

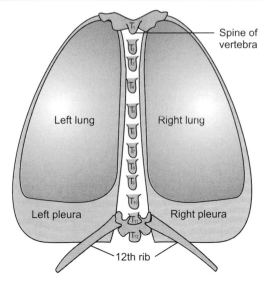

Fig. 12.31: Extent of pleura and lung (posterior aspect)

b. Pulmonary artery
c. Bronchus with its vessels
4. **Diaphragmatic Pleura:** It covers the base of lung, over the diaphragm and is reflected over the lateral surface of lung along the costo-diaphragmatic reflection.

Sites of Extension of Pleura Beyond the Thoracic Cavity (Fig. 12.31)

1. Right costo-xiphoid junction
2. Right and left costo-vertebral angles
3. Cervical pleura which extends into the root of neck
   At these sites it does not cover the lung and is not within the thoracic cage. Hence, is known as **naked pleura.**

Recesses of the Pleura (Fig. 12.30)

These act as reserve spaces for expansions of lungs.
1. **Costodiaphragmatic recess:** It is the potential space between the lower limit of pleural sac and the lower border of lung. The lower limit of lungs is however 6th rib in midclavicular line, 8th rib in midaxillary line and 10th rib posteriorly. However, along the costo diaphragmatic reflection the pleura extends upto 8th rib in midclavicular line, 10th rib in midaxillary line and 12the rib posteriorly. Therefore this provides a potential space for the expansion of lung during forceful respiration. It is the widest at the midaxillary line.
2. **Costomediastinal recess:** This recess is present along the anterior costomediastinal reflection of pleura. It is maximal in region of cardiac notch.

Blood Supply of Pleura

1. **Pulmonary pleura:** It is supplied by bronchial vessels.
2. **Parietal pleura:** It receives blood via intercostal, internal thoracic and musculophrenic arteries. Corresponding veins drain the pleura.

Lymphatic Drainage of Pleura

1. **Pulmonary pleura:** It is drained by bronchopulmonary lymph nodes.
2. **Parietal pleura:** The lymph drains into the intercostal, internal mammary, posterior mediastinal and diaphragmatic nodes.

Nerve Supply of Pleura

1. **Pulmonary pleura:** It has same nerve supply as lung
2. **Parietal pleura:** It is supplied by intercostal nerves and is pain sensitive.

Pleural Cavity

It is the potential space between the two pleurae which contains a thin layer of lubricating serous fluid. The intrapleural pressure is – 2 mm Hg during expiration and – 6 mm Hg during inspiration. This prevents collapse of lung parenchyma and also aids in the venous return of body.

THORACIC CAGE

It consists of an osseo-cartilaginous framework which encloses the thoracic cavity (Fig. 12.32).

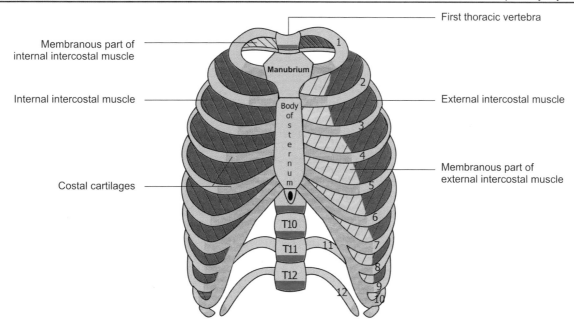

Fig. 12.32: Thoracic cage with intercostal muscles

Boundaries of Thoracic Cage

Anterior
1. Sternum made up of manubrium, body of sternum, xiphoid process.
2. Anterior part of ribs and their costal cartilages.

Posterior
1. Bodies of twelve thoracic vertebrae and their intervening discs.
2. Posterior part of ribs.

On each side
1. Twelve ribs, their cartilages.
2. Intercostal spaces.

Superiorly: Inlet of thorax is reniform in shape and is formed by upper borders of manubrium, first rib and first thoracic vertebra. It continues above with the neck.

Inferiorly: Thoracic outlet is wider than the inlet and is bounded by coastal margin, lower border of 11th and 12th ribs and lower border of 12th thoracic vertebra. It is separated from the abdomen by the muscular sheet known as diaphragm.

Functions of Thoracic Cage

1. This osseocartilaginous cage with its muscular attachments is responsible for the movements of respiration.
2. It protects the vital organs namely, lungs and heart.

Intercostal Spaces

The space between two adjacent ribs is known as intercostal space. There are 11 intercostal spaces on each side of the thorax. The 3rd, 4th, 5th and 6th intercostal spaces are typical in nature because their contents are limited within the thorax (Fig. 12.33).

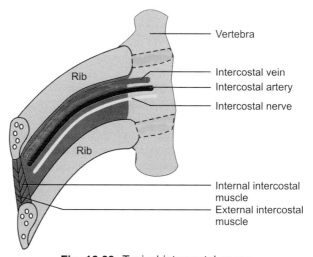

Fig. 12.33: Typical intercostal space

Contents of intercostal spaces
1. Intercostal muscles
2. Intercostal arteries: There are two anterior and one posterior intercostal arteries in each space.
3. Intercostal veins: The veins run along with the corresponding arteries.
4. Intercostal nerves: One intercostal nerve is present in each space and is the continuation of the ventral ramus of the corresponding thoracic spinal nerve.

Intercostal Muscles

Each is supplied by the corresponding intercostal nerve.

1. **External intercostal muscle:** Major part is fleshy. It arises from lower border of the rib above the space

and inserted on the outer lip of the upper border of the rib below.

Action: Helps in inspiration by elevating the ribs.

2. **Internal intercostal muscle:** It is fleshy anteriorly. It arises from the floor of the costal groove of the rib above and inserted on the inner lip of the upper border of the rib below.

Action: Helps in expiration by depressing the ribs.

3. **Inner intercostal:** It occupies the middle 2/4th of a typical inter-costal space and is absent in 1st and 2nd spaces. It arises from middle two-fourth of the ridge above the costal goove and inserted on inner lip of the upper border of the rib below.

Action: Helps in expiration by depressing the ribs.

Intercostal Arteries

There are anterior and posterior intercostal arteries in each space. They anastomose with each other at the junction of anterior 1/3rd and posterior 2/3rd (Fig. 12.34).

• There are two anterior intercostal arteries in each space. One is present along the lower border of upper rib and the other runs along the upper border of lower rib.

• 1st to 6th anterior intercostal arteries arise from internal thoracic artery.

• 7th, 8th and 9th anterior intercostal arteries arise from musculophrenic artery which is a terminal branch of the internal thoracic artery.

• The 1st and 2nd posterior intercostal arteries arise from the costocervical trunk of subclavian artery.

• The 3rd to 11th posterior intercostal arteries are branches of descending aorta.

Intercostal Veins

• Anterior and posterior intercostal veins are present alongwith the corresponding arteries.

• Anterior intercostal veins from 1st to 6th space drain into internal thoracic vein and from 7th to 9th space drain into the musculophrenic vein.

• 1st posterior intercostal veins drain into corresponding brachiocephalic vein. 2nd, 3rd, 4th left posterior intercostal veins join to form superior intercostal vein whcih drains into left brachiocephalic vein. 2nd to 11th right posterior intercostal veins drain into the azygos vein and 5th to 11th posterior intercostal veins drain into hemiazygos and accessory azygos veins.

Intercostal Nerves (Fig. 12.35)

One intercostal nerve is present in each space on each side. They arise as the ventral ramus of the corresponding thoracic nerve. Each nerve arises from the corresponding intervertebral foramina. It runs along with the vascular bundle in between the costal pleura and posterior intercostal membrane and then it lies in the costal groove. The neurovascular bundle consists of the vein superiorly and nerve inferiorly with the artery in between.

Branches

1. Collateral branch.
2. Lateral cutaneous branch.
3. Ganglionic branch: To sympathetic ganglion.
4. Anterior cutaneous nerve.
5. Muscular branches: These supply the corresponding intercostal muscles.

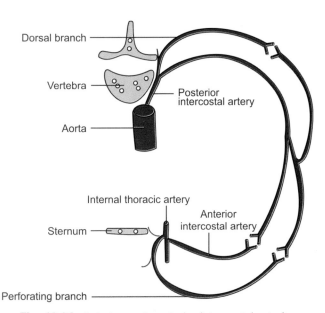

Fig. 12.34: Anterior and posterior intercostal arteries

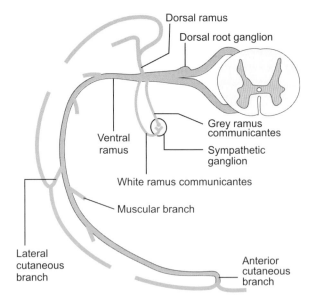

Fig. 12.35: Typical thoracic spinal nerve

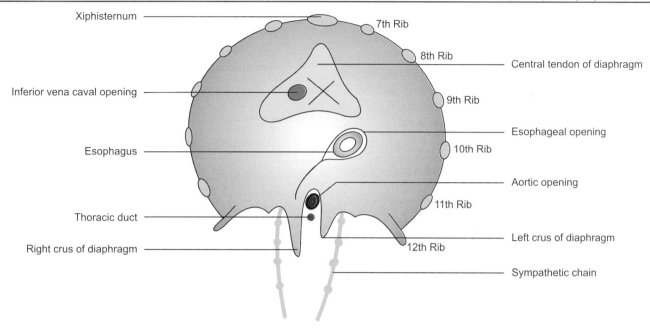

Fig. 12.36: Thoraco-abdominal diaphragm

DIAPHRAGM (FIG. 12.36)

Diaphragm is a dome shaped musculoaponeurotic structure which separates the thoracic and abdominal cavities. It also is an important muscle of respiration.
Origin: Diaphragm originates from sternum, ribs and vertebral column

1. **Sternal origin:** By two fleshy slips from the back of xiphoid process.
2. **Costal origin:** From inner surfaces of lower 6 ribs and costal cartilages.
3. **Vertebral origin:** It arises in the form of a pair of crura. Right crus extends from anterior surface of bodies of L_1, L_2 and L_3 vertebrae and their corresponding intervertebral discs. Left crus is attached to bodies of L_1 and L_2 vertebrae and the intervertebral disc. Both are united to each other in centre across aorta with the help of median arcuate ligament. Right crus is longer than the left.

Insertion: The fibres of diaphragm converge to form a central tendon.

It is shaped like a trefoil leaf and presents with median, right and left leaflets. The central tendon is fused to the pericardium above and is placed anteriorly, close to sternum.

Nerve Supply of Diaphragm

1. Motor supply is from phrenic nerve (C_3, C_4, C_5).
2. Sensory supply is from phrenic nerve and lower 6 intercostal nerves.
3. Sympathetic supply is via inferior phrenic plexus.

Openings in Diaphragm

Opening	Structures passing through
1. **Vena caval opening** It lies at the level of T_8 vertebra	1. Inferior vana cava 2. Right phrenic nerve 3. Lymph vessels of liver
2. **Esophageal opening** It lies at the level of T_{10} vertebra	1. Esophagus 2. Anterior and posterior vagal trunks 3. Esophageal branch of left gastric artery 4. Tributries of left gastric vein 5. Lymphatic from liver 6. Phrenico-esophageal ligament
3. **Aortic opening** It lies at the level of T_{12} vertebra	1. Abdominal aorta 2. Thoracic duct 3. Azygos vein
4. **Space of Larrey** *Opening*	Superior epigastric vessels *Structures passing through*
5. **Behind lateral arcuate ligament**	Subcostal nerve and vessels
6. **Behind medial arcuate ligament**	1. Sympathetic trunk 2. Lesser splanchnic nerve
7. **Piercing each crus**	1. Right crus–azygos vein 2. Left crus–inferior hemiazygos vein 3. Greater and lesser splanchnic nerves
8. **Left cupola of diaphragm**	Left phrenic nerve

CHAPTER-12

PHYSIOLOGY OF RESPIRATION

RESPIRATION

It is the process of exchange of gases in the lung where there is uptake of oxygen in exchange for carbondioxide. This is called external respiration. The exchange of oxygen and carbondioxide at tissue level is called internal respiration.

The first sixteen generations of dividing bronchi and bronchioles conduct air till terminal bronchioles. They form the conducting zone. The remaining seven generations consisting of respiratory bronchioles and alveoli form the respiratory zone, where exchange of O_2 and CO_2 occurs. At rest, human being breaths about 12-15 times per minute. 500 ml of air is taken in each breath which equals to 6-8 litres of air in 1 minute.

Composition of Air

The inspired air is composed of:

Oxygen (O_2)   :   21%
Carbondioxide (CO_2)   :   0.03%
Nitrogen (N_2)   :   78%
Other inert gases   :   about 1%

On breathing out (expiration) the air has 16% oxygen and 4% cabondioxide.

Respiratory Movements

These consist of two phases
1. **Inspiration:** Accompanied by expansion of lungs for uptake of air.
2. **Expiration:** Is the expulsion of air from lungs due to retraction of lungs.

These movements are accompanied by corresponding movements of the thoracic cage.

Inspiration

It is an active process. There is expansion of intrathoracic volume resulting in expansion of lungs. This creates a negative air pressure in the airway allowing the air to flow in. In normal conditions inspiration lasts for two seconds.

Muscles of Inspiration

1. **Primary muscles**
   a. **Intercostal muscles:** Contraction of external intercostal muscles; elevates the lower ribs and expands the thoracic cage.
   b. **Diaphragm:** Descent of diaphragm accounts for 75% change in intrathoracic pressure by increasing vertical diameter of thoracic cage.

2. **Accessory muscles (act during forced inspiration):** Erector spinae, scalene group of muscles, sternocleidomastoid, pectoralis major, serratus anterior, quadratus lumborum. They help to elevate thoracic cage in deep inspiration.

Expiration

It is a passive process in normal breathing. It occurs due to recoil of lungs at the end of inspiration. This pushes out air from lungs.

In forced expiration the following muscles are involved:
1. Anterior abdominal wall muscles namely; rectus abdominis, internal oblique, transversus abdominis. Contraction of these muscles increases the intra-abdominal pressure and pushes up the diaphragm.
2. Internal intercostal muscles: Contraction of these muscles pull upper ribs downwards. This decreases the intra-thoracic volume.
3. Accessory muscles: Adductor muscles of vocal cord. Their contraction is primarily protective, to prevent entry of food or fluid into trachea.

MECHANISM OF RESPIRATION

The expansion of thoracic cage creates a negative intra-thoracic pressure and allows the lung to expand during inspiration. Expiration is the reversal of inspiration.

The various movements of respiration occur at costovertebral and the manubriosternal joints and are described below
1. **Pump handle movement—in inspiration (Fig. 12.38)**
   — It increases the anteroposterior diameter of the thoracic cavity.
   — It occurs in the 2nd to 6th ribs. 1st rib is involved only during forced inspiration.
   — The fulcrum of the rib lies at its posterior end near the tubercle. Hence, a slight movement at the costo-vertebral joint increases the antero-posterior diameter to a great extent.
   — The axis of movement is oblique and runs from the costovertebral and costotransverse joints behind, to the opposite costochondral joint in front.
   — This is associated with an outward movement of the sternum because the anterior ends of the ribs are at a lower plane than posterior ends.
   — The upper 6 ribs also increase the transverse diameter of thorax though to a small extent.
2. **Bucket handle movement—in inspiration (Fig. 12.40)**
   — This increases the transverse diameter of the thoracic cavity.

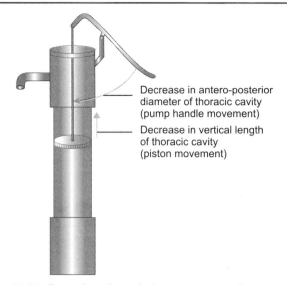

Fig. 12.37: Pump handle and piston movement in expiration

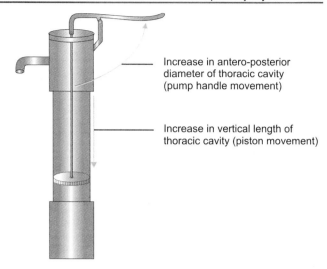

Fig. 12.38: Pump handle and piston movement in inspiration

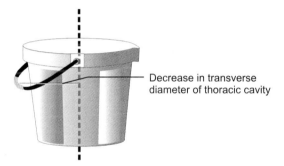

Fig. 12.39: Bucket handle movement in expiration

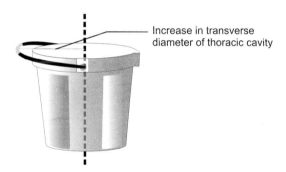

Fig. 12.40: Bucket handle movement in inspiration

— It occurs in the 7th to 10th ribs (vertebrochondral ribs).
— The axis of the movement passes antero-posteriorly from the costovertebral joints to same side costo-sternal joints.
— The elevation of 7th to 10th ribs results in an outward movement that resembles lifting of a handle of a bucket.

3. **Piston movement—in inspiration (Fig. 12.38)**
— This increases the vertical length of the thoracic cavity.
— It occurs due to the downward movement of the diaphragm.
— Maximal movement is seen in the recumbent position.

During expiration all three movements are reversed (Figs 12.37 and 12.39).

LUNG VOLUME AND CAPACITIES (FIG. 12.41)

Tidal volume (TV): Amount of air that is breathed into lungs in quiet respiration is tidal volume. It is 500 ml.

Inspiratory reserve volume (IRV): Is the maximal amount of air that can be inspired above the tidal volume with maximal inspiratory effort. Normal is 2000 to 3000 ml.

Expiratory reserve volume (ERV): Is the maximal volume of air expelled with maximum expiratory effort after passive expiration. Normal is 750 to 1000 ml.

Residual volume (RV): It is the volume of air which remains in the lung after maximal expiration. Normal is 1200 ml.

Inspiratory capacity (IC): It is the total amount of air that can be inspired on maximum inspiratory effort. It equals TV + IRV = 2500 to 3500 ml.

Expiratory capacity (EC): It is the maximum volume of air that can be expired after normal inspiration. It equals TV + ERV = 1250 to 1500 ml.

Vital capacity (VC): It is the maximum volume of air that can be expelled with maximum expiratory effort after maximal inspiration. VC = 1C + EC = 3750 to 5000 ml.

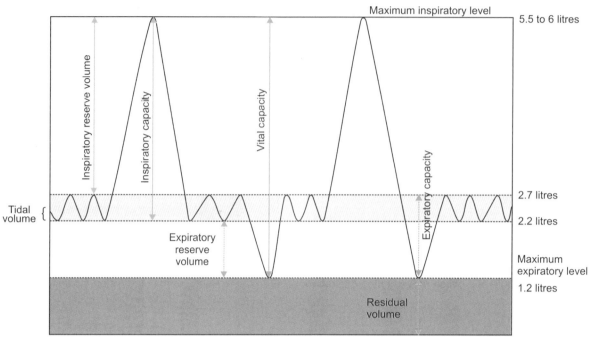

Fig. 12.41: Lung volumes and capacities

Respiratory minute volume: It is the amount of air inspired in one minute and it equals respiratory rate times tidal volume. 12 × 500 = 6000 ml.

Factors Affecting Vital Capacity

1. **Physiological**
   a. **Sex:** Vital capacity is higher in males due to larger chest size, muscle power and body surface area.
   b. **Age:** Vital capacity decreases with age due to gradual loss of elasticity or compliance of lungs.
   c. **Posture:** Vital capacity is maximum while standing due to position of diaphragm.
   d. **Pregnancy:** Vital capacity decreases because the diaphragm is pushed up by the pregnant uterus.
2. **Pathological**
   a. Diseases of lung parenchyma that decrease its compliance decrease vital capacity eg. pulmonary fibrosis, emphysema, pleural effusion etc.
   b. Ascites results in decreased vital capacity due to pressure on diaphragm.

Functional Residual Capacity (FRC)

It is the volume of air in the lungs at the end of normal expiration. It equals sum of residual volume and expiratory reserve volume and is 2500 ml. It is the reserve which allows exchange of gases to occur even during expiration. This avoids sudden changes in partial pressure of gases during inspiration.

Factors affecting FRC: It is increased in conditions associated with retention of air in lungs due to loss of elasticity or due to broncho-constriction.
1. Old age—Due to loss of elasticity
2. Emphysema—due to loss of elasticity
3. Asthma—due to bronchoconstriction leading to increase airway resistance

Forced Expiratory Volume In One Second (FEV_1)

It is the fraction of vital capacity that is expired during 1st second of forced expiration. Normal should be more than 80%.

Factors Affecting FEV_1

1. Restrictive lung disorders like kyphoscoliosis, pleural effusion lead to decrease expansion of chest. There is decrease in vital capacity but FEV_1 is nearly normal.
2. Obstructive lung disorders like asthma and emphysema, inspiration is usually unaffected while expiration is poor. The vital capacity is normal and FEV_1 is reduced.

Lung Compliance

It is defined as change in lung volume per unit change in airway pressure. It measures distensibility of the lung and chest wall. The lung and chest wall are elastic structures and hence have a tendency to recoil or collapse from the expanded position. The recoil depends on two factors namely

1. Recoil of elastic tissues and musculature of lungs and chest wall.
2. Alveolar surface tension: The alveoli tend to collapse due to surface tension between the fluid lining the alveoli and air.

Surfactant

- It is a mixture of dipalmitoyl phosphatidyl choline with other lipids and proteins.
- It is produced by type II epithelial cells (pneumocytes II) of alveoli.
- Role of surfactant: It plays an important role in the compliance of lung by
  — It reduces the alveolar surface tension by forming a layer between the lining fluid and air in alveoli. Thus, it prevents the collapse of alveoli, especially after expiration.
  — Prevents pulmonary edema by decreasing tension and intra-alveolar hydrostatic pressure.

VENTILATION AND PERFUSION OF LUNGS

Pulmonary ventilation is the amount of air inspired or expired in one minute. It equals about six litres per minute, i.e., tidal volume (500 ml) multiplied by respiratory rate (12 per minute). In standing position ventilation per unit lung volume is more in the base of lung than in apex. Alveolar ventilation is the volume of inspired air which is available for exchange of gases in alveoli.

Pulmonary vascular system is a low pressure system and pulmonary arterial pressures are 24 mm Hg systolic and 9 mm Hg diastolic with mean arterial pressure of 15 mm Hg. The pulmonary blood flow is equal to 5 to 5.5 litres per minute.

Dead Space

It is the volume of air in the lung which does not take part in the exchange of gases.

Anatomical Dead Space

This equals the volume of air in the conducting passages that is from nose to terminal bronchioles. It is about 150 ml.

Physiological Dead Space

It equals anatomical dead space plus the volume of air in alveoli which does not take part in gas exchange. This includes the air in alveoli which do not receive adequate blood flow.
In healthy state, anatomical and physiological dead space are identical.

In diseased conditions, the total dead space may be higher than this anatomical dead space either due to alteration in respiration or due to lack of perfusion of some parts of lung.
Factors affecting dead space volume
1. **Physiological:** Affects anatomical dead space
   a. **Sex:** It is more in males.
   b. **Height:** It is more in taller individuals.
   c. **Age:** It increases with age.
2. **Pathological**
   a. **Emphysema:** It is characterized by over inflated alveoli leading to excess ventilation in comparision to perfusion. This leads to wasted ventilation and increase in physiological dead space.
   b. **Bronchiectesis:** This is characterized by dilated bronchi and bronchioles leading to increase in anatomical dead space.
   c. **Pulmonary embolism:** It leads to lack of perfusion in a part leading to wasted ventilation and increase dead space.

Alveolar Ventilation

The volume of air reaching alveoli and available for gas exchange equals tidal volume minus dead space volume which is 350 ml. Hence, per minute alveoli ventilation is about 4200 ml.

Ventilation Perfusion Ratio (V/P ratio)

In normal conditions
1. Alveolar ventilation is about 4200 ml / minute (2000 ml/minute /lung).
2. Pulmonary blood flow is 5500 ml / minute (2500 ml / minute/ lung).
   Hence V/P ratio is 0.8

Factors Affecting VP Ratio

1. **Physiological:** Due to gravity negative pressure is higher in apex of lung as compared to base. Hence, the ventilation is higher at apex while perfusion is higher at base. The VP ratio is higher is apex while low at base.
2. **Pathological**
   a. Due to altered ventilation
      — Asthma
      — Emphysema
      — Pulmonary fibrosis
   b. Due to altered pulmonary circulation
      — Pulmonary embolism
      — Pulmonary hypertension due to congestive heart failure.

CHAPTER-12

Gas Exchange in Lungs (Fig. 12.42)

Gases diffuse from alveoli to blood circulation and vice versa passing through **alveolo-capillary membrane** consisting of:

1. Alveolar epithelium
2. Pulmonary capillary endothelium
3. Basement membrane of both lining cells.

Diffusion capacity of a gas is the amount of gas that crosses the alveolo-capillary membrane in a minute per mm Hg difference in the partial pressure of gas across the membrane. The diffusion capacity of oxygen (O_2) is 20 to 30 ml/minute/mmHg.

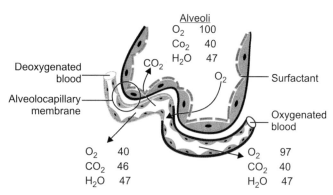

Fig. 12.42: Diagrammatic representation of exchange of gases from alveoli and pulmonary capillary

Factors Affecting Diffusion Capacity

1. Surface area of alveolo-capillary membrane: Higher the area more the diffusion.
2. Thickness of alveolo-capillary membrane: More the thickness less the diffusion.
3. Solubility and partial pressure difference across alveolo-capillary membrane: Diffusion capacity of carbon dioxide (CO_2) is 20 times higher than oxygen (O_2) because of its higher solubility.

Diffusion is increased during exercise especially of O_2 due to increase in circulation.

Diffusion is decreased in diseases like pulmonary fibrosis, sarcoidosis. It mainly leads to lack of O_2. However, retention of CO_2 is minimal as diffusion capacity of CO_2 is high.

Partial Pressure (P) of Various Gases

In alveoli	In pulmonary capillaries
$pO_2 = 100$	$pO_2 = 40$
$pCO_2 = 40$	$pCO_2 = 46$

The pO_2 of pulmonary blood is raised to 97 from 40 after inspiration and pCO_2 of blood leaving lungs is 40 mm Hg after exchange.

Pulmonary Circulation

— The pulmonary circulation system is a low pressure system with arterial pressures of 24mm Hg systolic and 9 mm Hg diastolic. The mean arterial pressure is 15 mmHg.

— Pulmonary capillary pressure is 10 mmHg and oncotic pressure is 25 mm Hg. This maintains fluid free alveoli. Increase in pulmonary capillary pressure as in congestive heart failure leads to pulmonary edema.

— Due to gravity, the blood flow to lung bases is higher than apices of lung.

— Ventilation perfusion ratio affects partial pressure of gases. If ventilation is reduced and perfusion is normal, pO_2 in alveoli is less and pCO_2 is higher. If perfusion is reduced however, pO_2 in alveoli is high as less is delivered to blood and pCO_2 is low as less is exchanged.

Transport of O_2 and CO_2 from Lung and Tissues

Oxygen Transport

Oxygen is carried from lungs to tissues via blood circulation in two ways:

1. **Bound to hemoglobin:** upto 99% O_2 entering pulmonary circulation binds to haemoglobin, an O_2 carrying protein.
2. **Dissolved in plasma:** only about 0.29 ml O_2 is transported, per 100 ml blood, in dissolved form.

Haemoglobin–O_2 reaction

• Hemoglobin is a protein made up of 4 subunits each having a haem moiety and a polypeptide chain. Each haem complex has one ferrous iron. Hence, each haemoglobin molecule has four iron atoms. Each ferrous ion can bind to one molecule of O_2. The oxygenation of haemoglobin is rapid and O_2 itself increases its binding affinity to haemoglobin.

• At 100% saturation each haemoglobin molecule contains 1.3 ml of O_2 which amounts to 20.1 ml / 100 ml blood when Hb count is 15 gm%.

• In arterial blood there is 97% saturation. Hence, each 100 ml blood has 19.5 ml O_2 bound to Hb.

• In venous blood, O_2 saturation is 75%, hence total oxygen content is about 15 ml / 100 ml. Thus for each 100 ml of blood about 4.5 ml O_2 is extracted by tissues.

O_2-haemoglobin Dissociation Curve (Fig. 12.43)

It presents the relation between pO_2 and oxygen saturation of Hb. It is a sigmoid curve. There is a linear increase in O_2 saturation of Hb with increase in pO_2.

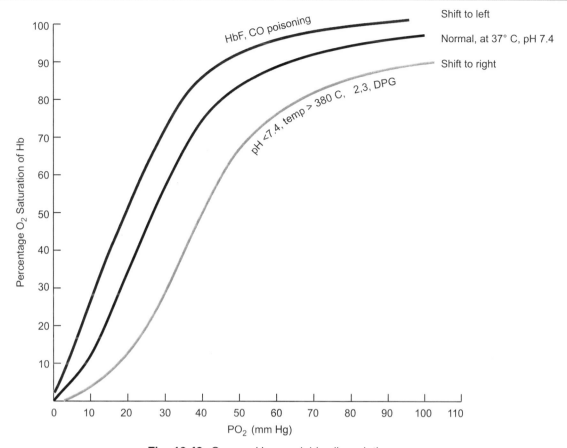

Fig. 12.43: Oxygen-Haemoglobin dissociation curve

This explains rapid uptake of oxygen into pulmonary capillaries.

Other factors affecting oxygen-Hb dissociation curve beside pO₂

1. **pH:** Decrease in pH shifts the curve to right. This is called **Bohr's effect.** As CO_2 increases in tissues due to cellular metabolism, the pH falls and more O_2 is released at tissues. The deoxygenated Hb binds to H^+ and allows more CO_2 to enter circulation, thus restoring local pH.

2. **Temperature:** Increase in temperature shifts the curve to right.

3. **2, 3 diphosphoglycerate levels (2, 3 DPG):** 2, 3 DPG is most abundant in RBCs. High 2, 3 DPG levels shifts the curve to right releasing O_2. High pH within red blood cells leads to increase in 2, 3 DPG. This releases the O_2 from Hb. 2, 3 DPG levels are increased in exercise, at high altitudes, in anemia and this facilitates delivery of O_2 to tissues.

4. **Fetal haemoglobin (HbF):** The Hb-O_2 curve shifts to left as HbF has a higher affinity for O_2. This is because HbF does not bind to 2, 3 DPG. Hence, its O_2 saturation is higher even at low pO₂ levels. This facilitates movement of O_2 from mother to fetus.

Transport of CO₂

CO_2 is transported in following ways:

1. Dissolved in blood, solubility of CO_2 is 20 times more than O_2.
2. By forming Carbamino compounds:
   a. With plasma protein in plasma
   b. With haemoglobin in red cells
3. Most, 75%, CO_2 rapidly diffuses into RBCs where in presence of carbonic anhydrase it forms H_2CO_3 that dissociates to H^+ and HCO_3^-. Deoxygenated Hb binds to H^+ easily and HCO_3^- diffuses out into plasma.

Chloride shift: HCO_3^- formed in RBCs enters plasma along its concentration gradient and Cl^- enters the cells in exchange. Because of this the Cl^- content of red cells in venous blood is higher than arterial blood.

CO₂ Transfer

About 4 ml of CO_2 is removed from tissues per 100 ml of blood passing through tissues. As the blood reaches lungs and O_2 binds to haemoglobin, affinity to CO_2 is reduced (Haldane effect) CO_2 release is facilitated. Cardiac output is 5 litre/minute. Hence $4/100 \times 5000 =$

200 ml of CO_2 is removed from tissues per minute and discharged in air.

REGULATION OF RESPIRATION

Rhythmic discharge of motor neurons in respiratory centre in brain results in normal breathing. This is controlled by the following (Figs. 12.44 to 12.47):
1. Neural mechanism of control
2. Chemical mechanism of control
3. Other mechanism of control

Neural Regulation

It occurs via two separate systems:
1. **Voluntary system**
   — It is located in cerebral cortex.
   — It passes impulses down to respiratory motor neurons in spinal cord (C_3, C_4, C_5 and thoracic segments) via corticospinal tract.
   — It is associated with conscious respiratory efforts, e.g., breath holding, forced inspiration and expiration.
2. **Involuntary system** or Automated system (Fig. 12.44)
   — It is located in the medulla and pons.
   — **Medullary respiratory centre:** Rhythmic discharges of neurons situated in respiratory centre in venterolateral medulla are mainly responsible for normal respiration:
   — The neurons are located in two groups, one dorsal and one ventral group.
   — Two types of neurons are present.
      a. **I-neurons** that discharge during inspiration.
      b. **E-neurons** that discharge during expiration.

— These neurons control activity in phrenic motor neurons and the inspiratory and expiratory motor neurons of intercostal muscles.
— **Pontine respiratory centre:** The rhythmic discharge of medullary centre is influenced by pons. It has two parts:
   a. **Apneustic centre:** Has neurons which are tonically active and activate I-neurons. It is inhibited by afferents from vagus nerve.
   b. **Pneumotaxic centre:** Has I and E neurons which are active in both phases of respiration.
— Vagal activity, stimulated by stretching of lungs during inspiration, is inhibitory to neurons in the apneustic centre of pons. They further inhibit I-neurons in medulla and limit the extent of inspiration.
— Hence, medulla is the primary respiratory centre with neural influences from:
   a. Reciprocal inhibitory impulses within medulla, between I and E neurons of medulla
   b. Pontine centre
   c. Vagal activity

Chemical Mechanism of Control

1. The increase in pCO_2 and H^+ concentrations in blood and decrease in pO_2 increases respiratory drive of respiratory centre of medulla while the opposite happens when these levels are reversed.
2. The effects of altered blood chemistry is mediated via chemoreceptors which are of two types:
   a. **Carotid and aortic bodies:** There are small rounded collection of cells situated at bifurcation of carotid, (carotid body) and arch of aorta (aortic body) (Fig. 12.45).
      — These cells are activated by drop in pO_2 (hypoxia) and stimulate the associated nerve

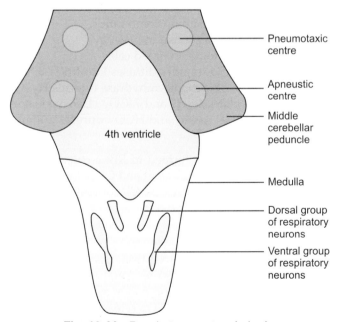

Fig. 12.44: Respiratory centres in brain

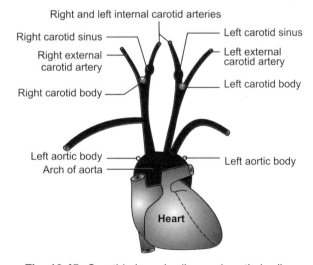

Fig. 12.45: Carotid sinus, bodies and aortic bodies

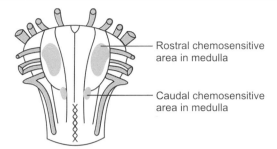

Fig. 12.46: Chemoreceptors in brain

endings. The principle transmitter here is dopamine.

— Carotid body is associated with glosso-pharyngeal nerve and aortic body with vagus nerve.

b. Chemoreceptors in brain stem (Fig. 12.46)

— These are located in medulla oblongata.

— They are stimulated by an increase in local levels of H^+ in the cerebrospinal fluid secondary to increase in pCO_2.

Effect of pCO_2 on Respiration

• Increase in pCO_2 results in increase formation of H_2CO_3 in red blood cells and CSF. H_2CO_3 dissociates to form H^+ and HCO_3^-.

• Increase H^+ ions stimulate medullary chemoreceptors which activate medullary respiratory centre.

• This increases pulmonary ventilation leading to increase CO_2 excretion by lungs resulting in normalization of pCO_2.

Effect of Hypoxia, Lack of Oxygen, on Ventilation

• Decrease in pO_2 stimulates aortic and carotid bodies which further stimulate the respiratory centre. However, this effect occurs only when pO_2 of arterial blood falls below 60 mmHg.

• When pO_2 falls there is shift of O_2-Hb curve to right. The deoxygenated Hb binds to H^+ ions and reduced levels of H^+ leads to inhibition of respiration. Further any slight increase in respiration reduces pCO_2 which also inhibits respiration. Thus, a slight fall in pO_2 does not have any effect on ventilation.

• Below pO_2 of 60 mm Hg the increasing strength of chemoreceptor response overcomes these inhibitions and increases ventilation response.

• Rise in pCO_2 levels is a potent stimulator of respiratory activity as compared to fall in pO_2 levels.

Effect of H^+ on Respiration

1. H^+ concentration may increase even when pCO_2 is normal as in metabolic acidosis, e.g., diabetes, renal failure, H^+ stimulates respiration and it washes out CO_2. pCO_2 falls leading to compensatory fall in H^+.

2. Reverse reaction occurs when there is metabolic alkalosis, as seen in cases of excess vomiting and loss of HCl.

3. In conditions where there is normal H^+ but ventilation is increased, as in voluntary hyperventilation, a fall in pCO_2 results in fall in H^+. This is called **respiratory alkalosis.**

4. In cases of emphysema or respiratory depression due to poisoning, accumulation of CO_2 leads to increase in H^+, known as **respiratory acidosis.**

Non-chemical Influences on Respiration

1. **Afferents from higher centres of brain to the respiratory centre in medulla**

   a. Fever, raised temperature leads to rapid breathing—is mediated via afferents from hypothalamus.

   b. Pain, fear, anxiety stimulate respiration – is mediated via afferents from hypothalamus and limbic system.

2. **Pulmonary and airway receptor response:** Receptors in lung and airways are innervated by vagal nerve fibers and are associated with:

   a. **Hering-Breuer reflexes:** Inflation of lung during inspiration stimulates local stretch receptors, afferents travel via vagal fibers to the pontine centres which inhibits further inspiration. Reverse occurs during expiration. These reflexes usually work during episodes of extra respiratory efforts like during exercise. They do not influence respiration at rest.

   b. **Juxta-capillary receptor responses:** Hyperinflation of lungs stimulate receptors in alveolar wall, J-receptors, afferents travels along vagal fibres and stimulate centre in pons leading to apnea followed by rapid breathing and associated bradycardia and hypotension.

3. **Coughing and sneezing reflexes:** Rapidly adapting irritant receptors present in trachea and bronchi are stimulated by inhalation of strong irritants or presence of foreign bodies. The afferents travel in vagal fibres. The reflex response consists of deep inspiration followed by forced expiration with a closed glottis resulting in an increased intrapleural pressure which opens the glottis with pressure and produces the sound of cough. In sneezing the glottis is open. These reflexes help clear the air passage of irritants to keep it clear.

4. **Bronchoconstriction reflex:** Irritant receptors in respiratory bronchioles when stimulated lead to the response of broncho-constriction and tachypnea

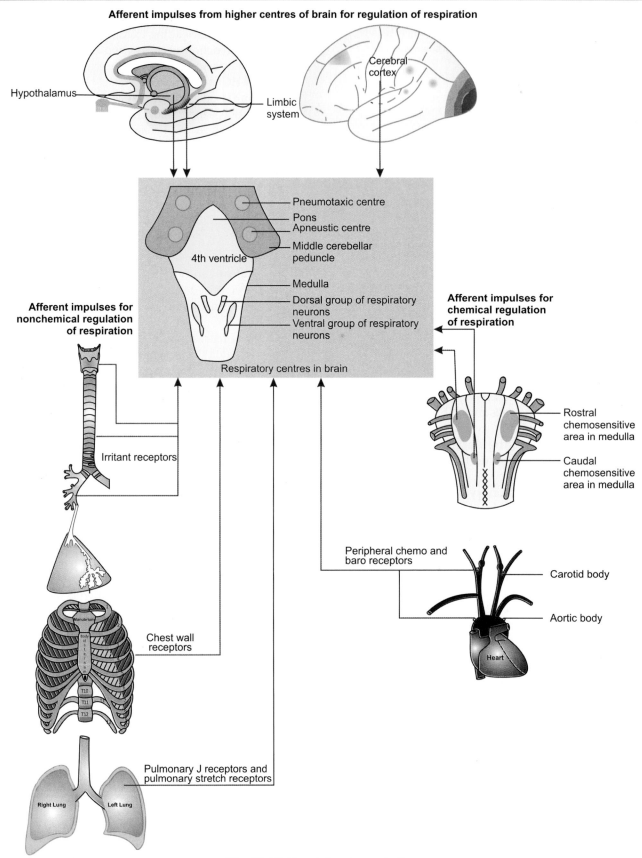

Fig. 12.47: Regulation in respiration

(increased shallow breathing). The aim is to protect the passage. However, in conditions like allergic bronchitis or asthma, an exaggerated response occurs and patient develops difficulty in breathing.

5. **Other respiratory responses**
   a. **Hiccup:** Spasmodic contraction of diaphragm and inspiratory muscles leading to a sudden short inspiration associated with sudden closure of glottis. This produces the characteristic sound.
   b. **Deglutition reflex or swallowing:** Respiration is inhibited during swallowing. This prevents entry of food into trachea. Inhibitory impulses travel along glossopharyngeal nerve.
   c. **Yawning:** Opening of mouth with deep inspiration. Physiological basis of yawning is not known.

Physiology of Exercise

Effect of Exercise on Respiration

To meet the extra O_2 requirements of body and remove excess CO_2 and heat from body during exercise, a number of respiratory and cardio-vascular responses occur. Respiratory responses are as follows:

1. Increase pulmonary ventilation: Increase respiratory rate + increase in depth of breathing (inspiratory capacity), which equals to providing upto 100 liters / min of ventilation.
2. Increase diffusion capacity of O_2 and increase O_2 consumption in lung. This is caused by
   a. Increased pulmonary circulation, due to increased cardiac output in exercise and opening up of entire capillary bed.
   b. Fall in pO_2 of pulmonary capillaries from 40 to 25 mHg, increases the O_2 gradient across the alveolo-capillary membrane. This increases diffusion of O_2 from alveoli into the circulation.

Total O_2 transfer increases from the normal of 250 ml / mt at rest, to 4000 ml/mt.

This is also associated in removal of excess CO_2, from 200 ml / mt at rest, to upto 8000 ml/mt.

Oxygen Debt or Oxygen Deficit

The rate of O_2 consumption in periphery increases rapidly during first few minutes of exercise but plateaus on reaching a maximum level (it is limited by the maximum blood flow to the tissue). After this the muscles gain energy (ATP) by anaerobic metabolism producing lactate. Hence, an O_2 debt is incurred.

At onset of exercise there is an increase in the rate and depth of respiration increasing the ventilation upto maximal levels for that individual. This helps to provide extra O_2 for exercise. However, even after cessation of exercise the minute ventilation remains high for a variable period, decreasing gradually to the normal pre-exercise levels. This extra O_2 consumption after stoppage of exercise pays for the oxygen debt to restore the ATP and O_2 levels to muscles.

CLINICAL AND APPLIED ASPECT

NOSE AND PARANASAL SINUSES

- The area on the antero-inferior part of the nasal septum is highly vascular. In this area the septal branches of anterior ethmoidal, sphenopalatine, greater palatine and superior labial arteries anastomose to form a plexus known as **Kesselbach's plexus.** This area is named as the Little's area and is the most common site of epistaxis or bleeding from nose. In children it is mostly due to nose picking or presence of a foreign body.
- The central septum of the nose may be deviated in some to the right or to the left side leading to varying degrees of obstruction of the respective nasal cavity. The deviation commonly involves the cartilaginous part and occasionally the bony part of septum. It can lead to recurrent attacks of nasal blockage and sinusitis. This condition is treated surgically by submucous resection of the deviated part of the septum.
- Maxillary sinus is the commonest site of infection amongst all sinuses. The infection is called maxillary sinusitis. This infection can occur from the following sources
  — Infection in the nose
  — Caries of upper molar teeth
  — Being the most dependant part it acts as a secondary reservoir of pus from frontal air sinuses through fronto-nasal duct and hiatus semilunaris.

The opening of the sinus is unfortunately present in the upper part of its medial wall. This results in inefficient drainage and persistence of infection leading to collection of pus in acute cases or formation of mucosal polyps in chronic cases. Surgical evacuation of maxillary sinus is performed in the following ways
  — Endoscopic sinus surgery
  — Antral punctue
  — Caldwell Luc operation

NASOPHARYNX AND LARYNX

- The nasopharyngeal tonsils are prominent in children but usually undergo atrophy at and after puberty. Enlargement of nasopharyngeal tonsils, usually due to repeated upper respiratory tract infections, is known as **adenoids.** Enlarged adenoids block the posterior nares and cause discomfort to the child as he will have to breath through the mouth. It is a common cause of snoring in children.

- The eustachian tube extends from middle ear to nasopharynx and helps to equalize pressure between the middle ear and the external ear. Infection in nasopharynx can cause swelling and blockage of the tube. This leads to decrease in pressure in the middle ear and the tympanic membrane is pulled towards it. There is a feeling of fullness in the ear and loss of hearing.
- Infection can also spread from the pharynx to middle ear via the tube. This is more common in children as the tube is short and straight. Hence. it is important to check the ears in children presenting with complaints of nasal congestion or tonsillitis.
- The vocal cords appear as pearly white avascular cords on laryngoscopy. This is because the mucosal lining consists of stratified squamous epithelium which is adherent to the underlying vocal ligament without an intervening submucosa.
- Laryngeal oedema is the collection of fluid in the vestibular folds which results in blockage of glottic area and inability to breath. Laryngeal oedema usually occurs due to severe allergic reactions As the vocal cords have no submucosa they are not involved in oedema.
- The posterior cricoarytenoid muscles are called the safety muscles of larynx. This is because they are the abductors of vocal cord. If they are paralyzed the unopposed action of adductors of larynx cut of air entry and can lead to death.
- The interior of larynx can be inspected directly by laryngoscope or indirectly through a laryngeal mirror.
  Following structures are viewed
  — Base of tongue
  — Valleculae
  — Epiglottis
  — Aryepiglottic folds
  — Piriform fossae
  — False vocal cords (red and widely apart)
  — True vocal cords (pearly white). These are seen medial to false vocal cords.
  — Sinus of larynx between false and true vocal cords.
- The following changes occur when recurrent laryngeal nerve is completely damaged:
  — In unilateral involvement, the ipsilateral vocal cord comes to lie in the paramedian position (between abduction and adduction). It does not vibrate. However, the other cord is able to compensate without any significant loss in phonation.
  — In bilateral involvement, the vocal cords come to lie in the cadaveric position. This leads to loss of phonation and difficulty in breathing.

TRACHEO-BRONCHIAL TREE

- X-ray of neck in lateral view shows a vertical translucent shadow in front of the cervico-thoracic vertebral column. This is the trachea filled with air. Compression of trachea due to an enlarged thyroid gland is visible on X-ray.
- Trachea can be felt in the suprasternal notch in the median plane. Any shift of trachea to right or left usually indicates a mediastinal shift which may be secondary to a lung pathology.
- The right principal bronchus is wider, shorter and more in line with the trachea. Hence a foreign body is more likely to be aspirated into the right lung.
- Apical segment of lower lobe of right lung is the commonest site of aspiration lung abscess and aspiration pneumonia (Mendelson's syndrome). Posterior segment of upper lobe is the second commonest.
- Knowledge of the position of bronchopulmonary segments and consequently the direction of the tertiary bronchus helps the doctors in obtaining natural drainage of secretions from the infected area of the lung by adopting different postures.
- Posterior segment of the right upper lobe is the most frequent site of tuberculosis.
- Anterior segment of upper lobe is the most frequent site of origin of carcinoma.

LUNG AND PLEURA

- Accumulation of air in pleural cavity is known as pneumothorax. It may be of following types
  - **Closed pneumothorax:** This occurs spontaneously due to rupture of a pulmonary bulla (expanded peripheral alveolar sac).
  - **Open pneumothorax:** It occurs due to a penetrating injury which results in communication of pleural cavity with atmosphere.
  - **Tension pneumothorax:** In this type of pneumothorax air enters into the pleural sac during inspiration but cannot move out with expiration. It constitutes a surgical emergency.
- **Naked pleura:** At places pleura is not covered by the skeletal framework of thoracix cage. This is termed as naked pleura. Thus, it can easily be injured resulting in pneumothorax. Example: Cervical pleura can be damaged while administering brachial plexus block.

- Accumulation of fluid in the pleural cavity is known as pleural effusion
  - **Hydrothorax:** It is the accumulation of transudative or exudative fluid.
  - **Pyothorax:** Accumulation of pus in pleural cavity is called pyothorax.
  - **Haemothorax:** It is the accumulation of blood in pleural cavity
  - **Chylothorax:** It is due to the rupture of thoracic duct and accumulation of chyle (lymph) in the pleural cavity.
- Inflammation of pleura is known as pleurisy or pleuritis. It may or may not be associated with effusion.
- Costodiaphragmatic recess is the most dependant part of the pleural sac. When any fluid appears in the sac, it first collects in the costo-diaphragmatic recess. This can be seen as obliteration of the costodiaphragmatic angle which is present on the infero-lateral sides of the lung shadow on X-ray chest.
- Paracentesis is the removal of fluid or air from the pleural cavity. In pneumothorax tapping is done by inserting a chest tube in the 2nd intercostal space just posterior to mid axillary line. In pleural effusion tapping is done by inserting a needle in the 6th intercostal space just posterior to mid axillary line.
- **Hyaline membrane disease:** Presence of surfactant in lungs at birth is important to keep the lungs in expansion after the baby takes its 1st few breaths. In premature babies where surfactant has not yet fully formed, the lung remains collapsed at certain areas leading to infant respiratory distress syndrome. It is associated with leakage of proteins into alveoli forming a membrane. It is known as hyaline membrane disease which can be fatal.
  Prevention: Administration of glucocorticoid injection to mother 24 hours prior to delivery may help some cases.
  Treatment: Is usually difficult but recently use of bovine surfactant and synthetic preparations have been used with some beneficial results in reducing severity of disease.

THORACIC WALL AND DIAPHRAGM

- Herpes Zoster infection is a viral infection caused by Herpes virus similar to chicken pox virus. The virus lies dormant. The most common site is the dorsal root ganglion of the inter-costal nerve. The other site is trigeminal nerve ganglion. Activation of virus leads to appearance of an erythmatous (red) vescicular rash which appears along the distribution of the nerve. This is associated with intense burning and pain in the dermatome supplied by the nerve. It is characteristically uni-lateral and doesnot cross the midline. Treatment with anti-virul drugs like acyclovir or famcyclovir decrease the intensity and duration of infection and reduce the risk of recurrence. Intercostal neuralgia is the most common complication of this infection.
- Diaphragm may fail to arise from the lateral arcuate ligament on one or both sides. This leads to congenital diaphragmatic hernia through this opening which is known as Bockdalek's hernia. The abdominal contents can herniate into the thoracic cavity leading to poor development of the lungs.
- Esophageal opening constricts during inspiration, venacaval opening dilates and there is no effect on aortic opening.
- In the lying down posture the height of diaphragm is maximum on the side of resting. Thus, the excursion of diaphragm during respiration would also be maximal on that side. Hence, a patient with one side lung disease is asked to rest on the opposite side so that maximal rest is given to the diseased side.

PHYSIOLOGY OF RESPIRATION

- **Tachypnea:** It is increase in respiratory rate.
  Bradyapnea: It is decrease in respiratory rate.
- **Dyspnea:** It is defined as difficulty in breathing when there is conscious effort involved in breathing which causes discomfort. It occurs due to the following condition:
  - Physiological dyspnea is seen after a bout of moderate to severe exercise because the pulmonary ventilation is increased to 4 to 5 times.
  - Pathological dyspnea occurs in various lung pathologies which decrease its vital capacity:
    i. Lung diseases like asthma, emphysema, pneumonia, pulmonary edema
    ii. Pneumothorax
    iii. Cardiac diseases, e.g., congestive heart failure which causes pulmonary edema.
  Apnea: It is the complete cessation or stoppage of respiration.
- **Asphyxia:** It is a condition in which there is decreased PO_2, i.e., hypoxia along with increase in PCO_2, i.e., Hypercapnia. It occurs, when there is blockage of air passages, e.g., in strangulation, drowning etc. or in chronic heart failure secondary to long standing lung diseases.
- **Pulmonary function tests:** Pulmonary function tests are broadly classified into three types:
  - Ventilatory function tests

— Tests to assess pulmonary diffusion on exchange of gases.
— Tests for PO_2, PCO_2 and acid-base status of blood.

Spirometry: It is a simple PFT that is a study of lung volumes.

- **Asthma:** It is a clinical condition characterized by hypersensitivity of brachial smooth muscles which leads to bronchoconstriction. Factors that parcipitate asthma can be cold air, cigarette smoking, air pollution, viral cold or pharyngitis, stress either emotional or physical. In this inspiration is usually not affected while air is retained due to bronchoconstriction and expiration is difficult leading to dyspnea and a characteristic whistling noise called wheeze or rhonchi.

- **Hypoxia:** It is deficiency of O_2 at tissue level. it can be due to:
  — Hypoxic hypoxia—is due to poor respiration and fall of pO_2 in blood.
  — Anemic hypoxia—is due to low Hb levels. pO_2 is normal.
  — Stagnant hypoxia—is due to stasis of blood resulting in poor blood flow even when pO_2 and Hb levels are normal.
  — Histotoxic hypoxia—is due to damage to tissues by toxins by which they can not take up O_2.

- **Cyanosis:** It is the blue discolouration of tissues which occurs due to excess deoxygenated Hb levels in circulation. When the deoxygenated Hb levels exceed 5 gm% cyanosis occurs and it is best seen in nail beds, ear lobes, lips, and tongue.

Chapter 13

Cardiovascular System

INTRODUCTION

Cardiovascular system consists of the heart which pumps blood for circulation and the blood vessels which carry the oxygenated blood (arteries) to the various organs and return the deoxygenated blood (veins) from various tissues and organs to the heart. It is responsible for the transport of nutritive substances from gastro-intestinal tract, transport of waste products for removal to liver and kidneys. It also distributes hormones and other agents that regulate various body functions and helps in regulation of temperature and the internal milieu (internal environment).

PERICARDIUM

Pericardium is a fibro-serous sac that encloses the heart and the roots of great vessels arising from it. The sac is conical in shape with apex upwards and base downwards. It extends from 2nd to 6th costal cartilages which corresponds to T_5 to T_8 vertebral levels.

Pericardium is made up of two parts
   1. Fibrous pericardium
   2. Serous pericardium

Fibrous Pericardium

It is a conical open sac made of fibrous tissue. The apex blends with the serous coat of great vessels at their origin and the pretracheal fascia. It lies at the level of sternal angle. The base is fused with upper surface of the central tendon of diaphragm. Anteriorly, it is attached to the body of sternum with the help of superior and inferior pericardial ligaments.

Serous Pericardium

It is a closed sac made up of mesothelium. It consists of parietal and visceral layers. Parietal layer is adherent to the fibrous pericardium while the visceral layer is adherent to the myocardium of the heart. Visceral layer is also known as epicardium. The visceral layer continues with the parietal layer at the site of origin (roots) of the great vessels. A potential space, called the pericardial space, is present between these two layers. It contains a thin capillary layer of fluid.

The posterior aspect of heart covered with pericardium presents with two spaces or sinuses (Fig. 13.1). These are
   1. Transverse sinus: It is present between the aorta, pulmonary trunk and left atrium.
   2. Oblique sinus: Cul-de-sac behind the left atrium is known as oblique sinus.

Arterial Supply of Pericardium
   1. Fibrous pericardium and parietal layer of serous pericardium are supplied by branches of internal thoracic artery and descending aorta.
   2. Visceral layer is supplied by branches of coronary arteries.

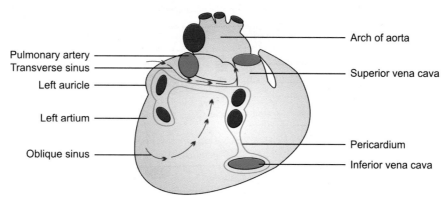

Pulmonary artery
Transverse sinus
Left auricle
Left artium
Oblique sinus

Arch of aorta
Superior vena cava
Pericardium
Inferior vena cava

Fig. 13.1: Base of heart-posterior view showing oblique and transverse sinuses of pericardium

Venous Drainage of Pericardium

1. Fibrous pericardium and parietal layer drain into azygos and internal thoracic veins.
2. Visceral pericardium drains into the coronary sinus.

Nerve Supply of Pericardium

1. Fibrous pericardium and parietal layer are supplied by phrenic nerve. Thus, they are sensitive to pain.
2. Visceral pericardium receives parasympathetic supply via vagus nerve and sympathetic supply via the coronary plexus (T_1 to T_5).

HEART

Heart is the organ that pumps blood into various parts of the body. It is a hollow, conical shaped, muscular organ which lies in the middle mediastinum. (Fig. 13.2 and 13.3).

Heart has four chambers, 2 atria and 2 ventricles which contract in an orderly fashion to pump blood into circulation. The 2 atria and the 2 ventricles are separated from each other by interatrial and interventricular septae respectively. The left atrium opens into the left ventricle and the right atrium opens into the right ventricle. Each of the opening is guarded by a valve to allow blood flow from atria to ventricle only and not reverse. Each ventricle has an outflow tract, right draining into pulmonary arteries and left draining into aorta. Each of these are also guarded by valves to allow unidirectional flow.

Measurements of Heart

Antero-posterior diameter	— 6 cm
Widest transverse diameter	— 8 to 9 cm
Length from apex to the base	— 12 cm
Weight (less in females)	— 230 to 340 gm

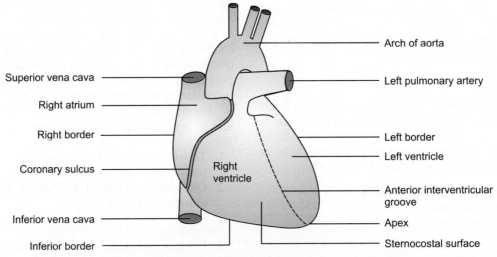

Fig. 13.2: Features of the heart (Sternocostal surface)

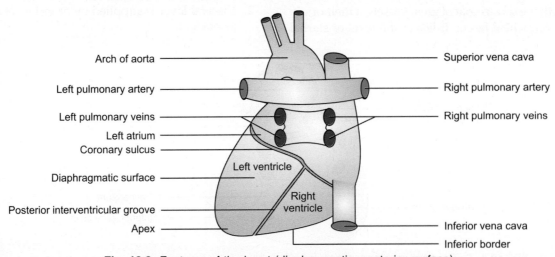

Fig. 13.3: Features of the heart (diaphragmatic, posterior surface)

External Features

The heart presents with an apex, a base, 3 borders and 3 surfaces.

Apex: It is entirely formed by the left ventricle. It is directed downwards, forwards and towards the left. It lies in the 5th intercostal space, just medial to mid clavicular line.

Base: It constitutes the posterior surface of heart and is directed backwards and to the right. It is formed by the posterior surfaces of right atrium (1/3rd) and left atrium (2/3rd). It is bounded by the pulmonary trunk above and posterior atrioventricular groove with coronary sinus below.

Right border: It is formed by the right atrium and extends vertically down from the right side of superior vena caval opening to the inferior vena caval opening. It separates the base of the heart from its sternocostal surface.

Inferior border: It extends horizontally from the opening of inferior vena cava to the apex of heart. It separates the sternocostal surface of heart from the diaphragmatic surface.

Left border: It is ill defined and extends from the left auricle to the apex of the heart. It separates sternocostal surface from left surface.

Sternocostal surface: This surface lies in relation to the posterior surface of the body of sternum and to the inner surfaces of 3rd to 6th costal cartilages of both sides. It is formed by

- Anterior surface of right ventricle which makes upto 2/3rd of this surface.
- Anterior surface of left ventricle which makes upto 1/3rd of this surface.

- It is also formed by anterior surface of right atrium, right auricle and part of left auricle.

It presents with anterior part of atrio-ventricular groove on the right which lodges the right coronary artery. On the left side it presents the anterior interventricular groove which indicates the anterior attachment of the interventricular septum. This groove lodges the anterior interventricular branch of left coronary artery and the great cardiac vein.

Diaphragmatic or inferior surface: It lies over the central tendon of the diaphragm. It is formed by

- Left ventricle, upto 2/3rd
- Right ventricle, upto 1/3rd.

It presents with the posterior interventricular groove. This indicates the posterior attachment of interventricular septum. The groove lodges the posterior interventricular branch of right coronary artery, branches of both coronary arteries and the middle cardiac vein.

Left surface: It is directed upwards, backwards and to the left and lies in relation to mediastinal pleura and left lung. It is formed by

- Left ventricle
- Part of left atrium and auricle

It presents with the left part of atrio-ventricular groove. It intervenes between the left auricle and left ventricle. It lodges the trunk of left coronary artery, beginning of coronary sinus and termination of great cardiac vein.

Anatomical Position of Heart

Heart lies in the middle mediastinum in such a fashion that the apex of heart faces downwards, forwards and towards the left just medial to the mid clavicular line, in

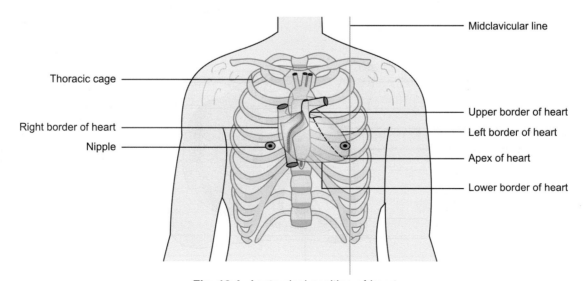

Fig. 13.4: Anatomical position of heart

the 5th intercostal space. Base of heart lies upwards and backwards on right side extending to the right 3rd costal cartilage (Fig. 13.4).

RIGHT ATRIUM

It is roughly quadrilateral in shape. It receives deoxygenated blood from the body. It extents from orifice of superior vena cava to the orifice of inferior vena cava. This corresponds to 3rd to 6th costal cartilages on the right side.

External Characteristics (Fig. 13.2)

1. The superior vena cava opens at its upper end and inferior vana cava at the lower end.
2. Right auricle: It is a hollow conical muscular projection from the antero-superior aspect of the atrium which covers the root of aorta.
3. Sulcus terminalis: Is a shallow vertical groove that runs along the right border of the heart. It corresponds with the crista terminalis of the interior of the atrium.

Interior of Right Atrium (Fig. 13.5)

It presents with the following two parts
1. Anterior rough part or atrium proper
2. Posterior smooth part or sinus venosus

Atrium Proper

- This rough part is separated from the posterior smooth part by a ridge of smooth muscle fibres called the crista terminalis.
- The ridge extends from the front of superior vena cava down to the right horn of valve of inferior vena cava.

- Muscle fibre bundles extend transversely from the crista terminalis to the atrioventricular orifice forming transverse ridges. These are called **musculi pectinati.**

Sinus Venosus

This is the smooth part and it receives the following tributaries:
1. **Opening of superior vena cava:** It conveys blood from upper part of body and opens at its upper end. It is not guarded by any valve.
2. **Opening of inferior vena cava:** It is present in the lower part close to the inter-atrial septum and is guarded by a rudimentary semilunar valve called the Eustachian valve.
3. **Opening of coronary sinus:** The coronary sinus opens at the lower part of the interatrial septum between opening of inferior vena cava and right atrio-ventricular orifice. It is guarded by a valve named Thebesian valve.
4. Foramina venarum minimarum
5. Opening of anterior cardiac vein
6. Intervenous tubercle of lower

Interatrial Septum

It is present between the two atria. The right side of septum presents the following features
1. **Fossa ovalis:** An oval depression lying above and to the left of opening of inferior vena cava. It is the site of embryonic septum primum.
2. **Limbus fossa ovalis/annulus ovalis:** It is the sickle shaped margin of fossa ovalis which forms the upper, anterior and posterior border of fossa. The anterior edge continues inferiorly with the valve of inferior vena cava. It is the remnant of free border of septum secundum.

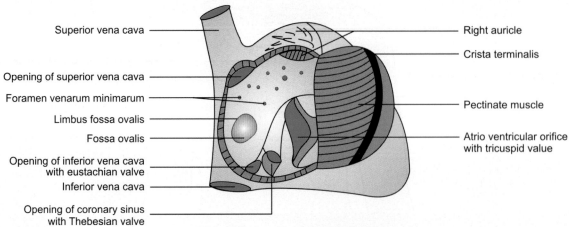

Fig. 13.5: Interior of right artium

RIGHT VENTRICLE

It is a triangular chamber situated to the left of right atrium. It receives blood from the right atrium and pumps it into the pulmonary trunk.

External Features

It has three surfaces (Figs 13.2 and 13.3)
1. Sternocostal or anterior surface: It is in relation to sternum and ribs
2. Inferior surface: It is in relation to diaphragm
3. Posterior surface: It is convex to the right and is formed by the inter-ventricular septum

Interior of Right Ventricle

It presents with two parts divided by a muscular ridge, known as the supraventricular crest (Fig. 13.6).
1. Ventricle proper or inflow tract
2. Infundibulum or outflow tract

Ventricle Proper

- Ventricle proper receives blood from right atrium via the right atrio-ventricular orifice.
- The interior is rough due to presence of muscular ridges known as trabeculae carnae.
- It develops from right part of primitive ventricle.

Trabeculae carnae: These are ridges made up of bundles of muscle fibres arranged in three forms:

1. **Ridges:** These present as linear elevations. **Supra-ventricular crest:** It is a ridge present between the pulmonary and atrioventricular orifices. It extends downwards in the posterior wall of the infundibulum.

2. **Bridges:** These are muscular elevations with fixed ends on ventricular walls. The centre is however free.

   Septomarginal trabecula: It is a specialized bridge which extends from the right of ventricular septum to the base of anterior papillary muscle. It contains the right branch of atrio-ventricular (A.V.) bundle.

3. **Papillary muscles:** These are concical projections of muscle fibre bundles. Their base is attached on the ventricular wall and the apex is attached to the chordae tendinae. The cordae tendinae are further attached to the cusps of the valves of atrio-ventricular orifices. The papillary muscles regulate closure of these valves and hence the blood flow across the orifices.
   There are three papillary muscles in the right ventricle
   a. Anterior: Is the largest
   b Posterior
   c. Septal: Is indistinct, may be absent.

Right Atrio-ventricular Orifice (Fig. 13.5)

- It is an oval to circular shaped opening present between the right atrium and right ventricle.
- It is directed ventrically downwards, forwards and to left making an angle of 45° with the sagittal plane.
- Circumference of the orifice is about 10 to 12 cm.
- It is guarded by the tricuspid valve complex. This consists of three cusps anterior, posterior and septal.

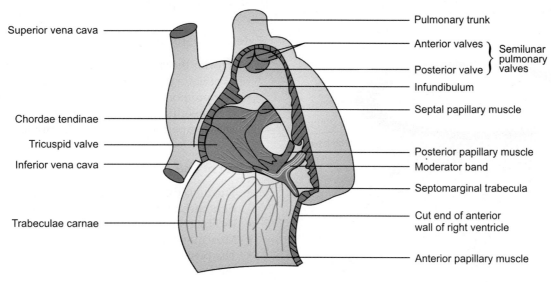

Fig. 13.6: Interior of right ventricle

- The cusps are separated by three commisures namely, anteroseptal, posteroseptal and anteroposterior.

Features of atrioventricular valves: Atrioventricular valves consist of following components (Fig. 13.7).

1. **Fibrous ring or annulus:** It is a collagenous ring to which the cusps are attached.
2. **Cusps of valve:** Are also known as leaflets.
   - They are flat leaf like structures with one margin attached to the fibrous annulus and other margin free extending into the ventricular cavity.
   - Each has an atrial surface which is smooth and a ventricular surface which is rough. This surface is attached to chordae tendinae.
   - They are made of 2 layers of endocardium with a central lamina fibrosa continuous with the fibrous ring.
   - Junction of these leaflets are called commissures.
   - The free margins of cusps show indentations. The posterior leaflet usually has 2 clefts. The cordae tendinae are attached to the clefts also.
   - Apposition of cusps of valve complex occurs in systole and prevents regurgitation of blood back into the atrium during ventricular contraction.
3. **Chordae tendinae:** These are thread like structures made up of collagenous fibres covered with endothelium which connect the papillary muscles to the rough and basal parts of the cusps. They are also attached to the commissures and clefts.

Infundibulum/Outflow Tract

- It is also called conus arteriosus and ejects blood from right ventricle to the pulmonary trunk.
- It is the remanant of right part of bulbus cordis.
- The infundibulum is conical, smooth walled and is directed upwards, backwards and to the left.

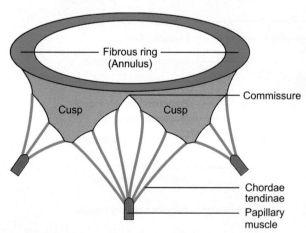

Fibrous ring
(Annulus)

Commissure

Cusp   Cusp

Chordae
tendinae
Papillary
muscle

Fig. 13.7: Feature of an atrioventricular valve

- It lies anterior to and above the inflow tract, towards left side of the atrioventricular orifice.
- The blood flowing from inflow tract makes an obtuse angle as it flows into the outflow tract.
- The upper end or apex presents with the pulmonary orifice.

Pulmonary Orifice

- It is circular in shape.
- It is guarded by three semilunar valves which are directly attached to the fibrous layer of vessel wall. There is no fibrous annulus.
- There are 2 anterior and one posterior valves.
- The free margin of cusps project into the pulmonary trunk.
- The valves consists of bilayered endocardium with a central lamina fibrosa.
- The pulmonary trunk at its origin presents with a dilatation above each cusp called the pulmonary sinus.
- The orifice is open during systole and closed during diastole. The valves meet in centre in a triradiate manner during diastole. This prevents flow into pulmonary trunk during ventricular filling phase.
- The infundibulum is separated from the ventricle proper below by the supraventricular crest and the septomarginal trabecula.

LEFT ATRIUM

It is also a quadrangular chamber which lies in a more posterior plane than the right atrium, separated from it by the interatrial septum. Left atrium receives oxygenated blood from the lung via pulmonary veins and pumps it to the left ventricle.

External Features (Fig. 13.3)

- It forms the base of heart and the anterior boundary of oblique pericardial sinus.
- The pulmonary veins open into its posterior wall.
- It presents with a conical projection on its anterosuperior aspect, the left auricle.

Interior of Left Atrium (Fig. 13.8)

- The muscular wall of left atrium is thicker than the right atrium. It is about 3 mm.
- Its inner surface is mostly smooth.
- Musculi pectinati are present within the auricle.
- The posterior wall presents with openings of four pulmonary veins.
- The anterior wall is formed by interatrial septum.

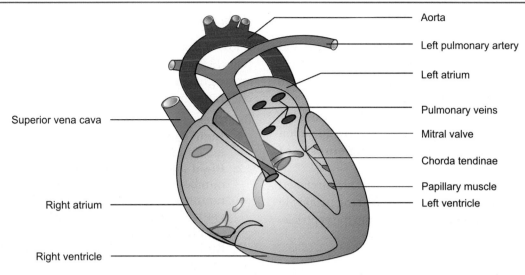

Fig. 13.8: Interior of heart

- The septal wall has a semilunar fold with concavity directed upwards. This is the upper margin of septum primum. Above this is present **fossa lunata** which corresponds to the fossa ovalis of right side.

LEFT VENTRICLE

Left ventricle is situated posterior to the right ventricle and is conical in shape. The musculature is 3 times thicker than right ventricle. It is about 8-12 mm thick. On cross section the cavity is circular. It receives oxygenated blood from left atria which is pumped out to the aorta.

External Features

It has three surfaces (Figs 13.2, 13.3)
1. Sternocostal or anterior surface
2. Diaphragmatic or inferior surface
3. Left surface

Interior of Left Ventricle

It presents with two parts (Fig. 13.8)
1. Ventricle proper or inflow tract
2. Aortic vestibule or outflow tract

Ventricle Proper/Inflow Tract

- Ventricle proper conducts blood across the atrioventricular orifice from left atrium to the apex. It lies below and behind the outflow tract.
- The interior is rough due to presence of trabeculae carnae which are more prominent than that in right

ventricle. Left ventricle has only two papillary muscles, anterior and posterior.
- It develops from the left part of primitive ventricle.

Left Atrioventricular Orifice

- It is smaller than the right orifice with a circumference of 7 to 9 cm.
- It is also directed downwards and forwards but lies postero-superior to the right orifice.
- It is guarded by the bicuspid or mitral valve complex. It consists of two cusps namely anterior and posterior separated by two deep indentations, anterolateral and posteromedial commissures.
- The characteristics of the valve complex is similar to the right atrio-ventricular valves.
- The free margin of anterior cusp has no indentation while the posterior cusp has two clefts.

Aortic Vestibule/Outflow Tract

- The vestibule is smooth walled and truncated with a conical shape. It ejects blood from left ventricle into the aorta.
- It is mostly made of fibrous tissue. There is very little muscle mass.
- It lies anterior to and above the inflow tract and towards the right side of mitral orifice. The blood flowing from the inflow tract makes an acute angle as it passes to the outflow tract.
- The summit of infundibulum presents with the aortic orifice.
- It is the remanant of left part of bulbus cordis.

Aortic Orifice

- It is circular in shape and is directed upwards and to the right.
- It is guarded by three semilunar cusps which are thicker than pulmonary cusps.
- There are one anterior and two posterior cusps.
- The aorta at its origin also presents with a dilatation above each cusps known as aortic **sinuses of Valsalva.**
- During systole the cusps open and are stretched along the aorta. They close during diastole preventing regurgitation of blood into the ventricle.

Interventricular Septum (Fig. 13.8)

- The septum that divides the two ventricles is directed obliquely and backwards. It bulges into the right ventricle.
- Externally the site of interventricular septum is indicated by presence of anterior and posterior interventricular grooves (Figs 13.2 and 13.3).
- It consists of two parts
  1. **Membranous part:** It is a small oval part which forms the posterosuperior part of septum.
  2. **Muscular Part:** Rest of the entire septum is muscular. The septal leaflet of tricuspid valve arises from the muscular part of septum on right side. The right branch of A–V bundle is conveyed via the septomarginal trabecula from the septum while the left branch pierces the membranous part of septum to appear on left side.

Crux of the Heart

It is the site of meeting of following structures
1. Inter-atrial septum
2. Posterior interventricular septum
3. Posterior part of atrio-ventricular groove

Arterial Supply of Heart

The heart is primarily supplied by the right and left coronary arteries. They are also known as vasa vasorum, as developmentally the heart is itself an artery. The coronary arteries behave as end arteries functionally. Anatomically however they do anastomose with each other. The inner 0.5 mm thickness of heart receives nutrition directly from the blood in its chambers.

Right Coronary Artery

It arises from the right aortic sinus of ascending aorta (Figs 13.9 and 13.10). It lies between the pulmonary trunk and right auricle. It ends by anastomosing with the circumflex branch of left coronary artery.

Branches
1. **Right conus artery:** It is the 1st branch. It supplies the infundibulum of right ventricle
2. **Right anterior ventricular rami:** These are 3-4 in number. The right marginal artery is the largest ramus and it supplies the adjoining surfaces of ventricle along the inferior border. Other rami supply the sternocostal surface of right ventricle
3. **Right atrial rami:** These supply the myocardium of right atrium
4. **Sino-atrial artery:** It supplies SA node in 65% individuals. In rest 35% S.A. node is supplied via left coronary artery
5. **Right posterior ventricular rami:** They supply diaphragmatic surface of ventricle.
6. **Right posterior atrial rami:** They supply posterior surface of right and left atria
7. **Posterior interventricular branch:** It supplies following areas:
   a. 1/3rd of interventricular septum, posterior-inferior part
   b. A-V node, in 90% individuals
   c. Diaphragmatic surface of right and left ventricles.

Left Coronary Artery

It is wider and larger than the right coronary artery. It arises from the left posterior aortic sinus of ascending aorta (Figs 13.9 and 13.10). It lies between the pulmonary trunk and the left auricle. It ends by dividing into anterior interventricular and circumflex branches.

Branches
1. Anterior interventricular artery: It runs in the anterior interventricular groove and gives following branches:
   a. **Anterior ventricular rami:** These supply sternocostal surface of both ventricles.
   b. **Septal rami:** Supply the major (about 2/3rd) part of interventricular septum.
2. **Circumflex artery:** It runs in the left atrioventricular groove, winds around left border of heart to reach the posterior atrioventricular groove and ends by anastomosing with the right coronary artery. It gives the following branches.
   a. Atrial rami, supply left atrium.
   b. Ventricular rami, supply left ventricle.

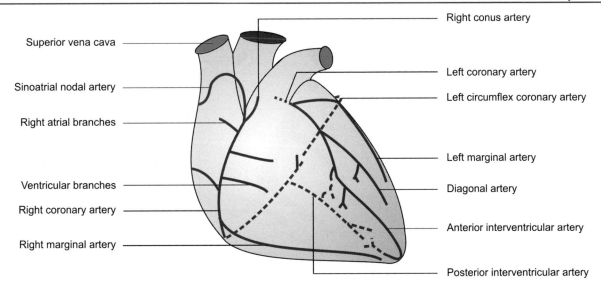

Fig. 13.9: Right and left coronary arteries (anterior view of heart)

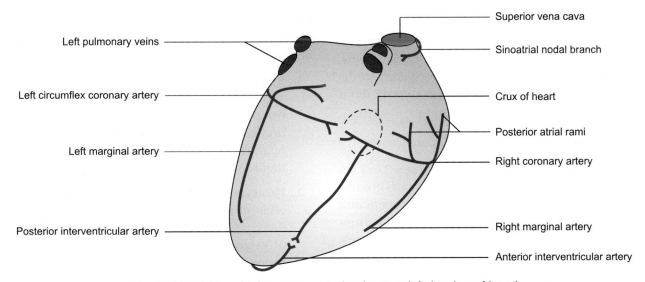

Fig. 13.10: Right and left coronary arteries (postero-inferior view of heart)

c. Left marginal artery.
d. SA nodal artery, in 35% individuals.
e. Posterior intercventricular artery, in 10% individuals.

Myocardial Circulation

The myocardial circulation presents with the following anastomosis which are important to maintain flow in minor blockages.

1. **Interarterial anastomosis:** The right and left coronary arteries anastomose at the precapillary level. These anastomosis increase with age.
2. Arterio-venous anastomosis

3. Arterio-sinusoidal anastomosis: Few terminal branches of coronary arteries end in sinusoids.
4. Sinu-sinusoidal and sinu-luminal: The sinusoids open into coronary sinus. Few directly open into lumen of atria
5. Arterio-luminal: Some terminal branches of coronary arteries open into lumen.

Collateral circulation: A potential communication exists between branches of coronary arteries and those which supply the fibrous and parietal pericardium namely
1. Internal thoracic artery.
2. Pericardial, bronchial and esophageal branches of descending aorta.
3. Phrenic arteries.

CHAPTER-13

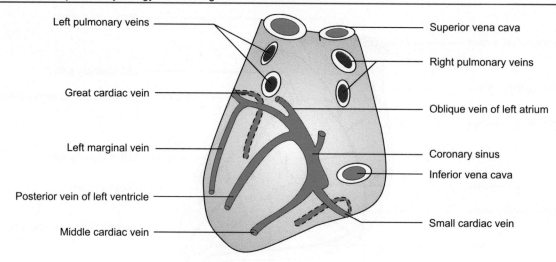

Fig. 13.11: Coronary sinus and its tributaries

Venous Drainage of Heart

The heart is primarily drained by coronary sinus and its tributaries. It is also drained by anterior cardiac veins, small cardiac veins or Thebesian veins (venea cordis minimi) and right marginal vein which directly drain into the right atrium.

Coronary Sinus

It is the largest venous channel of heart and is 2 to 3 cm in length. It lies in the posterior atrioventricular groove, also known as coronary sulcus (Fig. 13.11). It opens into the right atrium in the lower part of inter-atrial septum between the opening of inferior vena cava and atrio-ventricular orifice.

Tributaries

1. **Great cardiac vein:** Runs upwards in anterior interventricular groove.
2. **Middle cardiac vein:** Lies in posterior interventricular groove. Receives left marginal vein.
3. **Small cardiac vein:** Situated in atrioventricular groove on right side. Receives the right marginal vein.
4. **Posterior vein of left ventricle:** It drains the inferior surface of left ventricle.
5. **Oblique vein:** Drains posterior surface of left atrium.

Nerve Supply of the Heart

The heart is supplied by sympathetic and parasympathetic fibres. The sympathetic and parasympathetic fibres form a superficial cardiac plexus, which lies below the arch of aorta and a deep cardiac plexus, which lies in front of the bifurcation of trachea.

1. **Sympathetic supply:** These consist of both efferent and afferent fibres. Preganglionic fibres are derived from T_1 to T_5 segments of spinal cord. Postganglionic fibres arise from superior, middle and inferior-cervical sympathetic ganglia and T_1 to T_5 thoracic ganglia.

2. **Parasympathetic supply:** These consist of both efferent and afferents. Preganglionic fibres are derived from nucleus ambiguus and dorsal nucleus of vagus. Postganglionic fibres lie in the cardiac plexus.

Effect on Heart

1. **Sympathetic fibres supply the atria, ventricles and conducting system of the heart.**
   Sympathetic stimulation leads to
   a. Increase in heart rate.
   b. Increase in cardiac output.
   c. Vasodilation of coronary artery.
   d. Conveys painful sensation from heart.

2. **Parasympathetic fibres supply only the atria and conducting system of heart.**
   Stimulation of vagus nerve leads to
   a. Decrease in heart rate.
   b. Decrease in coronary blood flow.
   c. Visceral reflexes which depress cardiac activity.

CONDUCTING SYSTEM OF HEART

The musculature of heart consists of special cardiac myocytes that initiate and conduct the cardiac impulse from the pacemaker region of the heart to the atrial and ventricular myocardium (Fig. 13.12).

The conducting system of heart includes the following
1. **Sino-atrial node (SA-node)**
   — It is the pacemaker of the heart situated in the right atrium.
   — The node consists of special myocytes arranged in a flattened, ellipsoid form in the groove between right auricle and right side of opening of superior vena cava, above the crista terminalis.
   — It measures about 10 to 20 mm in length, 3 mm antero-posteriorly and 1 mm in thickness.
   — It is supplied by right vagal nerve and sympathetic fibers from right cervical sympathetic ganglia.
   — It consists of rhythmically discharging cells, P-cells (pacemaker cells).
2. **Atrio-ventricular node (AV-node)**
   — It is smaller than SA node.
   — AV node lies on right side of posterior part of atrial septum, just above the opening of coronary sinus.
   — It measures 8 mm in anteroposteriorly, 3 mm vertically and 1 mm transversely.
   — The impulse from SA node reaches the AV node via interatrial tracts or internodal tracts.
   — It is supplied by fibers from left vagus nerve and left side of cervical sympathetic chain.
3. **Internodal pathways:** These are modified atrial muscle fibers, present as three bundles which connect the SA node to AV node.
4. **Atrio-ventricular bundle (Bundle of His)**
   — This consist of a bundle of fibres that extend from the antero-inferior part of the AV node to the muscular part of ventricular septum passing along the postero-inferior border of membranous part of the septum.
   — It divides into right and left branches at the crest of muscular part of ventricular septum. They are distributed to the respective ventricles by breaking up into a network of Purkinje fibres.
4. **Purkinje fibres**
   — These are the terminal fibers originating from the right and left bundle branches.
   — These fibers are longer that the rest of musculature and spread to all parts of ventricular myocardium.
   — These consist of subendocardial plexuses of special myocytes which connect to the ventricular myocardium.

Origin and Spread of Cardiac Muscle Excitation

The contraction and relaxation of the cardiac muscle is brought about by specialized conduction tissue located in it which generates and propogates the electrical impulses.

Origin of cardiac excitation: Pacemaker action potentials originate in the sinoatrial node (SA node). Action potential in SA node is largely due to Ca^{2+} influx with little contribution of Na^+ influx. It has a relatively slow depolarization followed by slow repolarization. There is no rapid spike of depolarization. Vagal (cholinergic) stimulation causes hyper-polarization and decrease in spontaneous action potentials, that is decreased electrical activity. Sympathetic (adrenergic) stimulation, causes rapid depolarization phase and increases the rate of spontaneous discharges.

Spread of Cardiac Excitation (Fig. 13.12)
- The depolarization wave initiated from the SA node spreads from atrial fibers via the internodal pathways to converge on AV node.
- Atrial depolarization is complete in 0.1 second.
- AV node conduction is slower and presents a delay of 0.1 seconds before spread of depolarization to ventricles.
- The wave of excitation spreads from A–V node to Purkinje fibers via bundle branches.
- The Purkinje system is rapidly conducting and depolarization of ventricles is complete in 0.08–0.1 second.

Electrocardiogram (ECG)

ECG is the record of the changes in electrical potentials of the myocardium during the rhythmic discharge and spread of excitatory impulses. This record is obtained from external body surface as the body fluids are good conductors of electricity due to presence of numerous electrolytes.

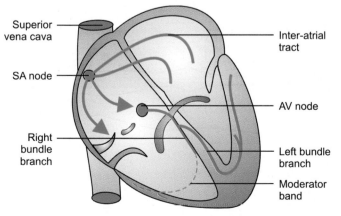

Superior vena cava
SA node
Right bundle branch
Inter-atrial tract
AV node
Left bundle branch
Moderator band

Fig. 13.12: Conducting system of heart

Procedure of Record of ECG (Fig. 13.13)

- ECG is recorded with the help of electrocardiograph machine.
- Patient is placed in supine position with arms on the side and told to relax. Upper chest is bared.
- A total of nine leads are placed. A conducting gel is applied in the interface between skin and helps to facilitate conduction.
- Three leads are placed respectively at the wrist of right arm (aVR), wrist of left arm (aVL) and just above ankle of left leg (aVF). This forms a triangle–Einthoven's triangle and the sum of potentials of the three equals zero.
- Six leads are placed on the chest at the following points:
  1. V_1: 4th intecostal space, to right of sternum.
  2. V_2: 4th intercostal space, to left of sternum.
  3. V_3: Midway between V_2 and V_4.
  4. V_4: 5th left intercostal space in midclavicular line.
  5. V_5: 5th left intercostal space in anterior axillary line.
  6. V_6: 5th left intercostal space in mid axillary line.
- The result is obtained on the ECG paper in the form of various waves which are: (Fig. 13.14)
  1. **P-wave**
     — It is produced due to atrial depolarization.
     — It is directed upwards (positive deflection) with duration of 0.1 sec.
  2. **PR segment:** It is a brief isoelectric period of 0.04 sec between end of P wave and beginning of R wave.
  3. **QRS complex**
     — It is produced due to ventricular depolarization.
     — It consists of small downward (negative) deflection, Q wave, then a prominent upward deflection, R-wave followed by another downward deflection, S-wave.

4. **ST segment:** It is an isoelectric segment from end of S-wave to beginning of T-wave, 0.04-0.08 second.
5. **T-wave:** It is produced due to ventricular repolarization and seen as a positive or upward deflection (except in aVR lead where T-wave is seen as a downward deflection normally).
6. **P-R interval:** It is the interval between beginning of P-wave and beginning of QRS complex. It denotes atrial depolarization and conduction across A-V node. Its normal duration is 0.13-0.16 seconds. P-R interval of more than 0.2 sec indicates delayed conduction.
7. **QT interval:** It is the interval between beginning of Q-wave to end of T-wave. It corresponds to ventricular depolarization and repolarization. Its normal duration is 0.4 sec.
8. **ST interval:** It is the interval between end of S-wave and end of T-wave. It represents ventricular repolarization and its normal duration is 0.32 sec.

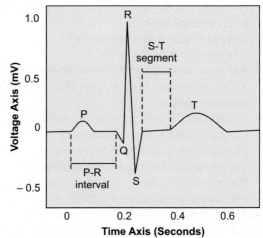

Fig. 13.14: Normal ECG

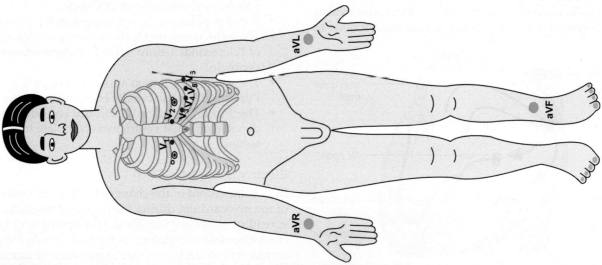

Fig. 13.13: Diagrammatic representation of position of various leads for ECG

CARDIAC CYCLE (FIG. 13.15)

The waves of excitation (depolarization) triggers contraction of myocardium leading to sequential changes in pressure and flow in heart chambers and blood vessels. The following events occur in one cardiac cycle.

1. **Late diastole:** It is the filling stage of heart with blood flowing into atria and from atria into ventricles. A-V valves are open while aortic and pulmonary valves are closed.
2. **Atrial systole:** It is the contraction of the atria.

— Both atria contract simultaneously to propel blood into the ventricles. It contributes to 30% of the ventricular filling.
— It starts after P-wave.
— Atrial systole lasts for 0.1 sec

3. **Ventricular systole:** Is the contraction of the ventricles, both contract simultaneously.
— Starts near the end of R-wave and ends just beyond the T-wave.
— At the onset, the AV valves close (1st heart sound occurs).

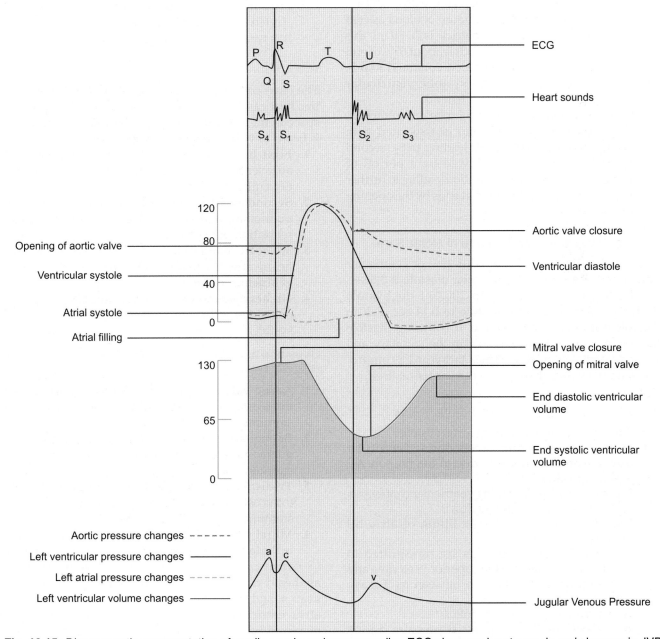

Fig. 13.15: Diagrammatic representation of cardiac cycle and corresponding ECG changes, heart sounds and changes in JVP

— It lasts for 0.3 second.
— The contraction has 2 phases:
  a. **Isometric or isovolumetric contraction:** The ventricles contract but the aortic and pulmonary valves are closed. The intra ventricular pressures rise above 80 mm Hg in left and 10 mm Hg in right. This is associated with bulging of AV valve into atria causing a small increase in atrial pressure. It lasts for 0.05 second.
  b. **Ventricular ejection:** With further ventricular contraction, the semilunar valves open and blood ejects out of ventricles. AV valves are pulled down and atrial pressure drops. It lasts for 0.25 second. The amount of blood ejected per contraction per ventricle is 70-80 ml, this is called stroke volume. It is about 65% of end diastolic ventricular blood volume (130 ml). About 50 ml of end systolic ventricular volume of blood is left behind.

4. **Early diastole:** At the end of ventricular contraction, ventricular pressure falls and is associated with closure of semilunar valves, leading to S_2 (second heart sound). This is followed by a period of isovolumetric ventricle relaxation leading to further fall in ventricular pressure that ends by the opening of AV valves.

Relation of Systole and Diastole to Heart Rate

At normal heart rate of 72/mt, duration of ventricular systole is 0.3 second and ventricular diastole is 0.5 sec. As the heart rate increases to 200/mt the systole decreases to 0.16 sec and diastole to 0.14 sec. Fall in diastole duration is more severe. It is during diastole that heart rests and there is flow in the coronary and subendocardial circulation. Thus, tachycardia compromises on the vascular supply to cardiac tissue itself.

Atrial Pressure Changes and Jugular Pulse

- Atrial pressure rises during atrial systole.
- Further rise in pressure occurs during ventricular isovolumetric contraction, due to bulging on AV valves into atria.
- Pressure falls rapidly during ventricular contraction as the AV valves are pulled down.
- Pressure again rises due to filling of atria till opening of AV valves.
- The atrial pressure changes are transmitted in retrograde manner into the superior vena cava and then jugular vein. This can be seen as 3-wave pattern of jugular pulse.
  a. **a-wave:** due to atrial systole.
  b. **c-wave:** due to rise in atrial pressure during isovolumetric ventricular systole.
  c. **v-wave:** due to rise in atrial pressure while filling before the opening of tricuspid valve.

Arterial Pulse

- The pressure of blood forced into aorta during systole leads to a pressure wave along the arteries.
- This expands the arterial wall and can be felt as a pulse in the periphery.
- Clinically, it is most often palpated in the distal forearm as the radial pulse. It is felt in the radial artery at the wrist 0.1 sec after the peak of systole.
- Intensity of pulse is determined by pulse pressure that is the difference between systolic and diastolic pressures. It is not related to mean arterial pressure. It is felt bounding during exercise and in fever while it is weak or thready in hypovolemia and shock.

Heart Sounds

The heart contracts (beats) at a rate of 72 to 80/mt and this beat can be felt on palpation in the 5th intercostal space in midclavicular line. On auscultation heart beat is heard as two distinct sounds namely:

1. **First heart sound, S_1:** It is due to closure of atrioventricular valves coinciding with contraction of ventricles.
2. **Second heart sound, S_2:** It is due to closure of pulmonary and aortic valves and coincides with relaxation of ventricles.
3. **3rd heart sound (S_3):** It is a very soft sound, usually heard after S_2. It coincides with period of rapid ventricular filling.
4. **4th heart sound (S_4):** It is heard just before S_1 and coincides with ventricular filling due to atrial systole.

Sites of Auscultation of Various Valve Sounds (Fig. 13.16)

1. **Aortic valve sound:** It is heard in the right 2nd intercostal space just next to the lateral margin of sternum.
2. **Pulmonary valve sound:** It is heard in the left 2nd intercostal space just next to the lateral margin of sternum.
3. **Tricuspid valve sound:** It is heard in the left 5th intercostal space just next to the lateral margin of sternum.
4. **Mitral valve sound:** It is heard at the apex of heart in the left 5th intercostal space in midclavicular line.

On auscultation of heart, primarily two heart sound are heard namely LUB (S_1) followed by DUB (S_2) First heart sound (S_1) occurs due to simultaneous closure of atrioventricular valves and second heart sound (S_2) occurs due to simultaneous closure of aortic and pulmonary valves.

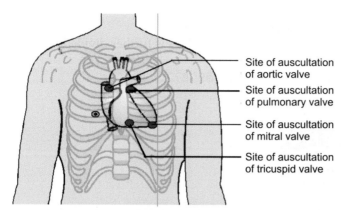

Site of auscultation of aortic valve
Site of auscultation of pulmonary valve
Site of auscultation of mitral valve
Site of auscultation of tricuspid valve

Fig. 13.16: Sites of auscultation of valve sounds

Cardiac Output (CO)

The amount of blood pumped out by each ventricle per minute into the circulation is cardiac output. It equals stroke volume (SV) times the heart rate (HR).

$CO = SV \times HR = 70$ ml/beat $\times 72$ beat/mt $= 5000$ ml/mt. The usual CO is 5 to 6 litres/mt.

Cardiac index is the cardiac output measured in relation to square meter of body surface area, It equals $3.2\ l/m^2$.

Factors Affecting Cardiac Output

These are factors affecting heart rate and stroke volume.

1. **Factors affecting heart rate:** Heart rate increases due to sympathetic stimulation and decreases due to parasympathetic stimulation.
   a. **Age:** At birth heart rate is normally 120 to 140/mt, in young children it is 80 to 100/mt and in adults it is 70 to 80/mt. This is due to increase in vagal tone.
   b. **Sex:** Heart rate is slightly higher in females. Further increase is seen in pregnancy.
   c. **Body temperature:** For every 1 degree F increase in temperature, heart rate increases by 10 beats fast.
   d. **Emotional stimuli:** Fear, anxiety and anger lead to increase in heart rate.
   e. **Exercise:** Increases heart rate.
   f. **Pain:** Is associated with increase heart rate.
   g. **Chronotropic drugs:** These increase the heart rate, e.g., sympathetomimetic drugs like epinephrine and norepinephrine.
   h. Diseases associated with increase heart rate are hyperthyroidism, hypoxia. Raised intra-cranial tension causes decrease heart rate.
2. **Factors affecting stroke volume:** The strength of cardiac muscle contraction determines the stroke volume. It is controlled by:

   a. **Neural mechanism:** Sympathetic stimulation causes increase contractibility while Vagal stimulation decreases atrial contractibility.
   b. **Drugs**
      Ionotropic drugs: These increase the strength of contraction.
      1. *Epinephrine:* Acts via cAMP which increases Ca^{2+} influx.
      2. *Glucagon:* Acts by increasing formation of cAMP.
      3. *Digitalis:* Acts via inhibiting $Na^+ K^+$ ATPase. This increases intracellular Na^+ which in turn increases the availability of Ca^{2+}.
      Drugs with negative ionotropic action
      1. Procainamide
      2. Quinidine
   c. Myocardial failure, infarction, hypoxia and acidosis depress contractility of cardiac muscle by decreasing cAMP levels.
   d. Relation of tension to length in cardiac muscle. Increase stretching of myocardium causes increase strength of contraction (Frank-starling Law). Preload or the end diastolic volume determines the degree to which myocardium is stretched. Hence, factors which affect preload will affect myocardial contractility.
      Preload is increased in
      1. **Inspiration:** Increases negative intra thoracic pressure and increases venous return to heart.
      2. Increased blood volume, e.g., pregnancy.
      3. **Increase capacity of venous system:** as in increased sympathetic stimulation.
      4. Increase skeletal muscle pumping, as in excercise.
      Preload is decreased in
      1. **Pericardial effusion:** Fluid in the pericardial space prevents adequate expansion and filling of cardiac chambers.
      2. Decrease ventricular compliance due to infarction, infiltrative diseases.
      3. Standing posture: 20% decrease in cardiac output occurs from lying down to standing position.
      4. Drugs like nitroglycerine and isosorbide dinitrate act by dilating peripheral veins and arteries leading to pooling of blood in the periphery. Thus, they reduce the venous return to the heart decreasing the end diastolic volume.

ARTERIAL SUPPLY OF BODY

The oxygenated blood pumped out of left ventricle is carried by the aorta and its branches to the entire body.

AORTA

Aorta is the arterial trunk of the body. It arises from the left ventricle of the heart and is divided anatomically into the following parts (Figs 13.17 and 13.18)

1. Ascending aorta
2. Arch of aorta
3. Descending aorta: This is further divided into
   a. Thoracic aorta
   b. Abdominal aorta

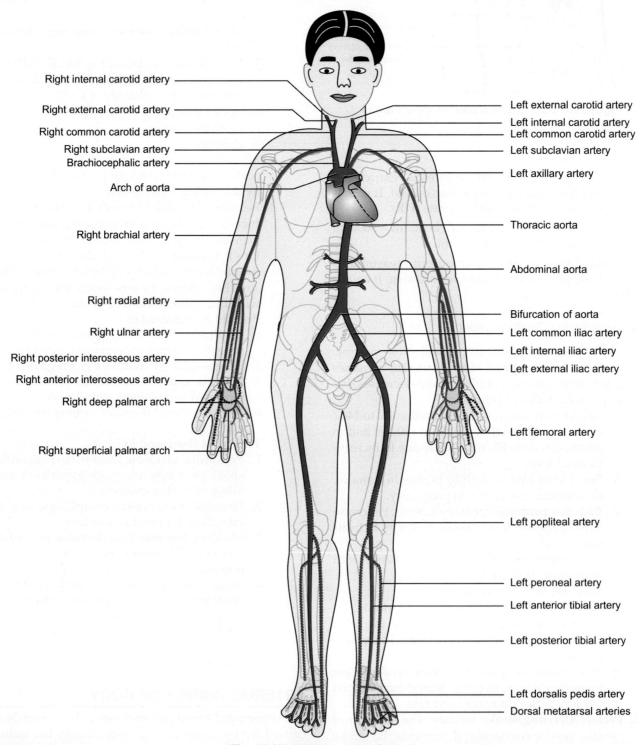

Right internal carotid artery

Right external carotid artery

Right common carotid artery

Right subclavian artery

Brachiocephalic artery

Arch of aorta

Right brachial artery

Right radial artery

Right ulnar artery

Right posterior interosseous artery

Right anterior interosseous artery

Right deep palmar arch

Right superficial palmar arch

Left external carotid artery

Left internal carotid artery

Left common carotid artery

Left subclavian artery

Left axillary artery

Thoracic aorta

Abdominal aorta

Bifurcation of aorta

Left common iliac artery

Left internal iliac artery

Left external iliac artery

Left femoral artery

Left popliteal artery

Left peroneal artery

Left anterior tibial artery

Left posterior tibial artery

Left dorsalis pedis artery

Dorsal metatarsal arteries

Fig. 13.17: Arterial supply of blood

Ascending Aorta

This is the first part of aorta which begins at the aortic orifice of the outflow tract of left ventricle. It ascends upwards, forwards and to the right till the right side of sternal angle. The aorta presents with three dilatations above the semilunar valves which are called the aortic sinuses of Valsalva.

Branches: These arise from the aortic sinuses

1. Right coronary artery
2. Left coronary artery

Arch of Aorta

Arch of aorta lies in the superior mediastinum behind the manubrium sterni. It begins at the level of 2nd costosternal joint on right side as a continuation of the ascending aorta. Here, it presents with a dilatation on the right known as bulb of aorta. It first arches upwards, backwards and towards left passing in front of trachea. Then it curves downwards over the left bronchus and passes behind it. Finally, it continues as the descending aorta at level of lower border of T_4 vertebra. This corresponds to the 2nd left costosternal joint.

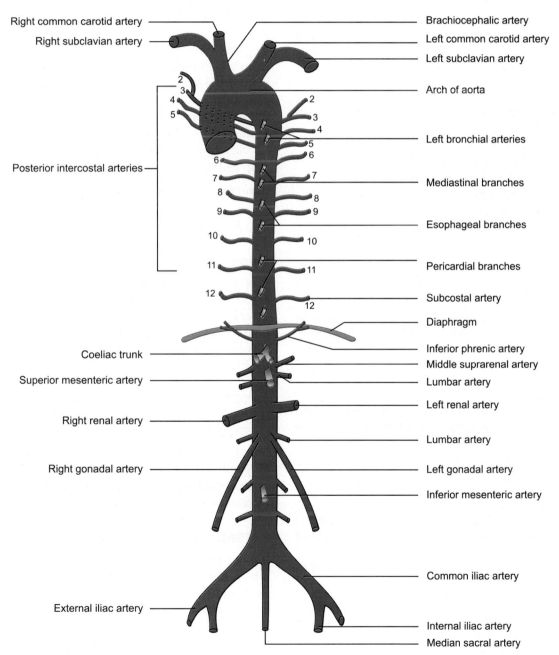

Fig. 13.18: Ascending aorta, arch of aorta, descending aorta, thoracic and abdominal aorta

Branches: It gives rise to three main branches to supply the upper extremities and head and neck.

1. Brachiocephalic trunk
2. Left common carotid artery
3. Left subclavian artery

It may also give rise to the following branches
1. Left vertebral artery
2. Inferior thyroid artery
3. Internal thoracic artery
4. Right subclavian artery

Descending Aorta (Thoracic Aorta)

The thoracic part of descending aorta extends from the level of lower border of T_4 vertebra to the aortic opening in the diaphragm at level of lower border of T_{12} vertebra. It lies in the posterior mediastinum.

Branches:
1. Posterior intercostal arteries: 9 pairs from 3rd to 11th intercostal spaces
2. Subcostal artery: 2 in number
3. Left bronchial artery: 2 in number
4. Oesophageal branches
5. Pericardial branches
6. Mediastinal branches
7. Superior phrenic arteries

Abdominal Aorta

It is the life line of the body below the level of diaphragm. It is the direct continuation of thoracic aort at the aortic opening of diaphragm. This corresponds to the level of lower border of T_{12} vertebra. It ends by dividing into right and left common iliac arteries at the lower border of L_4 vertebra (Fig. 41.3)

Length : About 11 cm
Breadth : 2 cm
Course : It descends downward in front of the vertebral column on the left side of inferior vena cava.

Branches: Total 22 branches are given. They are paired and unpaired

Unpaired are Ventral Branches
1. **Coeliac artery:** Arises at the level of T_{12} vertebra
2. **Superior mesenteric artery:** Arises at the level of L_1 vertebra
3. **Inferior mesenteric artery:** Arises at the level of L_3 vertebra

Paired Branches are divided into
4. **Lateral branches**
   a. Inferior phrenic artery
   b. Middle suprarenal artery
   c. Renal artery

d. Gonadal artery: Testicular artery in male, ovarian artery in female.
5. **Dorsolateral branches:** Four pairs of lumbar arteries.
6. **Terminal branches:** Right and left common iliac arteries.
7. **An unpaired median sacral artery** is the one which is the direct continuation of primitive aorta.

ARTERIAL SUPPLY OF HEAD AND NECK

COMMON CAROTID ARTERY

It is the chief artery supplying head and neck. There are two common carotid arteries, one on right and one on left side. The right common carotid artery originates from the brarchiocephalic trunk (innominate artery) behind the sternoclavicular joint in the neck. The left common carotid artery arises in the thorax directly from the arch of aorta. Each common carotid artery terminates at the level of the intervertebral disc between C_3 and C_4 vertebra by dividing into its terminal branches (Fig. 13.19).

Branches: It gives of only two terminal branches namely
1. External carotid artery
2. Internal carotid artery

Carotid Sinus

It is a dilatation at the terminal end of the common carotid artery or at the beginning of internal carotid artery. It has a rich innervation from the glosso-pharyngeal and sympathetic nerves. The carotid sinus acts as a **baroreceptor** (pressure receptor) and regulates the blood pressure.

Carotid Body

It is a small oval structure situated just behind the bifurcation of the common carotid artery. It is reddish-brown in colour and receives rich nerve supply from glossopharyngeal, vagus and sympathetic nerves. It acts as a **chemoreceptor** and responds to the changes in the oxygen and carbon dioxide contents of the blood.

EXTERNAL CAROTID ARTERY

It is one of the terminal branches of the common carotid artery. It supplies the structures present external to the skull and those in front of the neck. It arises from the common carotid artery at the upper border of lamina of thyroid cartilage. It ends by dividing into its terminal branches at the level of the neck of the mandible and behind the upper part of parotid gland (Fig. 13.19).

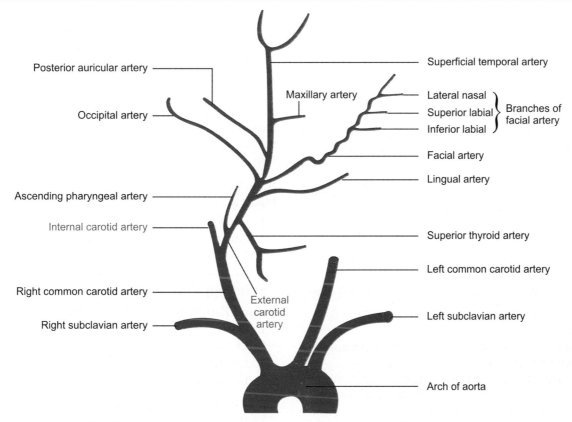

Fig. 13.19: Common carotid and external carotid arteries with their branches

Branches

1. **Ascending pharyngeal artery:** It is a slender artery which arises from the medial aspect of the external carotid artery near its lower end.
2. **Superior thyroid artery:** It arises from the anterior aspect of the external carotid artery just below the tip of the greater cornu of the hyoid bone. It gives of branches to thyroid gland, superior laryngeal artery and branches to sternocleiodomastoid muscle.
3. **Lingual artery:** It arises from the anterior aspect of external carotid artery opposite the tip of the greater cornu of the hyoid bone. It primarily supplies the tongue via: Suprahyoid branch, Dorsal lingual branches, Sublingual artery.
4. Facial artery
5. Occipital artery
6. Posterior auricular artery
7. Maxillary artery
8. Superficial temporal artery

FACIAL ARTERY (EXTERNAL MAXILLARY ARTERY)

It arises from the anterior aspect of external carotid artery just above the tip of greater cornu of hyoid bone. It ends at the nasal side of the eye as the angular artery. It is divided into two parts namely: cervical part and facial part (Fig. 13.19).

Branches
From cervical part (in the neck)
1. Ascending palatine artery
2. Tonsilar artery: main artery of tonsil
3. Glandular branches, to supply the submandibular gland.
4. Submental artery

From the facial part (in the face)
1. Inferior labial artery
2. Superior labial artery
3. Lateral nasal artery
4. Angular artery
5. Small unnamed branches

OCCIPITAL ARTERY

It arises from the posterior aspect of the external carotid artery at the same level as the facial artery. It supplies most of the back of the scalp (Fig. 13.19).

Branches
1. Sternomastoid branches
2. Mastoid artery

3. Meningeal branches
4. Muscular branches
5. Auricular branch
6. Descending branches
7. Occipital branches

POSTERIOR AURICULAR ARTERY

It arises from the posterior aspect of the external carotid artery a little above the occipital artery (Fig. 13.19).

Branches

1. Stylomastoid artery, which enters the stylomastoid foramen to supply the middle ear .
2. Auricular branch
3. Occipital branch

SUPERFICIAL TEMPORAL ARTERY

It is the smaller but a more direct terminal branch of the external carotid artery (Fig. 13.19).

Branches

1. **Transverse facial artery:** It runs forwards across the masseter below the zygomatic arch.
2. **Middle temporal artery:** It runs on the temporal fossa deep to temporal muscles and supplies temporal muscles and fascia.
3. Anterior and posterior terminal branches.

MAXILLARY ARTERY (SYN. INTERNAL MAXILLARY ARTERY)

It is the larger terminal branch of the external carotid artery. It begins behind the neck of mandible and runs horizontally forwards upto the lower border of lower head of lateral pterygoid. From here, it turns upwards and forwards and crosses the lower head of lateral pterygoid superficially (sometimes deep). After emerging between the two heads of lateral pterygoid it enters the pterygo-palatine fossa by passing through the pterygomaxillary fissure. Here, it ends by giving off its terminal branches. Thus the artery is divided into three parts by the lower head of lateral pterygoid muscle (Figs 13.19, 13.20).

Branches

First Part: It gives rise to five branches
1. Deep auricular artery
2. Anterior tympanic artery
3. Middle meningeal artery
4. Accessory meningeal artery
5. Inferior alveolar artery

Second Part: It gives rise to four branches
1. Deep temporal artery
2. Pterygoid branches
3. Masseteric artery
4. Buccal artery

Third Part: It gives rise to six branches
1. Posterior superior alveolar (dental) artery
2. Infra-orbital artery
3. Greater palatine artery
4. Pharyngeal artery
5. Artery of pterygoid canal
6. Spheno-palatine artery

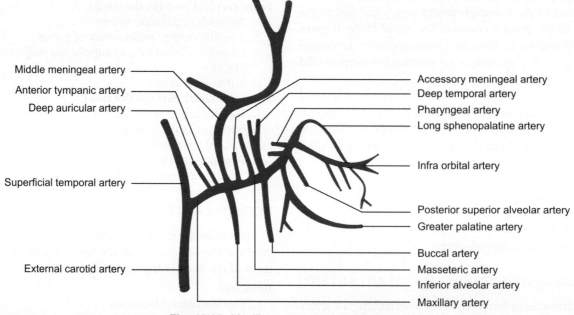

Fig. 13.20: Maxillary artery and its branches

Middle Meningeal Artery (Fig. 13.20)

Clinically, middle meningeal artery is the most important branch of the maxillary artery. It arises from the first part of maxillary artery. It ascends upwards deep to the lateral pterygoid muscle and behind the mandibular nerve. Then, it passes between the two roots of auriculotemporal nerve and enters the cranial cavity through the foramen spinosum along with the meningeal branch of mandibular nerve. After it emerges in the cranial cavity, it passes forwards and laterally on the squamous part of the temporal bone and divides into two branches

1. Frontal (anterior) branch
2. Parietal (posterior) branch

Distribution: The middle meningeal artery and its branches lie outside the dura and deep to the inner surface of skull and supply both. The area of distribution of frontal branch corresponds with the motor area of the cerebral cortex.

INTERNAL CAROTID ARTERY

The internal carotid artery is one of the two terminal branches of the common carotid artery and is more direct. It is considered as the upward continuation of the common carotid. **It supplies structures lying within the skull and in the orbit.** It begins at the upper border of the lamina of thyroid cartilage (at the level of inter-vertebral disc between C_3 and C_4) and runs upwards to reach the base of skull, where it enters the carotid canal in the petrous temporal bone. It enters the cranial cavity by passing through the upper part of the foramen lacerum. In the cranial cavity it enters the cavernous sinus and finally ends below the anterior perforated substance of the brain by dividing into the anterior cerebral and middle cerebral arteries. Hence it is divided into four parts namely cervical part, petrous part, cavernous part and cerebral part (Fig. 13.21).

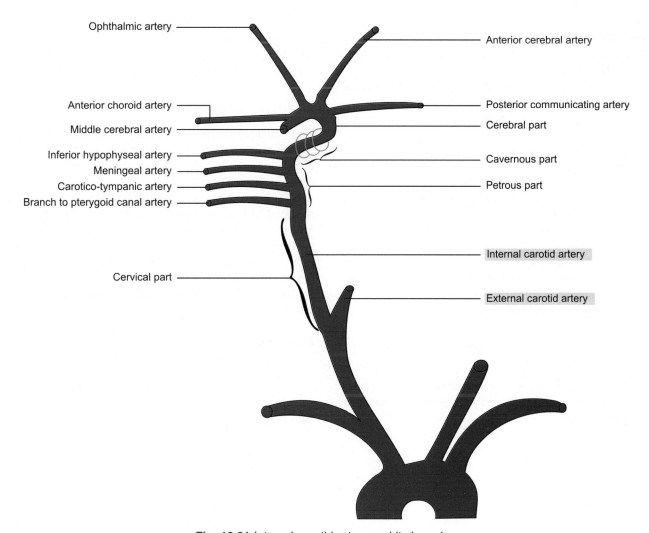

Fig. 13.21: Internal carotid artery and its branches

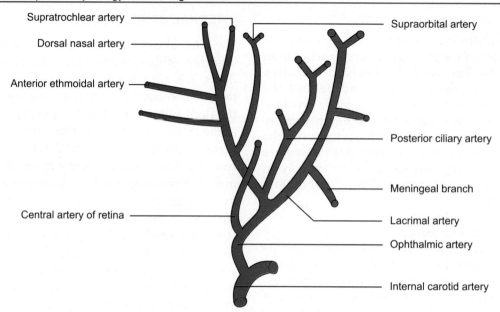

Fig. 13.22: Ophthalmic artery and its branches

Branches
1. **Cervical part:** The internal carotid artery gives no branches in the neck
2. **Petrous part:** It gives rise to the following branches:
   a. Carotico-tympanic branch to middle ear
   b. Pterygoid branch, a small and inconstant branch that enters the pterygoid canal.
3. **Cavernous part:** It gives rise to the following branches:
   a. Cavernous branches to the trigeminal ganglion.
   b. Superior and inferior hypophyseal arteries, to the hypophyseal cerebri (pituitary gland)
4. **Cerebral part:** It gives rise to the following branches:
   a. Ophthalmic artery
   b. Anterior choroidal artery
   c. Posterior communicating artery
   d. Anterior cerebral artery
   e. Middle cerebral artery

Ophthalmic Artery

It is a branch of internal carotid artery and arises from it, medial to the anterior clinoid process close to the optic canal (Fig. 13.22).

Branches
1. Central artery of retina
2. Lacrimal artery
3. Posterior ciliary arteries
4. Supra-orbital artery
5. Posterior ethmoidal artery
6. Anterior ethmoidal artery
7. Dorsal nasal artery
8. Supratrochlear artery
9. Medial palpebral branches

SUBCLAVIAN ARTERY

The subclavian artery supplies the upper limb, cranial cavity and structures in the neck. Right subclavian artery arises from the brachiocephalic trunk, behind the right sternoclavicular joint, at the root of neck. Left subclavian artery arises from the arch of aorta, in the thorax. The artery extends from the sternoclavicular joint on each side to the outer border of the first rib taking a curved course over the cervical pleura with convexity facing upwards. It continues as the axilliary artery beyond the outer border of Ist rib (Fig. 13.23).

Each artery is divided into three parts by the scalenus anterior muscle.

Branches
1. Vertebral artery
2. Internal thoracic artery
3. Thyrocervical trunk
4. Costocervical trunk (on left side only)
5. Dorsal scapular artery

Vertebral Artery (Fig. 13.23)

The vertebral artery arises from the upper aspect of the first part of the subclavian artery. It passes upwards through the foramina transverseria of cervical vertebrae on both sides (except C_7) and enters the cranial cavity

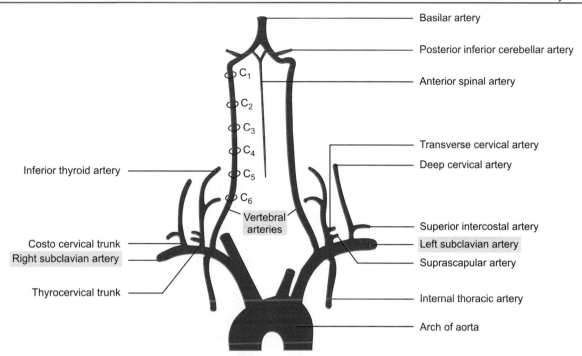

Fig. 13.23: Subclavian and vertebral arteries

via the foramen magnum. In the cranial cavity it unites with the vertebral artery of the other side at the lower border of the pons to form the basilar artery (Fig. 13.23).

Branches

In the neck (cervical branches)

1. Spinal branches: These enter the vertebral canal through intervertebral foramen to supply the upper 5 or 6 cervical segments of the spinal cord.
2. Muscular branches: They supply muscles of sub-occipital triangle.

In the cranial cavity (cranial branches)

1. Meningeal branches: They supply meninges of posterior cranial fossa.
2. Posterior spinal artery (sometimes it may arise from posterior inferior cerebellar artery). It passes downwards and divides into anterior and posterior branches. It first passes in front and later behind the dorsal roots of the spinal nerves to supply the spinal cord.
3. Posterior inferior cerebellar artery: It is the largest branch of the vetebral artery. It winds round the medulla and takes a tortuous course. It supplies:
   a. Lateral part of the medulla.
   b. Inferior vermis and infero-lateral surface of the cerebral hemisphere (see brain).

4. Anterior spinal artery
5. Medullar branches supply the medulla.

Internal Thoracic Artery (Internal Mammary Artery)

The internal mammary artery arises from the inferior aspect of the first part of the subclavian artery opposite the origin of thyro-cervical trunk. It runs vertically down to enter the thorax behind the sternal end of clavicle. Then it descends behind upper 6 costal cartilages 1 cm away from the lateral margin of sternum. It ends by dividing into musculophrenic and superior epigastric arteries in the 6th intercostal space.

Branches

1. Pericardicophrenic artery
2. Mediastinal artery
3. Pericardial artery
4. Sternal artery
5. Anterior intercostal arteries: 2 arteries are given off in each space from the 1st to 6th.
6. 5 or 6 perforating arteries in upper 5 or 6 intercostal spaces
7. Musculophrenic artery
8. Superior epigastric artery

Thyrocervical Trunk (Fig. 13.23)

The thyrocervical trunk arises from the upper aspect of the first part of subclavian artery lateral to the origin of vertebral artery.

Branches
1. **Inferior thyroid artery:** It supplies the thyroid and parathyroid glands. It further gives rise to following arteries:
   a. Ascending cervical artery
   b. Inferior laryngeal artery
   c. Tracheal and oesophageal branches
   d. Glandular branches
2. Superficial cervical artery
3. Supra-scapular artery

Costocervical Trunk (Fig. 13.23)

It arises from the posterior aspect of first part of the subclavian artery on the left side, second part of the subclavian artery on the right side. The artery arches backwards above the cupola of the pleura and on reaching the neck of first rib divides into deep cervical and superior intercostal arteries.

Dorsal Scapular Artery

It arises from the third part of the subclavian artery, sometimes from the second part. It passes laterally and backwards between the trunks of brachial plexus to reach underneath the levator scapulae. Now it descends along the medial border of the scapula along with the dorsal scapular nerve, deep to the rhomboids and takes part in the formation of arterial anastomosis around the sacpula.

CIRCLE OF WILLIS

It is a polygonal shaped arterial circle that lies in relation to the base of brain at the level of interpeduncular fossa (Fig. 13.24).
Formation: The circle is formed by branches of the two internal carotid and the two vertebral arteries as follows.

1. **Anteriorly:** Anterior communicating artery (between two anterior cerebral arteries
2. **Posteriorly:** Terminal part of the basilar artery, Proximal part of two posterior cerebral arteries
3. **Anterolaterally:** Two anterior cerebral arteries
4. **Posterolaterally:** Two posterior communicating arteries (between posterior cerebral and internal carotid artery on each side)
5. **Laterally:** Proximal part of both internal carotid arteries.

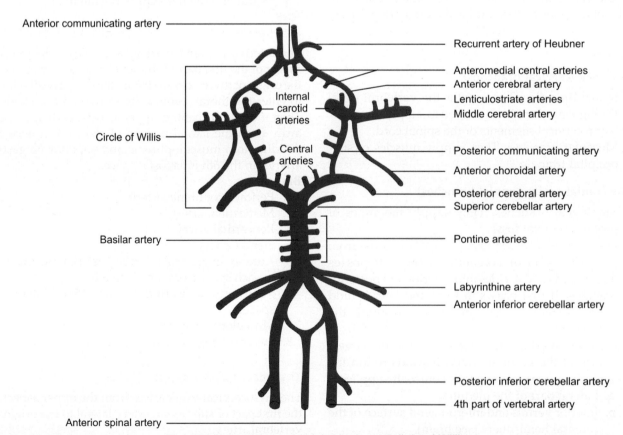

Fig. 13.24: Arterial supply of the brain and circle of Willis

Branches of Circle of Willis
1. Antero-medial branches of anterior communicating and anterior cerebral arteries.
2. Antero-lateral branches from middle cerebral artery.
3. Posteromedial branches from posterior cerebral and posterior communicating arteries.
4. Postero-lateral branches from posterior cerebral arteries.

Functions of Circle of Willis

1. It helps to equalize the blood flow during normal conditions to different parts of the brain.
2. Normally, there is no intermixing of blood between the internal carotid and vertebral arterial system.

ARTERIAL SUPPLY OF SCALP (FIG. 13.25)

The scalp is richly supplied by blood vessels. Each half of the scalp is supplied by five arteries. These are :

In front of the ear: 3 in number
1. Supra trochlear artery: Branch of ophthalmic artery
2. Supra orbital artery: Branch of ophthalmic artery
3. Superficial temporal artery: Branch of external carotid artery

Behind the ear: 2 in number
4. Posterior auricular artery: Branch of external carotid artery.
5. Occipital artery: Branch of external carotid artery

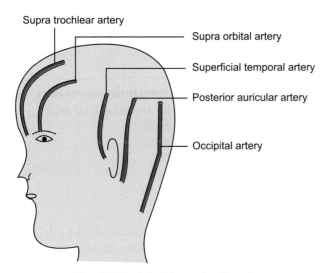

Fig. 13.25: Arterial supply of scalp

ARTERIAL SUPPLY OF FACE (FIG. 13.26)

The face has a rich blood supply.
1. Facial artery: This is the chief artery of face and arises from external carotid artery. It divides into following branches
   a. Superior labial
   b. Inferior labial
   c. Lateral nasal
2. Transverse facial artery, branch of superficial temporal artery.
3. Small arteries that accompany the cutaneous branches of trigeminal nerve.

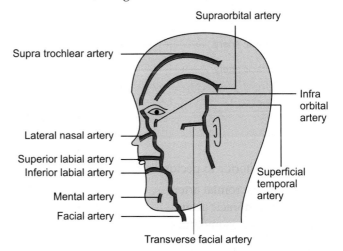

Fig. 13.26: Arterial supply of face

ARTERIAL SUPPLY OF UPPER LIMB

Upperlimb is supplied by the brachial artery and its branches. Brachial artery is a continuation of the axillary artery which supplies the axillary and pectoral areas.

AXILLARY ARTERY

It is the continuation of subclavian artery and it extends from the outer border of first rib to lower border of teres major muscle from where it continues as brachial artery. It enters axilla through the apex of axilla, enclosed in axillary sheath. It is accompanied inferomedially by axillary vein and is related to cords of brachial plexus in the axilla. It is divided into three parts by pectoralis minor muscle (Fig 13.27).

Branches

Ist part: Proximal to pectoralis minor muscle
1. Superior thoracic artery.

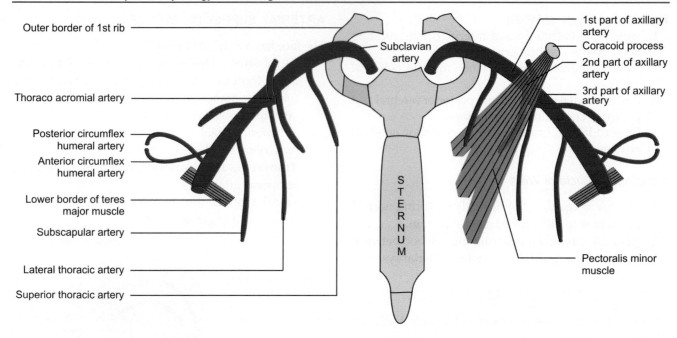

Fig. 13.27: Axillary artery and its branches

2nd part: Posterior to pectoralis minor muscle

1. Thoracoacromial artery.
2. Lateral thoracic artery.
3. Alar artery-sometimes.

3rd part: Distal to pectoralis minor muscle

1. Subscapular artery.
2. Anterior circumflex humeral artery.
3. Posterior circumflex humeral artery.

BRACHIAL ARTERY

It is the continuation of axillary artery and extends from the lower border of teres major to neck of radius where it divides into its terminal branches namely, ulnar and radial artery. It runs downwards and laterally from the medial side of arm to front of elbow. The artery is superficial and is accompanied by two vena comitantes. Median nerve crosses it anteriorly from lateral to medial side in the middle of arm (Fig. 13.28). In the cubital fossa it is related to

a. Bicipital aponeurosis—crosses above it.
b. Tendon of biceps lies lateral to it.
c. Median nerve lies medial to brachial artery.

Branches

1. Profunda brachii artery.
2. Nutrient artery to humerus.
3. Superior ulnar collateral artery.
4. Inferior ulnar collateral artery.

5. Muscular branches to anterior compartment.
6. Radial artery.
7. Ulnar artery.

RADIAL ARTERY

It is the smaller terminal branch of brachial artery. It begins at the neck of radius and runs under the superficial fascia of forearm. At the wrist it lies in anatomical snuff box and leaves it by passing through two heads of 1st dorsal interosseous muscle. It enters the palm between two heads of adductor pollicis. It terminates by forming the deep palmar arch with the help of deep branch of ulnar artery in palm (Fig. 13.28).

Branches

1. Radial recurrent artery
2. Muscular branches
3. Palmar carpal branch for palmar carpal arch
4. Dorsal carpal branch for dorsal carpal arch
5. Superficial palmar branch
6. Ist dorsal metacarpal artery
7. Arteria princeps pollicis
8. Arteria radialis indicis

ULNAR ARTERY

It is the larger terminal branch of brachial artery. It begins at the neck of radius and runs in the forearm lying deep in upper 1/3rd and superficial in lower 2/3rd. It enters the palm passing superficial to flexor retinaculum along

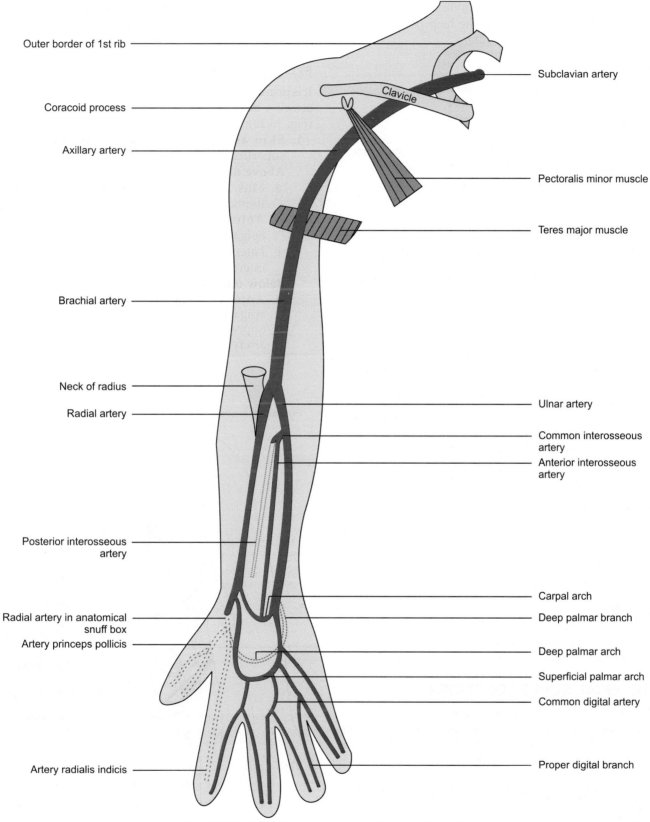

Fig. 13.28: Arterial supply of upper limb, anterior view

Outer border of 1st rib

Coracoid process

Axillary artery

Brachial artery

Neck of radius

Radial artery

Posterior interosseous artery

Radial artery in anatomical snuff box

Artery princeps pollicis

Artery radialis indicis

Subclavian artery

Clavicle

Pectoralis minor muscle

Teres major muscle

Ulnar artery

Common interosseous artery

Anterior interosseous artery

Carpal arch

Deep palmar branch

Deep palmar arch

Superficial palmar arch

Common digital artery

Proper digital branch

with the ulnar nerve. It terminates by forming the superficial palmar arch with the help of a branch of radial artery in palm (Fig. 13.28).

Branches
1. Anterior ulnar recurrent artery
2. Posterior ulnar recurrent artery
3. Common interosseous artery
4. Anterior interosseous artery
5. Posterior interosseous artery – It is the main artery for extensor compartment of the forearm
6. Palmar and dorsal carpal branches
7. Muscular branches

ARTERIAL SUPPLY OF HAND

Hand is supplied by a pair of arterial arches namely, superficial palmar arch, and deep palmar arch (Fig. 13.28).

Superficial Palmar Arch (Fig. 13.28)

It is an arterial arcade formed by superficial terminal branch of ulnar artery and completed on lateral side by one of the following arteries
a. Superficial palmar branch of radial artery
b. Arteria princeps pollicis, branch of radial artery
c. Arteria radialis indicis, branch of radial artery
   Superficial palmar arch lies beneath palmar aponeurosis

Branches
Four palmar digital arteries.

Deep Palmar Arch (Fig. 13.28)

It is formed by terminal end of radial artery and deep branch of ulnar artery.

Branches
1. Three palmar metacarpal arteries
2. Three perforating arteries
3. Recurrent branch

ARTERIAL SUPPLY OF THORAX

The thoracic wall is supplied by intercostal arteries (see page no. 378). The various viscera of the thorax are supplied by branches of thoracic aorta which are described along with the viscera itself.

ARTERIAL SUPPLY OF ABDOMEN AND PELVIS

The abdominal wall is supplied by branches of superior and inferior epigastric arteries and lumbar arteries. The various abdominal and pelvic viscera are supplied by branches of abdominal aorta. The pelvic structures are supplied by internal and external iliac arteries.

BLOOD SUPPLY OF ANTERIOR ABDOMINAL WALL

It is primarily supplied by superior and inferior epigastric arteries. Blood supply can be divided into two levels (Fig. 13.29):
1. **Skin and superficial fascia** are supplied by superficial branches of the following arteries:
   Above umbilicus
   a. Musculophrenic artery, branch of internal thoracic artery.
   b. Anterior cutaneous branches of superior epigastric artery.
   c. Lateral cutaneous branches of lower posterior intercostal arteries.
   Below umbilicus
   a. Anterior cutaneous branches of inferior epigastric artery.
   b. Superficial epigastric artery, branch of femoral artery.

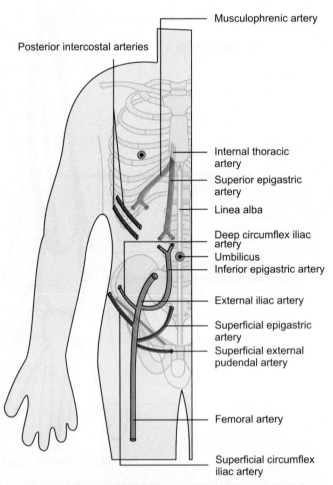

Fig. 13.29: Arterial supply of anterior abdominal wall

c. Superficial circumflex iliac artery, branch of femoral artery.

d. Superficial external pudendal artery.

2. **Muscles, fascia and parietal peritoneum**

   Above umbilicus

   a. Superior epigastric artery, branch of internal thoracic artery.

   b. 10th and 11th intercostal arteries.

   c. Subcostal artery.

   Below umbilicus

   a. Inferior epigastric artery, branch of external iliac artery.

   b. Deep circumflex iliac artery, branch of external iliac artery.

Superior Epigastric Artery (Fig. 13.29)

It is one of the terminal branches of internal thoracic artery. It enters the rectus sheath through a gap in the diaphragm between its sternal and costal origin at the 7th costal cartilage and runs vertically downwards.

Branches:

1. Muscular branches
2. Cutaneous branches
3. Hepatic branch
4. Terminal part anastomose with inferior epigastric artery

Inferior Epigastric Artery (Fig. 13.29)

It is a branch of the external iliac artery and arises just above the inguinal ligament. It passes medial to the deep inguinal ring where it is hooked by the vas deferens in front of the arcuate line. It pierces fascia transversalis and passes in front of arcuate line to enter the rectus sheath. It passes upwards and ends by anastomosing with superior epigastric artery

Branches

1. Cremasteric branch
2. Pubic branch – can replace obturator artery also known as **aberrant obturator artery**
3. Peritoneal branch
4. Muscular branches
5. Cutaneous branches
6. Anastomosing branches

COELIAC TRUNK

It is the artery of foregut, developmentally. It arises from abdominal aorta, opposite the intervertebral disc between T_{12} and L_1 vertebrae (Fig. 13.30).

Branches

a. **Left gastric artery:** It is the smallest branch of coeliac trunk, it supplies the major part of stomach. It gives esophageal branches.

b. **Splenic artery:** It is the largest branch of coeliac trunk. It is tortuous. It passes through the lienorenal ligament and reaches the hilum of spleen where it divides into 5 to 6 branches.

   Branches of splenic artery:

   1. Pancreatic
   2. Short gastric
   3. Left gastroepiploic

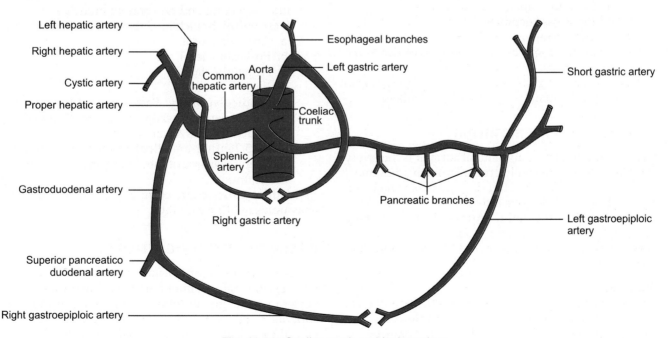

Fig. 13.30: Coeliac trunk and its branches

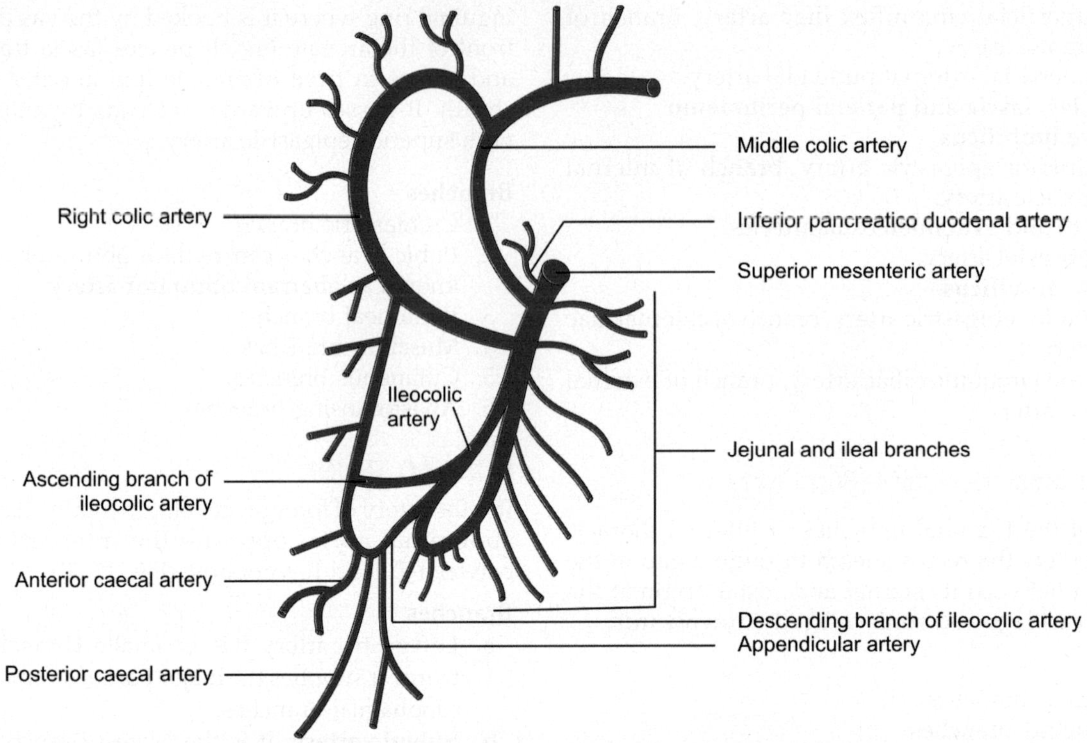

Fig. 13.31: Superior mesenteric artery and its distribution

c. **Common hepatic:** It enters the free margin of lesser omentum after passing through floor of epiploic foramen.
Branches
1. **Right gastric**
2. **Gastroduodenal:** It gives rise to
   i. Superior pancreaticoduodenal
   ii. Right gastroepiploic
3 **Hepatic proper:** It divides into right and left branches. Right hepatic artery gives rise to the cystic artery.
   Sometimes gastroduodenal artery gives rise to supraduodenal artery (Artery of Wilkie)

SUPERIOR MESENTERIC ARTERY

It is a ventral branch of abdominal aorta. It is the artery of midgut, developmentally. It arises from the abdominal aorta opposite L_1 vertebra. It ends by anastomosing with its own branch of ileocolic artery. It runs downwards, forwards and to the right, anterior to the uncinate process of pancreas where it crosses: 3rd part of duodenum, inferior vena cava, right psoas major, right ureter (Fig. 13.31).

Branches
1. **Inferior pancreaticoduoenal:** It is the first branch.
2. **Middle colic artery:** Given out at the lower border of pancreas divides into right and left branch.

3. **Right colic artery**
   a. Given at the middle of the convexity of superior mesenteric artery.
   b. Divides into ascending and descending branches.
4. **Ileo-colic artery:** It is the terminal branch. It divides into ascending and descending branches.
   Descending branch give rise to following arteries
   a. Anterior caecal
   b. Posterior caecal
   c. Appendicular
   d. Ileal
   Appendicular artery: Passes behind the terminal part of the ileum, reaches mesoappendix and tip of the appendix. It is an end artery.
5. 12 to15 Jejunal and ileal branches. They pass between the layers of mesentery and supply ileum and jejunum.
   Middle colic, right colic and ileocolic arteries anastomose with each other.

INFERIOR MESENTERIC ARTERY

It arises from the ventral aspect of aorta. Developmentally it is the artery of hind gut. It arises at the level of L_3 vertebra from the abdominal aorta. It continues as superior rectal artery in lesser pelvis which anastomose with the branches of inferior rectal artery (Fig. 13.32).

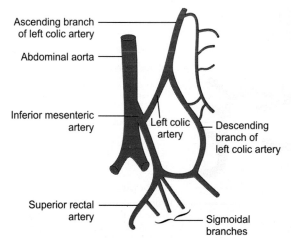

Fig. 13.32: Inferior mesenteric artery and its distribution

Branches

1. **Left colic artery:** divides into descending and ascending branches.
2. **Sigmoidal arteries:** 2 or 3 in number. They supply descending and sigmoid colon.
3. **Superior rectal artery:** It is the continuation of inferior mesenteric artery at the root of the sigmoid mesocolon over the left common iliac vessels. Opposite the S_3 vetebra, it divides into right and left branches which descend one on each side of rectum. These branches supply rectum and

communicate with inferior and middle rectal arteries in the mucosa of anal canal.

MARGINAL ARTERY OF DRUMMOND

Anastomoses of colic branches of superior mesenteric and inferior mesenteric arteries form the marginal artery of Drummond. This extends from the ileo-caecal junction to the rectosigmoid junction. This arterial arcade is situated along the concavity of colon. Following arteries contribute to form marginal artery (Fig. 13.33).
   a. Iliocolic artery
   b. Right colic artery
   c. Middle colic artery
   d. Left colic artery
   e. Sigmoidal arteries
   Vasa recta arising from the marginal artery supply the colon.

COMMON ILIAC ARTERY

The abdominal aorta terminates by dividing into a pair of common iliac arteries at the level of lower border of L_4 vertebra. The two arteries diverge and reach the respective sacro-iliac joints where the divide into external and internal iliac arteries. They give few branches to the surrounding structures (Figs 13.17 and 13.18).

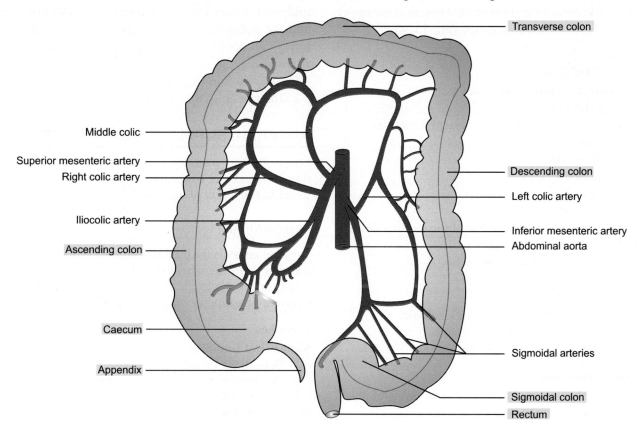

Fig. 13.33: Marginal artery of Drummond

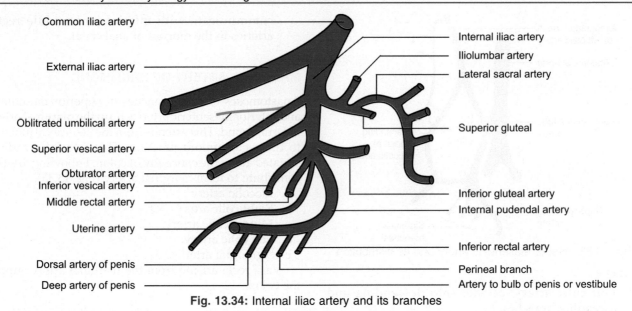

Fig. 13.34: Internal iliac artery and its branches

INTERNAL ILIAC ARTERY

It is also known as hypogastric artery. It arises from common iliac artery opposite the sacroiliac joint. It passes downwards anterior to sacroiliac joint, subperitoneally. Pelvic part of the ureter lies in front of the artery. Internal iliac vein and sacroiliac joint lie posterior to the artery. It divides into anterior and posterior division at the upper margin of greater sciatic foramen (Fig. 13.34).

Branches
Anterior Division
1. Obliterated umbilical artery
2. Superior vesical artery
3. Inferior vesical artery – equivalent to vaginal artery in female
4. Middle rectal artery
5. Obturator artery
6. Uterine artery
7. Vaginal artery
8. Inferior gluteal artery – one of the terminal branch
9. **Internal pudendal artery:** This artery further divides into following branches
   a. Inferior rectal artery
   b. Perineal branch
   c. Artery to bulb of penis or vestibule
   d. Deep artery of penis or clitoris
   e. Dorsal artery of penis or clitoris

Posterior Division
1. Iliolumbar artery: Passes upwards and laterally
2. Superior gluteal artery
3. Lateral sacral artery

EXTERNAL ILIAC ARTERY (FIGs 13.17, 13.28)

It is the terminal branch of common iliac artery given off at the level of sacro-iliac joint. Each artery descends along the medial border of psoas major muscle and enters into the thigh behind the inguinal ligament. At the level of inguinal ligament the artery lies at the midpoint of a line joining the anterior superior iliac spine and the pubic symphysis. It continues as the femoral artery and hence is the principal artery of lower limb.

Branches:
1. Deep circumflex iliac artery.
2. Inferior epigastric artery.

ARTERIAL SUPPLY OF LOWER LIMB

Lower limb is primarily supplied by femoral artery which is a direct continuation of external iliac artery distal to the inguinal ligament.

FEMORAL ARTERY

Femoral artery is the direct continuation of external iliac artery at mid inguinal point. It continues as popliteal artery at adductor hiatus or 5th osseoaponeurotic opening of adductor magnus (Fig. 13.35).

Branches
Superficial branches
1. Superficial epigastric artery
2. Superficial circumflex iliac artery
3. Superficial external pudendal artery
Deep branches
4. Deep external pudendal artery

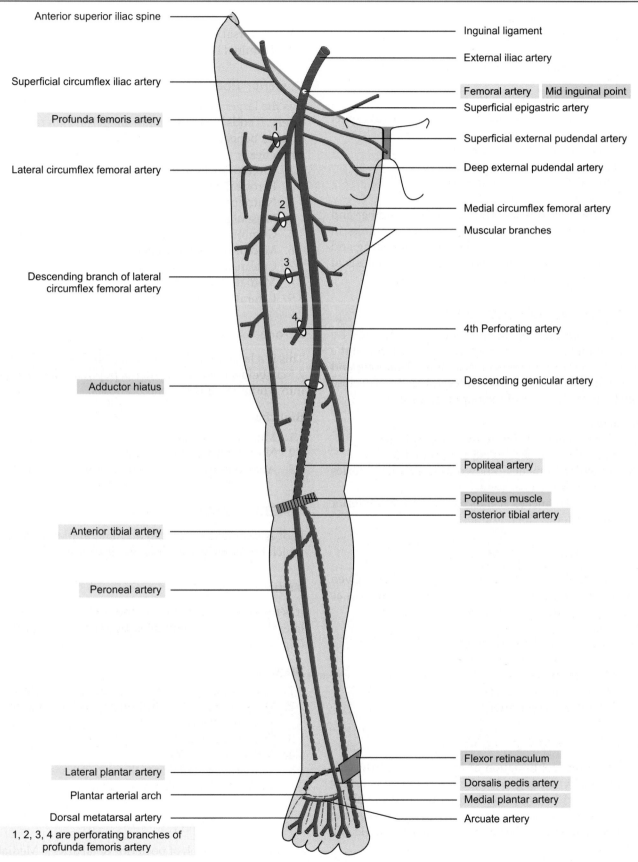

Anterior superior iliac spine

Superficial circumflex iliac artery

Profunda femoris artery

Lateral circumflex femoral artery

Descending branch of lateral circumflex femoral artery

Adductor hiatus

Anterior tibial artery

Peroneal artery

Lateral plantar artery

Plantar arterial arch

Dorsal metatarsal artery

1, 2, 3, 4 are perforating branches of profunda femoris artery

Inguinal ligament

External iliac artery

Femoral artery   Mid inguinal point

Superficial epigastric artery

Superficial external pudendal artery

Deep external pudendal artery

Medial circumflex femoral artery

Muscular branches

4th Perforating artery

Descending genicular artery

Popliteal artery

Popliteus muscle

Posterior tibial artery

Flexor retinaculum

Dorsalis pedis artery

Medial plantar artery

Arcuate artery

Fig. 13.35: Arterial supply of lower limb

CHAPTER-13

5. Muscular branches
6. Profunda femoris artery
7. Descending genicular artery: It is not given in femoral triangle. It arises in adductor canal.

Profunda Femoris Artery (Fig. 13.35)

Profunda femoris arises from the posterolateral aspect of the femoral artery in the femoral triangle.
    It gives of the following branches
1. Lateral circumflex femoral artery.
2. Medial circumflex femoral artery.
3. Muscular branches
4. **Perforating arteries:** They are four in number and pass through the four aponeurotic openings in adductor magnus. All of them give ascending and descending branches and form an anastomosis at the back of the thigh.

POPLITEAL ARTERY (FIG. 13.35)

It is the continuation of femoral artery. It ends by dividing into anterior and posterior tibial arteries at the lower border of popliteus muscle. It is 20 cm long and runs obliquely from medial to lateral side. It lies in close contact with the floor of the popliteal fossa.

Branches
1. Cutaneous branches to the back of the leg.
2. Muscular branches to adjacent muscles.
3. Articular branches, known as genicular arteries which supply knee joint.
4. Terminal branches: It ends by dividing into anterior and posterior tibial arteries.

Anterior Tibial Artery (Fig. 13.35)

It is one of the terminal branches of popliteal artery, given out at the lower border of popliteus muscle. It ends as the dorsalis pedis artery in front of ankle joint.

Branches
1. Posterior tibial recurrent artery
2. Anterior tibial recurrent artery
3. Muscular branches
4. Medial malleolar artery
5. Lateral malleolar artery

Dorsalis Pedis Artery (Fig. 13.35)

It is the direct continuation of anterior tibial artery. It terminates by joining with the lateral plantar artery (deep branch) to complete the plantar arch in sole. It enters the sole by passing through the gap between the **two heads of Ist dorsal interosseous** muscle (Fig. 45.12).

Branches
1. Lateral tarsal artery

2. Arcuate artery
3. Ist dorsal metatarsal artery
4. Terminal branch to plantar arch.

Posterior Tibial Artery (Fig. 13.35)

It is the larger of the two terminal branches of popliteal artery. It ends by dividing into medial and lateral plantar arteries beneath the flexor retinaculum.

Branches
1. Circumflex fibular artery
2. Peroneal artery
3. Nutrient artery
4. Muscular branches
5. Communicating branch
6. Medial malleolar branch
7. Calcanean branch
8. Medial plantar artery
9. Lateral plantar artery

Peroneal Artery (Fig. 13.35)

This is a large branch of posterior tibial artery. It begins 2.5 cm below the lower border of popliteus. It terminates into a number of calcanean branches.

Branches:
1. Muscular branches.
2. Nutrient artery to fibula.
3. Anastomotic branches to lateral malleolar network

ARTERIAL SUPPLY OF FOOT

Foot is supplied by medial and lateral plantar arteries which are branches of posterior tibial artery.

Medial Plantar Artery

It is the smaller branch of posterior tibial artery. On the lateral side it is accompanied by medial plantar nerve (Fig. 13.36).

Branches
1. Anastomosing branch to 1st metatarsal artery
2. Muscular branches to abductor hallucis and flexor igitorum brevis
3. Cutaneous branches
4. Articular branches
5. 3 superficial digital branches which anastmose with the 1st, 2nd, 3rd plantar metatarsal arteries

Lateral Plantar Artery

It is the larger branch of posterior tibial artery. Medially it is accompanied by lateral plantar nerve. It terminates

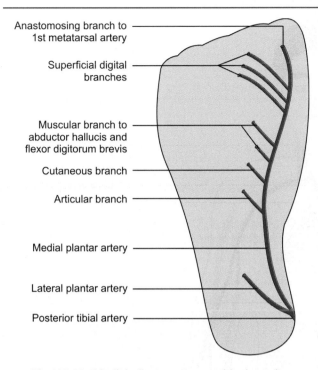

Fig. 13.36: Medial plantar artery and its branches

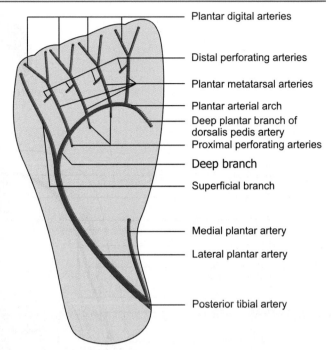

Fig. 13.37: Lateral plantar artery and plantar arterial arch

at the base of 5th metatarsal by dividing into a superficial and a deep branch (Fig. 13.37).

Branches

1. **Superficial branch** supplies lateral side of little toe both skin and muscles.
2. **Deep branch** supplies muscles, gives rise to articular branches and forms plantar arterial arch by anastomosing with terminal part of dorsalis pedis artery

Plantar Arterial Arch

It is formed by deep branch of lateral plantar artery and deep plantar branch of dorsalis pedis artery. It is situated across the base of 5th, 4th, 3rd and 2nd metatarsals between the 4th and 6th layers of the sole.

Branches of Plantar Arch

1. 3 proximal perforating arteries
2. 4 plantar metatarsal arteries: Metatarsal arteries give rise to
   a. Plantar digital arteries
   b. Distal perforating arteries

VENOUS DRAINAGE OF BODY

The blood from various parts of the body is ultimately drain into the superior and inferior vena cava. Superior vena cava receives blood mostly from the upper part of the body (above diaphragm) while the inferior vena cava drains the lower part of body (below diaphragm). The two veins finally open into the right atrium of the heart.

SUPERIOR VENA CAVA

It is one of the two venous channels which drains the blood from the body into the right atrium of the heart. It drains the blood from the upper part of the body. It is formed behind the lower border of right 1st costal cartilage by the union of right and left brachiocephalic veins. It pierces the fibrous pericardium opposite 2nd costal cartilage. It ends in the postero-superior smooth part of right atrium at level of 3rd costal cartilage (Fig. 13.38).

Features: It has no valves, It is 7 cm long and 2 cm wide, Lower half is covered by pericardium.

Tributaries

1. Right and left brachiocephalic veins
2. Azygos vein
3. Pericardial veins
4. Mediastinal veins

INFERIOR VENA CAVA

It is the venous channel which drains the blood from the body, below the diaphragm to right atrium of heart. It is formed in front of the body of L_5 vertebra by the

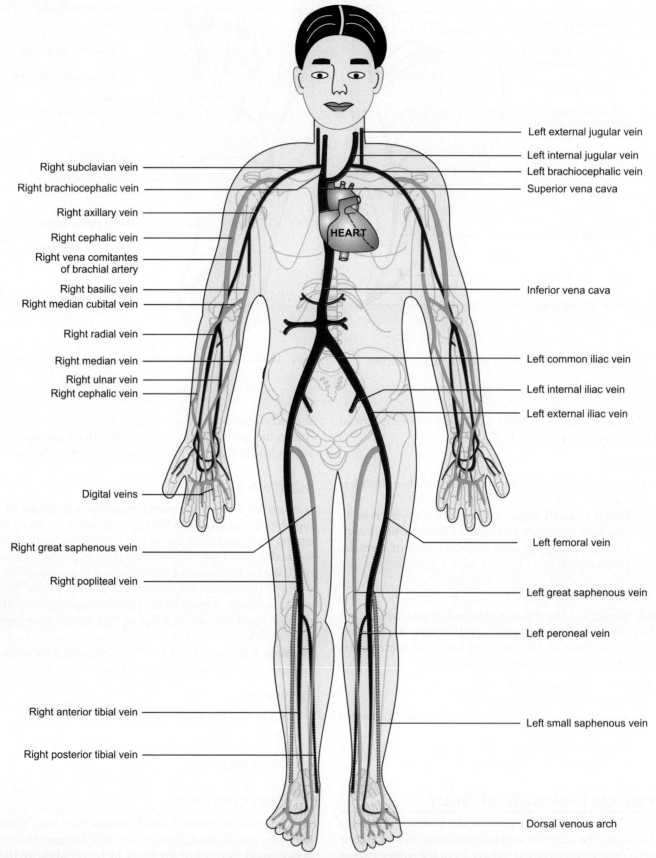

Right subclavian vein

Right brachiocephalic vein

Right axillary vein

Right cephalic vein

Right vena comitantes
of brachial artery

Right basilic vein

Right median cubital vein

Right radial vein

Right median vein

Right ulnar vein

Right cephalic vein

Digital veins

Right great saphenous vein

Right popliteal vein

Right anterior tibial vein

Right posterior tibial vein

HEART

Left external jugular vein

Left internal jugular vein

Left brachiocephalic vein

Superior vena cava

Inferior vena cava

Left common iliac vein

Left internal iliac vein

Left external iliac vein

Left femoral vein

Left great saphenous vein

Left peroneal vein

Left small saphenous vein

Dorsal venous arch

Fig. 13.38: Venous drainage of the body

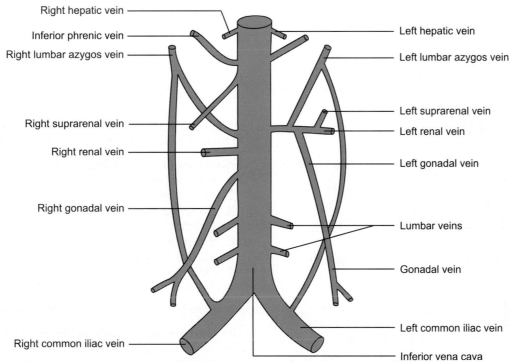

Right hepatic vein —
Inferior phrenic vein —
Right lumbar azygos vein —
Right suprarenal vein —
Right renal vein —
Right gonadal vein —
Right common iliac vein —

Left hepatic vein
Left lumbar azygos vein
Left suprarenal vein
Left renal vein
Left gonadal vein
Lumbar veins
Gonadal vein
Left common iliac vein
Inferior vena cava

Fig. 13.39: Inferior vena cava and its tributaries

union of left and right common iliac veins. It ends in the right atrium of heart through inferior vena caval opening (Figs 13.38, 13.39).

Length : 22 to 23 cm
Breadth : 2.5 cm

Tributaries: From below upwards

1. Left and right common iliac veins
2. Lumbar veins: There are four pairs of lumbar veins. The 1st and 2nd lumbar veins form anastomoses with azygos veins.
3. Right gonadal vein.
4. Right and left renal veins.
5. Right suprarenal vein.
6. Right and left inferior phrenic veins.
7. Right and left hepatic veins.
8. Lumbar azygos vein: It connects the inferior vena cava to superior vena cava.

BRACHIOCEPHALIC VEIN (FIG. 13.38)

The brachiocephalic vein is formed by union of subclavian vein and internal jugular vein. It begins on each side, behind the sternal end of clavicle and descends downwards. The two brachiocephalic veins join behind the sternal end of 1st right costal cartilage to form superior vena cava.

Tributaries
1. Vertebral vein
2. Internal thoracic vein
3. Inferior thyroid vein

4. 1st posterior intercostal vein
5. Superior intercostal vein on left side

VENOUS DRAINAGE OF HEAD, NECK AND BRAIN

SUBCLAVIAN VEIN

It is the continuation of axillary vein. It extends from the outer border of the first rib to the medial border of scalenus anterior where it joins the internal jugular vein to form the brachio-cephalic vein.

Tributaries
1. External jugular vein
2. Dorsal scapular vein
3. Thoracic duct on the left side and right lymphatic duct on the right side
4. Anterior jugular vein
5. Cephalic vein

External Jugular Vein (Fig. 13.40)

- External jugular vein is primarily the drainage channel of face and scalp.
- It is formed by the union of posterior division of retromandibular vein and posterior auricular vein just below the parotid gland, at angle of mandible.
- It descends under platysma and over the deep fascia covering sternocleidomastoid muscle.
- It passes slightly obliquely to reach the root of neck just posterior to the clavicular head of sterno-

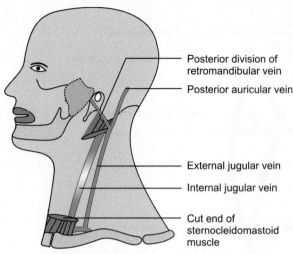

Fig. 13.40: External and Internal jugular vein

cleidomastoid muscle. Here, it pierces the deep fascia and drains into subclavian vein.

Tributaries
1. Posterior division of retromandibular vein
2. Posterior auricular vein
3. Anterior jugular vein
4. Posterior external jugular vein
5. Transverse cervical vein
6. Suprascapular vein

7. It communicates with internal jugular vein by and oblique jugular vein.

INTERNAL JUGULAR VEIN

It is the main venous channel of head and neck. It begins at the base of the skull in the jugular foramen as a direct continuation of the sigmoid sinus. It ends behind the sternal end of the clavicle by joining the subclavian vein to form the brachiocephalic vein (Fig. 13.41).

Tributaries of Internal Jugular Vein
1. Inferior petrosal sinus
2. Pharyngeal veins
3. Common facial vein
4. Lingual vein
5. Superior thyroid vein
6. Middle thyroid vein
7. Occipital vein

Venous Drainage of Scalp (Fig. 13.42)

The veins of scalp accompany the arteries and are named as:
1. **Supratrochlear and supraorbital veins:** They join to form the angular vein at the medial angle of eye and further continue as facial vein.
2. **Superficial temporal vein:** It forms the retromandibular vein after joining with maxillary vein.
3. **Posterior auricular vein:** Drains into external jugular vein.

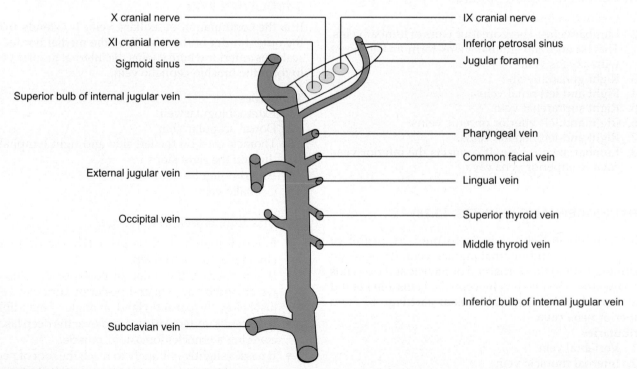

Fig. 13.41: Tributaries of internal jugular vein

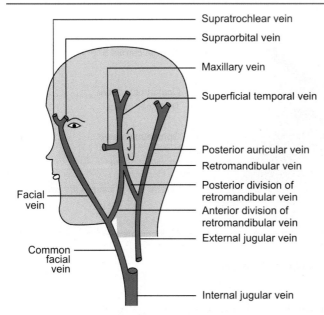

Fig. 13.42: Venous drainage of face

4. Occipital vein: Terminates into suboccipital plexus of veins.

Venous Drainage of Face

Venous drainage of face is by two veins (Fig. 11.7).

1. **Facial vein:** This is the main vein of the face. It begins as the angular vein at the medial angle of eye by the union of supratrochlear and supraorbital veins. It takes a straight course behind the facial artery. It pierces the deep fascia just below the mandible and joins the anterior division of the retromandibular vein to form the common facial vein which drains into the internal jugular vein.
2. Retromandibular vein
3. Supratrochlear vein
4. Supraorbital vein: This joins with the supratrochlear vein at the medial canthus of eye to form facial vein.

5. Tributaries of superficial temporal vein.
6. Tributaries of pterygoid of veins, e.g., infraorbital, buccal and mental veins.

INTRACRANIAL DURAL VENOUS SINUSES (FIG. 13.43)

These are venous channels enclosed within the cranial dura which drain the cranial cavity and the brain. They are present at either of the two sites:

1. Between the endosteal and meningeal layers of cranial dura.
2. Between the reduplicated meningeal layer of dura.

Characteristic features of intracranial dural venous sinuses:

1. They lie between the layers of duramater.
2. Are lined by endothelium only (muscular coat is absent).
3. Are valveless.
4. Receive venous blood and CSF.
5. Receive valveless emissary veins which regulate the intracranial blood flow and maintain equilibrium of venous pressure within and outside the skull.

Classification of Dural Venous Sinuses

They are classified as paired and unpaired sinuses (7 paired and 7 unpaired).

Unpaired:

1. **Superior sagittal sinus:** It is present in the attached superior margin of falx cerebri.
2. **Inferior sagittal sinus:** It lies in the posterior half of free margin of falx cerebri.
3. **Straight sinus:** It is present at the line of junction of falx cerebri with tentorium cerebelli.
4. **Occipital sinus:** It lies along the attached margin of falx cerebelli.
5. **Anterior intercavernous sinus**

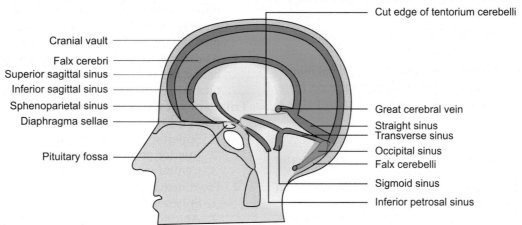

Fig. 13.43: Folds of duramater and dural venous sinuses (sagittal section of head and neck)

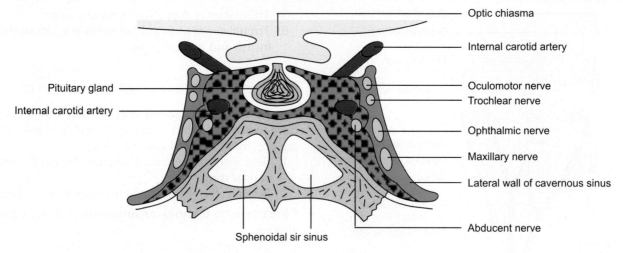

Fig. 13.44: Cavernous sinus (Coronal section)

6. Posterior intercavernous sinus
7. Basilar venous plexus (sinus)

Paired:
1. Cavernous sinus
2. Superior petrosal sinus
3. Inferior petrosal sinus
4. Transverse sinus
5. Sigmoid sinus
6. Spheno-parietal sinus
7. Petro-squamous sinus

Cavernous Sinus (Fig. 13.44)

- The cavernous sinus is an important venous channel and is situated in the middle cranial fossa, between the two layers of cranial dura, one on either side of the body of sphenoid.
- It is 2 cm long and 1 cm wide.
- Its interior is divided into a number of small spaces or caverns by various trabeculae.
- It consists of roof, floor and medial and lateral walls.
- Roof and lateral wall are formed by the meningeal layer of duramater. The medial wall and floor are formed by the endosteal layer of duramater.

Extent
Anterior: Upto the medial end of superior orbital fissure.
Posterior: Upto the apex of petrous temporal bone. Here, it drains into the transverse sinus via superior petrosal sinus.

Relations
Superior : Optic tract, internal carotid artery, anterior perforated substance.
Inferior : Foramen lacerum, junction of body and greater wing of sphenoid.
Medial : Pituitary gland (hypophysis cerebri), sphenoid air sinus.

Lateral : Temporal lobe (uncus) of cerebral hemisphere, cavum trigeminale containing trigeminal ganglion
Anterior : Superior orbital fissure, apex of the orbit.
Posterior : Crus cerebri of midbrain, apex of petrous temporal bone.

Structures Present within the Lateral Wall of the Sinus (Fig. 13.44)
From above downwards:
1. Oculomotor nerve
2. Trochlear nerve
3. Ophthalmic nerve
4. Maxillary nerve

The oculomotor and trochlear nerves enter the lateral wall of the sinus by piercing its roof while, ophthalmic and maxillary nerves pierce the lateral wall of the sinus.

Structures Passing Through The Sinus
1. **Internal carotid artery** surrounded by sympathetic plexus of nerves: It is present in the floor of the sinus. It enters from the apex of petrous temporal bone and runs forwards in the carotid canal. It emerges out from the anterior end of sinus by piercing the roof of sinus.
2. **Abducent nerve:** It enters the sinus by passing below the petrosphenoid ligament and accompanies the artery on its inferolateral aspect.

Tributaries of Cavernous Sinus
1. **From orbit**
    1. Superior ophthalmic vein
    2. Inferior ophthalmic vein
    3. Central vein of retina (sometimes)
2. **From meninges**
    1. Sphenoparietal sinus
    2. Anterior (frontal) trunk of middle meningeal vein

3. **From brain**
   1. Superficial middle cerebral vein
   2. Inferior cerebral veins (only few)

Communications of the Cavernous Sinus (Fig. 15.3)

The cavernous sinus communicates with the following:
1. Transverse sinus, via superior petrosal sinus.
2. Internal jugular vein, via inferior petrosal sinus.
3. Pterygoid venous plexus, via an emissary vein which passes through foramen ovale.
4. Facial vein via two routes:
   — Superior ophthalmic vein and angular vein.
   — Emissary vein $\longrightarrow$ pterygoid venous plexus $\longrightarrow$ deep facial vein.
5. Opposite cavernous sinus, via anterior and posterior inter cavernous sinuses.
6. Superior sagittal sinus, via superficial middle cerebral vein and superior anastomotic vein.
7. Internal vertebral venous plexus, via basilar venous plexus.

Transverse Sinus

On right side it is the continuation superior sagittal sinus while on left side it is the continuation straight sinus. The sinus lies in the attached margin of tentorium cerebelli on each side.

Sigmoid Sinus

It is the continuation of transverse sinus on each side. It further continues as the internal jugular vein at the jugular foramen.

VENOUS DRAINAGE OF THE BRAIN

The venous chanels of brain primarily consist of superior and deep cerebral veins.

Superficial Veins of the Cerebral Hemispheres

1. **Superior cerebral veins:** They are 8 to 12 in number and drain into the superior sagittal sinus. These veins drain blood from the superolateral and medial surface of the cerebral hemispheres.
2. **Superficial middle cerebral vein:** It runs along the posterior ramus and stem of lateral sulcus. It drains the blood from supero-lateral surface of the cerebral hemisphere into the cavernous sinus.
3. **Inferior cerebral veins:** These veins drain the inferior surface and lower part of superolateral surface. They drain into spheno-parietal, cavernous, superior petrosal and transverse sinuses.

Deep Veins of the Cerebral Hemispheres

1. **Internal cerebral veins:** These are formed by the union of thalamostriate and choroid veins. Right and left internal cerebral veins unite form great cerebral veins.
   Tributaries:
   a. Thalamostriate vein
   b. Choroid vein
   c. Septal vein
   d. Epithalamic vein
   e. Lateral ventricular vein
2. **Basal veins:** These are two in number. Each basal vein is formed by the union of
   a. Anterior cerebral vein
   b. Deep middle cerebral vein
   c. Striate vein
   Basal veins drain into the great cerebral vein.
3. **Great Cerebral Vein of Galen:** It is formed by the union of two internal cerebral veins. It is about 2 cm. long and drains into the straight sinus.
   Tributaries:
   a. Internal cerebral veins
   b. Basal veins
   c. Occipital veins
   d. Posterior callosal vein

Venous Drainage of Cerebellum

1. Superior cerebellar veins, drain into great cerebral vein.
2. Inferior cerebellar veins, drain into adjacent venous sinuses.

Venous Drainage of Brain Stem

Following veins drain the brain stem.

Mid brain: It is drained by the basal and great cerebral veins.

Pons: The veins of pons terminate into basal, transverse and petrosal sinuses.

Medulla: Veins from medulla drain into basilar plexus of veins and inferior petrosal sinus.

VENOUS DRAINAGE OF UPPER LIMB

Upper limb is mainly drained by a set of superficial veins which drain into the axillary vein and by the vena comitantes of brachial artery.

AXILLARY VEIN (FIGs 13.38 and 13.45)

Axillary vein is formed by union of basilic vein with the two vena comitantes of the brachial artery. It begins at the lower border of teres major muscle and it ends at

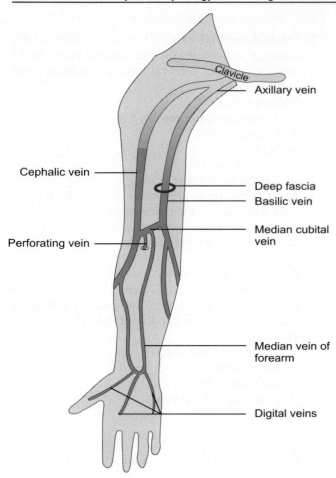

Fig. 13.45: Superficial veins of upper limb (anterior surface)

the outer border of 1st rib where it continues as the subclavian vein.

Tributaries
- Anterior circumflex humeral vein
- Posterior circumflex humeral vein
- Subscapular vein
- Lateral thoracic vein
- Thoracoacromial vein
- Cephalic vein
- Superior thoracic vein

SUPERFICIAL VEINS OF UPPER LIMB (FIG. 13.45)

Superficial veins of upper limb have following characteristic features:
a. Most superficial veins join together give rise to larger veins namely, **basilic and cephalic veins.**
b. They are absent in palm, ulnar boder of fore arm, and back of arm.
c. Superficial veins are accompanied by lymphatics and cutaneous nerves.

d. The superficial lymph nodes lie along the superficial veins
e. Cephalic vein and basilic vein are interconnected with the each other through **medial cubital vein.**

Dorsal Venous Arch

It is a plexus of veins present in the dorsum of the hand. It is formed by three metacarpal veins which receives two dorsal digital vein from thumb and one dorsal digital vein from lateral side of index finger. It continues as cephalic vein.

Cephalic Vein (Figs 13.38 and 13.45)

Cephalic vein arises from the lateral end of dorsal venous network, in the anatomical snuff box of hand. It runs along the lateral border or radial border of forearm and curves forwards to the anterior aspect of forearm below the elbow. In front of the elbow it is connected with the basilic vein with the help of median cubital vein. It passes upwards in the arm upto the infraclavicular fossa. Then it pierces the clavipectoral fascia and drains into the axillary vein.

Basilic Vein (Figs 13.38 and 13.45)

It begins from the ulnar side of dorsal venous network and runs along the medial border of the forearm. It curves to the anterior surface of forearm below the elbow and runs upwards in front of the arm. It pierces the deep fascia of middle of the arm. Here, it is accompanied by venae comitantes of the brachial artery. The two venae comitantes and basilic vein join together and form the axillary vein.

Median Cubital Vein (Figs 13.38 and 13.45)

It is an anastomotic channel connecting cephalic vein to basilic vein in front of the elbow.

Median Antebrachial Vein (Figs 13.38 and 13.45)

It arises from the anastomotic channels of the superficial palmar plexus. It ascends in front of forearm and ends in the cubital vein or basilic vein.

DEEP VEINS OF UPPER LIMB (FIG. 13.38)

They consist of
1. **Brachial veins:** These are the vena cominantes of the brachial artery.
2. **Vena comitantes of radial and ulnar arteries:** Radial veins are formed by deep dorsal veins of hand. Ulnar veins are formed by the deep palmar venous arch.

VENOUS DRAINAGE OF THORAX

The thoracic wall is drained by anterior and posterior intercostal veins (see page no. 378). The venous drainage of various viscera of thorax is described in the corresponding chapters. The final pathway of venous drainage of this region is via the azygos system of veins which is described below.

AZYGOS SYSTEM OF VEINS (FIG. 13.46)

Azygos means unpaired. These veins are not accompanied with the corresponding arteries. Following are the characteristic features of azygos system of veins
1. They are straight veins.
2. These venous channels are situated in the posterior mediastinum and are paravertebral in position.
3. They are provided with valves.

4. These veins have communicating channels with the vena caval system, in front and the vertebral venous plexus, behind.
5. Thehy drain blood from the back, thoracic wall and abdominal wall.

The three main venous channels of azygos system are
1. Azygos vein
2. Hemi-azygos vein
3. Accessory azygos vein

Azygos Vein

The trunk of azygos vein is formed by the union of lumbar azygos vein, right subcostal vein and right ascending lumbar veins near the leve of right renal veins. It enters the thorax either through a separate opening in the right crus of diaphragm or along with aorta in the aortic opening. In the thorax, it lies in front of the lower eight thoracic   vertebrae. It ends by opening into the superior vena cava opposite 4th thoracic vertebra.

Tributaries
1. All right posterior intercostal veins except 1st posterior intercostal vein
2. Right subcostal vein
3. Right ascending lumbar veins
4. Hemiazygos vein
5. Accessory azygos vein
6. Right bronchial vein
7. Oesophageal veins
8. Pericardial and mediastinal veins

Hemiazygos Vein

It is formed by the union of left ascending lumbar and left subcostal veins. It enters the thorax by piercing the left crus of diaphragm and ascends on left side of vertebral column. The descending aorta is present in front of it. It turns to the right and ends into the azygos vein opposite T_8 vertebra.

Tributaries
1. Lower three or four left posterior intercostal veins.
2. Left lumbar veins.
3. Left subcostal vein.

Accessory Azygos Vein

It begins as the continuation of 4th left posterior intercostal vein. It runs downwards infront of the vertebral column. It turns to the right opposite T_7 vetebra and ends into the azygos vein.

Tributaries
Left 5th, 6th, 7th posterior intercostal veins.

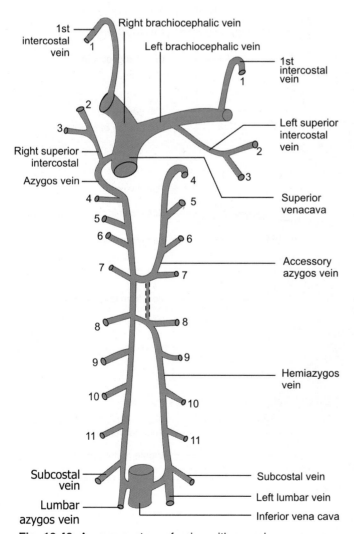

Fig. 13.46: Azygos system of veins with superior vena cava

VENOUS DRAINAGE OF ABDOMEN AND PELVIS

The abdomen and pelvis is drained by two sets of venous drainage system:

1. **Caval system:** It consists of the veins draining into the inferior vena cava. These are on each side
   a. **Common iliac vein:** It is formed by the union of internal and external iliac veins.
   b. **Internal iliac vein:** It is formed by convergence of various tributaries which are vena cominantes of the corresponding branches of internal iliac artery.
   c. **External iliac vein:** It is the proximal continuation of femoral vein. It receives inferious epigastric vein, deep circumflex iliac vein and pubic vein.
2. **Portal system:** It consists of the portal vein which drains most of the viscera of abdomen and pelvis.

PORTAL VEIN

Portal vein is formed behind the neck of pancreas, at level of L_2 vertebra, by the union of superior mesenteric vein and splenic vein in front of inferior vena cava. It is 8 cm in length and runs upwards in the right border of lesser omentum. It divides into right and left branches at the porta hepatis and enters the liver. Its branches end into the hepatic sinusoids (Fig. 13.47).

Tributaries of Portal Vein

1. Superior mesenteric vein
2. Splenic vein
3. Right gastric vein
4. Left gastric vein
5. Cystic vein, from gall bladder
6. Paraumbilical veins
7. Obliterated left umbilical vein (ligamentum teres)
8. Superior pancreaticoduodenal vein
9. Prepyloric vein (sometimes)

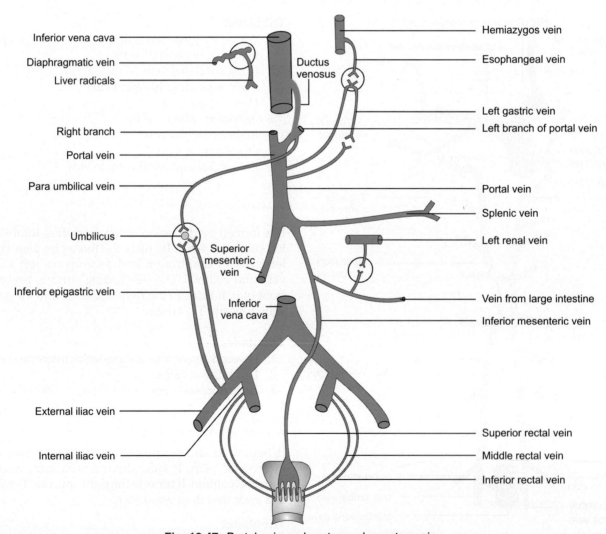

Fig. 13.47: Portal vein and portocaval anastomosis

Special Features of Portal Vein

Portal vein is a part of the portal system which has capillaries at both the ends and vein in between.
1. It begins as a vein and ends as an artery.
2. It is devoid of valves.
3. Portal system can store 1/3rd of total blood in body.
4. In the portal vein, the blood streams of superior mesenteric vein and of splenic vein remain segregated.

Portocaval Anastomosis

The portal vein divides into smaller branches which end in sinusoids of the liver along with the blood from hepatic arteries. The blood drains ultimately via hepatic veins into the inferior vena cava.

Normally veins drain into the caval system. But in case of portal system, veins of gastrointestinal tract drain into the portal vein. There are areas of anastomosis between the portal and the caval system that provide collateral circulation, for the drainage of gastrointestinal tract directly to caval system when there is portal obstruction.

Following are the sites of the portocaval anastomosis (Fig. 13.47)
1. **Lower end of rectum and anal canal**
   Portal system: Superior rectal vein
   Caval system: Middle and inferior rectal vein
2. **Lower end of esophagus**
   Portal system: Esophageal branches of left gastric vein
   Caval system: Esophageal vein (Hemiazygos vein)
3. **At Umbilicus**
   Portal system: Paraumbilical vein
   Caval system:
   — Superior epigastric vein
   — Lateral thoracic vein
   — Superficial epigastric vein
   — nferior epigastric vein
   — Posterior intercostal vein
   — Lumbar veins vein
4. **In the falciform ligament**
   Portal system: Paraumbilical vein
   Caval system: Diaphragmatic veins
5. **Bare area of liver**
   Portal system: Radiating veins of liver
   Caval system: Diaphragmatic vein
6. **Posterior abdominal wall**
   Portal system: Splenic vein, Colic vein
   Caval system: Left renal vein
7. **In intra uterine life:** At the fissure for ductus venosus (via ductus venosus).
   Portal system: Left branch of portal vein
   Caval system: Inferior vena cava

SUPERIOR MESENTERIC VEIN

It is a relatively large vein which drains blood from small intestine, caecum, appendix, ascending colon and right 2/3rd of transverse colon. It begins in right iliac fossa by union of tributaries of ileocaecal veins. Here, it lies on the right side of superior mesenteric artery. It terminates behind neck of pancreas by joining with splenic vein to give rise to portal vein.

Tributaries
1. Tributaries corresponding to the branches of superior mesenteric artery namely, jejunal, ileal, ileocolic, right colic and middle colic veins.
2. Right gastroepiploic vein.
3. Inferior pancreaticoduodenal vein.

INFERIOR MESENTERIC VEIN

It begins as the continuation of superior rectal vein and terminates in splenic vein or sometimes at the junction of superior mesenteric vein and splenic vein.

Tributaries
These correspond to branches of inferior mesenteric arteries and consists of sigmoid, middle and left colic veins.

SPLENIC VEIN

It is formed in the splenorenal ligament by the confluence of veins arising from spleen at its hilum. It passes medially and downwards to join the superior mesenteric vein behind the neck of pancreas to form the portal vein.

Tributaries
1. Short gastric veins
2. Left gatro epiploic vein
3. Posterior gastric veins
4. Small tributaries from pancreas
5. Inferior mesenteric vein

VENOUS DRAINAGE OF LOWER LIMB

Three distinguishable sets of veins are present in the lower limb. These are (Figs 13.48 and 13.49)
1. **Superficial veins:** They lie in the superficial fascia and superficial to deep fascia.
   Characteristic features
   — They are thick walled
   — Numerous valves are present distally
   — They drain into deep veins
   Superficial veins are:
   a. Great saphenous vein
   b. Short saphenous vein

2. **Deep veins:** They lie in deep structures under cover of deep fascia.

   Characteristic features:
   — They accompany arteries and their branches as vena comitantes
   — Have more valves than superficial veins
   — They usually run deep to muscles

   Deep Veins are (from below upwards)
   a. Posterior tibial vein, formed by medial and lateral plantar veins from deep plantar venous arch.
   b. **Anterior tibial vein:** continuation of vena comitantes of dorsalis pedis artery.
   c. Peroneal vein
   d. **Popliteal vein:** Formed by joining of tibial and peroneal veins. Continues as femoral vein.
   e. Femoral vein

3. **Perforating veins:** They Connect the superficial veins with the deep veins by piercing fascia. They follow intermuscular septae.

   Characteristic features: They are provided with valves which direct blood from—superficial to deep. They are of two types:
   a. **Direct:** Form a direct connection between superficial and deep veins.
   b. **Indirect:** Connect superficial vein to deep vein via the veins which pass through the muscles.

GREAT SAPHENOUS VEIN

(Longest vein in the body) (Figs 13.48 and 13.49)
It is the upward continuation of medial end of dorsal venous arch of the foot supplemented by medial marginal vein. It ascends in front of medial malleolus and runs upwards and backwards along the medial surface of tibia reaching medial aspect of knee. It passes to the posteromedial aspect of knee joint, runs along the medial side of thigh to reach saphenous opening and passes through cribriform fascia and drains into femoral vein, 3 cm below inguinal ligament and little below and lateral to pubic tubercle. It contains about 15 to 20 valves.

In leg: It is accompanied by saphenous nerve

In thigh: Medial femoral cutaneous nerve runs along with it.

Tributaries

Leg
1. Posterior arch vein.

Calf
2. Anterior leg vein.
3. Few veins from calf communicate with short saphenous vein.

Thigh
4. Anterolateral vein.
5. Posteromedial vein.

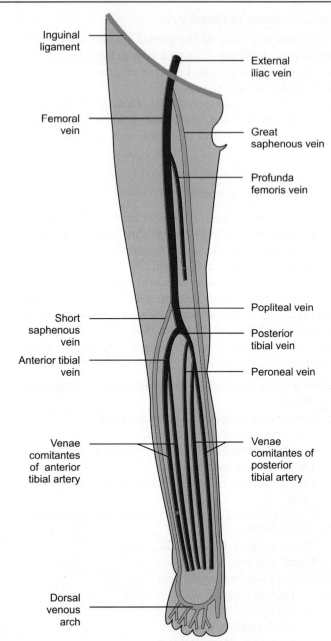

Fig. 13.48: Veins of lower limb

6. Superficial epigastric vein.
7. Superficial circumflex iliac vein.
8. Superficial external pudendal vein.
9. Deep external pudendal vein.

SHORT SAPHENOUS VEIN (FIGs 13.48 and 13.49)

It is an upward continuation of dorsal venous arch supplemented by lateral marginal vein. It begins behind the lateral malleolus. It terminates into the popliteal vein. It usually has 5 to 10 valves. In leg it is accompanied by sural nerve. It is connected with peroneal vein through lateral ankle perforator.

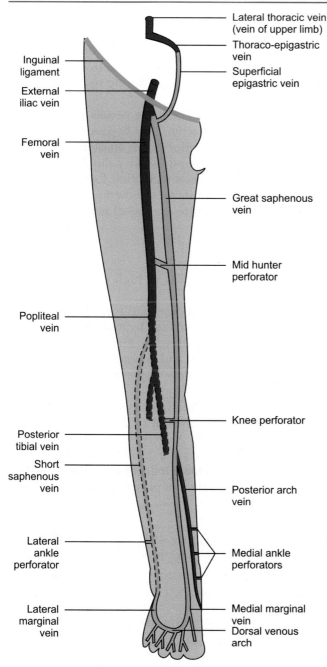

Fig. 13.49: Venous drainage of lower limb

FEMORAL VEIN

It is the upward continuation of popliteal vein at the lower end of adductor canal. In thigh, it lies lateral to femoral artery in lower part posterior to femoral artery in middle part and medial to femoral artery in upper part. It continues as external iliac vein behind inguinal ligament.

Tributaries
1. Great saphenous vein
2. Lateral and medial circumflex femoral veins
3. Descending genicular vein
4. Muscular veins
5. Veins accompaning profunda femoris artery and deep external pudendal artery.

PERFORATING VEINS OF LOWER LIMB

There are six main venous perforators. They are generally fixed in position. These perforators are described below (Fig. 13.49).
   1. **Mid hunter perforator**
      Location: Adductor canal
      Connecting veins: Great saphenous with femoral
   2. **Knee perforator**
      Location: Just below knee
      Connecting veins: Great saphenous with posterior tibial
   3. **Three medial ankle perforators**
      Location
         a. Upper one, at the junction of middle and lower third of leg.
         b. Lower one, below and behind the medial malleolus
         c. Middle, present between them
      Connecting veins: All are interconnected to **posterior arch vein** which connects great saphenous vein with posterior tibial vein.
   4. **Lateral ankle perforator**
      Location: Situated at the junction of middle and lower third of leg.
      Connecting veins: Short saphenous with peroneal.

Factors Affecting Venous Drainage from Lower Limb

   1. **Calf pump:** Contraction of soleus muscle helps in pumping blood from below upward. Hence, it acts like a pump. **Therefore soleus is known as the peripheral heart.**
   2. **Contraction of heart:** In resting supine position this helps in venous drainage.
   3. **Suction pressure of diaphragm:** Contraction of diaphragm opens the inferior vena caval opening. The negative intrathoracic pressure helps in venous drainage from inferior vena cava, hence from the lower limb.
   4. **Valves:** Prevents back flow of blood into the distal part of lower limb.
      Direction of flow of blood: In the veins of lower limb flow is from superficial to deep veins except in the foot where it is from deep to superficial.

DYNAMICS OF CIRCULATION OF BLOOD AND LYMPH

The blood vessels carry blood from the heart to various tissues supplying oxygen, nutrients and endocrinal inputs. The blood flows back from the tissues to the heart carrying deoxygenated blood and waste products of tissue metabolism.

VASCULAR SYSTEM

It consists of the following:

1. **Arteries and arterioles:**
   — Larger arteries like aorta and its branches have larger amount of elastic tissue. The flow in these is governed by pumping of the heart, and the elastic recoil during diastolic phase.
   — Arterioles contain more muscular fibers and are richly innervated with sympathetic nerve fibres. They are the site for resistance to blood flow. Hence, are known as **resistance vessels.** A small change in their caliber due to neural or hormonal stimulation leads to large changes in total peripheral vascular resistance.

2. **Capillaries**
   — These are the **exchange vessels** which allow exchange of gases and nutritive substances across, to and fro from tissues.
   — They are made up of a single layer of endothelial cells, being only 1mm thick.
   — Capillaries provide channels between small arterioles and venules. They have a diameter of 5 mm at arterial end and 9 mm at venous end.
   — The flow in capillaries is regulated by precapillary sphincters which determine the size of capillary exchange area. The factors controlling precapillary sphincters and hence blood flow are:
      a. Neural: Sympathetic stimulation causes vasoconstriction.
      b. Hormonal: Serotonin (5HT) causes vaso-constriction.
      c. Local factors: Hypoxia, hypercapnia, increase in temperature and pH cause vaso-dilatation. Hypothermia causes vasoconstriction.

3. **Venules and veins**
   — They are called **capacitance vessels.**
   — They have thinner walls than arteries with little muscle fibers. Hence, they easily distend to accommodate large volumes of blood. However, they collapse easily also.
   — The intima of veins is folded at intervals to form valves which allow flow in one direction only, that is towards the heart.
   — There are no valves in small veins, very large veins, in cerebral and visceral veins.
   — Flow in veins is determined by compression of veins by skeletal muscle action, negative intrathoracic pressures during respiration and pumping of heart.

Thoroughfare vessels: These are vessels that connect an arteriole to vein directly. They bypass the capillary network forming an arterio-venous anastomosis. These are present in skin extremities like palm and toes, ear lobes, lips. They help in heat regulation. Exposure to heat leads to dilatation and increase flow to dissipate heat while at low temperature the vessel is constricted to conserve heat.

Blood Flow Dynamics

- Blood flows from area of high pressure to low pressure.
- Flow through a particular part is equal to effective perfusion pressure divided by resistance. Effective perfusion pressure is the difference between intraluminal arterial and venous pressures.
- Velocity of blood flow depends mainly on two factors
   a. Radius of resistance vessels. Resistance is inversely proportional to the fourth power of radius. $R \propto 1/r^4$. A decrease in radius by factor of 2, increases resistance by factor of 16.
   b. **Viscocity of blood:** It depends on the haematocrit, concentration of plasma proteins and flow rates.

ARTERIAL BLOOD FLOW AND BLOOD PRESSURE

Arterial flow is phasic, velocity being higher in systole and zero or negative at diastole. It is the elastic recoil of arteries which propels blood forwards during diastole.

Laminar and Turbulent Blood Flow

- The flow in blood vessels in laminar, that is streamlined.
- The layer of blood just next to vessel wall hardly moves while the velocity of flow increases towards the centre of the vessel.
- As the velocity of blood flow is increased the flow becomes turbulent. Above a critical velocity the turbulence of flow of blood produces sounds. For example, abnormal heart sounds or murmurs are heard in cases with aortic valve stenosis. This is because during systole the blood flow across stenosis produces turbulence. Murmurs are also heard in anemia where velocity of blood is higher due to lowered viscocity.

Blood Pressure

It is the force exerted by blood on the vessel wall. The pressure of blood in the vessels varies with the cardiac cycle.

- **Systolic blood pressure:** It is the pressure produced in the aorta and large arteries during ventricular systole. The peak systolic blood pressure (SBP) in adults is 120 mm Hg.
- **Diastolic blood pressure:** It is the pressure in the arteries during ventricular diastole and it is around 70-80 mm Hg.
- **Pulse pressure (PP)** is difference between systolic and diastolic pressures (DBP).
- **Mean blood pressure (MBP)** is the average pressure in the arteries throughout cardiac cycle. It is denoted by the formula: MBP = DBP + 1/3 PP.
- Pressure in small arteries and arterioles is lower, mean pressure being 30 to 35 mmHg and pulse pressure being 5 mm Hg.
- The pressures in vessels below heart are higher than those above the heart due to effect of gravity.

Factors affecting blood pressure (mainly systolic)

Blood pressure is governed by two factors:

1. **Cardiac output:** Increase cardiac output leads to increase SBP with little or no effect on DBP.
2. **Peripheral resistance:** DBP increases with increase in resistance as in atherosclerosis.
   - **Age:** Increase rigidity of arteries with aging increases the blood pressure. For adults above 50 years blood pressure of 140/90 is normal.
   - **Sex:** Blood pressure is generally lower in females.
   - **Body build:** Systolic blood pressure is higher in obese patients.
   - **Diurnal variation:** Systolic blood pressure is lower during sound sleep by 15 to 20 mm Hg and peaks around noon. Slight increase of 5 mm Hg is seen after meals.
   - **Exercise:** Transient increase in systolic blood pressure occurs during exercise.
   - **Emotions:** Fear, anxiety, stress increase systolic blood pressure by 5 to 10 mm Hg.
   - **Posture:** Pressure in lower limb arteries is higher than upper limb while standing. Also, diastolic pressure increases transiently from lying down to standing position.

Methods of Measuring Arterial BP

Instrument used to measure BP is called sphygmomanometer (Fig. 13.50).

1. **Palpation method**
   - The patient is in sitting or supine position with arm kept about the level of heart.

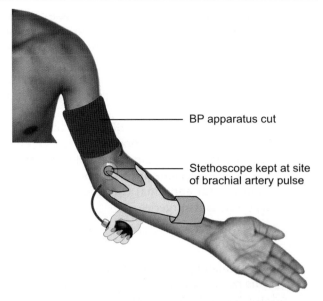

Fig. 13.50: Measurement of blood pressure in left arm

BP apparatus cut

Stethoscope kept at site of brachial artery pulse

- The sphygmomanometer cuff is wrapped around the arm and inflated.
- Radial artery pulsations are palpated: The pressure is raised 15 to 20 mm Hg above the pressure at which the pulsations disappear and then the cuff is gradually deflated. The pressure at which the pulsations are first felt is the systolic blood pressure.
- This does not measure diastolic pressure.

2. **Auscultatory method (Fig. 13.50)**
   - After inflation of cuff to a pressure at which radial pulse disappears, a stethoscope is placed over the site of brachial artery pulsations.
   - The pressure in the cuff is then lowered slowly and at the point where systolic pressure just exceeds cuff pressure, tapping sounds are heard known as Korotkoff sounds. This is due to sudden passage of blood with high velocity (turbulent flow).
   - As the pressure is lowered the sounds becomes dull and muffled and finally disappear (stream line flow attained).
   - Systolic BP is the pressure at which 1st sound is heard and diastolic BP is the pressure when the sound completely disappears.
   - Palpatory method usually records systolic pressure 5 mm Hg lower than the auscultatory method.
   - Prerequisites to be kept in mind before taking BP are:
     a. Cuff must be at the level of heart to avoid effect of gravity.

    b. In measuring BP in thigh or in obese patients, cuff should be of wider width to give accurate reading. False high readings are obtained with standard cuff.

    c. Transient rise in BP due to continuous inflation of cuff or fall on standing have to be kept in mind.

    d. Important to compare BP in both limbs at the time of 1st examination.

3. Direct arterial cannulation: Cannulation of arteries can be done to measure arterial pressure. It is done only in certain abnormal conditions like shock, heart transplant surgeries.

Capillary Circulation

- 5% of circulating blood is in capillaries.
- It is the most important component of blood which allows for exchange of nutrients, O_2 and waste products to and fro from tissues.
- Flow in capillaries is slow as the total cross sectional area is large. This allows for adequate exchange.
- Exchange across capillary walls depends on following factors:
  1. **Hydrostatic pressure gradient:** It is determined by the difference in
     a. Capillary hydrostatic pressure
     b. Interstitial tissue pressure
  2. **Osmotic pressure gradient:** It is determined by the difference in
     a. Capillary colloid osmotic pressure
     b. Interstitial tissue colloid osmotic pressure
- Fluid moves out of capillaries at the arteriolar end where filtration pressure is more than osmotic pressure and moves into capillaries at venous end when osmotic pressure is higher than filtration pressure.
- Exceptions:
  1. Fluid moves out of entire length of glomerular capillaries.
  2. Fluid moves into the capillaries in the entire length of intestines.

Venous Circulation

- The pressure in venules is 12 to 18 mm Hg and falls steadily in bigger veins to 5.5 mm Hg.
- **Central venous pressure:** The pressure in great veins at entry into atrium is around 4 to 6 mm Hg. This is termed central venous pressure.
- **Peripheral venous pressure:** It is 7 to 10 mm Hg. It depends on the central venous pressure and the pressure of surrounding tissues on veins. It is affected by gravity and is 0.77 mm Hg higher in

veins present each cm below level of heart and 0.77 mm Hg lower for each cm above level of heart.
- CVP (Central venous pressure) is increased in the following conditions:
  1. Expansion of blood volume
  2. Positive pressure breathing
  3. Straining: It results in raised intra-abdominal pressure
  4. Heart failure
- CVP is reduced in hypovolemic shock due to excess bleeding
- The flow of venous blood is governed by:
  1. **Thoracic pump:** Intrapleural pressures fall from – 2.5 to – 6 mm Hg during inspiration and aids in flow towards heart.
  2. **Effect of heart beat:** The blood is sucked into atria from great veins during ventricular contraction. As already mentioned during ventricular systole, A-V valves are pulled into the ventricles. This increases the capacity of atria and creates negative pressures in them. This aids the venous flow towards heart.
  3. **Muscle pump:** Contraction of skeletal muscles surrounding the limb veins leads to pumping of blood towards heart.

LYMPHATICS

- It is an alternative system of vessels which carries the interstitial fluid through channels that coalesce to form lymph vessels which drain into the corresponding side subclavian veins.
- The lymph vessels are lined with endothelium with minimal basal lamina. There are no fenestration but intercellular gap junctions are open to allow easy flow of molecules.
- The vessels have lymph nodes in their path at regular intervals. These nodes contain lymphocytes that help in immunological defence mechanism of the body.

Lymphatic Circulation

- Extra fluid that has filtered into tissues is carried back to blood via lymphatics.
- Small lymph channels have endothelial lining with loose junctions which allow passage of macro-molecules also.
- The flow in these lymphatic channels is aided primarily by muscular contractions.
- The smaller lymphatics drain into collecting lymphatics which have an endothelial lining with valves and a muscular wall. Flow in these is aided primarily by contraction of muscular wall, skeletal

muscle contraction, blood flow in veins associated with lymphatics and negative intrathoracic pressure.

- Lymphatic circulation helps to:
  — Maintain the interstitial fluid pressure.
  — Transport of nutrient macromolecules especially free fatty acids and cholesterol from intestines to portal circulation of liver for assimilation.
  — They have immunological function due to presence of lymph nodes along the path.

REGULATION OF CARDIOVASCULAR FUNCTION

Regulation of cardiovascular function is required to maintain blood supply to tissues, to help in redistribution of blood flow for regulation of body temperature and to readjust perfusion in various physiological situations like exercise and clinical conditions like blood loss (e.g., due to haemorrhage).

Mechanisms of Cardiovascular Adjustments
1. Alteration of cardiac output by affecting heart rate and stroke volume.
2. Altering diameter of arterioles.
3. Altering the amount of blood pooled in venous circulation.

Local Regulatory Mechanisms

The factors that regulate these mechanisms are:
1. **Autoregulation** is the capacity of tissues to regulate their own blood flow. This is brought about by:
   a. Change in vascular resistance in response to change in perfusion pressure.
      — Increase blood pressure leads to stretching of the vascular wall which responds by contraction of its muscles to reduce blood flow to normal. This is **myogenic theory of autoregulation.**
   b. Metabolite theory of autoregulation
      — Metabolic activities of cells and tissues lead to local accumulation of metabolites. These mainly effect arterioles and precapillary sphincters. Local metabolites that lead to vasodilatation are:
      — Decrease pCO_2
      — Decrease pH
      — Increase pCO_2: Direct vasodilator effect is mostly seen in skin and brain
      — Increase lactate levels
      — Increase potassium, K^+ levels
      — Increase local temperature
      — Histamine: It is produced locally in response to inflammation and injury.

Local metabolites causing vasoconstriction are:
a. **Serotonin:** It is released from platelet at site of injury and causes contriction of injured vessel. Helps to prevent blood loss.
b. **Decrease in local temperature:** Helps to prevents heat loss.

2. **Regulation by endothelial cells:** Endothelial cells produce the following substances that effect local blood flow :
   a. **Endothelium derived relaxing factor:** It is nitric oxide **(NO).** NO is synthesized from arginine and rapidly diffuses into smooth muscle cells. It causes vasodilatation. NO levels maintain normal blood pressure. The vasodilator action of bradykinin and acetylcholine is mediated by production of NO.
   b. **Endothelins:** Endothelin-2 produced by endothelial cells is a potent vasoconstrictor and is produced in response to hypoxia, angiotensin II, catecholamines, insulin, and shear stress. It is inhibited by NO, atrial natriuretic peptide and prostacyclin.
   c. **Prostacyclin (PGI2a):** It is usually produced during injury. It causes vasodilatation. In association with thromboxane A2 from platelet cells which causes vasoconstriction and platelet aggregation, it regulates clot formation and flow in the vessel.

Systemic Regulatory Mechanisms

The systemic regulation of cardiovascular function is by circulating hormones and neural control.
1. **Hormonal regulation**
   a. **Vasodilator hormones:** These include:
      — **Kinins – Bradykinin** causes vasodilation via NO and increases capillary permeability. They are found in sweat glands, salivary glands and pancreas and may regulate blood flow to skin and GIT.
      — **Atrial natriuretic peptide:** Is secreted by heart and causes vasodilatation. Has a role in glomerular filtration.
   b. **Vasoconstrictor hormones**
      — **Catecholamines:** They are produced by adrenal gland. Norepinephrine produces generalized vasoconstriction. Epinephrine causes vasodilation in skin and coronary arteries.
      — **Angiotensin II:** It is produced in response to renin which is secreted by the kidneys secondary to a fall in ECF volume. Angiotension II causes vasoconstriction to regulate BP.

CHAPTER-13

— **Vasopressin:** Vasopressive response of vasopressin is seen during acute haemorrhage and hypotension. It normally acts to control ECF volume by its action on renal tubules (see page no. 555).

2. **Neural regulation**
   — Blood vessels throughout the body are innervated with sympathetic nerve fibers. The resistance vessels namely arterioles and precapillary sphincters are most densely innervated. Veins on the other hand have a scanty innervation. The noradrenergic discharge in these nerves leads to vasoconstriction. The sympathetic activity has a base line tone maintaining the vessel caliber.
   — The heart receives both sympathetic and parasympathetic (Vagal) innervation. Sympathetic stimulation leads to increase heart rate (positive chronotropic action) and increase stroke volume (positive ionotropic action) while vagal stimulation causes bradycardia and decrease muscle activity. Both sympathetic and vagal supply have a basal tone with vagal tonic activity predominating under normal conditions.

Regulation by Medulla Oblongata

1. **Vasomotor centre (VMC)**
   a. It is the collection of neurons in the reticular system of medulla oblongata.
   b. It integrates impulses reaching from various pathways and regulates the tonic discharge of spinal sympathetic neurons.
   c. Stimulation of vasomotor centre primarily leads to increase sympathetic activity resulting in increase heart rate, stroke volume and cardiac output. It also causes vasoconstriction leading to rise in blood pressure and venoconstriction leading to increase venous return.
2. **Vagus nerve nuclei:** Vagal nerve nuclei namely dorsal motor nucleus of vagus, nucleus of tractus solitarius and nucleus ambiguus are present in the medulla. Fibers arising from motor nucleus and nucleus ambiguus nuclei descend to converge on:
   a. Preganglionic sympathetic neurons of spinal cord and inhibit their activity
   b. **Cardiac muscle:** Inhibit SA node activity and decrease heart rate and force of myocardial contraction.

Factors Influencing Medullary Centres

1. Afferents that produce excitatory response in vasomotor centre are:
   a. From cerebral cortex and hypothalamus: In response to emotional stimuli e.g., sexual stimulus and anger.
   b. From pain pathways via reticular activating system.
   c. From carotid and aortic chemoreceptors.
2. Afferents that produce inhibitory responses by inhibiting VMC and stimulating vagal centres are:
   a. From cerebral cortex and hypothalamus – Example is stimulation of vagal centre and inhibition of VMC due to fear and anxiety leading to bradycardia and fainting
   b. From lungs: Inflation of lungs stimulates vagal afferents that decrease sympathetic activity of VMC leading to vasodilatation and fall in BP
   c. From baroreceptors

Chemoreceptors

- These receptors are sensitive to changes in pO_2, pCO_2 and pH levels of blood.
- Their primary role is regulation of respiration. They also send afferents to VMC.
- Chemoreceptors consist of carotid bodies situated at bifurcation of common carotid artery (supplied by glosopharyngeal nerve) and aortic bodies situated at origin of aortic arch (supplied by vagus nerve).
- Stimulation of chemoreceptors by hypoxia primarily stimulates respiration. Their effect on cardiovascular function is slight and only when there is severe hypoxia due to severe hypotension do they stimulate sympathetic activity via VMC.

Baroreceptors (Mechanoreceptors)

- These are receptors sensitive to stretch.
- They are present in carotid sinus, arch of aorta and walls of right and left atria, and left ventricle.
- They are stimulated by increase in blood pressure or cardiac pressure.
- The afferents travel via vagus nerves and from carotid sinus in glossopharyngeal nerve to the nucleus tractus solitarius.
- This stimulates inhibitory pathway of VMC that decreases sympathetic activity and increases the vagal tone to heart resulting in vasodilatation, venodilatation, fall in blood pressure, bradycardia and decrease cardiac output.

CIRCULATION IN SPECIAL REGIONS OF BODY
Coronary Circulation

The blood supply of heart is described on pages 400 to 402. Heart is supplied by right and left coronary arteries which are functionally end arteries. However, anastomotic channels are present between the two arteries, which open up with age and presence of coronary artery disease. Flow pattern in coronary vessels during cardiac cycle is described below:

- Normal coronary blood flow at rest in adults is 250 ml/ mt (5% of cardiac output).
- O_2 consumption per unit blood flow by myocardium is 70% as compared to 25% in peripheral body tissues.
- As the muscle (myocardium) contracts, it compresses its own blood supply.
- Since the ventricular pressures are high during systole, coronary blood flow primarily (80%) occurs during diastole.
- This phasic variation of blood flow in coronary vessels is specially true for left ventricle and practically no blood flow occurs in the subendocardial region of left ventricle during systole.
- As heart rate increases, diastolic phase decreases. Thus, the blood flow to left ventricle is compromised in tachycardia.
- Hence, subendocardial region of left ventricle is more prone to myocardial infarction in conditions such as coronary artery diseases.

Regulation of Coronary Blood Flow

Blood flow in coronary arteries increases with increase in metabolic activity of myocardium. This auto regulation is brought about by following factors:

1. **Chemical factors:** Increase metabolic activity of myocardium results in local hypoxia, low O_2 and increase local CO_2, H^+, K^+, lactate levels which regulate local adenosine levels and prostaglandin levels. These bring about coronary vasodilatation and increase the flow.
2. **Neural factors**
   a. **Sympathetic stimulation:** Noradrenergic activity increases myocardial contraction and hence its metabolism leading to coronary vasodilatation. Besides stimulation of β receptors on arterioles causes vasodilatation.
   b. **Parasympathetic activity (stimulation of vagus nerve):** Acetylcholine is the neuro-transmitter and it causes coronary vaso-dilatation.

Factors Affecting Coronary Blood Flow

1. Factors which increase myocardial metabolism due to increase in contractions result in increase blood flow. These are:
   a. Exercise

   b. Emotional excitement
   c. Hypotension: due to reflex sympathetic discharge
   d. Hyperthyroidism
   e. Hyperthermia
   f. Anemia
2. Factors which decrease coronary blood flow are:
   a. Hypothermia decreases O_2 consumption of heart and hence decreases coronary blood flow.
   b. **Aortic stenosis:** The left ventricle has to push blood into aorta with a greater effort due to stenosis and this leads to increase ventricular pressure during systole. Thus it compromises coronary blood flow.
   c. In conditions with low aortic diastolic pressures like severe haemorrhage, coronary artery blood flow is reduced.
   d. In congestive cardiac failure, coronary artery blood flow is compromised due to poor contraction of heart.
   e. **Coronary artery disease:** In this condition there is thickening of subendothelial part of arteries due to deposition of atherosclerotic plaques and narrowing of lumen of arteries. This leads to reduced flow in the arteries. When blood flow is reduced to a large extent, hypoxia leads to production of 'P' factor that stimulates pain nerve endings and causes angina pectoris (pain of heart attack). If block is about 70-75%, only angina occurs specially during activity that increases heart rate like exercise. If blood flow due to obstruction is > 85% then hypoxia leads to damage to myocardium which is called myocardial infarction (heart attack).

Cerebral Circulation

The vascular supply of brain is derived from circle of Willis and its branches formed by bilateral internal carotid arteries and vertebral arteries (page nos 413, 414, and 416). 80% of the blood is derived from internal carotid arteries. Venous drainage is via cerebral dural sinuses which primarily terminate in internal jugular vein (page no. 430).

- The blood vessels receive noradrenergic supply from superior cervical ganglion, parasympathetic supply (acetylcholine) from sphenopalatine ganglion and in addition sensory supply from trigeminal nerve which produce substance P.
- The brain receives around 750 ml blood per minute which is equal to 54 ml / 100gm/mt. Average blood flow in grey matter is 69 ml / 100 gm / mt while in white matter is 28 ml /100 gm/mt.

- Blood flow is maximum in premotor and frontal regions. Flow increases in the part of brain in which activity is stimulated.

Blood Brain Barrier (BBB)

- The concentration of various ions like Na^+, K^+, H^+, Mg^+ etc are maintained within a close range for proper functioning of neurons. This is achieved by presence of blood brain barrier that allows selective passage of ions and substances while prevents entry of toxins and exit of neurotransmitters.
- The barrier is formed by presence of tight junctions between capillary endothelial cells in brain. In choroid plexus where capillary endothelium has fenestrations, the barrier is formed by presence of tight junctions between epithelial cells of choroids.
- CO_2, O_2 and water penetrate the brain easily. O_2 consumption by brain at rest is about 20% of the total body consumption.
- Lipid soluble substances like steroid hormones also cross barrier easily.
- Proteins, polypeptides, urea, bile salts cannot cross while H^+, HCO_3^-, Na^+, K^+ etc have low penetration across the blood brain barrier.
- Glucose is taken up by facilitated diffusion by glucose transporters (GLUT). It is the major source of energy for the brain under normal conditions.

Regulation of Cerebral Blood Flow

- The cerebral blood flow shows auto-regulation.
- The changes in CO_2 levels and H^+ levels are important in regulating blood flow. Any decrease in perfusion with accumulation of CO_2 and hypoxia leading to accumulation of H^+ cause vasodilatation.
- Local neural reflexes also have some role.
- A constant blood flow is maintained at blood pressures of 65-140 mmHg by auto regulation. The flow is markedly reduced at BP< 65 mm Hg and unconsciousness can occur within 10 sec. of cutting of the blood supply to brain.
- Effect of intra cranial pressure on systemic BP: The normal CSF pressure is upto 7 mm Hg. An increase in intracranial pressure leads to increase in systemic blood pressure. This helps to maintain flow to brain. This reflex is called **Cushing's reflex**. The decrease in blood flow due to raised intracranial pressure results in lowered pO_2 and raised pCO_2 levels at the vasomotor area. VMC gets stimulated leading to increase in BP. However, if CSF pressure rises above 33 mm Hg, this mechanism fails leading to sudden fall in cerebral circulation.

Splanchnic Circulation

Splanchnic blood flow describes blood flow to and from GIT, liver, pancreas and spleen. The arterial supply to the organs are described in the respective chapters.

Intestinal Circulation

- The blood flow is regulated by local metabolic activity. Increase metabolic activity produces metabolites that themselves stimulate local vasodilatation. They also result in release of local GIT hormones and stimulate the vagal activity which increases local blood flow. Hence, blood flow to intestine shows extensive auto regulation. It is the reason for an increase in blood flow after meals.
- Sympathetic activity causes vasoconstriction and decrease in blood flow.

Hepatic Circulation

- Liver receives 80% blood from portal vein which has pressure of 10 mm Hg and 20% from hepatic arteries with mean pressure 90 mm Hg and drains into hepatic veins (pressure of 5 mm Hg).
- The local myogenic response and presence of metabolites maintain a high pre capillary arteriolar tone of hepatic arteries to lower its capillary pressure. However, when portal flow decreases, flow in hepatic artery increases. This is regulated by adrenergic response.
- The primary nervous supply to portal veins and hepatic arteries is by sympathetic nerves. Stimulation of noradrenergic fibers cause vasoconstriction.
- Portal vein radicles dilate passively in response to pressure changes like an increase systemic BP or back pressure by congestive cardiac failure. This can cause hepatic congestion.

Blood Circulation in Skin and Skeletal Muscle

- The rate of flow of blood in skin has an important role to play in regulation of body temperatures.
- The blood vessels to skin are supplied by noradrenergic sympathetic fibers which maintain a constant tone and flow at rest. Sympathetic over activity as in exposure to cold or stress causes vasoconstriction and decrease flow to skin.
- Vasodilatation is not a direct neural response but occurs in response to lowered sympathetic activity or accumulation of metabolites, low pO_2 levels and local chemicals like bradykinin.
- A rise in body temperature due to fever or exercise increases sympathetic discharge in body but also

stimulates hypothalamus which decreases vaso-constrictor activity in skin and effective result is vasodilatation and sweating.

- The vascular supply to muscles is also maintained by the sympathetic tone of the arterioles and precapillary sphincters.
- Increase sympathetic discharge as in hemorrhage leads to pre and post capillary sphincter constriction. This diverts the blood from skin and muscles to heart.

- Sympathetic noradrenergic supply to arterioles causes vasodilatation. This is responsible to increase blood flow to muscles in response to local metabolites.

Fetoplacental Circulation (Fig. 13.51)

Blood flow to uterus is increased during pregnancy by about 20 times normal. O_2 uptake by uterus is markedly increased and the actual O_2 saturation of maternal blood

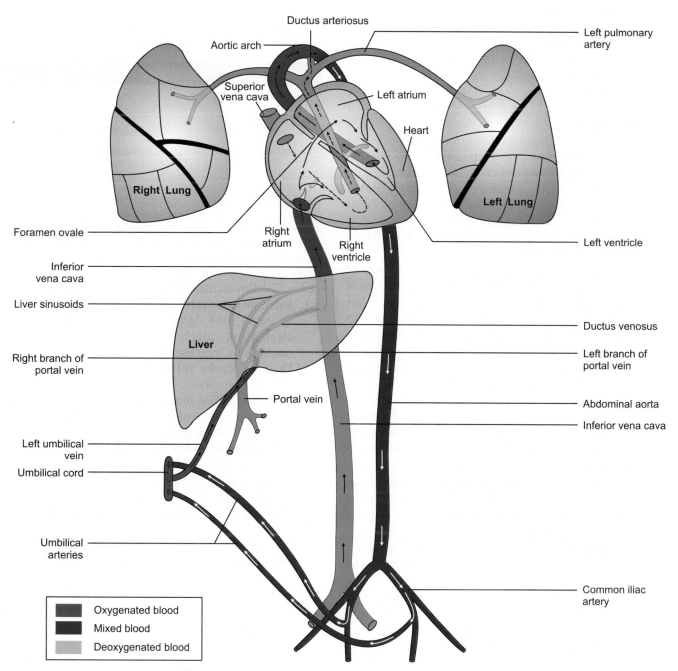

Fig. 13.51: Fetal circulation (Diagrammatic representation)

- Oxygenated blood
- Mixed blood
- Deoxygenated blood

is reduced. However, high affinity of HbF to O_2 in fetus allows for adequate supply to fetus.

Fetal Circulation

- The placenta provides oxygen and nutrients to the fetus and is the site of excretion of toxic substances from fetus to mother.
- A pair of umbilical veins carry oxygenated blood from placenta to fetus. The right umbilical vein disappears very early in fetal life and only one umbilical vein is left.
- The umbilical vein passes into fetus at the umbilicus and runs along the anterior abdominal wall in the falciparum ligament towards liver. It opens into left branch of portal vein. At this point it gives of a larger branch, ductus venosus.
- The ductus venosus opens directly into the inferior vena cava delivering a large part of oxygenated blood to it.
- Part of blood draining into portal vein supplies the liver. Blood from liver is drained by the hepatic veins into inferior vena cava.
- The inferior vena cava also receives deoxygenated blood from lower half of body. Thus the blood in inferior vena cava is mixed and is less oxygenated (67% O_2 saturation) than the blood in umbilical vein (80% O_2 saturation).
- The inferior vena cava opens into right atrium of heart and this blood is directed to the left atrium of heart via foramen ovale and hence to the left ventricle. Blood from left ventricle passes into ascending aorta and coronary arteries to supply heart. It further flows to arch of aorta and its branches namely common carotid arteries to supply the head (brain) and neck.
- The right atrium also receives deoxygenated blood from superior vena cava returning from upper half of body that flows into right ventricle, hence pulmonary artery. The lungs are collapsed in intrauterine life resulting in high pulmonary pressure. A very small percentage of blood enters pulmonary circulation while the majority drains into aorta directly via ductus arteriosus, a channel connecting pulmonary trunk to arch of aorta.
- This pattern of blood flow ensures well oxygenated blood to brain and heart while less oxygenated blood flows to the extremities.
- The mixed blood (oxygenated + deoxygenated '60% O_2 saturation') courses down from arch of aorta supplying rest of the body via its branches. It passes back to the placenta via right and left umbilical arteries, branches of anterior trunk of internal iliac arteries.
- At birth when umbilical cord is clamped and cut, umbilical circulation is obliterated. The pressure in inferior vena cava and right atrium falls closing foramen ovale. The high pulmonary vascular pressure also falls due to first breath of baby leading to expansion of lungs thus further closing foramen ovale and causing closure of ductus arteriosus also. Adult circulation is thus established.
- The umbilical arteries and veins, ductus venosus, ductus arteriosus undergo gradual atrophy and obliteration and result in formation fibrous cords, seen as remnants in adults.

Fetal vessel	Remnants in adult
Umbilical vein	Ligamentum teres
Umbilical arteries	Medial umbilical ligaments
Ductus venosus	Ligamentum venosum
Ductus arteriosus	Ligamentum anteriosum

PHYSIOLOGY OF EXERCISE

Effect of exercise on cardiovascular system

To meet the extra O_2 requirements of body and remove excess CO_2 and heat from body during exercise, a number of respiratory and cardiovascular responses occur. Cardiovascular responses are as follows :

1. **Increase heart rate:** Initially occurs due to decrease in vagal tone, later on occurs due to increase circulating catecholamines and stimulation of medulla by increase levels of pCO_2.
2. **Increase stroke volume:** It is marked in isotonic muscle exercises.
3. **Increase cardiac output:** This is due to increase in heart rate and stroke volume and it may increase upto 5 to 6 times of normal.
4. **Blood pressure changes:** Systolic blood pressure increases during exercise while diastolic blood pressure is maintained in mild to moderate exercise and rises only in severe exercise.
5. **Increase venous return:** This is brought about by increase muscular contractions, increase activity of negative thoracic pressures, mobilization of blood from splanchnic circulation and venoconstriction by catecholamines.
6. **Circulatory changes:** There is increased blood flow in muscular, coronary, pulmonary and cutaneous arteries while visceral blood flow is reduced specially in severe exercise.

CLINICAL AND APPLIED ASPECTS

PERICARDIUM

- Inflammation of pericardium is known as pericarditis
- Paracentesis of pericardial fluid or aspiration of pericardial effusion is done by two routes
  - Parasternal route: A needle is inserted close to the sternal margin in the 4th or 5th intercostal space on the left side to prevent injury to left pleural sac and internal thoracic artery.
  - Subcostal route: The patient is placed in a slightly propped up position. Aspiration is performed through the left costoxiphoid angle with an upward inclination of the needle of 45°.
- Intracardiac injection of adrenaline is given through the parasternal route described above during the process cardio-pulmonary resuscitation.

SURFACE ANATOMY OF HEART

Sterno-costal Surface

- Right border
  - Put a point 1.2 cm. lateral to the margin of sternum on the upper border of the right 3rd costal cartilage.
  - Put a point in the right fourth intercostal space 3.7 cm. lateral to the median plane.
  - Mark the sternal end of the right sixth costal cartilage.
    Draw a line joining these points with a gentle convexity to the right.
- Lower border
  - Put a point on the sternal end of the right sixth costal cartilage.
  - Mark the xiphisternal junction.
  - Locate the apex beat.
    Draw a line joining these points.
- Left border
  - Mark the apex beat.
  - Put a point 1.2 cm. lateral to the sternal margin on the lower border of the left second costal cartilage.
    Join these points by a line with an upward convexity.
- Upper border: Join the upper ends of the right and left borders.

HEART

- The 1st heart sound (Lub) occurs due to closure of atrioventricular valves. The 2nd heart sound (Dub) occurs due to closure of semilunar valves.
- In an adult, normal heart rate is 72 to 80 beats per minute. This is normal rhythm of S.A. node.

Increased heart rate is known as **tachycardia** and decrease in heart rate is **bradycardia.** An alteration in regularity is known as **arrythmia.**

- **Murmurs:** These are abnormal sounds heard with a stethoscope, over the precordium in relation to heart beats. When the blood flow is smooth, normal heart sounds are heard but any turbulence brought about by narrowing of passages like mitral valve stenosis or aortic valve stenosis or incompetence of valves leading to regurgitation of blood leads to production of additional sounds. The presence of various murmurs in common clinical conditions are tabulated below:

Valve defects	Type of murmurs
Mitral/tricuspid stenosis	Diastolic murmur
Mitral/tricuspid regurgitation	Systolic murmur
Aortic/pulmonary valve stenosis	Systolic murmur
Aortic/pulmonary valve incompetence	Diastolic murmur

- **Rheumatic heart disease:** It is an endocardial inflammation of heart. It is known to occur after a bout of pharyngitis caused by a particular strain of streptococcus bacteria. The most common site of inflammation is the valves of heart. The inflammation heals and results in scarring leding to fibrosis or destruction of the valves. This leads to stenosis or incompetance of the valves resulting in malfunction of heart.
- **ASD or atrial septal defect** is a congenital defect of ostium primum or ostium secundum.
- **VSD or ventricular septal defect** is a congenital defect usually in the development of membranous part of ventricular septum. This defect leads to mixing up of oxygenated blood from left side of heart with deoxygenated blood of right side of heart.
- **Co-arctation of aorta** is the congenital stenosis of the arch of aorta usually, distal to the origin of left subclavian artery. This results in high blood pressure in upper extremities and low blood pressure in lower extremities.

ABNORMAL ECG

- **Atrio-ventricular block:** This can be caused by coronary artery disease which affects A–V node or bundle of His. On ECG it is seen as :
  - **1st degree heart block:** All atrial impulses reach ventricles but with a delay. This is seen as prolonged PR interval.
  - **2nd degree heart block:** Not all atrial impulses reach ventricles, ratio of atrial to ventricular beats may be 2: 1, or 3: 1. This is seen as more P

waves than QRS complexes. PR interval is also prolonged.
  — **3rd degree or complete heart block:** Ventricles beat independently of atria and at a lower rate of < 45 beats / minute. This is seen as multiple P waves and occasional QRS complexes.
- **Ectopic excitation:** Focus of excitation is in atria or ventricle and not SA or AV node. This leads to an extra systole – It is seen as an abnormal P-wave (atrial extra systole) or abnormal QRS – complex without P-wave (ventricular extra systole) which interrupts the normal rhythm.
- **Atrial arrythmias:** In this condition there is an increase in atrial depolarization waves due to presence of ectopic focus of excitation or due to abnormal conduction. Atrial arrhythmias are seen in conditions of electrolyte imbalance, following a myocardial infarction, etc. It is of three types depending upon heart rate:
  — Atrial tachycardia: Beats upto 200 / mt
  — Atrial flutter: Beats between 250 to 350 / mt
  — Atrial arrthymias: Beats more than 350 / mt
  Ventricular rate in such cases is from 80 to 160 / mt
- **Ventricular arrythmias:** This occurs due to rapid ventricular depolarizations leading to tachycardia or fibrillation.
- **Myocardial infarction (MI):** It is a clinical condition which occurs due to interruption of blood supply to a portion of myocardium leading to ischemic changes. The following ECG changes are seen:
  — Elevation of ST segment in electrodes over infracted area in acute phase.
  — Appearance of deep Q-waves.
  — Appearance of various arrythmias.
- **Effect of changes in concentration of extra cellular fluid potassium**
  — **Hyperkalemia:** Leads to prolonged QRS complex and tall T-waves.
  — **Hypokalemia:** Leads to prolonged PR interval and ST segment depression.

REGIONAL ARTERIAL SUPPLY

- Abdominal aorta can be felt per abdomen in thin person. It can be an important differential diagnosis of lump abdomen.
- The middle meningeal artery is sometimes torn in fracture of side of skull. This results in the formation of an extradural haematoma that overlaps the motor area of the cerebral cortex. Consequently there is compression of the brain leading to paralysis of the movements of the opposite half of the body. The pressure due to haematoma can be relieved by drilling a burr hole in skull through the pterion.

- The central artery of retina is an end artery and obstruction of this artery by an embolism or pressure results in sudden total blindness.
- Subclavian steal syndrome: If there is obstruction of subclavian artery proximal to the origin of vertebral artery, some amount of blood from opposite vertebral artery can pass in a retrograde fashion to the subclavian artery of the affected side through the vertebral artery of that side to provide the collateral circulation to the upper limb on the side of lesion. Thus there is stealing of blood meant for the brain by the subclavian artery of the affected side.
- Tests to evaluate coronary blood flow are:
  — Radioactive tracer scan
    a. Radionucleotide of thalium ^{201}Tl is taken up by the actively functioning myocardial cells and its uptake is directly proportional to the blood flow. Infusion of ^{201}Tl is used to assess blood flow pattern in the myocardium.
    b. Radionucleotide of technetium, ^{99m}Tc is selectively taken up by myocardial tissue damaged by hypoxia, and is used to locate myocardial infarcts.
  — **Coronary angiography:** Radioopaque contrast media is injected into coronary arteries after cannulating them to see blood flow pattern by X-rays.

VEINS OF HEAD AND NECK

- In case of obstruction of inferior vena cava a collateral circulation between inferior vena cava and superior vena cava opens up and provides an alternative channel.
  Important collateral veins are
  1. Azygos venous system
  2. Internal vertebral venous plexus
  3. Epigastric – superior and inferior
  4. Circumflex Iliac – deep and superficial
  5. Lateral thoracic
  6. Thoraco-epigastric
  7. Internal thoracic
  8. Posterior intercostal veins
- The internal jugular vein acts as a guide for surgeons during removal of deep cervical lymph nodes.
- The internal jugular vein can safely be cannulated in cases of cardio vascular collapse by introducing the needle in a backward and upward direction in the triangular space between the two heads of origin of sternocleidomastoid. However it can lead to hematoma formation or inadvertant puncture of cupola of pleura in this position leading to pneumothorax.

- **Air embolism:** The venous pressure in vessels above the level of heart in sitting or standing positions are lower and usually reach zero. The neck veins are generally collapsed. However, since the intracranial dural sinuses have rigid walls they do not collapse. Hence, the pressures in these systems are negative. It is important for a neurosurgeon to be careful while performing surgeries in seated position as an inadvertent injury to these sinuses can suck in the air into circulation leading to air embolism. On reaching the heart, air cannot be pumped out as it is compressible and thus may block circulation leading to death.
- CVP can be measured directly by placing a catheter into subclavian veins or indirectly by placing a catheter in external jugular vein (EJV). Peripheral pressure in EJV corresponds to CVP. CVP measurement and monitoring is important in managing shock as it determines the rate of IV fluid infusion.

VEINS OF UPPER LIMB

- Median cubital vein is connected to the deep veins of the upper limb through a perforator which fixes it. Hence, it does not slip away when intravenous injections are given. It acts as lifeline in emergency conditions to give intravenous injections and fluids. **It is also used for cardiac catheterization.**
- Cephalic vein is used to form internal areterio-venous fistulae for hemodialysis in chronic renal failure. A fistulae is established between cephalic vein and radial artery.
- In case of axillary vein obstruction, the venous drainage of upper limb is maintained through a communication present between the cephalic vein and external jugular vein in neck.
- Thoraco epigastric vein connects superficial epigastric vein which is a tributary of great saphenous vein to lateral thoracic vein, a tributary of axillary vein. Great saphenous vein drains into femoral vein at the saphenous opening. Hence, femoral vein is connected to the axillary vein.

VEINS OF LOWER LIMB

- In 80% individuals, external iliac vein presents a valve which protects the saphenofemoral junction against high pressure.
- **Varicose veins:** Dilatation and tortuocity of superficial veins of lower limb is known as varicose veins. The main factor leading to varicose vein is incompetencey of valves at different levels namely
  — Valves in perforating veins
  — Sapheno femoral valve
  — Valves in superficial veins

The following is the sequence of events in the development and complications of varicose veins.
  — Incompetence of valves
  — Dilatation of veins
  — Tortuocity of veins - varicose veins
  — Stasis of blood, local ischemia.
  — Formation of varicose ulcer with infection or bleeding from the ulcer.
  — Thrombosis of vessels and embolism
- **Tourniquet test:** Tourniquet test is performed by applying a tourniquet at various levels of leg and thigh. It helps to identify the level at which there is incompentance of the valves.
- Femoral vein is used for venous blood sampling and occasionally used for intravenous infusion in cases of peripheral circulatory collapse. The femoral vein is localized by feeling the pulsations of the femoral artery which is lateral to it, below the inguinal ligament.

PORTAL CIRCULATION

- Portal vein has no valves.
- Portal system accommodates 1/3 of blood of circulation. Portal vein is formed by splenic and superior mesenteric vein. If there is any obstruction to portal vein, it leads to back flow to the splenic vein and superior mesenteric vein and opening up of portocaval anastomosis. Backflow of blood in splenic vein leads to stasis of blood in spleen and accumulation of blood. This leads to enlargement of spleen.
- In case of portal obstruction or hypertension, portocaval anastomosis at different sites open up and provide collateral circulation. If portal hypertension is severe, it leads to enlargement of anastomotic channels at the lower end of esophagus and causes their dilatation and tortuocity. These are known as esophageal varices. They can rupture if they are very large.
- Internal piles can occur due to the opening up of portocaval anastomosis at the lower end of rectum and anal canal at the level of the pectinate line.
- Paraumbilical veins anastomose with six systemic veins namely,
  — Superficial epigastric
  — Superior epigastric
  — Lateral thoracic
  — Posterior intercostal
  — Lumbar vein
  — Inferior epigastric
In case of portal hypertension this collateral circulation opens up and forms a spoke wheel appearance on the anterior abdominal wall with the umbilicus as the centre. This is known as caput medusae.

CHAPTER-13

PHYSIOLOGY OF CARDIOVASCULAR SYSTEM

- **Cardiac failure (heart failure):** This is a clinical condition is characterized by failure of pumping action of heart which results in decreased cardiac output and hence poor circulation of blood with poor tissue perfusion. It can be:
  a. Acute cardiac failure: This sudden onset occurs due to poor myocardial contractility. Example in myocardial infarction.
  b. Chronic cardiac failure: It occurs gradually and is also called congestive cardiac failure. It occurs due to poor filling of ventricles. Example in valvular defects.
- **Shock:** It is a clinical condition which is characterized by sudden fall in cardiac output resulting in severe hypotension and impairment of tissue perfusion. It can be classified according to cause as:
  — Hypotensive shock, e.g., Hemorrhage or severe bleeding due to injury or surgery.
  — Vasogenic shock: Usually due to diffuse peripheral vasodilatation resulting in poor venous return to heart, e.g., neurogenic shock, anaphylactic shock (severe allergy) or septic shock (severe infection).
  — Cardiogenic shock: Due to acute cardiac failure
  — Obstructive shock: Due to obstruction of ventricles, e.g., severe pericardial effusion, pulmonary artery embolus.
- **Ischemic heart disease:** It is a clinical condition which arises due to deficient coronary circulation leading to damage to myocardium of heart. It can cause mild attack of pain known as angina or can lead to acute myocardial infarction or heart attack and death.
- **Hypertension:** It is defined as a sustained increase in peripheral arterial blood pressure taken as blood pressure > 140 / 90 mm Hg.
- **Hypotension:** It is defined as fall in blood pressure leading to feeling of dizziness, sweating and occasionally fainting.
- **Orthostatic hypotension:** Hypotension occurring due to standing posture is known as orthostatic hypotension.
  - Blood brain barrier develops during infancy and therefore is more permeable to various most substances in children. In newborns with jaundice bile pigments easily cross the blood brain barrier and damage sensitive structures like basal ganglia leading to a condition called kernicterus. Thus, jaundice in newborn, even if physiological needs to be carefully monitored and treated.

  During sudden loss of blood as in hemorrhage there is an increase in sympathetic activity which leads to vasoconstriction in splanchnic circulation. Thus most of the blood gets diverted to systemic circulation to maintain systemic BP and perfusion of vital organs like brain and heart.

- **Edema:** It is accumulation of interstitial fluid in abnormally large amounts. The various causes of edema are:
  — Increase in hydrostatic capillary pressure-**This can occur due to:**
  a. Arteriolar dilatation: Example, in excess heat.
  b. Increase venous pressure leading to stasis of blood. Examples are: Heart failure, incompetent venous valves, venous obstruction due to thrombo-embolism effect of gravity as in continuous standing, increase in ECF due to salt and water retention as in pregnancy etc.
  — **Decreased capillary oncotic pressure:** Hypoproteinemia as seen in liver cirrhosis and nephrosis results in lowered plasma osmolality. This causes extravasation of fluid out of capillaries.
  — **Increase capillary permeability:** This occurs due to presence of local substances like kinins, and histamine as in allergic reactions.
  — **Lymphatic blockade:** This leads to accumulation of fluid which is rich in proteins. It is called lymphedema. Examples are:
  a. **Filariasis:** In this condition infestation with filarial worms blocks the lymphatic channels.
  b. **Radical mastectomy:** Mastectomy is removal of breast which is usually performed in cases of breast cancer. The surgery involves removal of axillary lymph nodes. This leads to block in drainage and lymphedema in the corresponding side upper limb.

Chapter 14

Blood and Its Components

INTRODUCTION

Blood forms 8% of total body weight, that means, in an adult weighing 60 to 70 kg circulating blood volume would be 4800 to 5600 ml (5 to 6 liters). It primarily has two components:

1. **Cellular elements:** These consists of red blood cells, white blood cells and platelets. It is 45% of total blood volume (Fig. 14.1).
2. **Plasma:** It is the clear fluid component of blood which suspends the cellular elements. It forms 55% of total blood volume.

Functions of Blood

1. Blood carries O_2 from lungs to tissues and CO_2 from tissues to lungs.
2. It carries various nutritive substances absorbed from gastrointestinal tract to the tissues.
3. It transports products of metabolism for excretion from kidneys.
4. It helps in circulation of various hormones and chemical agents from their site of secretion to the effector organ and tissues.

5. It helps in regulation of temperature.
6. Blood forms an important buffer to control the pH, temperature and electrolyte content of the body.
7. The white blood cell component of blood is responsible for providing defence, i.e., immunity both against infections and foreign bodies.
8. It contains platelets and other complex factors that regulate haemostasis, i.e., clotting of blood on injury.
9. Plasma protein component maintains the intra-vascular oncotic pressure and helps in transport of various substances like iron, thyroid hormones etc. to various sites.

RED BLOOD CORPUSCLES OR CELLS (RBCs)/ ERYTHROCYTES (FIGs 14.1 and 14.2)

- RBCs are biconcave, disc like cells with a diameter of 7.5 m and thickness of 2 m. This shape allows them to easily fold upon themselves and pass through capillaries. The surface area of these cells is also increased to allow proper exchange of gases.

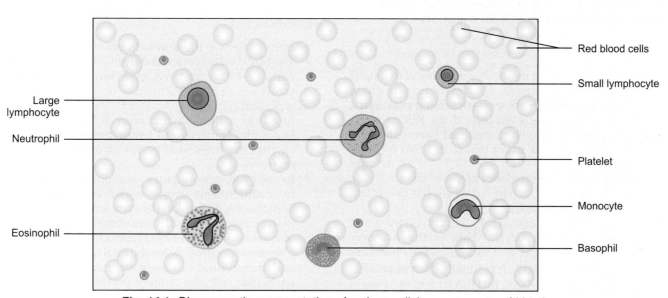

Fig. 14.1: Diagrammatic representation of various cellular components of blood

Large lymphocyte
Neutrophil
Eosinophil
Red blood cells
Small lymphocyte
Platelet
Monocyte
Basophil

Fig. 14.2: Erythrocyte (RBC)

- Mature RBCs do not have nucleus and lack important organelles like mitochondria. RBCs mainly contain haemoglobin. They depend entirely on glucose metabolism for energy supply.
- Total RBC count in blood varies from 4.0 to 6.5 million/ml.
- The old RBCs are removed from circulation by tissue macrophage system of spleen and liver. Life span of RBCs in blood is 120 days.
- The primary function of RBCs is transport of O_2 which is bound to hemoglobin.

Erythrocyte Sedimentation Rate (ESR)

When blood is collected in a tube with anticoagulant and allowed to stand upright, it gets separated into two layers. The RBCs pile on each other forming aggregates (known as rouleaux formation). The aggregates settle down leaving a clear pinkish layer on top. ESR is defined as the rate of settling down of RBCs at the end of one hour and is expressed in millimeters. ESR is higher in females especially during pregnancy. It is increased in anaemia, acute infections, chronic conditions like tuberculosis, arthiritis and malignancies.

Packed Cell Volume (PCV)

It is also known as the haematocrit. It is the percentage of cellular component of blood which include WBCs, RBCs and platelets. As mentioned it is normally 45%. Practically, PCV denotes RBC content of blood as these cells are the most predominant of the cellular component.

Haemoglobin (Hb)

- It is a large protein molecule consisting of two pairs of polypeptide chains. Each polypeptide chain forms a complex with iron containing porphyrin, haeme. This imparts red color to the RBCs.
- The adult haemoglobin is named haemoglobin A (Hb A). It is made up of two α and two β chains $(\alpha_2\beta_2)$.
- Other types of hemoglobin are:
  a. Haemoglobin A_2 (Hb A_2) which has two α and two δ chains $(\alpha_2\delta_2)$.
  b. Fetal haemoglobin (HbF) which has two α and two γ chains $(\alpha_2\gamma_2)$. This is the primary haemoglobin present in fetus which has very high affinity for O_2. It gradually disappears after birth and is replaced by HbA by end of 1 year of life.

- Each haeme moiety has one Fe^{2+} ion (ferrous form of iron) and each Fe^{2+} binds to one molecule of O_2. Hence, each molecule of Hb carries 4 molecules of O_2.
- Hb binds to O_2 to form oxyhaemoglobin. When O_2 is removed from Hb it is termed deoxygenated Hb. O_2 dissociates from Hb in tissues due to fall in pH and rise in temperature which happens secondarily to cellular metabolism. Lack of O_2 also releases O_2 into tissues from Hb. The O_2-Hb dissociation curve is described on page 384, 385. The deoxygenated Hb is transported via circulation to the lungs where it combines with O_2 again as the levels of O_2 are high there.
- Hb also binds to CO_2 in blood to form carbamino-Hb.
- Normal levels of hemoglobin :

In Newborn	20 to 22 gm%
In Infants	10.5 to 12.5 gm%
In Adult males	14 to 16 gm%
In Adult females	12 to 14 gm%

- Synthesis hemoglobin requires adequate protein and iron in diet. Copper and vitamin C in diet are essential to promote iron absorption.
- Hemoglobin is released from RBCs when they are destroyed by tissue macrophage system and protein part is re-utilized. Iron is also re-utilized or stored as tissue ferritin. Haeme is metabolized to biliverdin that is converted to bilrubin in liver. Bilirubin is excreted in bile and urine and imparts yellow color to stool and urine.

Functions of Hb

- It primarily transports O_2. It also transports little CO_2.
- It provides for 70% of buffering capacity of blood (binds to H^+ ions).

HEMOPOIESIS

- Hemopoiesis is the development of cells of blood.
- The blood cells are derived from pleuripotent stem cells of bone marrow also known as hemocytoblasts. Active bone marrow or red bone marrow is present in marrow cavities of all bones in children. In adults active bone marrow is limited to long bones like humerus and femur, the rest of marrow cavities get infiltrated by fat forming the yellow marrow.
- In fetal life, upto infancy, hemopoeisis occurs in liver and spleen. This is called extra-medullary hemopoesis. In adults it is seen only in conditions that are associated with destruction or replacement of bone marrow like blood cancer or myelofibrosis.
- The stem cells provide for the pool of precursor cells and differentiate to form progenitor cells of a particular cell line namely erythroid, lymphoid, granulocyte or megakaryocyte progenitor cells.

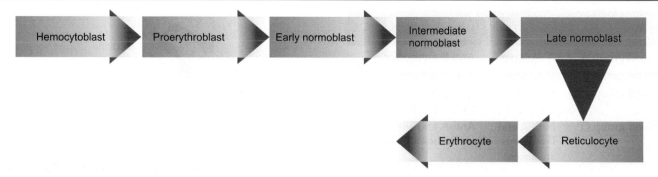

Erythropoiesis

- It is the orderly development of mature RBCs from stem cells. The steps are shown above.
- The proerythroblast is the earliest appearing differentiated cell of erythroid series.
- As the cell matures there is reduction in cell size, due to decrease in cytoplasm and nuclear size. The decrease in nucleus is associated with decrease in RNA and ribosomal content of cell making it more acidophilic from the initial basophilic staining.
- Hemoglobin appears in the intermediate normoblasts. In final stages (late normoblast) there is condensation and degeneration of nucleus. the nucleus is seen as a small dot, which is known as pyknotic nucleus. The nucleus finally degenerates. Reticulocytes contain fragments of RNA and no definite nuclear material. Mature RBCs have eosinophilic cytoplasm since they do not have any DNA, RNA or cytoplasmic organelles.
- The mature RBCs or erythrocytes are released into circulation. Only 1% circulating RBCs are reticulocytes. Immature form of RBCs are not seen in circulation normally.

Regulation of Erythropoiesis

- The primary stimulus of erythropoiesis is hypoxia, lack of O_2 to tissues and low RBC levels (due to bleeding or destruction of RBCs).
- Hypoxia stimulates secretion of erythropoietin hormone from kidney which stimulates production of proerythroblasts in the marrow. Thus, the total number of circulating RBCs are maintained within a narrow range by this feedback mechanism.
- Increase RBC synthesis occurs at high altitudes due to low O_2 levels in air. Other factors controlling erythropoietin production are hormones like thyroxine, androgens, TSH, GH which increase its levels. It is also stimulated by catecholamines and adenosine.
- Chronic liver diseases, kidney diseases and other conditions leading to hypoproteinemia decrease production of erythropoietin and are associated with anemia.
- Other factors necessary for RBC synthesis:
  - **Protein:** Protein is needed for synthesis of globin chains of hemoglobin.
  - **Trace elements:** Trace elements are minerals that are required in trace amounts for the normal functioning of body. **Iron** is needed for synthesis of haeme moiety of haemoglobin. Other trace elements like copper, cobalt and manganese also help in heme formation.
  - **Vitamins:** Vitamin B_{12} and folic acid are required for synthesis of DNA of dividing cells. Vitamin C is required for iron absorption and synthesis of nucleotides (important cofactor for haemoglobin synthesis).

Haemolysis

- Breakdown or destruction of RBCs is called haemolysis.
- Under normal conditions life span of RBCs is 120 days after which they are destroyed by phagocytic tissue macrophage system of spleen, liver and bone marrow.

Blood Groups

- The cell membrane of RBCs have a specific oligosaccharide-lipid complex which are known as blood group antigens. The expression of the antigen is genetically determined. There are primarily two types of antigens which have been named, type A and type B.
- Circulating plasma contains antibodies against these RBC antigens. It is seen that in individuals with type A blood antigen, anti-B antibodies are present and vice versa.
- Four blood types are identified according to antigens present. These are:

Blood group type	Type of surface antigen	Type of circulating antibodies
Blood group A	A Antigen	Anti-B antibodies
Blood group B	B Antigen	Anti A antibodies
Blood group AB	A and B	No antibodies to antigens either A or B
Blood group O	Both A and B antigens are absent	Anti-A and anti-B antibodies are present

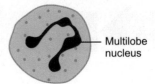

Fig. 14.3: Neutrophil

- If blood of one individual is transfused to another individual having a different blood group from the donor, immediate antigen antibody reaction takes place due to presence of antibodies in circulation. There is destruction of donor RBCs. This is called **transfusion reaction.** The reaction can vary from mild skin eruptions to severe anaphylactic shock and death.
- Other minor blood group antigens have also been identified now. These are Rh, MNS, Lutheran, Kell, Kidd etc. Out of which Rh antigen is of greatest clinical importance after A and B types.
- Rh-group of antigens is named after the rhesus monkey in which it was first studied. It consists of C, D and E antigens which are also present on the red cell membrane. D antigen is the most important component. Rh positive individuals have D antigen on their RBCs while Rh negative individuals do not have D antigen. Exposure of Rh negative individuals to Rh positive blood results in production of anti-D antibodies. The Rh antibodies (IgG) can cross placenta.

WHITE BLOOD CELLS (WBCs)/LEUCOCYTES

- The white blood cells are responsible in providing defense against infections like viral or bacterial, worm infestations and provide immunity even against tumors.
- WBCs are larger, rounded nucleated cells with a diameter of 10 to 14 μm.
- The normal WBC count in blood is 4000 to 11000 per ml of blood.
- They are broadly grouped into two types:
  1. Granulocytes: These cells have cytoplasmic granules which contain vesicle bound bio-logically active substances in them. They are further of three types
     a. Neutrophils
     b. Eosinophils
     c. Basophils
  2. Agranulocytes: They are of two types
     a. Lymphocytes
     b. Monocytes

Neutrophils

They form 50 to 70% of toal WBC population. They have a multilobed nucleus. Cytoplasm has neutrophilic cytoplasm, granules take up both acid and basic stains on staining. Neutrophils are mainly responsible for phagocytosis and destruction of microbes (Fig. 14.3).

The following steps in neutrophil action are seen:
- Invasion by microbes, mainly bacteria, leads to production of an inflammatory response by plasma which releases chemotaxins. Chemotaxins are substances that attract leukocytes to the infected area. They consist of leukotrines, complement system factors and other proteins from plasma.
- Neutrophils are mobile cells. They attach to the endothelial surface and pass through them into the tissues by a process called **diapedesis.**
- The movement of neutrophils towards infected site is called **chemotaxis** and they form clumps at that site.
- The bacteria are engulfed by neutrophils by endocytosis and are presented to the intracellular lysosomes and peroxisomes that hydrolyse the contents of endosomes. This is called **phagocytosis.**

Neutrophilia: Increased neutrophil count is seen in:
- Acute bacterial infections.
- Tissue injury due to burns, surgery etc.
- Leukemia (blood cancer).
- Miscellaneous causes like smoking, acute inflammation like gout, arthritis.
- In normal conditions like after exercise, later half of menstruation, pregnancy.

Neutropenia: Low neutrophil count is seen in
- Infants: Neutophils form 30 to 40% of toal WBCs
- Typhoid fever
- Viral fever
- Suppression of bone marrow.

Eosinophils

They form 1 to 6% of total WBC count. They have a bilobed nucleus which stains with acidophilic dyes, appear pink with esosin stain. They are less motile and hence less phagocytic. They also undergo diapedesis and

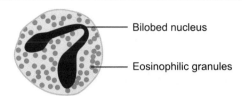

Fig. 14.4: Eosinophil

chemotaxis. They are mostly involved in providing mucosal immunity as are maximally present in respiratory, gastrointestinal and urinary tracts. (Fig. 14.4).

Eosinophilia: Eosinophil count is increased in allergic conditions like asthma, worm infestations and allergic skin conditions.

Eosionopenia: Eosionophil count is suppressed by use of corticosteroids.

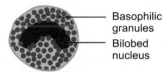

Fig. 14.5: Basophil

Basophils

They are < 1% of total circulating WBC. They also have a bilobed nucleus with cytoplasm which is granular but the granules take up basic stains. They appear bluish with hematoxylin stain. They have mild phagocytic activity. The granules contain histamine and heparin which are responsible for acute allergic (hypersensitivity) reactions and anticoagulation of blood respectively (Fig. 14.5).

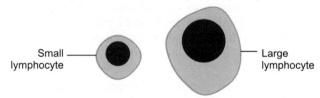

Fig. 14.6: Lymphocytes

Lymphocytes

They form 20 to 40% of circulating WBCs. They are primarily part of lymphatic system and are present in large number in lymph nodes, spleen and thymus. They

are further of two types T-lymphocytes and B-lymphocytes and are responsible in providing the acquired immunity (Fig. 14.6).

Lymphocytosis: Increase in lymphocytes is seen in:
- Chronic infections like tuberculosis
- Viral infections
- Leukemia
- Normally in children lymphocytes are 60% and form most of circulating WBC.

Lymphopenia: Low counts of lymphocytes are seen in immunosupressed patients, either taking steroids or suffering from AIDS.

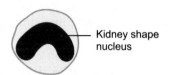

Fig. 14.7: Monocyte

Monocytes

They form 1 to 8% of total circulating WBCs. These are relatively larger cells with irregular shape. They have a single kidney shaped nucleus. They enter circulation form bone marrow and remain there for 72 hours after which they enter tissues and become tissue macrophages. Examples of tissue macrophages are Kupffer cells in liver, pulmonary alveolar macrophages, microglia in brain. They have the same phagocytic action as neutrophils and appear at the site of infection after neutrophils providing for long term defence. They also secrete more than 100 substances that are responsible for inflammatory responses, reparative responses, anti-tumorigenic responses and immunological responses (Fig. 14.7).

Leucopoiesis

It is the orderly development and formation of WBCs from pleuripotent stem cells of bone marrow. There is a slight difference in synthesis of granular WBCs versus agranulocytes as shown below.

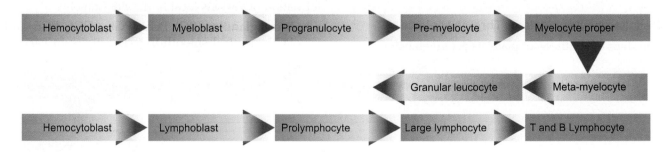

- Lymphoblasts and myeloblasts are the first identifiable precursors of WBC series. As the cell matures the cell size reduces, cytoplasm becomes granular and nucleus takes its characteristics appearance.
- The final maturation of lymphocytes to T-lymphocytes occurs in thymus and to B-lymphocytes occurs in bone marrow.

Factors Regulating Leucopoiesis

Leucopoesis is regulated by colony stimulating factors produced by monocytes, fibroblasts and endothelium. Interleukin produced by T-lymphocytes also stimulate leucopoesis. These factors stimulate mitosis of stem cells committed to leucocytes and also release of mature leucocytes from bone marrow into circulation.

PLATELETS

Platelets are small, 2 to 4 µ in diameter, rounded, granulated cells. The normal circulating platelet levels range from 1.5 to 4 lacs per ml of blood. Platelets have a half life of 4 days.

Characteristics features of platelets are:

- The cell membrane shows extensive invaginations creating a fine system of canals with ECF in them.
- The cell membrane has specific receptors for Von Willie brand factor, collagen and fibrinogen.
- Phospholipids of cell membrane produce arachidonic acid which is a precursor for prostaglandins and thromboxane.
- Cytoplasm shows characteristic arrangement of microtubules in periphery responsible for invagination of cell membrane.
- Cytoplasm has contractile filaments namely, actin and myosin. It also has endoplasmic reticulum, golgi apparatus and mitochondria which stores Ca^{2+} ions and provides ATP.
- Two types of cytoplasmic granules are present:
  — Dense granules which contain non protein substances like serotonin, ADP, ATP etc.
  — α-granules which contain proteins namely the clotting factors, and platelet derived growth factor (PDGF). PDGF promotes wound healing by stimulating mitosis of vascular smooth muscle cells.

Megakaryocytopoiesis or Thrombopoiesis

The steps of synthesis of platelets are given below.

Megakaryocytes are giant multinucleated cells and each megakaryocyte gives rise to 3000 to 4000 platelets by pinching off bits of cytoplasm.

Regulation of Platelet Synthesis

Synthesis of platelets is controlled by colony stimulating factors and a circulating plasma protein named thrombopoietin. Low levels of platelet stimulate these factors which increases megakaryocytosis.

Functions of Platelets

The primary function of platelets is **haemostasis.** Platelets help in arresting the bleeding from an injured vessel by stimulating vasoconstriction, forming a haemostatic plug and stimulating the intrinsic clotting pathway. This is brought about by:

- An injury to vessel wall exposes underlying collagen and Von Willie brand factor. Platelets adhere to these by their receptors. Platelet adhesion does not require energy. Collagen, Ca^{2+} and thrombin aid in adhesion.
- Platelet adhesion leads to platelet activation which is characterized by:
  — Change in shape, formation of pseudopodia
  — Platelet aggregation
  — Degranulation: Release of contents of granules
  This process utilizes energy in form of ATP.
- Platelet activation factor is produced by neutrophils and monocytes during injury and this further stimulates platelet aggregation.
- Aggregation and agglutination of the platelets forms a temporary hemostatic plug.
- The net effect of the above reactions also stimulates release of arachidonic acid from cell membrane of platelets.
- Platelet also stimulate the intrinsic pathway of clotting mechanism that leads to formation of definitive fibrin clot.
- The platelets are responsible for clot retraction by function of their contractile proteins.

Arachidonic acid It is a polyunsaturated fatty acid which on release from cell membrane acts as a precursor to formation of various local hormones namely:

1. **Prostaglandins (PG):** PGE_2, $PGF_{2\alpha}$, PGI_2. PGE_2 and $PGF_{2\alpha}$ control smooth muscle activity in various

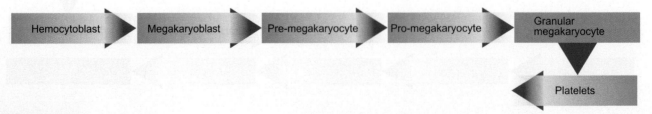

organs. PGI$_2$ or prostacyclin inhibits platelet aggregation and is a local vasodilator.

2. **Thromboxanes:** Thromboxane A$_2$ is the classic thromboxane. It is produced from platelets and stimulates platelet aggregation.

3. **Leukotrienes:** They are mediators of allergic and inflammatory responses.

Hormones and synthetic steroid preparations inhibit release of arachidonic acid thus limiting an inflammatory response.

PLASMA

Plasma is the acellular fluid part of blood, which constitutes 55% of blood volume and 5% of total body weight. It contains 90% water. The rest is made up of inorganic molecules like Na$^+$, Ca^{2+}, HCO$_3^-$, K$^+$, PO$_3^{3-}$, Fe^{2+} etc. and organic molecules like plasma proteins and other non protein nitrogenous substances, sugars, fats, enzymes and hormones.

Serum is the fluid remaining after the blood clots. It is similar to plasma but does not have clotting factors especially fibrinogen, factor II, V and VIII.

Plasma Proteins

Normal plasma proteins values are 6.5 to 8.0 gm%. They are primarily of three types namely:

1. **Albumin:** It forms 55% of total plasma proteins. It is synthesized in liver. The two primary functions of albumin are
   a. It acts as a carrier protein for various hormones, aminoacids, ions, drugs etc.
   b. It helps to maintain the plasma oncotic pressure.
2. **Globulin:** It is produced by liver, plasma cells, lymphocytes and tissue macrophages. It forms a part of plasma lipoprotein complexes that helps in transport of fatty acids, triglycerides and cholesterol. Derivates like transferrin and ceruloplasmin are involved in transport and storage of iron and copper ions respectively. Immunoglobulins are derivatives of γ-globulin fraction of plasma protein. Albumin to globulin ratio in blood is usually 1.5 to 1.7 : 1.
3. **Fibrinogen:** It is synthesized in liver and is responsible for clotting of blood.

Functions of Plasma Proteins

1. Maintainance of intravascular colloidal oncotic pressure.
2. Act as carriers for various substances for their storage and action at appropriate sites.
3. Regulate clotting of blood.
4. **Act as an accessory blood buffer:** Plasma proteins provide for 20% of buffering capacity of blood to maintain acid-base balance.

5. **Immunological function:** γ-globulin fraction of plasma proteins gives rise to antibodies.

CLOTTING OF BLOOD

The process of formation of clot to arrest bleeding from an injured vessel is hemostasis. It is brought about by the following mechanisms:

1. Constriction of injured blood vessels
2. Platelets aggregation (see text)
3. Clotting of blood

Clotting Factors

These are soluble protein molecules present in the plasma. These are 13 clotting factors named from factor I to factor XIII.

Clotting Mechanism

It is the process of formation of insoluble fibrin from the soluble plasma protein fibrinogen. Fibrin consists of polypeptide strands that get associated with each other to form a mesh like structure, the definitive clot (Fig. 6.2).

Fibrinogen is a soluble plasma protein (factor I). It is converted to fibrin by the action of thrombin (activated factor II). Thrombin is derived from prothrombin by the action of prothrombin activator. The activator is formed by a series of reactions that result in formation of active factor X (Xa). There are two pathways by which activation of factor X takes place.

Anticlotting Mechanism in Blood

The blood does not clot unless there is injury to vessels. Also the clotting tendency after injury is regulated to limit the process to the affected site only. This is brought about by (Fig. 14.8):

1. **Antithrombin III:** It is a protease inhibitor present in blood that blocks the proteases that activate clotting factors.
2. **Thrombomodulin:** It is a thrombin binding protein produced by endothelial cells. The thrombin binds to thrombomodulin and activates protein-C which functions as anticoagulant by inhibiting factor V and VIII.
3. **Fibrinolytic mechanism: Plasminogen-plasmin system:** Plasminogen is an inactive protein produced by liver and circulating in the plasma. It gets activated by thrombin and tissue plasminogen activator released by damaged tissues and gets converted to the active enzyme, plasmin. Plasmin is responsible for degradation of fibrin and fibrinogen.

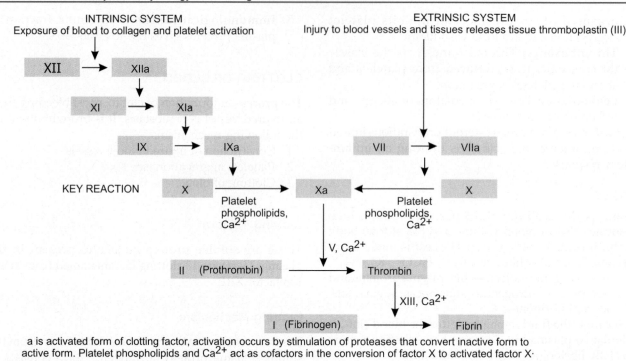

a is activated form of clotting factor, activation occurs by stimulation of proteases that convert inactive form to active form. Platelet phospholipids and Ca^{2+} act as cofactors in the conversion of factor X to activated factor X.

Fig. 14.8: Diagrammatic representation of mechanisms of clotting

CLINICAL AND APPLIED ASPECTS

ANEMIA

Anemia is defined as the decrease in circulating levels of RBCs below 4 million per ml or decrease in Hb below 12 gm%.

Etiology of anemia: Anemia can occur due to any one of the following causes:

- **Impaired production of RBCs/ haemoglobin**
  1. Deficiency of nutritional factors: Iron deficiency, vitamin B_{12} and folic acid deficiency.
  2. Destruction or depressed function of bone marrow due to tumors like leukemia, fibrosis, drugs like anti-cancer drugs, antibiotics like sulphonamides, radiation exposure and viral diseases.

  Hypoplastic anemia: In this condition bone marrow function is reduced.

  Aplastic anemia: In this condition bone marrow function is absent.

- **Increase destruction of RBCs—Haemolytic anemias:** These are seen in following conditions:
  1. **Congenital causes—Due to:**
     a. Haemoglobinopathies, e.g., sickle cell anemia.
     b. Altered cell structure, e.g., spherocytosis. This is characterized by cytoskeletal defects in cells leading to spherical shape of cells. These cells do not compress easily and are destroyed by spleen and liver.
     c. Hemolytic disease of newborn: Due to transfer of antibodies from mother to fetus which destroy fetal cells.

  2. **Acquired causes:** Due to damage to RBCs by:
     a. Antibodies to RBCs as seen in autoimmune diseases.
     b. Mismatched blood transfusion.
     c. Infections like malaria.
     d. Drugs like aspirin, quinine.
     e. Enlarged spleen.
     f. Damage by artificial heart valves, kidney dialysis machines.

- **Loss of blood:** This can be acute or chronic due to:
  1. Injury
  2. Worm infestation–Hook worm
  3. Diseases of GIT like ulcer, piles
  4. Excess menstruation (in females)

Iron Deficiency Anemia

This is the most common form of anemia in India. The normal requirement of iron is 1 to 2 mg, in females the requirement is upto 3 mg to replace iron loss in menstruation. Etiology of iron deficiency anemia:
  1. Deficient diet
  2. Increase demand: Pregnancy, excess menstruation
  3. Defective absorption: Diseases of stomach associated with loss of acid secretion, diseases or surgery of duodenum.
  4. Loss of blood: Acute or chronic hemorrhage.

Clinical features: These occur mainly due to deficiency in O_2 carrying capacity of blood.
  1. Easy fatigue
  2. Breathlessness (dyspnea) on exertion
  3. Palpitations on exertion
  4. Generalized weakness

5. Loss of concentration, irritability
6. In severe cases it leads to congestive heart failure which is associated with generalized edema
7. Associated changes: Dry and brittle nails, hair loss.

Changes in Blood Picture
- Hb and RBC are low
- RBCs show following changes:
  a. **Microcytosis:** Decrease in size of RBCs
  b. **Hypochromia:** Decrease in staining of RBCs (due to low haemoglobin)
  c. Alteration of size of RBCs **(anisocytosis)** and shape of RBCs **(poikilocytosis).**
- White blood cell count and platelet is normal, except in anemias caused by bone marrow depression.
- Serum iron and ferritin levels are low but total iron binding capacity is high.

Bone marrow changes: Erythpoesis is stimulated and there is normobastic hyperplasia of bone marrow.

Management
1. Improve diet: Encourage intake of green leafy vegetables, fruits. Avoid excess tea and coffee (these interfere in iron absorption).
2. Iron therapy: Iron tablets are administered and response is noted by improvement in Hb levels.

Folic Acid Deficiency Anemia

Folic acid helps in DNA synthesis for cell division and in maturation of erythrocyte series in bone marrow. It is normally stored in liver, RBCs and WBCs. Daily requirement is 100 to 200mgm (increases to 400 to 500 mgm in pregnancy).

Dietary sources: Folate is available in sufficient quantities in all green vegetables and liver.

Causes of deficiency of folic acid
1. Dietary causes: Overcooking of vegetables leads to destruction of folic acid due to heat.
2. Alcohol intake increases the requirement for folic acid.
3. Increase demand: In infancy, pregnancy.
4. Malabsorption diseases of small intestine like celiac disease.
5. Drugs which interfere in folic acid uptake – anticonvulsant drugs, anticancer drugs.

Clinical features are similar to anemia. In addition there is inflammation of tongue, glossitis.

Changes in Blood Picture
- Hemoglobin and RBCs levels are low.
- RBCs show a characteristic increase in size, they are macrocytic but staining is normal (normochromic).
- Abnormal cell maturation leads to presence of increase number of nucleated RBCs in circulation, reticulocytes count may increase to 5%.
- Altered shape of RBCs leads to decrease life span and increase in destruction which is seen as increase serum iron levels and irregular shaped RBCs.
- WBCs and platelet count is normal though the size of platelets is increased (megakaryocytosis).

Bone marrow changes: Erythropoesis is stimulated but the normoblasts increase in size and form **megaloblasts**, hence it is also called **megaloblastic anemia.** This increase in size is due to delayed maturation of cells due to defective DNA synthesis.

Management
1. **Dietary changes:** Improve intake of fresh fruit and vegetables.
2. Folic acid tablets can be given.

Vitamin B$_{12}$ Deficiency Anemia

This is another form of megaloblastic anemia since vitamin B$_{12}$ is required for nucleic acid synthesis and cell maturation. The clinical features and blood picture is similar to folic acid deficiency. Additional features are presence of neurological deficits called subacute combined degeneration of spinal cord as vitamin B$_{12}$ is required for normal myelination of neurons. Vitamin B$_{12}$ deficiency usually occurs due to defect in absorption. Hence, treatment is usually by giving injections of vitamin B$_{12}$.

HEMOGLOBIN (Hb)
- Hb binds to carbon monoxide (CO) to form **carboxyhaemoglobin.** Hb has high affinity for CO and O$_2$ gets displaced. CO poisoning leads to reduction in O$_2$ carrying capacity of blood and causes severe hypoxia.
- **Abnormal hemoglobin synthesis:** These are genetic disorders that result in faulty protein synthesis. There are primarily two types of disorders of hemoglobin synthesis namely:
  a. **Hemoglobinopathies:** In this the polypeptide chains are abnormal. Examples are:
  — Sickle cell anemia: In this condition there is mutation in gene coding for b chains leading to formation of abnormal β chains. Hemoglobin is named HbS. In presence of low O$_2$ tension the HbS polymerizes and alters shape of RBCs leading to increased destruction of RBC. The abnormal RBCs also clump together and block small blood vessels causing pain in areas where the blood supply gets blocked.
  — Other abnormal Hb described are HbC, HbE, HbJ etc.
  b. **Thalassemias:** In these conditions the polypeptide chains are normal but are either produced in very low number or not produced at all. According to the polypeptide chain affected they are named α-thalassemias or β-thalassemias. These conditions are associated with high levels of Hb A$_2$ or persistence of Hb F in circulation.

JAUNDICE
It is the clinical condition which is associated with excess circulating levels of bilirubin in blood leading to yellow discoloration of eyes and skin.

Bilirubin metabolism: Bilirubin is produced when the red blood cells are destroyed. The haemoglobin of RBCs splits into globin and haeme. Haeme is converted to biliverdin which is further converted to bilirubin in the tissue macrophage system. Bilirubin is takenup by the liver from circulation and conjugated with glucoronides. The conjugated bilirubin is secreted by hepatocytes into bile which passes into the intestine. Action of intestinal bacteria converts it into urobilinogen. This is partly reabsorbed and partly excreted in faeces. The bilirubin levels in circulation are only 0.2 to 1 mg% (circulating bilirubin is conjugated bilirubin with small quantity of unconjugated bilirubin and urobilinogen). Any excess is secreted into urine and in stools. Clinically, jaundice is visible when plasma bilirubin levels are above 2 gm%.

Causes of Jaundice

- **Damage to liver:** This leads to destruction of hepatocytes and release of bilirubin into circulation. Hepatitis or inflamation of liver can occur due to viral infections or due to liver toxins like alcohol.
- **Excess formation of bilirubin:** Due to excess breakdown of RBCs **(haemolytic jaundice)**. This is seen in hemolytic anemias.
- Obstruction of secretion of bile due to liver disease or gall bladder stone.

POLYCYTHEMIA

This is a condition associated with increase levels of RBCs in blood. This leads to increase viscosity of blood which favours stasis and clotting of blood.

Etiology of Polycythemia

- **Physiological:** This is seen in patients living at high altitudes due to chronic exposure to low O_2 levels.
- **Pathological:** Usually it is secondary to tumors of bone marrow and can be idiopathic (whose cause is unknown).

ERYTHROBLASTOSIS FETALIS

Haemolytic disease of the new born (erythroblastosis fetalis). This condition occurs when an Rh negative mother is carrying an Rh positive baby. At the time of delivery small amount of fetal blood passes into the maternal circulation and induces production of anti-D antibodies. In subsequent pregnancies these anti-D antibodies cross the placenta and destroy the RBCs of the second Rh positive baby. This leads to haemolysis and jaundice in the baby.

PLATELET DISORDERS

- **Thrombocytopenia:** It is the decrease in platelet count and occurs due to:
  — Bone marrow depression
  — Increase destruction of platelets due to
   a. Viral infections like dengue
   b. Drug reactions
   c. Increase splenic activity as seen in spleno-megaly.
   d. **Idiopathic:** In which the cause of platelet destruction is not known. It may be due to autoimmune lysis of cells.

Clinical features: Thrombocytopenia is characterised by pin point subcutaneous haemorrhages known as purpura. There is deficient clot retraction and constriction of vessels after an injury. It can be treated by giving platelet transfusions or removing the spleen (spleenectomy).

- **Thrombocytosis:** It is a condition characterised by increase platelets levels of more than $5,00,000/mm^3$ of blood. It is often seen after removal of spleen or (spleenectomy), or as a response to stress.

CLOTTING OF BLOOD

- **Anticoagulants:** These are substances that inhibit clotting of blood by various mechanisms. Drugs and their action are shown below.
  a. **Heparin:** Stimulates antithrombin III, antithrombin III is a circulating protease inhibitor that prevents activation of factors IX, X, XI and XII.
  b. **Warfarin and dicoumarol:** These act by blocking action of vitamin K. Vitamin K helps in the synthesis of clotting factors in liver.
  c. **Ca^{2+} chelators:** In vitro, addition of salts like EDTA (ethylene diamino tetra acetic acid) to blood prevents blood clotting. This is because EDTA binds to Ca^{2+} in blood. Ca^{2+} is an important cofactor in activation of factor X and conversion of fibrinogen to fibrin.
- **Disorders of coagulation:** These are characterised by defective coagulation due to deficiency of one or more clotting factors in the plasma. They are mostly congenital due to genetic defects. Common causes of acquired coagulation defects are vitamin K deficiency and liver diseases.
  Hemophilia A: It is the most common clinical condition of deficiency of clotting factors. It is caused by deficiency of clotting factor VIII. This is an X-linked genetic defect and hence manifests only in males while females are carriers. It is characterised by spontaneous bleeding tendencies. It is associated with prolonged coagulation time.
- **Thrombosis:** It is a clinical condition characterized by clotting of blood within intact blood vessels. The important causes are:
  a. **Stasis or stagnant blood flow:** This is an important cause of venous thrombosis of lower limb in patients with obesity, prolonged immobilization.
  b. Damage to vascular endothelium that trigger clotting cascade. This is the most important cause of thrombosis in arteries due to hypertension, deposition of cholesterol plaques especially in coronary and cerebral arteries.
  c. **Increase coagulability of blood:** This usually occurs in condition associated with deficiency of coagulation inhibition.
  Emboli: These are small pieces of clotted blood that get detached from main thrombus and enter circulation. Thrombus and emboli block the blood vessel and cut off the blood supply to the region causing ischemia.

Chapter 15

Lymphatic System

INTRODUCTION

Lymphatic system is a closed system of vessels which draws the extra tissue fluid into the blood vascular system (Fig. 15.1).

Components of Lymphatic System

1. Lymph and lymph vessels
   a. Lymph
   b. Lymph capillaries

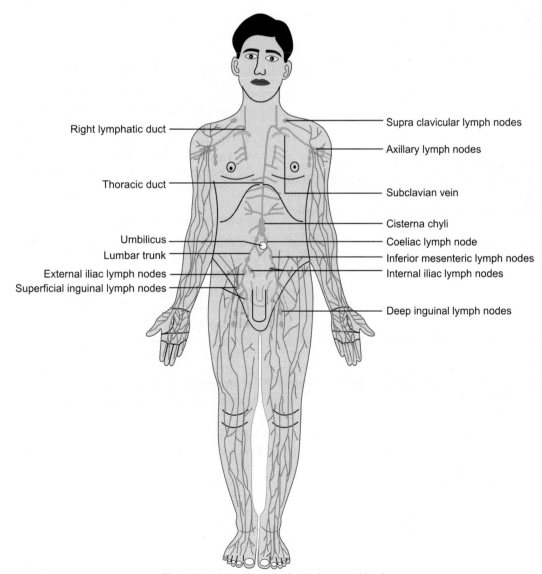

Right lymphatic duct

Thoracic duct

Umbilicus
Lumbar trunk
External iliac lymph nodes
Superficial inguinal lymph nodes

Supra clavicular lymph nodes

Axillary lymph nodes

Subclavian vein

Cisterna chyli
Coeliac lymph node
Inferior mesenteric lymph nodes
Internal iliac lymph nodes

Deep inguinal lymph nodes

Fig. 15.1: Main lymphatic drainage of body

    c. Lymph vessels proper
    d. Terminal lymph ducts (trunks)
  2. Lymphoid tissue
    a. Primary lymphatic follicles
    b. Lymph nodes
    c. Haemolymph nodes
    d. Thymus
    e. Bone marrow

Functions of Lymph and Lymphatic System

- It helps to maintain interstitial tissue pressure
- Lymph carries protein molecules, electrolytes and other macromolecules back from interstitial fluid to circulation.
- It helps to transport lymphocytes, red blood cells, antigens and antigen presenting cells to the secondary lymphoid organs.
- Lymph nodes and spleen help to destroy any foreign particles and microorganisms in circulation, thus guarding against them.
- The digested fats in small intestines are absorbed into the lymph vessels and carried to the liver and the circulation.
- It supplies oxygen and nutrients to selected parts of the body.

LYMPH

The tissue fluid which enters the lymphatic system is known as lymph. Protein concentration of lymph fluid is equal to tissue fluid but lower than the plasma. Lymph carries particulate material, colloids and macromolecules from tissue fluid. This helps to maintain the low protein concentration of tissue fluid. Lymph also clots on standing due to presence of clotting factors. Lymphocytes are the most abundant cellular component of the lymph.

LYMPH CAPILLARIES

These begin blindly in the extracellular spaces and communicate freely with adjacent lymph capillaries. Lymph capillaries are numerous in mucous membrane specially in the intestines, serous surfaces, dermis of skin and skeletal muscles.

Characteristics of Lymph Capillaries

  1. They are lined by single layer of endothelial cells which do not have any definite basal lamina. Pericytes and muscle layer are absent.
  2. Endothelial cells are not connected with tight junctions and the intercellular gaps allow free flow of fluid into the lumen of capillaries.
  3. They do not have any valves.
  4. Capillary wall is anchored to connective tissue. Hence the capillary lumen remains patent.

Places Where Lymph Capillaries are Absent

  1. Avascular structures like epidermis, cornea, cartilage
  2. Brain and spinal cord
  3. Splenic pulp
  4. Bone marrow
  5. Liver lobule
  6. Lung units
  7. Superficial fascia

LYMPH VESSELS PROPER

They are formed by the convergence of lymph capillaries.

Characteristics of Lymph Vessels

  1. They consists of single layer of endothelium surrounded by smooth muscle fibres and elastic tissue in their walls. Large trunks have three distinct layers, tunica intima, tunica media and tunica adventitia.
  2. Valves are present that give them a beaded appearance. This ensures that the lymph flows in one direction only.
  3. They accompany the blood vessels supplying the area and are more numerous than the vessels and form plexuses.
  4. The lymphatic vessels are connected to and traverse various lymph nodes in their path.
  5. Retrograde flow may take place if the vessels are obstructed.

TERMINAL LYMPH DUCTS

These are formed by convergence of lymph vessels.

Cisterna Chyli

It is a dilated, sac like structure present at level of L_1 vertebra and lies between the right and left crura of diaphragm, just behind the right side of aorta. It is formed by the confluence of various lymph trunks (vessels) namely (Fig. 15.1):
  a. Right and left lumbar lymph trunks
  b. Intestinal lymph trunks
It continues upwards as the thoracic duct.

Thoracic Duct (Figs 15.1, 15.2)

It is a common lymphatic trunk which begins at upper end of the confluence of lymphatics or the cysterna chyli, at the level of lower border of T_{12} vertebra. It enters thorax along with the aorta through aortic opening of diaphragm. It passes up in posterior mediastinum to right of midline between azygos vein and thoracic aorta, behind esophagus. Above the level of T_5 vertebra it shifts gradually to the left side of mid-line. It runs in the posterior part of superior mediastinum along the left margin of esophagus. It enters the neck and runs up 3 to 4 cm above the level of clavicle. Then it arches down behind the internal carotid artery and internal jugular vein and comes to lie infront of origin of subclavian artery. It ends by opening into the junction of subclavian vein and internal jugular vein. It may be duplicate or divide at its termination and end in internal jugular vein or brachiocephalic vein.

Features

Length   : 45 cm
Breadth   : 0.5 cm
Appearance : Beaded due to presence of numerous valves in its lumen.

Tributaries of Thoracic Duct: Thoracic duct drains the lymphatics from the entire body except, the right side of head and neck, right upper limb, right lung, right thoracic wall, right half of heart and the convex surface of liver (Fig. 15.2).

1. A pair of ascending lymph trunks: Each drains the upper lumbar lymph nodes.
2. A pair of descending lymph trunks: Each drains the posterior intercostal lymph nodes of right and left lower six intercostal spaces.
3. Vessels which drain posterior mediastinal lymph nodes.
4. Posterior intercostal lymph nodes of upper six intercostal spaces of the left side.
5. Left jugular lymph trunk.
6. Left subclavian lymph trunk.
7. Left broncho-mediastinal lymph trunk.

Right Lymph Duct

This is also a large terminal lymphatic trunk. It may be single, double or plexiform, formed by lymphatic vessels of right side of head and neck (right jugular trunk), right upper limb (right subclavian trunk), posterior intercostal lymph nodes of upper six intercostal spaces of right side, thorax and lung (right bronchial and broncho-media-stinal trunk) (Figs 15.1 and 15.2).

LYMPHOID TISSUE

The lymphoid tissues are part of tissue macrophage system (also known as reticulo-endothelial system) that plays an important role in immunological surveillance. They are formed by aggregation of lymphocytes, macrophages, plasma cells and dendritic cells arranged on a background framework of reticular fibers. They help to destroy bacteria, foreign bodies, old RBCs and WBCs. They also process foreign antigens and act as antigen presenting cells to the lymphocytes.

Tissue macrophages are scattered at the following sites in the body:

1. Kupffer cells of liver.
2. Reticulum cells of red and white pulp of spleen.

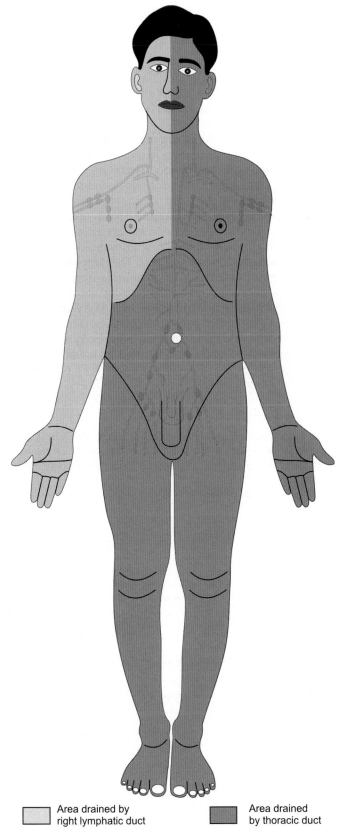

| | Area drained by right lymphatic duct | | Area drained by thoracic duct |

Fig. 15.2: Diagrammatic representation of area drained by thoracic duct and right lymphatic duct

CHAPTER-15

3. Lymph nodes.
4. Pulmonary alveolar macrophages.
5. Cells lining bone marrow.
6. Osteoclasts of bone.
7. Microglia of brain.
8. Dendritric or Langerhan's cells in skin.

The Lymphoid tissues can be grouped into two type of organs:

1. **Primary lymphoid organs:** These generate new lymphocyte population from stem cells which are released into circulation. There are two primary lymphoid organs in our body, bone marrow and thymus.
2. **Secondary lymphoid organs:** These contain mature B and T-lymphocytes with antigen presenting cells and hence help in initiating immunological response to an infection or trauma. The lymphocytes and antigen presenting cells originate from the stem cells of bone marrow and reach the organs via circulation. They enter the organs by migrating across blood or lymph-capillaries. The various secondary lymphoid organs in the body are lymph nodes, spleen and various mucosal lymph aggregates, e.g., Palatine tonsil, Peyer's patches in small intestine etc.

Lymph Nodes

These are small oval to bean shaped bodies that are present along the path of lymphatic vessels. There are about 800 lymph nodes present in human body. The nodes may be aggregated in groups or chains at certain areas like axilla, neck, around coeliac trunk etc.

Structure of Lymph Nodes

Grossly, they appear bean shaped with an indentation on one side, that is the hilum. Hilum is the site of entry and exit of blood vessels and efferent lymphatic vessels. A number of afferent vessels traverse through the periphery of lymph node. Each lymph node consists of a capsule and the gland substance (Fig. 15.3).

1. **Capsule:** A fibrous capsule invests the entire node and is separated from the gland substance by a subcapsular space known as **subcapsular sinus.** A number of connective tissue trabeculae extend radially into the substance of the node from the capsule dividing it into lobules.

2. **Gland substance:** It is made up of an outer cortex and an inner medulla. Cortex is cellular and consists of densely packed B lymphocytes with plasma cells, macrophages and dendritic cells arranged on a background of reticular fibres. The cells are arranged in the form of lymphatic follicles. Primary follicles consist of densely packed lymphocytes while secondary follicles have a lighter staining germinal center consisting of stimulated B lymphocytes and large plasma cells surrounded by a zone of densely packed lymphocytes. The inner cortex is madeup of a zone of T-lymphocytes and dendritic

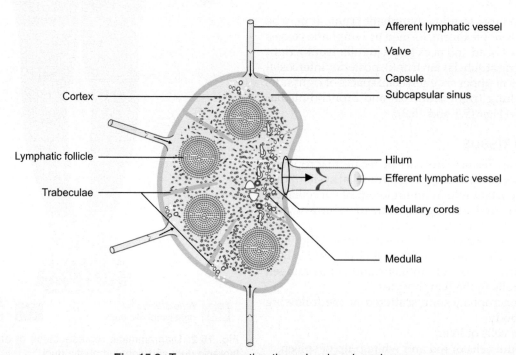

Fig. 15.3: Transverse section through a lymph node

cells. Medulla is madeup of irregular cords of lymphocytes known as medullary cords with intervening network of lymphatic channels or sinuses. Macrophages and plasma cells are present in medulla.

Functions of Lymph Nodes

1. They filter lymph and remove particulate matter and noxious agents.
2. They are made up of numerous lymphocytes which provide for the immune response of the body. Plasma cells produce antibodies and provide immunity against the antigens.

SPLEEN

It is the organ of reticuloendothelial system lying in the abdominal cavity. It is a haemo-lymph organ as it filters blood by taking out worn out RBCs, leucocytes, platelets and microbial antigens from circulation. Spleen lies in left hypochondrium, partly extending into epigastrium (Fig. 15.4).

Dimensions: It is 1 inch thick, 3 inches in breadth, 5 inches in length, and weighs 7 oz (150 gm). It extends from 9 to 11th rib. This is easy to remember with the help of Harris dictum – 1, 3, 5, 7, 9, 11.

Presenting Parts

It is oblong in form and presents with
1. **Anterior or lateral end:** It is expanded
2. **Posterior or medial end:** It is rounded and is directed backward and medially
3. **Inferior border:** It is rounded
4. **Superior border:** It is notched and indicates lobulated origin of spleen.
5. **Intermediate border:** It is rounded and directed to the right
6. **Diaphragmatic surface:** This surface is convex and smooth and is related to diaphragm,left lung and pleural sac with 9th, 10th and 11th ribs and respective intercostal spaces.

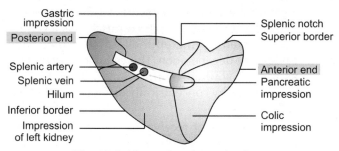

Fig. 15.4: Visceral surface of spleen

7. **Visceral surface:** It is irregular and presents with the following impressions (Fig. 15.4).
   a. **Gastric impression:** It is created by the fundus of stomach.
   b. **Renal impression:** It is due to left kidney.
   c. **Colic impression:** The splenic flexure of colon is related to spleen near the anterior end.
   d. **Pancreatic impression:** It lies between hilum and the colic impression, due to tail of the pancreas.
   e. **Hilum:** It is a cleft present along the long axis of spleen which transmits splenic vessels and nerves and also provides attachment to gastrosplenic and lienorenal ligaments.

Peritoneal Relations of Spleen

Spleen is covered by the peritoneum and is suspended by two ligaments namely:
1. **Lienorenal ligament:** It is a peritoneal fold which attaches the left kidney to the posterior lip of the hilum of the spleen. It is made up of 2 layers and contains splenic artery, splenic vein, nerves and lymphatics, tail of pancreas.
2. **Gastro-splenic ligament:** It extends from hilum of spleen to greater curvature of stomach. It contains short gastric vessels, nerves and lymphatics.
3. **Other ligaments related to spleen**
   — Phrenico-colic ligament
   — Phrenico-splenic ligament

Arterial Supply of Spleen

Splenic artery. It is a tortuous artery and is the largest branch of coeliac trunk.

Venous Drainage of Spleen

Splenic vein. It joins the superior mesentric vein to form portal vein.

Lymphatic Drainage of Spleen

Subcapsular and perivascular lymph drains into pancreatico-splenic lymph nodes. **Red pulp has no lymphatics.**

Nerve Supply of Spleen

Sympathetic fibres are derived from coeliac plexus. They are vasomotor.

Structure of Spleen (Fig. 15.5)

- It is the largest lymphoid organ of the body. It has an outermost serous layer derived from peritoneum.

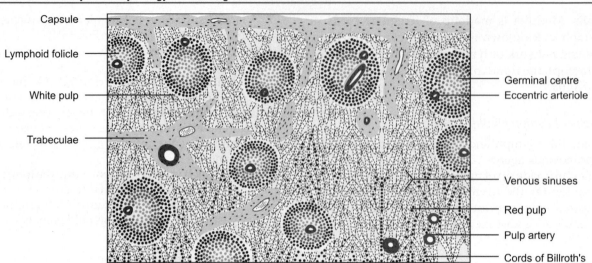

Capsule
Lymphoid folicle
White pulp
Trabeculae
Germinal centre
Eccentric arteriole
Venous sinuses
Red pulp
Pulp artery
Cords of Billroth's

Fig. 15.5: Microscopic appearance of transverse section of spleen

- Below the serous layer the spleen is enclosed by a fibrous capsule. The capsule gives rise to a number of connective tissue trabeculae into the substance of the spleen.
- Parenchyma of spleen contains two components namely, red pulp and while pulp. The red pulp provides for 75% of splenic volume and gives it the spongy texture while the white pulp is seen as specks scattered within the red pulp. Following features are seen on microscopy.
  — The red pulp is made up of a network of reticular fibres which enclose spaces containing blood derived from terminal pencil branches of splenic arterioles. The intervening area is made up of irregular cords of cells containing lymphocytes and macrophages these cords are known as **Bilroth's cords.** Numerous venous sinusoids are present within the red pulp which drain into splenic veins.
  — The white pulp is made up of collection of lymphocytes and plasma cells in the form of follicles which surround the small splenic arterioles. The arterioles are present eccentrically in the follicle.

Functions of Spleen

- It is a store house of T and B-lymphocytes and plays an important role in the immune response of the body.
- It contains numerous macrophages which are responsible for the removal of old RBCs, WBCs and platelets from the circulation.
- Spleen is the site of haemopoesis in fetal life.

THYMUS

It is a symmetrical bilobed structure present in the superior and anterior mediastinum. At birth, it is prominent and weighs about 10 to 15gm, it is about 20 gm at puberty. It rapidly diminishes after puberty (Fig. 15.6).

Structure of Thymus (Fig. 15.7)

- It is made up of two lobes. Each lobe is covered by a fibrous capsule. Fibrous septae extend inwards from the capsule into the substance of the gland and divide it into lobules.
- The framework of thymus is formed by epithelio-cytes instead of reticular fibres. This framework is packed with lymphocytes.
- Each lobule has an outer cortex and inner medulla.
- Cortex consists of numerous closely packed small thymocytes or thymic (T) lymphocytes and macro-phages, dendritic cells and epithelioid cells. Typical lymphatic follicles are not present in the thymus.
- Medulla contains loosely arranged lymphocytes and epithelioid cells. The epithelioid cells are larger than lymphocytes and contain vesicular nucleus. Characteristic feature of medulla is the presence of Hassall's corpuscles. Each corpuscle has a central core formed by the epithelioid cells that have undergone degeneration. This cellular debris is seen as a pink stained hyaline mass. This mass is surrounded by concentrically arranged epithelioid cells.
- Thymus does not receive any lymph vessels but gives off efferent lymph vessels which lie along the blood vessels supplying it.

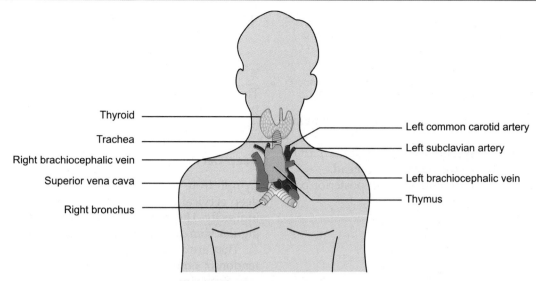

Fig. 15.6: Thymus and its relations

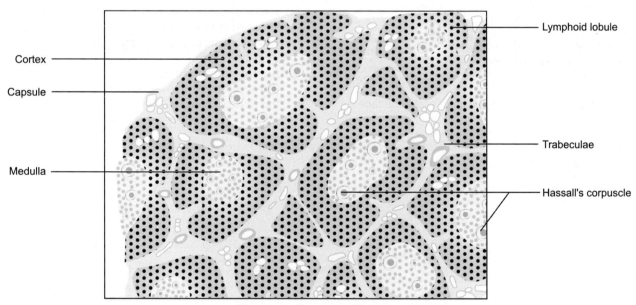

Fig. 15.7: Histology of Thymus

- After puberty the gland undergoes atrophy and the thymic tissue is replaced by adipose and aerolar tissue.

Functions of Thymus

- It is the central organ of lymphatic system, one of the primary lymphoid organ of our body.
- It is essential in the early weeks of neonatal life and regulates the functioning of peripheral lymphoid tissues.
- It provides the mature T-lymphocytes population of the body.

Mucosa Associated Lymphoid Tissue (MALT)

- These are aggregates of B and T-lymphocytes present under various mucosal surfaces.
- They are supported within a fine network of reticular fibres. However, they are not covered by capsule. They do not have afferent vessels but are drained by efferent lymphatic channels. Hence they do not filter lymph but provide local immunity.
- They are seen in the mucosal walls of intestine (Payer's patches), respiratory, reproductive and urinary tracts.

- Larger collections form the various tonsils in the body namely: Palatine tonsil, lingual tonsil, etc.

LYMPHATIC DRAINAGE OF BODY

LYMPHATIC DRAINAGE OF SCALP AND FACE

Lymphatics from scalp and face drain into the following lymph nodes (Fig. 15.8):

- **Pre-auricular lymph nodes:** Drain anterior part of scalp, except below the centre of forehead.
- **Post auricular lymph nodes:** Drain posterior part of scalp.

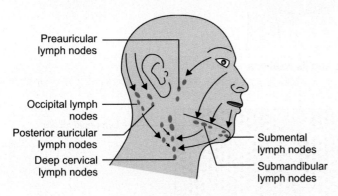

Fig. 15.8: 2 Lymphatic drainage of scalp and face

- **Occipital lymph nodes:** Part of the posterior part of scalp is also drained by these nodes.

LYMPHATICS OF HEAD AND NECK

The head and neck has about 300 lymph nodes out of a total of 800 present in the body. They are made up of deep and superficial cervical lymph nodes (Fig. 15.9).

Deep Cervical Lymph Nodes

Lymph from head and neck drains ultimately into the deep cervical group of lymph nodes either directly or indirectly. These nodes lie along and around the internal jugular vein deep to the sternocleidomastoid (Fig. 15.9).

They are divided into two groups by the intermediate tendon of omohyoid.

1. **Superior group:** These lie above the omohyoid muscle. They are known as **jugulo-digastric nodes** and receive lymph primarily from palatine tonsils. Hence they are also named as node of tonsil. The superior group drains into the inferior group
2. **Inferior group:** These lie along the internal jugular vein below the omohyoid muscle. It consists of **jugulo-omohyoid node.** This node receives lymph primarily from the tongue. Hence, it is also called the node of tongue.

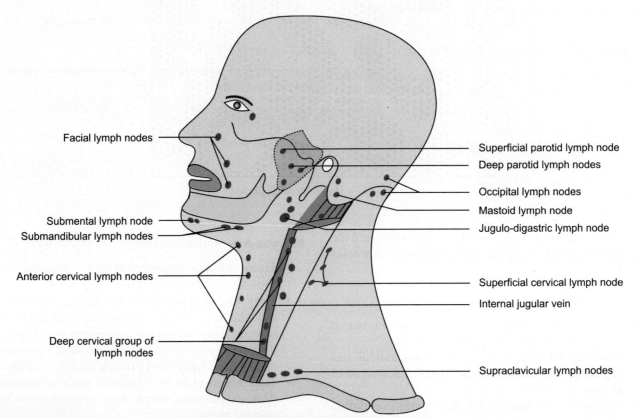

Fig. 15.9: Lymph nodes of head and neck

Deep Cervical Nodes Receives Afferents from

a. Superficial cervical lymph nodes: (discussed below).
b. Lymph nodes related to the viscera of head and neck.
c. Palatine tonsils.
d. Tongue
e. Larynx above the vocal folds

Efferents from Deep Cervical Nodes

The lymphatics from deep cervical lymph nodes form the right and left jugular lymph trunks.

The right jugular lymph trunk joins at the junction of subclavian and internal jugular vein either directly or via the right lymphatic duct.

The left jugular lymph trunk joins with the terminal part of thoracic duct or may directly enter left subclavian vein.

Superficial Cervical Lymph Nodes (Fig. 15.9)

These nodes are arranged in a circular fashion like a pericervical collar, at the junction base of skull with neck. They form an outer circle of lymphatics. They consist of the following lymph nodes as discussed in table below:

Superficial cervical lymph nodes	Afferents from	Efferents to
1. Submental nodes — Four in number — Present in submental triangle	1. Tip of tongue 2. Floor of mouth 3. Central part of lower lip 4. Chin	1. Submandibular node 2. Jugulo-omohyoid node
2. Submandibular nodes — Three in number — Lie in the submandibular triangle along the submandibular gland	1. Centre of forehead 2. Medial angle of eye 3. Side of nose 4. Cheek 5. Angle of mouth 6. Upper lip and lateral part of lower lip 7. Anterior 2/3rd of tongue 8. Gums 9. Frontal and maxillary sinuses 10. Submental lymph nodes	Deep cervical lymph nodes
3. Parotid/Preauricular lymph nodes — Superficial group lie over the gland — Deep group lie with in the gland	1. Forehead 2. Temporal region 3. Auricle, lateral surface 4. Anterior wall of external acoustic meatus 5. Eyelids, lateral half	Deep cervical lymph nodes
4. Retroauricular/Mastoid nodes Lie over upper part of sternocleidomastoid muscle	1. Auricle, cranial surface 2. Adjoining scalp 3. Posterior wall of external acoustic meatus	Superior group of deep cervical lymph nodes
5. Occipital nodes Situated at the apex of occipital triangle along the occipital artery	1. Posterior part of scalp	Supraclavicular nodes
6. Buccal nodes — Lie on the buccinator muscle, along the facial vein — Are an upward extension of submandibular nodes	1. Part of cheek 2. Lower eyelid	Superior group of deep cervical lymph nodes
7. Superficial cervical nodes — Are present over the sternocleido-mastoid muscle, along the external jugular vein — Are off shoots of parotid nodes	1. Floor of external acoustic meatus 2. Lobule of ear 3. Angle of jaw 4. Lower parotid region	Inferior group of deep cervical nodes
8. Anterior cervical nodes Lie along anterior jugular vein, are a downward extension from submental nodes	Anterior triangle of neck, below hyoid bone	Inferior group of deep cervical nodes

Lymphatics along the Viscera of Head and Neck

These form an inner circle of lymphatics of head and neck. They consist of the following:

1. **Infrahyoid nodes:** are present anterior to thyrohyoid membrane.
2. **Prelaryngeal nodes:** These are situated in front of conus elasticus membrane of larynx.
3. **Pretracheal nodes:** They lie in front of trachea, above the isthmus of thyroid gland.
4. **Paratracheal nodes:** These are present on either side of trachea and oesophagus, along the recurrent laryngeal nerve.

These four groups drain lymph from the larynx (below the vocal folds), trachea, oesophagus and thyroid gland.

5. **Retropharyngeal nodes:** They lie in the retropharyngeal space in front of the prevertebral fascia. These drain the pharynx, palatine tonsils, palate, part of nasal cavity, auditory tube, tympanic cavity, sphenoidal and ethmoidal sinuses.

Efferents from visceral cervical nodes drain into deep cervical group of lymph nodes.

WALDEYER'S LYMPHATIC RING

It consists of submucosal collection of lymphoid tissue around the commencement of air and food passages arranged in a ring like pattern (Fig. 15.10).

From posterior to anterior it is made up of the following

1. **Pharyngeal (nasopharyngeal) tonsils:** These lie postero-superiorly under the mucus membrane of the roof and adjoining posterior wall of naso pharynx.
2. **Tubal tonsils:** They are present on each side around the opening of eustachian tube into nasopharynx.
3. **Palatine tonsils:** They are present in the tonsillar fossa on each side of the oropharyngeal isthmus.
4. **Lingual tonsil:** This is present anteroinferiorly, in the submucosa of posterior 1/3rd of dorsum of tongue.

This ring of lymphatics prevents invasion of microorganisms into the air and food passages. The lymph from the Waldeyer's ring drains into the superficial and deep cervical group of lymph nodes.

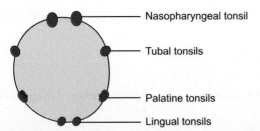

Fig. 15.10: Inner Waldeyer's ring

PALATINE TONSIL

The palatine tonsil is a collection of lymphoid tissue situated in the tonsillar fossa (see page 359), one on each side, in the lateral wall of the oropharynx (Fig. 15.11, 15.12). It is almond shaped. It has a rich arterial supply derived from the tonsillar branch of facial artery (it is the principal artery of tonsil) and branches from lingual artery, ascending palatine, ascending pharyngeal and greater palatine arteries. The veins drain into the pharyngeal plexus of veins through the paratonsillar vein.

Lymphatics from tonsil drain into the jugulodigastric lymph nodes. It is often called as the 'tonsillar lymph node' because it is enlarged in infections of the tonsil (tonsillitis).

Tonsils are supplied by glossopharyngeal nerve.

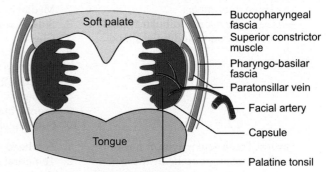

Fig. 15.11: Palatine tonsils

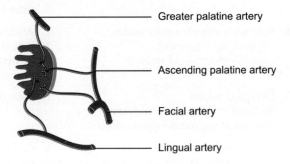

Fig. 15.12: Arterial supply of palatine tonsil

LYMPHATIC DRAINAGE OF UPPER LIMB

Upper limb is primarily drained by axillary group of lymph nodes. Other lymph nodes identified are infraclavicular lymph nodes, present below clavicle and supratrochlear lymph nodes, present behind the medial epicondyle of humerus (Figs 15.13 and 15.14).

The lymphatics of upper limb are arranged in superficial and deep lymphatic vessels.

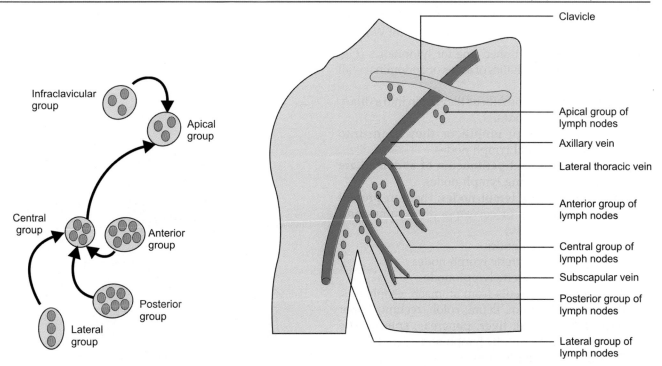

Fig. 15.13: Flow of lymph in axillary lymph nodes

Fig. 15.14: Axillary group of lymph nodes

Superficial Lymphatics: These run along cephalic vein and basilic vein. Vessels running along cephalic vein drain into infraclavicular and apical group of lymph nodes. Vessels along the basilic vein drain into supra-trochlear group of lymph nodes.

Deep lymphatic vessels: These run along the radial, ulnar and brachial arteries. They drain into lateral group of axillary lymph nodes.

Axillary Group of Lymph Nodes

They are 20 to 30 in number and are divided into five groups.
1. **Anterior group:** Lie along lateral thoracic vein.
2. **Posterior group:** Lie along subscapular vein.
3. **Lateral group:** Lie along axillary vein.
   Upper limb is mainly drained by lateral group of axillary lymph nodes.
   — Anterior group of axillary lymph nodes drain skin and muscles of anterior and lateral walls of trunk upto level of umbilicus and part of mammary gland.
   — Posterior group of axillary lymph nodes drain the skin and muscles of back of the trunk from iliac crest below to upper part of neck above
   — Lateral group of axillary lymph nodes drain upper limb.
4. **Central group:** Are embedded in the fat of axilla. The anterior, posterior and lateral groups of lymph nodes drain into central group. Efferents from

central group are given to apical group of lymph nodes.
5. **Apical group:** Lie at the apex of the axilla, medial to axillary vein. Receive afferent vessels from lymphatics that accompany the cephalic vein, upper margin of mammary gland, efferents from central group. Efferents from apical group form the sub-clavian trunk which drains into circulation at the junction of subclavian and internal jugular vein.

LYMPHATIC DRAINAGE OF THORAX

Superficial lymph nodes of thorax consist of intercostal, parasternal and superior diaphragmatic lymph nodes. The deep group of lymph nodes are present along the various viscera of thorax and form the lymphatic channels draining the thorax. These ultimately join the thoracic duct (see page nos 464, 465). The lymphatic vessels of thorax are
1. Left upper intercostal lymph trunks, from left upper six intercostal spaces.
2. Lower intercostal lymph trunks, from lower six intercostal spaces of both sides.
3. Mediastinal and Bronchomediastinal trunks.
4. Lymphatics from pretracheal and paratracheal lymph nodes.
5. Right upper six intercostal spaces are drained by right upper intercostal lymph trunk which ends into the right lymphatic duct (see page no. 465).

LYMPHATIC DRAINAGE OF ABDOMEN AND PELVIS

Lymphatic Drainage of Anterior Abdominal Wall

Umbilicus acts as water shed line for lymphatics (Fig. 15.15). Superficial lymphatics of anterior abdominal wall drain as follows:

1. Above the level of umbilicus they drain into axillary group of lymph nodes.
2. Below the level of umbilicus they drain into superficial inguinal lymph nodes.

The various viscera and peritoneum of abdomen are drained by the following lymph nodes

1. **Pre-aortic group of lymph nodes:** These are present along the arteries of corresponding names and consist of (Fig. 15.16)
   a. Coeliac lymph nodes
   b. Superior mesenteric lymph nodes
   c. Inferior mesenteric lymph nodes
   They receive afferents from stomach, esophagus, duodenum, jejunum, ileum, colon, rectum, upper part of anal canal, liver, pancreas, spleen. The efferents from pre-aortic lymph nodes join to form the **intestinal lymph trunk.**

2. **Para-aortic lymph nodes:** These are situated on both sides of abdominal aorta, anterior to the crura of diaphragm on the medial margins of psoas major muscle. They receive afferents from common iliac, internal iliac, external iliac, circumflex iliac, epigastric, sacral lymph nodes. Hence they drain lower limb, pelvis and perineum, infra-umbilical abdominal walls, pelvic viscera, gonads, kidneys and suprarenal glands. Efferents from para-aortic lymph nodes form the **right and left lumbar lymph trunks.**

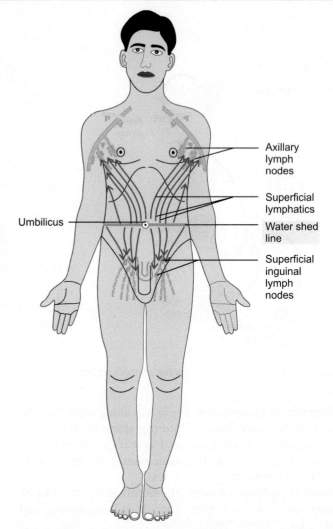

Fig. 15.15: Superficial lymphatics of anterior abdominal wall

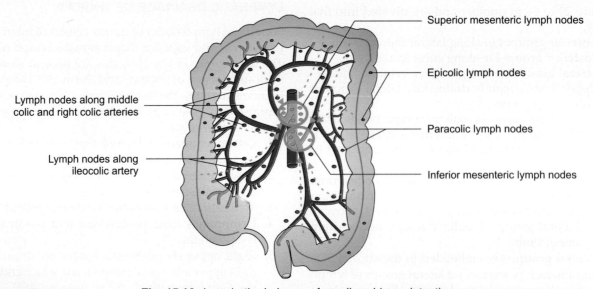

Fig. 15.16: Lymphatic drainage of small and large intestine

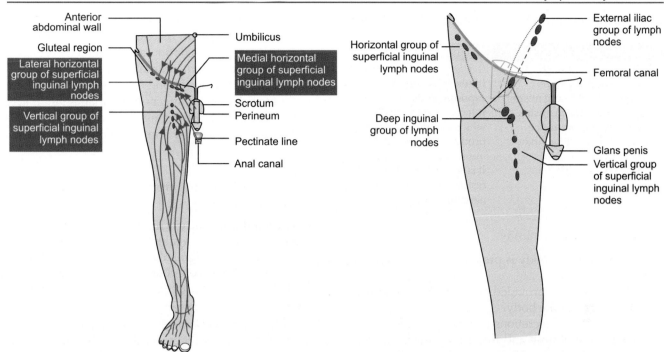

Fig. 15.17: Superficial group of inguinal lymph nodes

Fig. 15.18: Deep inguinal group of lymph nodes

LYMPHATICS OF LOWER LIMB

Lymph from lower limb is primarily drained by inguinal group of lymph nodes. Only few peripheral nodes are present in the leg, mainly in popliteal fossa.

Inguinal Lymph Nodes

Inguinal lymph nodes are divided into two groups
1. Superficial inguinal lymph nodes
2. Deep inguinal lymph nodes

Superficial Inguinal Lymph Nodes

They are distributed in a T-shape manner and are divided into an upper horizontal group and a lower vertical group (Fig. 15.17).
1. Upper horizontal group: It consists of 5–6 nodes present below the inguinal ligament. It is further divided into
   a. **Lateral group:** Drains gluteal region, and the adjoining anterior abdominal wall.
   b. **Medial group:** Drains anterior abdominal wall below umbilicus, perineum, anal canal below pectinate line.
      In males, it also drains penis, prepuce and scrotum.
      In females, it also drains vulva, vagina below hymen, cornu of uterus.
2. Lower vertical group is made up of 4-5 lymph nodes which lie along the great saphenous vein. All superficial lymph vessels from the lower limb

except along the short saphenous vein territory, drain into this vertical group. **Vertical group is the main lymphatic drainage of the lower limb.**

Deep Inguinal Lymph Nodes

They are 1 to 3 in number and lie on the medial side of femoral vein. Lymph node that lies in femoral canal is known as **Cloquet's gland** (Fig. 15.18). Deep lymph vessels accompany femoral vessels. They drain glans penis in male, glans clitoris in female and receive efferents from superficial inguinal lymph nodes.

Efferents from deep inguinal group of lymph nodes drain into the external iliac group of lymph nodes.

IMMUNITY

It is the ability of the body to protect itself against invasion by organisms like bacteria, viruses and parasites; against foreign particles and against tumors. Immunity is classified into two types:
1. **Innate immunity:** This type of immunity is present at birth by virtue of the genetic and constitutional development of the body. It is independent of any previous exposure to the organism. It hence provides the first line of defense against infections.
2. **Acquired immunity:** This type of immunity is acquired by the body after it is exposed to an organism or an immunogenic substance during the lifetime. It is brought about by activation of specific lymphocytes.

Differences between innate and acquired immunity

Innate immunity	Acquired immunity
1. It is present at birth	It is acquired during life
2. It is independent of exposure of an organism	It develops only after exposure to the organism
3. It involves mechanisms already present in the body. Hence, there in no latent period.	It has a latent period which is requied to produce the desired immunological response.
4. It is non-specific.	It is specific and results in resistance only against the particular stimulus.

Innate or Natural Immunity

Innate immunity of body is provided by the following factors:
1. Physical barrier provided by intact skin and mucus membrane of the body.
2. Barrier due to secretions produced by the mucus membrane of nose and respiratory tract, saliva of the mouth, hydrochloric acid of stomach, mucus lining the intestinal lumen.
3. Natural anti-bacterial and antiviral substances in various parts of body like lysozymes in saliva and lacrimal fluid, mucopolysaccharidases in nasopharyngeal secretions, normal bacterial flora of distal ileum and colon.
4. Antimicrobial molecules in circulation.
   a. Complement system
   b. Cytokines (interferons)
   c. Antibacterial peptides
5. Cellular defences:
   a. Presence of phagocytic cells in the body like macrophages present in alveoli of lung, tissue fluids etc. and polymorphonucleocytes (neutrophils) present in the circulation. These cells accumulate at the site of injury or invasion and ingest and destroy the foreign particles or organisms.
   b. **Natural killer cells:** These are large lymphocytes present in the circulation that are specially active against viral particles, few bacteria and fungi and also tumor cells without any prior sensitization. They activate complement system, secrete cytokines and causes lysis of cells by damaging cell membrane.
   c. **Eosinophils:** These are a type of WBC which contain toxic granules that are active against few parasites.
6. **Inflammatory responses of the body:**
   a. Injury or infection at a site leads to vasodilatation, leaking of phagocytes from capillary circulation into the tissues and the destruction of the organism. Increase in local temperature due to vasodilatation also is directly lethal to the invading microorganisms.
   b. Fever: Increase in body temperature is usually seen during an infection or inflamation. It acts by directly inhibiting the growth of microorganisms and by stimulating interferons.

Acquired Immunity

It is the immune response brought about by an antigenic stimulus. It is of two types:
1. **Humoral immunity:** This is mediated by production of antibodies against an antigen. The antigen is usually a foreign substance (protein molecule) for example cell components of bacteria or viruses. Antibodies are produced by activated B-lymphocytes or plasma cells.
2. **Cellular or cell mediated immunity:** This is mediated primarily by action of T-lymphocytes. It not only is active against microorganisms but has a function is immunity against cancer, graft reaction and few autoimmune diseases.

Acquired immunity can be obtained in two ways:
1. **Active acquired immunity:** This immunity is acquired after being exposed to an antigen. The immunological machinery of the body is activated and results in production of antibodies or immunocompetent cells against the antigen. It can be further acquired in two ways:
   a. **Natural active immunity:** This immunity develops after an apparent infection, e.g., after an episode of chicken pox the individual acquires immunity against the infection which protects him against any second attack.
   b. **Artificial active immunity:** This immunity develops after exposure to an antigen administered by way of vaccines.
   Examples of vaccines:
   — Bacterial vaccines: These can be live attenuated antigens, e.g., BCG for tuberculosis or killed antigens, e.g., Typhoid vaccine.
   — Viral vaccines: These can be live attenuated antigens, e.g., oral polio vaccine, measles and chicken pox vaccine or killed antigens, e.g., injectable polio vaccine.
   — Vaccines madeup of bacterial products, e.g., toxoid vaccines of Tetanus and diphtheria.
2. **Passive acquired immunity:** This immunity is acquired by the passive administration of antibodies to an individual. The immunological machinery of the individual is not stimulated. It can also be acquired in two ways:

a. **Natural passive immunity:** It is the immunity acquired by the fetus/baby by the transmission of antibody across placenta/milk from the mother to the baby during intra uterine life and lactation respectively.

b. **Artificial passive immunity:** It is the immunity acquired by an individual by the administration of antibodies directly into circulation, e.g., Use of hyperimmune serum in the treatment of tetanus, diphtheria and gas gangrene infections.

LYMPHOCYTES

These are the second most common type of circulating white blood cells or leucocytes. Lymphocytes are broadly divided into B-lymphocytes and T-lymphocytes.

B-Lymphocytes

These develop and differentiate from haemopoetic stem cells of bone marrow.

- They are transported via blood to secondary lymphoid organs like lymph node and spleen.
- Mature B-lymphocytes have antigen receptor sites on their cell membrane.
- Activated B-lymphocytes are called plasma cells. They produce antibodies in response to antigenic stimulus.
- Some activated B-lymphocytes do not form plasma cells and instead remain as memory B-cells.

Antibodies (Immunoglobulins)

Antibodies are also termed as immunoglobulins (Ig). They are produced by plasma cells. Immunoglobulins are glycoprotein molecules and are made up of two pairs of polypeptide chains, two small or light and two large or heavy chains. They are classified into five classes namely:

1. **IgG:** It is the most abundant of immunoglobulins. IgG acts as an opsonin and promotes phagocytosis. It binds to the antigen and forms antigen-antibody complex which stimulates complement system. IgG can cross placenta and confers immunity to newborn.

2. **IgA:** IgA is responsible for providing local immunity on mucosal and body surfaces. Besides plasma, it is produced in saliva, tears, intestinal secretion, breast milk. It cannot cross placenta.

3. **IgM:** IgM is predominantly intravascular in location. It is the first immunoglobulin produced in an immunogenic response. It does not cross placenta. It acts by promoting phagocytosis and stimulating complement system.

4. **IgE:** It usually coats mast cells and basophils and leads to degranulation of these cells when they combine with antigen. This results in release of histamine and other chemical mediators. It is responsible for allergies, hypersensitivity reactions and inflammatory responses against parasites.

5. **IgD:** It is concerned with antigen recognition.

Mechanism of action of antibodies:

- They neutralize bacteria toxins by binding to them
- They bind to viral cell membranes and prevent intracellular invasion of viruses. Since viral replication needs incorporation into host DNA, it ultimately leads to viral death.
- Antibodies bind to bacterial cells and favours their phagocytosis (opsonization)
- Antibody-antigen complexes stimulate complement system.

Primary Immune Response

When the body is exposed to an organism for the 1st time there is production of antibodies which help limit the infection. The first antbody to appear is IgM. The immune response has a lag phase of 1–4 weeks because there is initiation of immunological response for the first time. Also, the antibody levels decline gradually by four weeks. Hence, it is usually a short lived response.

Secondary Immune Response

This is brought about when there is a second exposure to same organism. The response is mediated via memory B-lymphocytes and occurs immediately against the organisms. This is mediated by production of IgG antibodies. The level of antibody production is higher and also the level of IgG antibodies decline slowly and usually persist for many years or throughout life.

T-lymphocytes

- They originate from bone marrow but first migrate to thymus where they become immunologically mature thymic lymphocytes or T-lymphocytes.
- They then re-enter circulation and are distributed to the secondary lymphoid organs namely: lymph nodes and spleen.
- T-lymphocytes are further divided into three subgroups
  — Helper T-lymphocytes
  — Suppressor T-lymphocytes
  — Cytotoxic T-lymphocytes
  — Memory T-lymphocytes

T-lymphocytes are responsible for cell mediated immune response against an antigen.

Function of Helper T-lymphocytes

T-helper cells act in two ways:

a. Stimulate proliferation of B-lymphocytes, producing memory B cells and plasma cells in response to an antigen. They help in humoral immunity.

b. Produce IL-2 and interferons to mediate cellular immunity

Function of Suppressor T-lymphocytes

They help to regulate the immune response by suppressing the production of antibody production from B-lymphocytes and suppressing the action of cytotoxic cells.

Function of Cytotoxic T-lymphocytes

Cytotoxic T-cells mediate allergic reaction, destruction of transplanted or foreign tissues and aid lysis of tumor cells.

T-lymphocytes have glycoproteins receptors on their cell surfaces which are primarily of two types:
1. CD8 receptors: Present in cytotoxic T-cells
2. CD4 receptors: Present in helper T-cells

Function of Memory T-lymphocytes

They are a subset of cytotoxic lymphocytes that are stimulated by exposure to an antigen and remain in the circulation for a number of months to years. On second exposure to the same antigen they mount a quicker and stronger immune response against the same.

Pathway of Immunological Response

Antigen Recognition

For an immune response to occur the B and T-lympho-cytes should be able to recognise the presence of a foreign antigen. The antigen is taken up and phagocytosed by specialized cells in body like Langerhan's cells of skin, dendritic cells of lymph node and spleen, the B-lymphocytes and macrophages in plasma. It is then recognised by the antigen recognizing cells which are T and B-lymphocytes and macrophages. These cells produce cell surface proteins coded by major histocompatibility complex (MHC) genes. MHC genes are present on chromosome 6. There are two classes of MHC proteins known as:

- **MHC-I proteins:** They are present on all nucleated cells of the body (absent on RBCs). These recognise endogenous antigens, e.g., viral infected host cells or tumor cells.
- **MHC-II proteins:** These are present only on B-lymphocytes and T-lymphocytes. These recognise foreign antigens, like cell components of bacteria and bind to them.

The antigen MHC complex is finally transported to the lymph node or spleen via the lymphatic circulation and it activates the immune response.

Pathway of Antigen Destruction (Immune response)

The various mechanisms of immune response are:
1. Phagocytosis
2. Activation of cytokines
3. Activation of complement system
4. **Direct cell lysis by cytotoxic T-cells:** The cytotoxic T-cells recognise MHC-I proteins bound to endogenous antigens like viral infected cells, tumor cells, cells of tissue transplant and bind to them. Activation of cytotoxic T-cells results in release of proteins that damage the cell membrane or activate intracellular enzymes and destroy them.

Cytokines

These are a group of hormone like molecules produced by lymphocytes. Other cells producing cytokines are macrophages, somatic cells etc. They consist of the following molecules:
1. Interleukins (IL)-13 types have been identified, named IL-1 to IL-13
2. Tumor necrosis factor (TNFa and TNFb)
3. Interferons (INFa, INFb and INFg)
4. Tumor growth factor (TGFb)

They act in a paracrine fashion to stimulate leucopoesis. IL-1 is responsible for B lymphocyte proliferation, immunoglobulin (Ig) production, phagocytic stimulation and inflammatory response. It also causes fever. TNF produces actions similar to IL-1. It also stimulates vascular thrombosis and tumor necrosis. Interferons are prime stimulators of cell mediated immunity. They are most active against viral invasion.

Complement System

The complement system consists of nine plasma enzymes designated numbers from C1 to C9. The activation of complement system is brought by binding of C1 to antigen antibody complex (acquired immunity) or binding of circulating protein called factor 1 to cell membrane of bacteria or virus (innate immunity).

This leads to a cascade of reactions that result in:
1. **Opsonization of bacteria:** The bacteria get coated with factors that make them easy targets of phagocytosis by neutrophils and macrophages.
2. The C-factors act as chemotactic agents attracting neutrophils and macrophages.
3. Stimulate inflammatory response by causing release of histamine.
4. The activated complement complex formed at end of reaction forms perforations in cell membrane of organisms resulting in their death.

CLINICAL AND APPLIED ASPECT

LYMPH VESSELS AND LYMPH NODES

- **Chylothorax:** Injury to thoracic duct may result in accumulation of fluid in thoracic or pleural cavities known as chylothorax.
- **Chyluria:** Thoracic duct obstruction leading to backflow of intestinal lymph into the lymphatic capillaries of kidney may produce chyluria.
- **Filariasis** is infestation by microfilaria parasites. These have predilection for lymphatics and may block the thoracic duct and other lymphatic channels causing oedema of the limbs. Bursting of thoracic duct into pleural cavities can cause a chylous pleural effusion.
- Enlargement of lymph nodes can occur due to various causes like
  — Acute infections, e.g., jugulodigastric lymph nodes are enlarged in tonsillitis, infection of toe nail of greater toe leads to enlargment of lower vertical group of superficial inguinal lymph nodes.
  — Chronic infections, e.g., tuberculosis
  — Malignancies, e.g., lymphomas, metastasis from visceral cancers. Virchow's nodes: These are enlarged lymph nodes which can be felt just above the medial end of clavicle, lateral to the insertion of sternocleidomastoid. They are usually enlarged in patients with advanced cancers mainly involving the stomach and pelvic structures.
- The tissues and organs devoid of lymphatics are:
  — Central nervous system
  — Bone marrow
  — Eye ball
  — Intralobular portion of the liver
  — Internal ear
  — Red pulp of spleen
  — Fetal-placenta
  — Areas devoid of capillaries

SPLEEN

- Spleen is palpable per abdomen only when it is enlarged to atleast twice its normal size.
- Spleen is identified by splenic notch.
- While ligating splenic vessels, damage to the tail of the pancreas should be prevented as it lies in the lienorenal ligament along with splenic vessels.
- Patient with ruptured spleen, occasionally complain of pain in the left shoulder because of haemorrhage of ruptured spleen irritates the diaphragm which is supplied by the phrenic nerve (C_3, C_4, C_5). Pain is referred to shoulder because the supraclavicular nerve (which supplies skin over the shoulder) also has the root value of C_3 C_4. There is involvement of same spinal segment.

PALATINE TONSILS

Tonsils are larger in children and atrophy by adulthood. They are known to increase in size in childhood due to repeated infections causing tonsillitis. Tonsillectomy i.e. superficial removal of tonsils is necessary if they become a site of repeated infections or there is a tonsillar abscess or they enlarge so much that they block the passage. Injury to paratonsillar vein during surgery is an important cause of haemorrhage which is usually controlled by applying pressure.

ABNORMAL IMMUNE RESPONSES

Autoimmune Diseases

During intrauterine life the antigens presented to the immune system of fetus are recognised as self antigens and tolerance to them is produced. However later in life the immune system may start producing antibodies against self antigens and results in autoimmune diseases. Examples are:
1. **Rheumatoid arthiritis:** In this the body produces antibodies against the synovial membrane of the joints.
2. **Haemolytic anemia:** Antibodies are produced against one's own RBCs.
3. **Grave's disease:** In this condition there is hyperthyroidism due to antibodies in the body that stimulate receptors of thyroid gland cells.

Hypersensitivity Reaction

It is an abnormally exaggerated immune response to an antigen that causes harm to the body of host. There are four types of hypersensitivity reactions namely:
1. **Type 1:** This occurs due to exaggerated IgE mediated immune response which results in release of histamine from the mast cells and basophils. It can be mild which presents in the form of itching, hives or urticaria. It can be severe leading to anaphylactic shock associated with bronchoconstriction and systemic vasodilatation with severe hypotension and occasional death.
2. **Type 2:** This type of hypersensitivity reaction is a result of antibody mediated toxicity.
3. **Type 3:** This type of reaction occurs due to excess production of antigen-antibody complexes in circulation.
4. **Type 4:** It occurs due to excess stimulation of memory T-lymphocytes. Example of this is graft rejection.

CHAPTER-15

Immuno Deficiency Diseases

These diseases are associated with decreased or absent activity of various immunological mechanisms of the body. Thus, they result in an increased risk of infection and occasionaly tumor formation. They can be:

1. **Congenital**, which means present by birth. This is due to genetic abnormality.
2. **Acquired**, which is acquired during life it can be due to
   a. Infections, e.g., HIV infection leading to AIDS
   b. Malignancies of WBCs, e.g., leukemias.

AIDS

AIDS means acquired immunodeficiency syndrome. It is caused by the virus named HIV (human immuno deficiency virus). The virus can enter the body in the following ways:

1. Sexual contact with infected person.
2. Transmission across placenta from infected mother to the baby.
3. Innoculation of virus by using contaminated needles, blood, etc.

HIV has a high affinity for the CD4 receptors of T-lymphocytes resulting in their destruction. This leads to deficiency in CD4 helper T-lymphocytes. There is an increase in opportunistic infections in the body like tuberculosis, systemic viral and fungal infections. It is also associated with increase in formation of malignant tumors like lymphomas.

Digestive System

INTRODUCTION

Digestive system or gastrointestinal system is responsible for intake, digestion and absorption of food.

Ingestion, digestion and absorption of various components of food provide for the daily nutritive requirements of the body (Fig. 16.1).

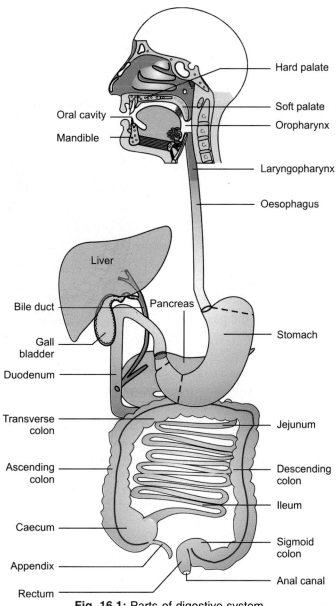

Oral cavity

Mandible

Hard palate

Soft palate

Oropharynx

Laryngopharynx

Oesophagus

Liver

Bile duct

Gall bladder

Duodenum

Transverse colon

Ascending colon

Caecum

Appendix

Rectum

Pancreas

Stomach

Jejunum

Descending colon

Ileum

Sigmoid colon

Anal canal

Fig. 16.1: Parts of digestive system

Ingestion

The food is placed in mouth; it mixes with secretions of salivary glands. Mastication (chewing) involves breaking down of large food particles into smaller pieces by movement of jaws, brought about by muscles of mastication and by action of teeth. A bolus of food is thus formed and then swallowed (Deglutition).

Digestion

It is an orderly process that involves breaking down of various constituents of food like starch, protein and fat to absorbable units by the various digestive enzymes of gastro intestinal tract (GIT) aided by saliva in mouth, hydrochloric acid of stomach and bile from liver.

Absorption

It is the process of passage of various nutritive components of food like protein, carbohydrates and fats besides water, minerals and vitamins from intestinal lumen across mucosal cells into the blood or lymphatic circulation. These components are made available to various parts of the body for proper functioning of tissues. Absorption primarily occurs in small intestine. Some amount of water and electrolyte absorption takes place in large intestine.

Elimination

The undigested food particles are removed from the distal end of GIT or anus by the process of defecation.

ANATOMY OF GASTROINTESTINAL TRACT

Gastrointestinal tract is a tubular tract for the passage of food. It consists of the following parts:
- Oral cavity
- Pharynx
- Oesophagus
- Stomach
- Small intestine
- Large intestine
- Rectum and anal canal

It is associated with various organs that help in digestion and absorption of food. These are
- Three pairs of salivary glands
- Liver and biliary tract
- Pancreas

ORAL CAVITY (MOUTH)

It is the first part of digestive tract (Fig. 16.2). It is divided into two parts:

1. Oral cavity proper
2. The vestibule

Oral Cavity Proper

It is the larger part of the oral cavity (Figs 16.2). It is mostly occupied by the tongue posteriorly.

Boundaries

Anteriorly	:	Alveolar arches with teeth and gums on each side.
Roof	:	Hard and soft palate
Floor	:	Two mylohyoid muscles and other soft tissues.
Posteriorly	:	Palatoglossal arch.

The oral cavity communicates posteriorly with the pharynx through the **oropharyngeal isthmus also called isthmus of fauces.** The isthmus is bounded superiorly by the soft palate, inferiorly by the tongue and on each side by the palatoglossal arches.

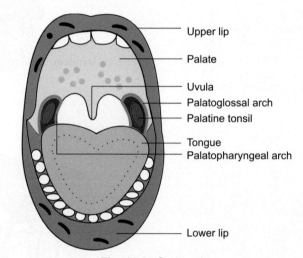

Fig. 16.2: Oral cavity

Vestibule

Vestibule of mouth is a narrow space that lies outside the teeth and gums and inside the lips and cheeks (Fig. 16.3) . When the mouth is open, it communicates with the oral cavity proper but when the mouth is closed, i.e., when the teeth are occluded it communicates with the oral cavity through a small gap behind the third molar tooth The vestibule is lined by mucous membrane except in the area of teeth.

Openings in the Vestibule of the Mouth

1. **Opening of parotid duct:** The parotid duct opens into the lateral wall of vestibule opposite the crown of upper second molar tooth.

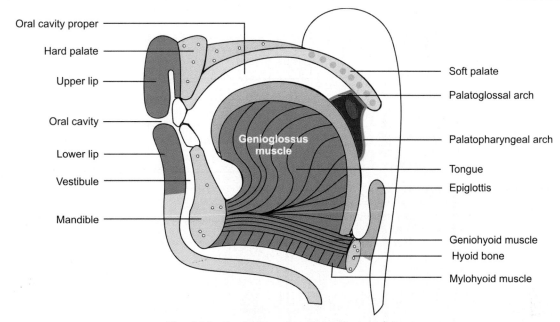

Fig. 16.3: Sagittal section through oral cavity

2. Openings of labial and buccal mucous glands.
3. Openings of 4 to 5 molar glands (mucous) situated on the buccopharyngeal fascia

Lips

Lips are a pair of mobile musculo-fibrous folds that surround the opening of the mouth. Upper and lower lips meet laterally, on each side, at an angle called angle of mouth. The lips are lined externally by skin and internally by mucous membrane (Fig. 16.3).

Cheeks

Cheeks are fleshy flaps which lie over the maxilla and mandible and form a large part of the face. Each cheek is continuous in front with the lip. Like the lips the cheeks are lined externally by skin and internally by mucous membrane. The cheek is largely composed of the buccinator muscle present under the skin. It overlies the buccal pad of fat (best developed in infants) and is internally lined by buccopharyngeal fascia.In addition it also contains buccal glands, blood vessels and nerves.

Oral Mucosa

The mucosal lining of oral cavity continues with the skin of lips anteriorly and mucosa of oropharyx posteriorly. It can be divided into three types according to the anatomical location and function:

1. **Lining mucosa:** It lines most of the oral cavity. It consists of non-keratinized stratified squamous epithelium present over lamina propria and sub-mucosa.

2. **Masticatory mucosa:** It is the mucosa that lines the upper part of alveolar process, neck of teeth and the hard palate. It consists of keratinized stratified squamous epithelium with minimal lamina propria and no submucosa.

   Gingiva (Gum): Gingiva is the masticatory mucosa that covers the alveolar processes of maxilla (upper jaw) and mandible (lower jaw) and surrounds the neck of teeth.

3. **Specialised mucosa:** It is the mucosa covering the dorsal surface of tongue. It is directly adherent to the underlying muscles. There is no submucosa. It gives rise to a number of projections called **lingual papillae.**

TEETH

Teeth are mineralized or horny structures projecting from the jaws. Study of teeth, strictly speaking, forms the subject of 'odontology' and the science concerned with diagnosis and treatment of diseases of the teeth and its associated structures is called 'dentistry' (L.dens, dentis, = tooth) (Fig. 16.4).

Anatomical Features of Teeth

Each tooth consists of the following three parts:

1. **Crown,** which projects above the gum.
2. **Root,** which is embedded within the socket of jaw beneath the gum.
3. **Neck,** it is the constricted part of tooth present between the crown and root. It is encircled by the gum.

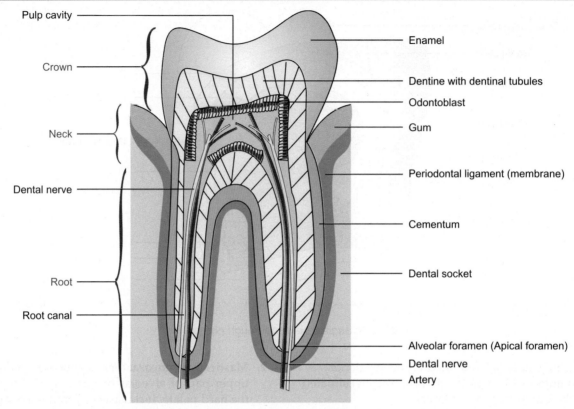

Fig. 16.4: Structure of a tooth

Structure of a Tooth

Each tooth is composed of:

1. **Pulp cavity:** It is the inner soft tissue core containing blood vessels, nerves and lymphatics in a specialized connective tissue called pulp. The pulp is covered by a layer of tall columnar cells called odontoblasts.
2. **Dentine:** It is a calcified material surrounding the pulp cavity produced by odontoblasts. It forms a major part of the tooth.
3. **Enamel:** It consists of densely calcified white material covering the crown of the tooth. It is the hardest substance in the body.
4. **Cementum:** It is the bony covering over the neck and root of the tooth. It commonly overlaps the lower part of the enamel
5. **Periodontal membrane or ligament:** It is present between the cementum and the socket of a tooth. It acts as the periosteum. It holds the tooth in the socket and is therefore often termed as periodontal ligament.

Arterial Supply of Teeth

The upper teeth are supplied by superior alveolar arteries which are branches from the maxillary artery.

The lower teeth are supplied by the inferior alveolar artery, a branch of maxillary artery (Fig. 16.4).

Nerve Supply of Teeth

1. The upper teeth are supplied by the **superior dental plexus** of nerves formed by posterior superior, middle superior and anterior superior alveolar nerves. These are branches of the maxillary division of fifth cranial nerve.
2. The lower teeth are supplied by the **inferior alveolar** nerve or dental nerve, branch of mandibular division of fifth cranial nerve.

Type of Teeth

The teeth are classified into four groups
1. **Incisors:** There are four incisors in each jaw, two on each side of the median plane. The central four are called medial while the one lateral to them are called lateral incisors. As the name suggests incisors cut food by their cutting edges. They are chisel like. The upper and lower incisors overlap each other like blades of a pair of scissors, when mouth is closed.
2. **Canines:** There are two canines in each jaw, one on each side, present lateral to the incisors. They are

so named because they are prominent in dogs. Canines are long and have conical and rugged crowns that help in holding and tearing food.

3. **Premolars:** There are four premolars in each jaw, two on each side of the canines. They assist in crushing of food. They have two cusps and therefore are also called as bicuspid teeth.

4. **Molars [L molar(s) = grinders]:** There are six molars in each jaw, three on each side of the premolars. They help to crush and grind the food. They possess three to five tubercles on their crowns. While the rest of teeth have a single root, the upper molars have three roots and the lower molars have two roots.

Eruption of Teeth

Most of the teeth in an adult are 'successional' that is, they have succeeded the corresponding number of milk teeth. The permanent molars however are 'accessional' that is they have been added behind the milk teeth during development.

Eruption of deciduous teeth: The deciduous teeth begin to erupt at about 6 months of age. A complete set erupts by the end of 2nd year. The teeth of lower jaw erupt somewhat earlier than the corresponding teeth of upper jaw.

Teeth	Time of Eruption
Lower central incisors	6 months
Upper central incisors	7 months
Lateral incisors	8 to 9 months
First molar	12 months (1 year)
Canines	18 months (1½ year)
Second molars	24 months (2 years)

Eruption of permanent teeth: The sequence of eruption of permanent teeth is tabulated below:

Teeth	Time of Eruption
First molar	6 years
Medial incisors	7 years
Lateral incisors	8 years
First premolar	9 years
Second premolar	10 years
Canines	11 years
Second molars	12 years
Third molar (Wisdom tooth)	17 to 25 years

Functions of the Teeth

1. To incise and grind the food material during mastication.
2. To perform (sometimes) the role of weapon of defense or attack.

3. To provide beauty to the face and means for facial expression.

TONGUE

Tongue is a mobile muscular organ present in the oral cavity (Figs 16.3, 16.5 and 16.6).

Anatomical Features

It is conical in shape and presents with following features.

1. **Tip:** It is the anterior end of the tongue and lies in contact with the incisor teeth.

2. **Base:** It is formed by the posterior 1/3rd of tongue. The posterior part of tongue is connected to the epiglottis by three folds of mucus membrane namely one median glosso-epiglottic fold and two lateral glosso-epiglottic folds. On either side of the median fold is present a depression called vallecula.

3. **Root:** The part of tongue attached to the floor of mouth is called the root. The lower fibres of genioglossus attach it to the mandible and hyoid bone.

4. **Two lateral margins** present on either side of tongue are free. The palatoglossal fold merges with these margins at the junction of anterior 2/3rd with posterior 1/3rd on each side.

5. **Dorsal surface:** It is convex on all sides and is divided into two parts by an inverted V-shaped sulcus known as sulcus terminalis. The apex of the sulcus is directed backwards and is marked by a shallow depression called **foramen caecum** which represents the site of the embryological origin of thyroid gland. The surface is lined by non-keratinized stratified squamous epithelium. The two parts of the dorsal surface are.

   a. **Presulcal or oral part:** It constitutes anterior 2/3rd of the dorsal surface. It usually presents a median furrow. Which represents the bilateral origin of tongue. The mucus membrane does not have submucosa. Numerous papillae or projections are present on the surface. These are
   1. Vallate papillae
   2. Fungiform papillae
   3. Filiform papillae
   4. Foliate papillae
   5. Papillae simplex

   b. **Post sulcal or pharyngeal part:** Mucus membrane of this area overlies a loose submucosa containing numerous mucus and serous glands. A large number of lymphoid follicles known as lingual tonsils are also present under the lining epithelium. There are no papillae.

Human Anatomy and Physiology for Nursing and Allied Sciences

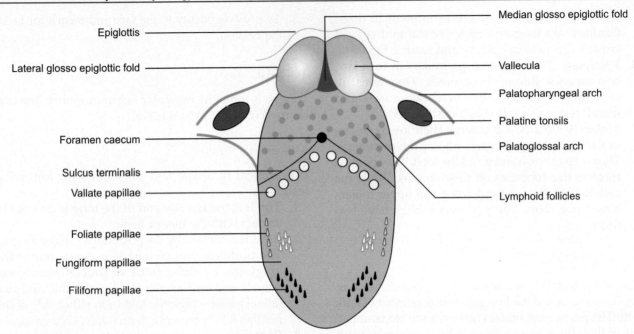

Fig. 16.5: Dorsum of the tongue

Taste buds: Taste buds are modified epithelial cells arranged around a gustatory cell. The base of each bud is penetrated by the afferent gustatory fibres. All papillae except filiform papillae contain taste buds. Taste buds are present at the following sites:
— Anterior 2/3rd of dorsum of tongue
— Inferior surface of soft palate
— Palatoglossal arches
— Posterior surface of epiglottis
— Posterior wall of oropharynx

Four type of taste sensations are projected on to the tongue namely, salty, sweet, sour, bitter.

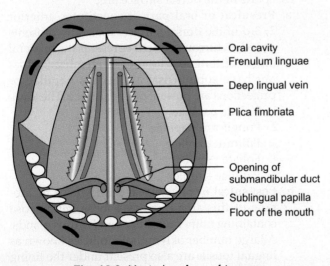

Fig. 16.6: Ventral surface of tongue

6. **Ventral or inferior surface (Fig. 16.6):** The ventral surface is lined by a thin mucus membrane which gets reflected on to the floor of the mouth. It does not contain papillae. It presents with the following features:
   a. **Frenulum linguae:** It is a median fold of mucus membrane connecting the tongue to the floor of mouth.
   b. **Lingual veins:** These are seen on either side of the frenulum. Lingual nerve and artery lie medial to the veins on each side but are not visible.
   c. **Plica fimbriate:** It consists of a ringed fold of mucus membrane present lateral to the lingual vein.
   d. **Sublingual papilla:** It is present on each side of the base of frenulum linguae as an elevation which has the opening of the duct of submandibular gland at its summit.

Muscles of the Tongue

The tongue is divided into two symmetrical halves by a median fibrous septum. Each half contains 4 intrinsic and 4 extrinsic muscles. Intrinsic muscles alter the shape of the tongue while the extrinsic muscles alter the position of the tongue (Figs 16.3, 16.7 and 16.8).

1. **Extrinsic muscles:** These attach the tongue to the surrounding bones (Fig. 16.7).
   a. Hyoglossus
   b. Genioglossus

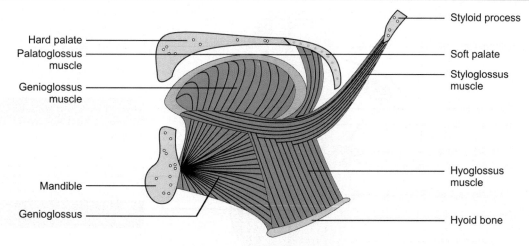

Fig. 16.7: Extrinsic muscles of the tongue

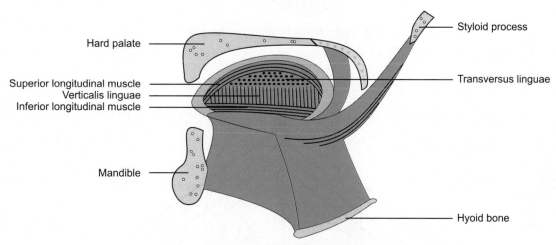

Fig. 16.8: Intrinsic muscles of the tongue

c. Styloglossus
d. Palatoglossus

2. **Intrinsic muscles:** They occupy the upper part of tongue and are attached to the submucus layer and the median fibrous septum (Fig. 16.8).
   a. Superior longitudinal lingual muscles
   b. Inferior longitudinal lingual muscles
   c. Transversus linguae
   d. Verticalis linguae

Nerve Supply of Tongue

Tongue receives motor and sensory supply.

1. **Motor supply**
   a. **Somato-motor supply:** It supplies the muscles of tongue.

   i. **Hypoglossal nerve:** It supplies all extrinsic and intrinsic muscles of tongue except palatoglossus.
   ii. **Cranial part of accessory nerve (via vagus nerve)** supplies palatoglossus.

   b. **Secretomotor supply to lingual glands:** Preganglionic fibres arise in superior salivatory nucleus and postganglionic fibres arise from submandibular ganglion and are conveyed via lingual nerve.
   c. **Vasomotor supply:** It supplies the blood vessels and is derived from the sympathetic plexus around lingual artery

2. **Sensory supply (Fig. 16.9)**
   a. **Lingual nerve:** Receives general sensation from anterior 2/3rd of the tongue.
   b. **Chorda tympani:** Receives taste sensations from anterior 2/3rd except from vallate papillae.

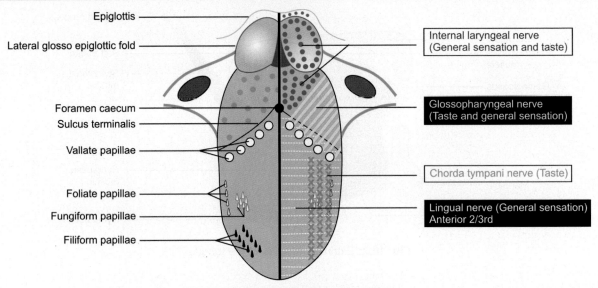

Fig. 16.9: Sensory supply of tongue

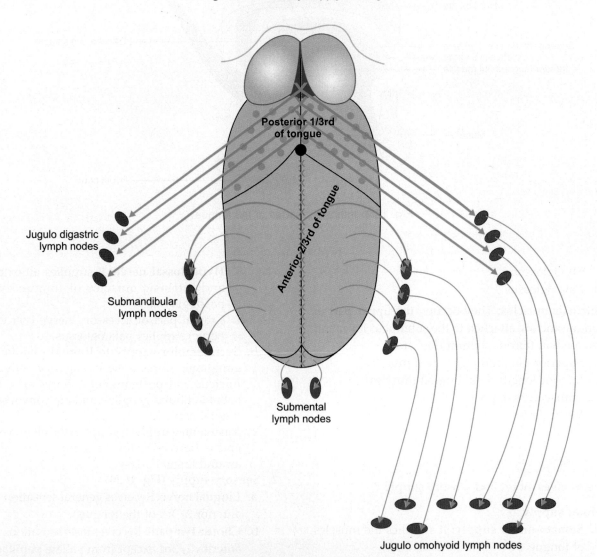

Fig. 16.10: Lymphatic drainage of tongue

c. **Glossopharyngeal nerve:** Conveys all sensations from posterior 1/3rd. of the tongue. Carries taste sensation from vallate papillae.

d. **Internal laryngeal branch of superior laryngeal nerve** from vagus. It conveys taste sensation from posterior most part of tongue and vallecula.

Arterial Supply of Tongue

1. Lingual artery, branch of external carotid arterty is the chief artery of tongue
2. Ascending palatine artery, branch of facial artery
3. Tonsillar artery, branch of facial artery

Venous Drainage of Tongue

It consists of superficial and deep veins. These veins unite at the posterior border of hyoglossus to form the **lingual vein** which terminates into the internal jugular vein.

Lymphatic Drainage of Tongue

The drainage zones of tongue can be grouped into three (Fig. 16.10):
1. Tip and inferior surface of tongue drain into submental lymph nodes
2. Anterior 2/3rd of dorsum of tongue
   a. Each half drains into ipsilateral submandibular lymph nodes and thence to lower deep cervical lymph nodes.

b. Few lymphatics from the central region, with in ½ inch of midline, drain bilaterally into submandibular lymph nodes.
3. Posterior 1/3rd of dorsum of tongue: Drains bilaterally into the upper deep cervical lymph nodes, the jugulo-digastric nodes.

Functions of Tongue

It helps in the following functions
   a. Speech
   b. Taste
   c. Mastication
   d. Deglutition
   e. Facial expression
   f. Pasting postage stamp
   g. Pattern of papillae has medicolegal importance

PALATE

It is an osteomuscular partition between nasal and oral cavities.It also separates nasopharynx from oropharynx (Fig. 16.11). It consists of two parts:
   1. **Hard palate,** forms the anterior 2/3rd of the palate.
   2. **Soft palate,** forms the posterior 1/3rd of the palate.

Hard Palate

Hard palate forms a partition between the nasal and oral cavities. Anterior 3/4th is formed by the palatine processes of the maxillae and the posterior 1/4th by the horizontal plates of the palatine bones. The superior

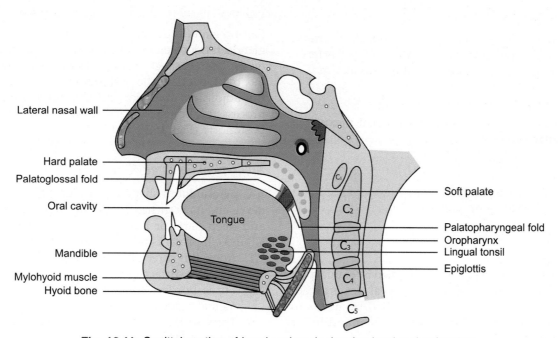

Fig. 16.11: Sagittal section of head and neck showing hard and soft palate

surface forms the floor of nasal cavity and the inferior surface forms the roof of the oral cavity. Anteriorly and laterally, the hard palate becomes continuous with the alveolar arch (formed by alveolar process of bilateral maxillae) and gums. The posterior margin of hard palate is free and provides attachment to the soft palate.

Soft Palate

Soft palate is a mobile muscular fold suspended from the posterior border of the hard palate like a curtain or velum. It separates the nasopharynx from oropharynx. Inferior border is free and forms the anterior boundary of the pharyngeal isthmus. A conical, small tongue like projection hangs from its middle and is called the uvula. On each side, from the base of uvula, two curved folds of mucous membrane extend laterally and downwards.

1. **Palatoglossal fold:** It is the anterior fold which merges inferiorly with the sides of the tongue at the junction of its oral and pharyngeal parts. The palatoglossal fold contains the palatoglossal muscle. It forms the lateral boundary of the oropharyngeal isthmus and the anterior boundary of tonsillar fossa.
2. **Palatopharyngeal fold:** It lies posterior to the palatoglossal fold and merges inferiorly with the lateral wall of the pharynx. The palatopharyngeal fold contains the palatopharyngeus muscle and forms the posterior boundary of the tonsillar fossa.

The soft palate consists of five pairs of muscles namely tensor palati, levator palati, musculus uvulae, palatoglossus, palatopharyngeus.

Arterial Supply of Palate

1. Greater palatine artery, branch of maxillary artery.
2. Ascending palatine artery, branch of facial artery.
3. Palatine branch of ascending pharyngeal artery.

Venous Drainage of Palate

Venous blood drains into the pharyngeal plexus via paratonsillar veins

Lymphatic Drainage of Palate

1. Retropharyngeal nodes
2. Deep cervical lymph nodes

Nerve Supply of Palate

1. **Motor supply**
   a. All muscles of palate are supplied by cranial part of accessory nerve via pharyngeal plexus except tensor palati which is supplied by nerve to medial pterygoid, a branch of mandibular nerve.

   b. **Secretomotor supply to palatine glands:** preganglionic fibres arise in superior salivatory ganglion and post-ganglionic fibres arise from pterygopalatine ganglion and run in the greater and lesser palatine nerves to supply the palatine glands.
2. **Sensory supply:** It is via greater and lesser palatine nerves, sphenopalatine nerves and glossopharyngeal nerves.

Functions of Palate

1. Hard palate separates the oral cavity from nasal cavity.
2. Soft palate separates the oropharynx from nasopharynx. During swallowing food does not enter the nose.
3. Soft palate isolates the oral cavity from oropharynx during chewing so that breathing is unaffected.
4. Soft palate helps to modify the quality of voice, by varying the degree of closure of the pharyngeal isthmus.

SALIVARY GLANDS

A number of salivary glands are scattered throughout the oral cavity. There are primarily three pairs of large salivary glands nemely (Fig. 16.12):

1. Parotid gland, beside the ear
2. Submandibular gland, below the mandible
3. Sublingual gland, below the tongue

Secretions from all these glands help keep the oral cavity moist and begin the process of digestion.

Parotid Gland (G:Para = near, Otis = ear)

Parotid gland is the largest of the three pairs of salivary glands. It is located under the skin and superficial fascia on the lateral aspect of face, below the external acoustic meatus. It overlaps the posterior ramus of mandible and the adjoining masseter muscle, anteriorly, mastoid process and upper part of sternocleidomastoid muscle, posteriorly (Figs 16.12 and 16.13).

Anatomical Features

It is pyramidal in shape and weighs 25 gm. The facial nerve and its branches divide the gland into superficial and deep parts or lobes which are connected by an isthmus. It presents with following features:

1. Apex: It is directed downwards
2. Superior surface or base
3. Three borders namely, anterior, posterior and medial border.
4. Three surfaces namely superficial or lateral surface, anteromedial and anterolateral surface.

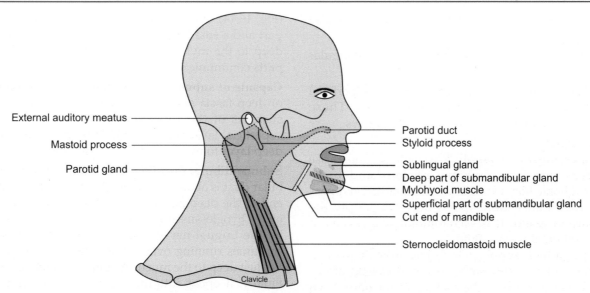

Fig. 16.12: Diagrammatic representation of location of salivary glands

The following structures emerged out of the anterior border of parotid gland in a radiating manner.
a. Zygomatic branch of facial nerve
b. Transverse facial vessels
c. Upper buccal branch of facial nerve
d. Parotid duct
e. Lower buccal branch of facial nerve
f. Marginal mandibular branch of facial nerve

Capsules of parotid gland: Parotid gland is enclosed in two layers of capsule:
1. **False capsule:** It is formed by the tough investing layer of deep cervical fascia.

2. **True capsule:** It is formed by the condensation of fibrous tissue of parotid gland.

Structure of Parotid Gland

It is a compound tubulo-alveolar gland. The acini are lined by seromucinous cells which open into collecting ducts. A number of collecting ducts unite and form the parotid duct.

The parotid duct: It is 5 cm long. It emerges from the middle of the anterior border of the gland and runs forwards over the masseter. It opens into the vestibule of mouth opposite the second upper molar tooth.

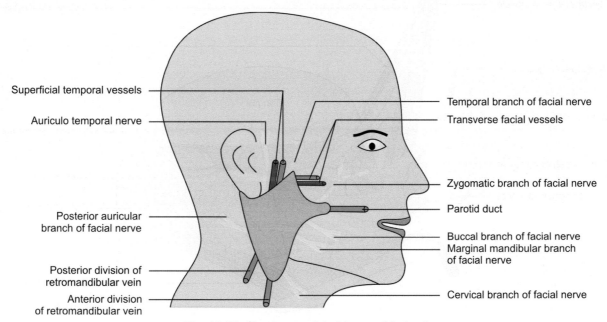

Fig. 16.13: Structures related to parotid gland

Arterial supply: It is derived from branches of external carotid artery.

Venous drainage: Veins drain into the external jugular vein.

Lymphatic drainage: Lymphatics drain into superficial and deep parotid group of lymph nodes. These ultimately end in the deep cervical lymph nodes.

Nerve Supply

1. **Parasympathetic supply:** Preganglionic fibres arise from inferior salivatory nucleus and post-ganglionic fibres arise from otic ganglion and pass through auriculotemporal nerve to supply the parotid gland. It is secretomotor and results in secretion of watery fluid.
2. **Sympathetic supply:** It is derived from the sympathetic plexus around the external carotid artery which is formed by the postganglionic fibres from superior cervical sympathetic ganglion. It is secretomotor and results in production of mucus rich sticky secretion. It is also vasomotor to the gland.
3. **Sensory supply:** It is derived from
   a. Auriculotemporal nerve.
   b. Great auricular nerve.
   c. C_2 is sensory to parotid fascia.

Submandibular Salivary Gland

It is about half the size of the parotid gland and lies below the mandible, in the anterior part of the digastric triangle (Fig. 16.14). It consists of two parts, a large superficial part and a smaller deep part, which lie superficial and deep to the mylohyoid muscle respectively. The two parts communicate with each other posteriorly.

Capsule of submandibular gland: The investing layer of deep fascia splits to cover the inferior and medial surfaces of the superficial part of the gland. The superficial layer gets attached to base of mandible and deep layer to mylohyoid line on mandible.

Submandibular duct (Wharton's duct): The submandibular duct is about 5 cm long. It emerges at the anterior end of the deep part and runs forwards and medially on the hyoglossus muscle under mylohyoid. It is crossed by the lingual nerve from lateral to medial side. It continues running over the sublingual gland. Here, it lies just deep to the mucus membrane of the oral cavity. Finally, it opens into oral cavity on the summit of a sublingual papilla at the side of the frenulum of tongue.

Arterial supply: It is supplied by branches of facial and lingual arteries.

Venous drainage: Veins run along with corresponding arteries and drain into the internal jugular vein.

Lymphatic drainage: Lymphatics drain into submandibular lymph nodes and then into jugulodigastric lymph nodes.

Nerve Supply

1. **Parasympathetic or secretomotor supply:** Preganglionic fibres arise from superior salivatory nucleus.

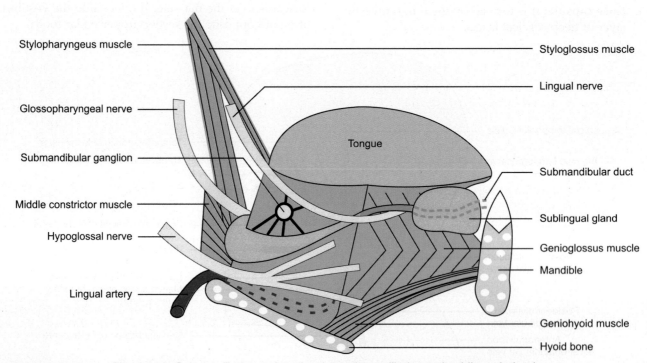

Fig. 16.14: Submandibular region showing submandibular and sublingual glands

They pass successively through the facial nerve, chorda tympani nerve, lingual nerve and relay into the submandibular ganglion. Postganglionic fibres arise from cells of the ganglion and directly supply the gland. It is secretomotor and causes secretion of watery fluid.

2. **Sympathetic supply:** It is derived from the sympathetic plexus around facial artery formed by postganglionic fibres from superior cervical sympathetic ganglion. It is secretomotor and results in secretion of mucus rich fluid. It is also vasomotor.

3. **Sensory supply:** Lingual nerve.

Sublingual Salivary Gland (Fig. 16.4)

This is the smallest of the three pairs of salivary glands. It lies immediately below the mucosa of the floor of the mouth. It is almond-shaped and rests in the sublingual fossa on the inner aspect of the body of mandible. It is separated from the base of the tongue by the submandibular duct. The gland pours its secretion by a series of ducts, about 10 to 15 in number, into the oral cavity on the sublingual fold. The vascular and nerve supply is similar to that of submandibular salivary gland.

Histology of Salivary Glands

- Salivary glands are tubulo-alveolar type of glands. The secretory element may be acinar, alveolar, tubulo-acinar, tubular or tubulo-alveolar type (Fig. 16.15).
- Each gland is enclosed by a connective tissue capsule which send numerous septae into the substance of the gland forming lobules. Each lobule has two parts:

1. **Secretory part:** Secretory component contains either mucous cells or serous cells. At places mucous alveoli are covered by a group of serous cells on one side which are known as demilunes. Serous acini are formed by pyramidal cells with a spherical nucleus located at the base. Secretory granules are present towards the apices of the cells. Mucous acini are formed by columnar cells with flattened nuclei present at the base of cell. Mucus acini are larger that serous acini.

2. **Conducting part:** Each acini is drained by intercalated ducts which join together to form intralobular and then inter-lobular ducts.

- **Other components of salivary gland**
  a. **Myoepithelial cells:** These cells are present between the basal lamina and epithelial cells of the alveoli and intercalated ducts. They are contractile in nature and help in pouring out the secretion.
  b. Ig A secreting plasma cells are present in the alveolar connective tissue.

Characteristics of Different Salivary Glands

- Parotid gland is predominantly serous.
- Submandibular gland is mixed and contains both serous and mucinous components. Demilunes are characteristically present in this gland.
- Sublingual glands are predominantly of mucous type.

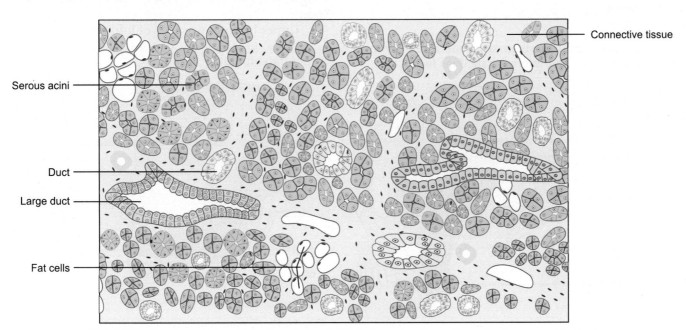

Serous acini

Duct

Large duct

Fat cells

Connective tissue

Fig. 16.15: Section of Parotid (salivary gland) (Stain-hematoxylin-eosin under low magnification)

Muscles of Mastication

Four pairs of muscles move the mandible during mastication. They are (Figs 16.16 and 16.17):
1. Temporalis
2. Medial pterygoid
3. Lateral pterygoid
4. Masseter

They present with the following features:
a. All muscles except masseter are located in the infratemporal region.
b. They are inserted in the ramus of mandible.
c. All four muscles are innervated by branches of the anterior division and trunk of mandibular nerve which is the branch of trigeminal nerve.
d. Their vascular supply is derived from branches of maxillary vessels.
e. All act on the temporomandibular joint.

Temporalis

It is fan shaped, anterior fibers are verticle while posterior fibers are almost horizontal with intermediate fibers of variable degrees of obliquity (Fig. 16.16).

Origin: Floor of temporal fossa upto inferior temporal line, under surface of temporal fascia.

Insertion: The fibres converge to form a tendon which passes down from temporal fossa, medial to anterior part of zygomatic arch and inserts on tip, anterior and posterior borders and medial surface of coronoid process of mandible and adjoining anterior border of ramus of mandible.

Actions: The two muscles act together
1. Anterior and middle fibres elevate mandible to occlude the teeth.
2. Posterior fibres retract the mandible after protrusion.

Masseter

It is quadrilateral in shape and has three layers—superficial, deep and intermediate (Fig. 16.16).

Origin: Lower border and inner surface of zygomatic arch.

Insertion: Large central area on outer surface of ramus of mandible and adjoining surface of coronoid process of mandible.

Actions: Both muscles act together
1. Elevation of mandible to approximate the teeth.
2. Retraction of mandible.
3. Superficial fibres help in protrusion of mandible.

Medial Pterygoid

It is a thick quadrilateral muscle (Fig. 16.17).

Origin: It originates from two heads:
1. **Superficial head:** Maxillary tuberosity on infratemporal surface of maxilla and adjoining surface of pyramidal process of palatine bone.
2. **Deep head:** It is larger and arises from medial surface of lateral pterygoid plate of sphenoid bone.

Insertion: Medial surface of ramus of mandible postero-inferior to the mylohyoid groove and adjoining inner aspect of angle of mandible.

Actions: The two muscles act together
1. Assist in elevation of mandible.
2. Along with lateral pterygoid muscles they cause protrusion of mandible.
3. Help in side to side movements of the jaw and grinding of food between teeth on each side.

Lateral Pterygoid

It is the key muscle of the pterygopalatine fossa (Fig. 16.17).

Origin: It is a short thick muscle which arises from two heads:
1. **Upper head:** Lower part of infratemporal surface of the greater wing of sphenoid and adjoining infratemporal crest.

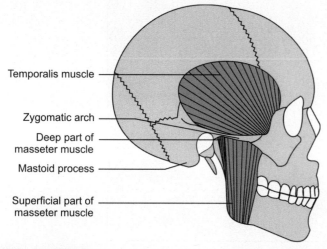

Fig. 16.16: Attachment of temporalis and masseter muscles

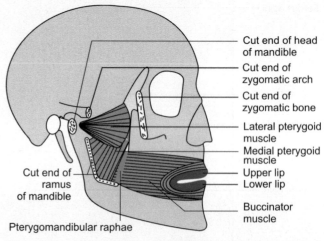

Fig. 16.17: Diagrammatic representation of attachment of lateral pterygoid, medial pterygoid and buccinator muscles

2. Lower head: It is larger and arises from lateral surface of lateral pterygoid plate of sphenoid bone.

Insertion: Both heads converge as a single tendon to insert on the pterygoid fovea in the anterior surface of neck of mandible and adjoining articular disc and capsule of temporomandibular joint.

Actions: The two muscles act together
1. Assist in depression of mandible to open jaw.
2. Protrusion of mandible.
3. Help in side to side movements of the jaw and grinding of food between teeth on each side.

Accessory Muscle of Mastication: Buccinator

Origin: Upper fibres arise from outer surface of the alveolar process of maxilla opposite the molar teeth, middle fibres arise from pterygomandibular raphe and lower fibres arise from outer surface of alveolar process of mandible, opposite the molar teeth.

Insertion: Upper fibres pass straight to the upper lip, lower fibres pass straight to the lower lip, middle fibres decussate and then pass to both the upper and lower lips.

Nerve supply: Buccal branch of the facial nerve.

Actions:
1. Flattens the cheek against the gum and teeth.
2. Prevents accumulation of food in the vestibule of mouth and helps to push it back between the teeth of upper and lower jaws. This is why it is named as accessory muscle of mastication.
3. Helps to expel the air between the lips from inflated vestibule as in blowing the trumpet.

PHARYNX

Pharynx is a musculo-fascial tube extending from the base of skull to the oesophagus. It is situated behind the nose, mouth and larynx with which it communicates. It acts as a common channel for both deglutition and respiration (Fig. 16.18).

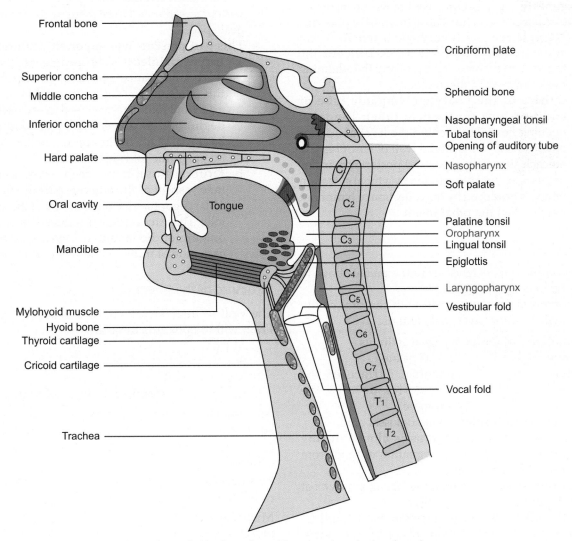

Fig. 16.18: Sagittal section of head and neck showing pharynx

Measurements

Length : 12 to 14 cm
Width : Upper part—3.5 cm, Lower part—1.5 cm

The pharynx is divided into three parts. From above downwards these are

1. Nasopharynx
2. Oropharynx
3. Laryngopharynx

Nasopharynx

- The nasopharynx lies above the soft palate.
- Superiorly, it is limited by the body of sphenoid and basi-occiput.
- It communicates anteriorly with the nasal cavities through posterior nasal aperture
- Inferiorly, it communicates with the oropharynx at the pharyngeal (nasopharyngeal) isthmus.

    Boundaries of Pharyngeal Isthmus
    Anteriorly : Soft palate.
    Posteriorly : Posterior wall of the pharynx.
- Two important structures lie in this part of pharynx.
    a. **Nasopharyngeal (pharyngeal) tonsil:** It is a collection of lymphoid tissue beneath the mucous membrane of the roof and the adjoining posterior wall of this region.
    b. **Orifice of the pharyngotympanic tube or auditory tube (Eustachian tube):** The tubal opening lies 1.2 cm behind the level of inferior nasal concha in the lateral wall of nasopharynx on each side. The upper and posterior margins of this opening are bounded by a tubal elevation which is produced by the collection of lymphoid tissue called the **tubal tonsil.**

Oropharynx (Fig. 16.18)

- The oropharynx extends from the palate above to the tip of epiglottis below.
- It communicates anteriorly with the oral cavity through the oropharyngeal isthmus.

    Boundaries of Oropharyngeal Isthmus
    Above : Soft palate.
    Below : Dorsal surface of the posterior third of the tongue.
    Lateral (on each side) : Palatoglossal arch.
    The oropharyngeal isthmus is closed during deglutition to prevent regurgitation of food from pharynx into the mouth.
- Inferiorly, it continues with the laryngopharynx at the upper border of epiglottis.
- Posteriorly oropharynx lies over the C_2 and C_3 vertebrae separated from them by the retro-pharyngeal space and its contents.

- The lateral wall on each side presents with
    a. **Tonsillar fossa:** A triangular fossa which lodges the palatine tonsil.
    b. **Palato-glossal arch:** Fold of mucus membrane which forms the anterior wall of the fossa.
    c. **Palato-pharyngeal arch:** Fold of mucus membrane which forms the posterior wall of the tonsillar fossa.

Laryngopharynx (Fig. 16.18)

- Laryngopharynx extends from the upper border of epiglottis to the level of C_6 vertebra from where it continues caudally as the esophagus.
- In its upper part, it communicates anteriorly with the laryngeal cavity through the laryngeal inlet. Below the inlet, its anterior wall is formed by the posterior surfaces of arytenoids and lamina of cricoid cartilages.
- Posteriorly it overlies the bodies of C_4, C_5 and C_6 vertebrae, separated from them by the retropharyngeal space.
- **This part presents two important features**
    a. **Laryngeal inlet:** It is the opening into the larynx. It is bounded antero-posteriorly on each side by the epiglottis, aryepiglottic folds and inter-arytenoid fold. The laryngeal inlet closes during deglutition to prevent entry of food into the laryngeal cavity by the approximation of the two aryepiglottic folds in midline.
    b. **Piriform fossa:** It is a deep recess seen in the inner aspect of the anterior part of lateral wall of laryngopharynx, on each side of the laryngeal inlet. These recesses are produced due to inward bulging of the lamina of thyroid cartilage on each side of midline into this part of pharynx.

Structure of the Pharynx

The wall of the pharynx consists of following layers. From within outwards these are

1. Mucosa
2. Submucosa
3. Muscular coat
4. Loose areolar sheath or the buccopharyngeal fascia

Mucosa: The mucosa of pharynx is made up of stratified squamous epithelium except, in the region of naso-pharynx where it is lined by ciliated pseudo stratified columnar epithelium.

Submucosa: The submucosa is thick and fibrous. It is called the pharyngobasilar fascia.

Muscular coat: The muscular coat consists of striated muscles which are arranged in an outer circular layer and an inner longitudinal layer.

1. Circular layer also known as constrictor muscle layer forms the main bulk of the muscular coat of Pharynx. It consists of three constrictor muscles which are arranged like flower pots placed one inside the other but are open in front for communication with the nasal, oral and laryngeal cavities. These are
   a. Superior constrictor
   b. Middle constrictor
   c. Inferior constrictor

   They aid in deglutition by the coordinated contractions.
2. The longitudinal coat comprises of three pairs of longitudinal muscles
   a. Stylopharyngeus
   b. Palatopharyngeus
   c. Salpingopharyngeus

   They elevate the larynx and shorten the pharynx during swallowing. At the same time palatopharyngeal sphincter closes the pharyngeal isthmus.

Loose areolar sheath of the pharynx: A loose areolar membrane also called the 'buccopharyngeal fascia' covers the outer surface of the muscular coat of pharynx. It extends anteriorly across the pterygomandibular raphe to cover the outer surface of the buccinator also.

Nerve Supply of the Pharynx

1. **Motor supply:** All the pharyngeal muscles are supplied by the cranial root of accessory nerve via pharyngeal branch of vagus and pharyngeal plexus except the stylopharyngeus which is supplied by the glossopharyngeal nerve.
2. **Sensory supply**
   a. Nasopharynx, by pharyngeal branch of the pterygo-palatine ganglion which carries fibres from maxillary division of trigeminal nerve
   b. Oropharynx, by glossopharyngeal nerve
   c. Laryngopharynx, by the internal laryngeal nerve.

Pharyngeal Plexus of Nerves

The pharyngeal plexus of nerves lies between the buccopharyngeal fascia and the muscular coat of middle constrictor. It is formed by the following nerves
1. Pharyngeal branch of vagus carrying fibres from cranial part of the accessory nerves.
2. Pharyngeal branch of the glossopharyngeal nerve.
3. Pharyngeal branch from superior cervical sympathetic ganglion.

ESOPHAGUS

It is a muscular tube of the gastrointestinal tract. It extends from the lower end of pharynx (lower border

of C_6 vertebra) to the cardiac orifice of stomach (T_{11} vertebra) (Fig. 16.19).

Measurements
Length : 25 cm
Width : 2 cm

The lumen is flat anteroposteriorly and opens up only to allow passage to bolus of food.

Anatomical Features

- It has three parts
  1. **Cervical part (4 cm):** Esophagus passes behind the trachea, in front of prevertebral fascia over C_6 and C_7 vertebrae in the neck
  2. **Thoracic part (20 cm):** It runs through the posterior part of superior mediastinum behind the trachea and arch of aorta. Then it passes through posterior mediastinum, in front and to the right of descending aorta.
  3. **Abdominal part (1.25 cm):** It pierces the diaphragm at level of T_{10} vertebra to end in the cardiac end of stomach. This lies at level of T_{11} vertebra, 2.5 cm to the left of median plane.
- It presents with slight curvatures externally and constrictions internally. There are four curvatures:
  1. The esophagus curves in the anteroposterior planes corresponding to the curvatures of the cervical and thoracic spine.
  2. It also presents with two lateral curves both on left side which are seen at the following sites:

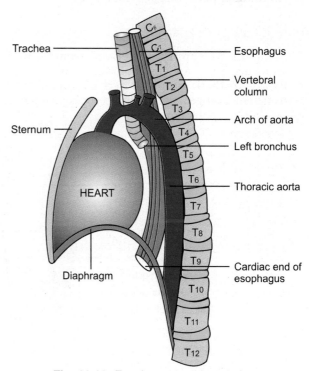

Fig. 16.19: Esophagus and its relations

a. At the upper end, at its beginning (C_6 vertebra)
b. Near the lower end, opposite T_6 to T_7 vertebra.

There are four constrictions of esophagus seen at the following sites:
1. At its origin.
2. At the site of crossing of arch of aorta over it.
3. At the crossing of left bronchus over it.
4. At its opening in the diaphragm.

Arterial Supply of Esophagus

Esophagus is supplied by branches of following arteries:
1. Inferior thyroid artery
2. Descending thoracic aorta
3. Bronchial artery
4. Left gastric artery
5. Inferior phrenic artery

Venous Drainage of Esophagus

The various parts of esophagus are drained as follows:
1. **Cervical part:** Inferior thyroid vein
2. **Thoracic part:** Azygos vein and hemiazygos vein
3. **Abdominal part:** Left gastric vein (belongs to portal system)

Lymphatic Drainage of Esophagus

The various parts of esophagus are drained as follows:
1. **Cervical part:** Deep cervical and retropharyngeal lymph nodes.
2. **Thoracic part:** Paratracheal, tracheobronchial, posterior mediastinal lymph nodes.
3. **Abdominal part:** Coeliac lymph nodes.

Nerve Supply of Esophagus

1. **Sympathetic supply:** Is derived from T_5 to T_9 segments. These are vasomotor in function.
2. **Parasympathetic supply:** Is derived from bilateral recurrent laryngeal nerves and oesophageal plexus from vagus nerves. These nerves are sensory, motor and secretomotor to esophagus.

STOMACH

It is also called as ventriculus. It is a muscular bag which acts as a reservoir for food (Fig. 16.20). It extends from lower end of esophagus to beginning of small intestine that is duodenum.

Location : It lies in epigastrium, umbilical region and left hypochondrium

Shape : It is variable

Capacity : 30 ml at birth, 1000 ml at puberty, 1500 ml in adults.

Anatomical Features

Stomach can be studied in three parts (Fig. 16.20):
1. **Fundus of stomach:** It is the part of stomach that lies above the level of cardiac orifice. It is filled with air when stomach is empty. On X-ray abdomen, in erect posture, the air is seen as a black shadow in the form of a bubble just below left costal margin.
2. **Body:** It extends from fundus to pylorus.
3. **Pyloric part:** It is a relatively narrow part which extends from lower end of body of stomach to pyloric orifice. It is about 10 cms long. It consists of pyloric antrum, 7.5 cms, which further leads to the pyloric canal, 2.5 cms. They are separated from each other by sulcus intermedius. Pyloric canal ends in pyloric orifice. At the orifice a thick band of circular muscle fibres is present forming a sphincter. It is known as the pyloric sphincter. This regulates entry of food from stomach to duodenum.

Stomach presents with the following external features:
1. **2 openings:** Cardiac orifice, pyloric orifice.
2. **2 curvatures:** Greater curvature, lesser curvature.
3. **2 surfaces:** Anterosuperior and posteroinferior surfaces.

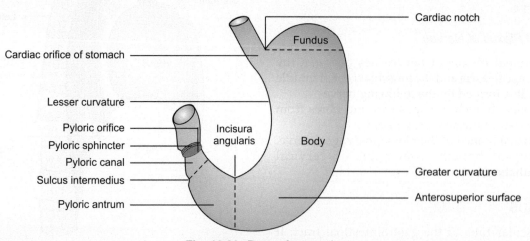

Fig. 16.20: Parts of stomach

Cardiac Orifice

It is present at the junction of esophagus and stomach. It lies on the left of mid line, behind 7th costal cartilage, 2.5 cm lateral to the sternal margin. This corresponds to the level of T_{11} vertebra. **Cardiac notch or incisure** is the acute angle formed between esophagus and greater curvature of stomach, present in relation to cardiac orifice.

Pyloric Orifice

Stomach opens into duodenum via the pyloric orifice. It lies 1.25 cm to the right of midline on the transpyloric plane which passes through L_1 vertebra (when body is supine and stomach is empty). A circular pyloric constriction is present at this end. It is identified with the help of presence of **prepyloric vein.**

Lesser Curvature

It is the posterosuperior or medial border which extends from medial aspect of greater curvature cardiac orifice to pyloric orifice. The most dependent part of lesser curvature is **incisure angularis.**

Greater Curvature

It lies anteroinferiorly and is 4 to 5 times longer than lesser curvature. It extends from cardiac incisure to pyloric orifice. From cardiac orifice the curvature arches upwards posterolaterally upto the 5th costal cartilage on left side to form the **fundus.** It then curves downwards, medially and anteriorly with convexity to the left side to end at pyloric orifice. It presents with a bulge called **pyloric antrum** at the lower end opposite the incisura angularis.

Anterosuperior Surface

It is covered with peritoneum and lies behind the left 6th to 9th ribs and the intervening intercostal spaces which separates it from the anterior abdominal wall. It is related to liver on the upper right side and diaphragm laterally which separates it from left pleura, base of left lung and pericardium superiorly.

Posteroinferior Surface

It is covered with peritoneum and lies on the following structures which form the **stomach bed** (Fig. 16.21).
- Left crus of diaphragm
- Left suprarenal gland
- Anterior surface of left kidney
- Splenic artery

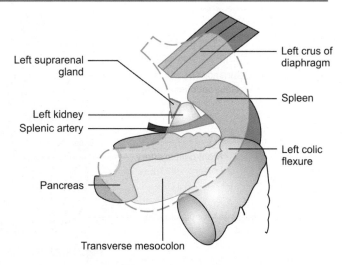

Fig. 16.21: Structures forming stomach bed

- Anterior pancreatic surface
- Left colic flexure
- Transverse mesocolon
- Anterior surface of spleen

Peritoneal Relations of Stomach

Stomach is an intraperitoneal organ and is covered on both surfaces with peritoneum.
1. **Lesser omentum:** Formed by upward continuation of the anterior and posterior layers of peritoneum from lesser curvature of stomach.
2. **Greater omentum:** Along the greater curvature the two peritoneal layers meet and continue downwards as the greater omentum.
3. **Gastrosplenic ligament:** At the cardiac end of greater curvature the two layers of peritoneum meet and extend toward spleen. This forms the gastrosplenic ligament
4. **Gastrophrenic ligament:** At the upper end of posterior surface, the posterior layer of peritoneum gets reflected onto the diaphragm as the gastrophrenic ligament. This small area of posterior surface of stomach above the ligament is the bare area of stomach, which lies in direct contact with diaphragm.

Blood Supply of Stomach (Fig.16.22)

Stomach is supplied by following arteries
1. Left gastric artery, branch of celiac trunk
2. Right gastric artery, branch of hepatic artery proper
3. Short gastric arteries, branch from splenic artery
4. Right gastroepiploic artery, branch of splenic artery
5. Left gastroepiploic artery, branch of gastroduodenal artery
6. Posterior gastric arteries, branches of splenic artery.

CHAPTER-16

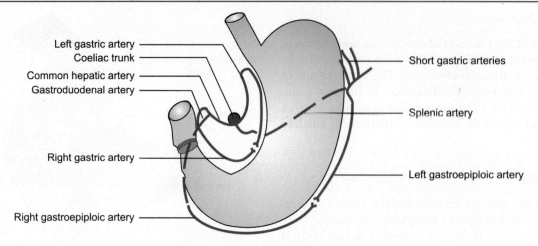

Fig. 16.22: Arterial supply of stomach

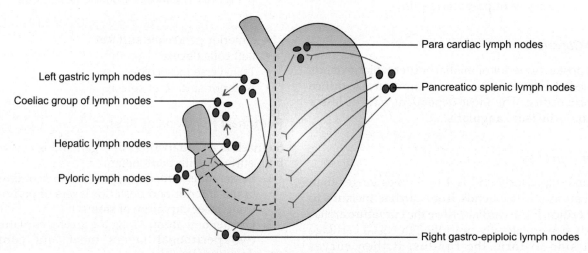

Fig. 16.23: Lymphatic drainage of stomach

Veins of Stomach

The veins run along with the corresponding arteries
1. Right gastroepiploic vein, drains into superior mesenteric vein.
2. Right and left gastric veins, drain into portal vein.
3. Short gastric vein, left gastroepiploic vein and posterior gastric vein, drain into splenic vein.

Lymphatic Drainage of Stomach

A line is drawn from the cardiac orifice vertically downwards (Fig. 16.23).
The part right to this line drains into
1. Hepatic group of lymph nodes
2. Pyloric group of lymph nodes
3. Right gastroepiploic group of lymph nodes
4. Left gastric group of lymph nodes
The part of the stomach left to this line drains into
1. Paracardiac group of lymph nodes
2. Pancreaticosplenic group of lymph nodes

Efferents drain into coeliac group of pre-aortic lymph nodes

Nerve Supply of Stomach
1. **Sympathetic supply:** Preganglionic fibres are derived from T_6 to T_9 segments of spinal cord.
2. **Parasympathetic supply:** It is derived from gastric branches of vagus nerve which form anterior and posterior vagal trunks.

SMALL INTESTINE

It is the primary site of digestion and absorption of food. It extends from the pylorus of stomach to the ileo-caecal junction and is 6 metres long (Fig. 16.24). It is divided into three parts:
1. **Duodenum:** It is 25 cm long and is retroperitoneal.
2. **Jejunum:** It is the second part of the small intestine. It is mobile and intraperitonal.
3. **Ileum:** It is the last part of the small intestine. It is also intraperitoneal.

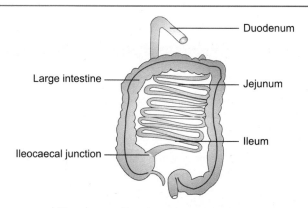

Fig. 16.24: Small and large intestine

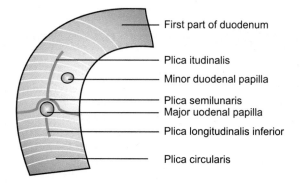

Fig. 16.26: Interior of second part of duodenum

Duodenum

It means equal to twelve fingers. It is devoid of mesentery. It forms a C-shaped curve (Fig. 16.25).

Anatomical Features
Duodenum has four parts:
1. **First part of duodenum:** It is 2 inches or 5 cm long. It is 2.5 cm on surface projection. It is directed upwards, backwards and towards the right. It lies at the level of L_1 vertebra.
2. **Second part of duodenum:** It is 3 inches or 8 cm long. It lies at the level of L_1 to L_3 vertebrae in the right paravertebral gutter. Interior of 2nd part of duodenum presents the following features (Fig. 16.26)
   a. **Plica circularis:** These are permanent circular folds of mucosa. They are not seen in Ist part of duodenum.
   b. **Major duodenal papilla:** It lies 8 to 10 cm caudal from the pylorus. Ampulla of Vater which is the common opening of pancreatic duct and common bile duct opens at its summit.
   c. **Minor duodenal papilla:** It lies 2 cm above the major papilla. Accessory pancreatic duct opens at this level.
   d. **Plica semicircularis:** It is a semilunar fold present above major duodenal papilla.
   e. **Plica longitudinalis:** It is a longitudinal fold of mucus membrane and indicates the course of bile duct in duodenal wall.

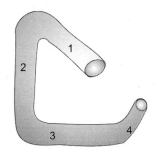

Fig. 16.25: Parts of duodenum

3. **Third part of duodenum:** It is 4 inches or 10 cm long. It lies at the level of L_3.
4. **Fourth part of duodenum:** It is 1 inch or 2.5 cm long. It lies 1.25 cm below the transpyloric plane and 1.5 cm to the left of median plane. It lies at the level of L_3, L_2 vertebrae.

Suspensory Ligament of Treitz

It is a fibro muscular band which extends from the right crus of diaphragm to duodenojejunal flexure.

Arterial Supply of Duodenum

Duodenum is supplied by following arteries
1. Supraduodenal branch of gastroduodenal artery
2. Retroduodenal branch of gastroduodenal artery
3. Infraduodenal branch of right gastroepiploic artery
4. Superior and inferior pancreaticoduodenal arteries.

Lymphatic Drainage of Duodenum

Lymphatics of duodenum drain into pancreatico-duodenal group of lymph nodes

Nerve Supply of Duodenum

1. **Sympathetic supply:** Preganglionic fibres are derived from T_6 to T_9 segments of spinal cord.
2. **Parasympathetic supply:** It is through vagus.

Jejunum and Ileum

Jejunum forms the upper 2/5th and ileum forms the lower 3/5th of mobile part of small intestine (Fig. 16.24).

Blood Supply of Jejunum and Ileum

Jejunum and ileum are supplied by superior mesenteric artery, branch of abdominal aorta. They are drained by the corresponding veins.

Lymphatic Drainage of Jejunum and Ileum

The lymphatics pass via the mesentery to superior mesenteric lymph nodes.

Differences between Jejunum and Ileum

Character	Jejunum	Ileum
Gross features:		
1. Wall	Thicker	Thinner
2. Lumen	Wider (4 cm diameter) and often found empty.	Narrower (3.5 cm diameter) and often found full.
3. Vascularity	More vascular.	Less vascular.
4. Circular folds (plicae circulares)	Large and closely set.	Small and sparsely set.
5. Mesentery	i. Thinner near the gut. ii. Jejunal arteries are wider. iii. Arterial arcades are 1 or 2 in number. iv. Vasa recti are longer and fewer. v. Presence of peritoneal windows between the vasa recti due to paucity of fat near the gut.	i. Thicker near the gut. ii. Ileal arteries are narrower. iii. Arterial arcades are 5 or 6 in number. iv. Vasa recti are shorter and numerous. v. No peritoneal windows due to presence of abundant fat between the vasa recti.
Microscopic features:		
6. Villi	More in number, larger, thicker and leaf like.	Less in number, shorter, thinner and finger like.
7. Aggregates of lymphatic follicles (Peyer's patches)	Small, circular and few in number.	Large, oval and more in number.

LARGE INTESTINE

It extends from ileocaecal junction to the anus (Fig. 16.27). It is responsible for reabsorption of water and solutes from the undigested food particles and the final expulsion of faeces. It is about 1.5 metres long and is divided into

1. Caecum
2. Appendix
3. Ascending colon
4. Transverse colon
5. Descending colon
6. Sigmoid colon
7. Rectum
8. Anal canal

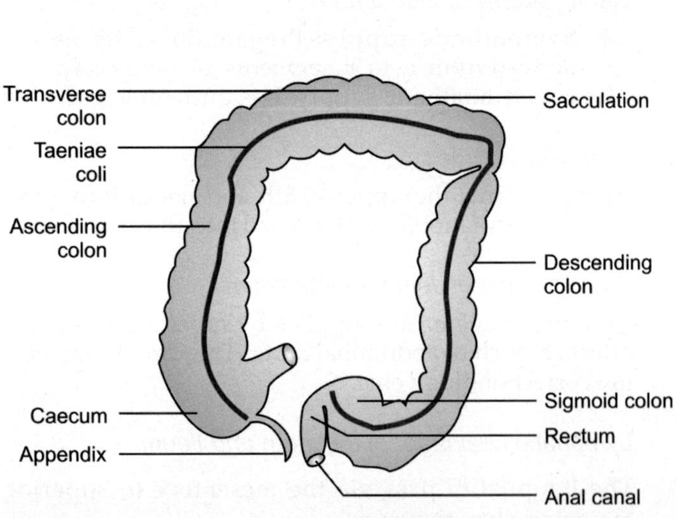

Caecum

Caecum means blind end. Caecum is the beginning of large intestine. It lies in the right iliac fossa (Fig. 16.28).

Size: 6 cm in length and 7.5 cm in width.
It is covered by peritoneum from all sides.

Interior of Caecum

Two orifices open into caecum (Fig. 16.28). These are
1. **Ileocaecal orifice:** It is 2.5 cms in diameter. It opens into the posteromedial wall of the caecum and is guarded by a valve.
2. **Appendicular orifice:** It is a small circular opening present 2 cm below and slightly behind the ileocaecal orifice.

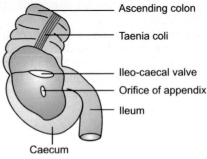

Fig. 16.28: Interior of caecum

Arterial supply of caecum: It is supplied by anterior and posterior caecal arteries, branches of inferior division of ileocolic artery (Fig. 16.30).

Venous drainage of caecum: Veins drain into ileocolic vein hence in portal system.

Fig. 16.27: Large intestine

Lymphatic drainage of caecum: Lymphatics drain into ileocolic group of lymph nodes.

Nerve supply of caecum
1. **Sympathetic supply:** Preganglionic fibres are derived from T_{10} to L_1 segments of spinal cord.
2. **Parasympathetic supply** is from vagus nerve.

Appendix (Figs 16.29 and 16.30)

It is also known as **vermiform** (worm like) **appendix**. It is a tubular structure that extends from the postero-medial wall of caecum.
Length: It is variable, between 2 to 20 cm.

Presenting Parts

It has a base, body and tip. It is covered with a peritoneal fold known as mesoappendix.
1. **Base:** It is attached to the postero-medial wall of caecum about 2 cm below ileo-caecal junction.
2. **Body:** It is long, narrow with a lumen. Lumen opens into the caecum
3. **Tip:** It is directed in various positions. It is least vascular part of the appendix.

Positions of Appendix

Base of the appendix is fixed but the position of tip varies. Therefore, position of appendix is defined in respect of position of tip (Fig. 16.29).
1. **Retrocaecal:** It is the commonest position of appendix. It is found in 60% population. It lies at 12'o clock position and is present behind the caecum.
2. **Pelvic position:** It is second commonest position found in 30%. It lies at 4'o clock position.
3. **Splenic:** Present in 1 to 2%. Tip of the appendix passes upwards and medially anterior or posterior to terminal part of ileum.
4. **Subcaecal or paracolic:** 2% appendix lies below the caecum. It is 11'o clock in position.
5. **Mid inguinal:** Very rare, it is at 6'o clock position
6. **Promontoric:** Very rare again, it is at 3'o clock position.

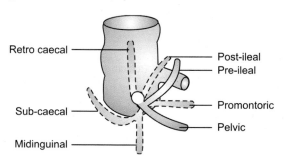

Fig. 16.29: Positions of appendix

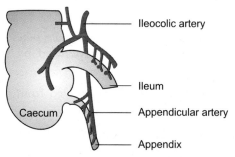

Fig. 16.30: Arterial supply of appendix

Arterial supply of appendix: It is supplied by appendicular artery a branch from inferior division of ileocolic artery. Artery passes behind the terminal part of ileum. Appendicular artery is an end artery (Fig. 16.30).

Venous drainage of appendix: Appendicular vein drains into superior mesenteric vein.

Lymphatic drainage of appendix: Drains into the superior mesenteric lymph nodes.

Nerve Supply of Appendix
1. **Sympathetic supply:** Preganglionic fibres are derived from T_{10} spinal cord segment. Post ganglionic fibres are derived from superior mesenteric plexus.
2. **Parasympathetic supply** is from both vagus nerves.

Ascending Colon

It is about 15 cms long and extends from the caecum to the hepatic flexure which is related to inferior surface of the right lobe of liver (Fig. 16.27).

Transverse Colon

It is 45 cms long and extends from hepatic flexure of colon to splenic flexure of colon. In fact, it is not transverse. It hangs down as a loop. It is suspended by the transverse mesocolon. It has a wide range of mobility (Fig. 16.27).

Descending Colon

It is about 25 cms long, It extends from splenic flexure of colon to the beginning of sigmoid colon. It is narrower than the ascending colon (Fig. 16.27).

Flexures of Colon

The junction of transverse colon with ascending and descending colon is seen as right and left bends or flexures. The ascending colon forms right colic flexure (hepatic flexure) and descending colon forms the left colic flexure (splenic flexure) respectively (Fig. 16.27).

Sigmoid Colon

It is about 35 cm long and extends from pelvic brim to 3rd piece of sacrum. It is suspended by sigmoid mesocolon.

Arterial supply to colon: It is derived from marginal artery (see page no. 423).

Lymphatic drainage of colon: Lymphatics from colon drain into the following lymph nodes :
1. Epicolic lymph nodes
2. Paracolic lymph nodes
3. Lymph nodes along the sides of superior and inferior mesenteric vessels.

Nerve supply of colon
1. **Sympathetic supply:** Preganglionic fibres are derived from T_{11} to L_1 spinal segments. Postganglionic fibres are derived from coeliac and superior mesenteric ganglia.
2. **Parasympathetic supply:** It is from both vagus nerves and pelvic splanchnic nerves. Ascending colon and upto right 2/3rd of transverse colon is supplied by vagus nerve. Rest of the colon is supplied by pelvic splanchnic nerve.

RECTUM (FIGs 16.31 and 16.32)

Rectum means straight. However, at the ano-rectal junction it is bent by the pubo-rectalis muscle (a part of levator ani muscle). It extends from the sigmoid colon (S_3 vertebra) to anal canal, which lies 2 to 3 cm below the tip of coccyx.

Length: 12 cm long

Anatomical Features

It can be divided anatomically into three parts:
1. **Upper 1/3rd:** It is directed downwards and back-wards.
2. **Middle 1/3rd:** It is directed vertically downwards.
3. **Lower 1/3rd:** It is directed downwards and for-wards.

It has two **anterioposterior curvatures**
1. Sacral curve: convex backwards
2. Perineal curve: convex forwards

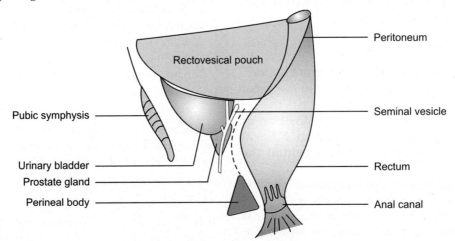

Fig. 16.31: Rectum in male

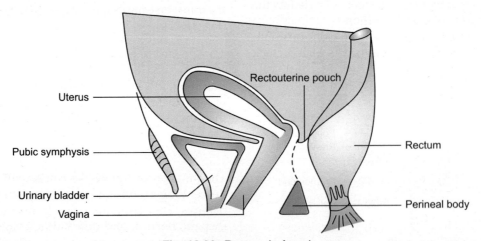

Fig. 16.32: Rectum in female

There are **three lateral curvatures** in rectum
1. Upper curvature: convex towards right
2. Middle curvature: convex towards left
3. Lower curvature: convex towards right

Peritoneal Relations (Figs 16.31 and 16.32)

- Upper 1/3rd of rectum is covered by the peritoneum from three sides.
- The middle 1/3rd has peritoneal covering only anteriorly. It forms rectovaginal pouch in female and rectovesical pouch in male.
- Lower 1/3rd of the rectum is not covered by peritoneum.

Interior of Rectum

The mucosal lining of rectum presents with temporary longitudinal folds that disappear on distention of rectum and few permanent folds. These permanent folds form Houstan's valves. They are semilunar in shape and lie horizontally along the concavity of lateral curves of rectum. Four such valves are present (Fig. 16.33).
1. **1st valve:** It lies opposite S₃ vertebra about 12 cm above anus on the left or right side. It is constant and always present.
2. **3rd valve:** It is always present. It lies anteriorly and in the right wall of the rectum in relation to the middle rectal curve at the level of S₅ vertebra about 5 cm above anus. It divides rectum into upper and lower chambers. The presence of faeces in the upper chamber does not stimulate reflex of defecation while presence of faeces in lower chamber stimulates the defecation reflex. The differentiation between flatus and faeces is done by the degree of tension in the rectum.
3. **2nd valve:** It lies 2.5 cm above the third valve, in relation to left rectal wall.
4. **4th valve:** It is 2.5 cm below the third valve, in relation to left wall of rectum.

Arterial Supply of Rectum
1. **Superior rectal artery:** Principal artery of rectum. It is a branch from inferior mesenteric artery.

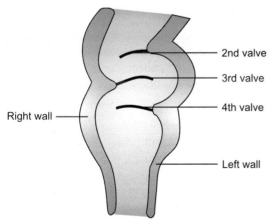

Fig. 16.33: Interior of rectum

2. **Middle rectal artery,** branch from anterior division of internal iliac artery.
3. **Inferior rectal artery,** branch from internal pudendal artery.

Venous Drainage of Rectum

Venous plexus of rectum is known as annulus haemorrhoidalis. It encircles lower part of rectum and anal canal. It has got two sets of venous plexus.
1. **Internal venous plexus:** It lies above the Hilton's line between mucous membrane and sphincter ani and drains into portal system.
2. **External venous plexus:** It lies between the perianal skin and subcutaneous tissue. It drains via pudendal veins into iliac veins (caval system).

Lymphatic Drainage of Rectum

The lymphatics are arranged in two plexuses namely, intramural plexus and external mural plexus. Upper part drains into left common iliac lymph nodes and para rectal lymph nodes. Middle and lower part drain into left internal iliac group of lymph nodes.

Nerve Supply of Rectum

1. **Sympathetic supply:** Preganglionic fibres are derived from L₁ L₂ spinal segments.
2. **Parasympathetic supply:** Preganglionic fibres are derived from S₂ S₃ S₄ spinal segments.

ANAL CANAL

It is the terminal part of the gastro-intestinal tract. It extends from anorectal juction to anal orifice which lies 4 cm below and in front of tip of coccyx (Fig. 16.34). It is separated anteriorly from lower vagina (in female) or bulb of penis (in male) by the perineal body. It is surrounded on each side and posteriorly by the fatty tissue of ischiorectal fossa. A dense connective tissue layer known as anococcygeal ligament attaches the posterior surface of anus to the tip of coccyx.

Length: 3.8 cm

Interior of Anal Canal

It is divided into three parts with help of pectinate and Hilton's lines.

Pectinate line is the muco-cutaneous junction.

Hilton's line: This line indicates the lower end of internal sphincter muscle.
1. **Upper area:** It lies above the pectinate line and is about 1.5 cm in length. It is lined by simple columnar epithelium and presents with the following features:
   a. **Anal columns:** These are also known as columns of Morgagni. These are permanent

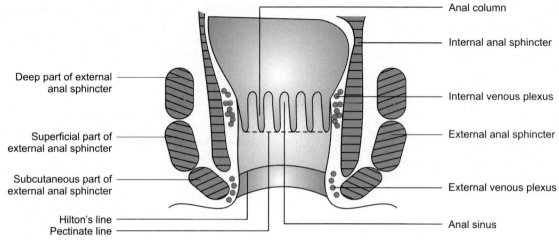

Fig. 16.34: Anal canal

longitudinal folds of mucosa made up of reduplication of mucous membrane containing radicles of superior rectal veins.

  b. **Anal valves:** Anal columns are connected by cresentric, horizontal mucous folds. These folds are known as anal valves. The free margin of these valves is directed upwards.

  c. **Anal papillae:** Epithelial processes projecting from anal valves are known as anal papillae. These present remnants of cloacal membrane.

  d. **Anal sinuses:** Recesses above the anal valves are known as anal sinuses.

  e. **Anal glands:** Floor of the sinuses receives the ducts of tubular glands.

2. **Intermediate area:** It lies between pectinate and Hilton line. It is known as the transitional zone. It is 1.5 cm in length and surrounded by internal rectal venous plexus. This area is lined by stratified squamous epithelium.

3. **Lower area:** 8 mm in length. It is the area below Hilton's line. It is lined by true skin.

Arterial Supply of Anal Canal

Middle and inferior rectal arteries.

Venous Drainage of Anal Canal

1. Upper part drains into the portal system.
2. Lower part, below pectinate line, drains into the caval system.

Lymphatic Drainage of Anal Canal

1. Upper area drains into the internal iliac group of lymph nodes
2. Area below pectinate line drains into superficial group of inguinal lymph nodes.

Nerve Supply of Anal Canal

1. **Above pectinate line:** Sympathetic preganglionic fibres are derived from L_1 and L_2 spinal segments. Parasympathetic preganglionic fibres are derived from S_2, S_3 and S_4 spinal segments.
2. **Below pectinate line:** Inferior rectal nerve provides the somatic supply.

Differences between large and small intestine

	Character	Large intestine	Small intestine
1.	**Length**	1.5 metres	6.5 metres
2.	**Fixity**	For the most part, it is fixed in position. Hence, less mobile.	For the most part, it is less fixed in position. Hence, greater mobility.
3.	**Calibre**	Greater	Lesser
4.	**Sacculations (haustrations)**	Present	Absent
5.	**Taenia coli**	Present	Absent
6.	**Appendices epiploicae**	Present	Absent
7.	**Mucous membrane**		
	a. Circular folds (plicae circulares)	Present	Present
	b. Villi (microscopic feature)	Absent	Present

STRUCTURAL ORGANIZATION OF GASTROINTESTINAL TRACT (GIT)

The gastrointestinal tract from the esophagus to anal canal is a fibromuscular tube made up of the following four layers:

1. Mucus membrane
2. Submucosa
3. Muscularis externa
4. Adventitia or serosa

Mucus Membrane

It further consists of:

1. Epithelium with basement membrane: It is modified according to the function of the part.

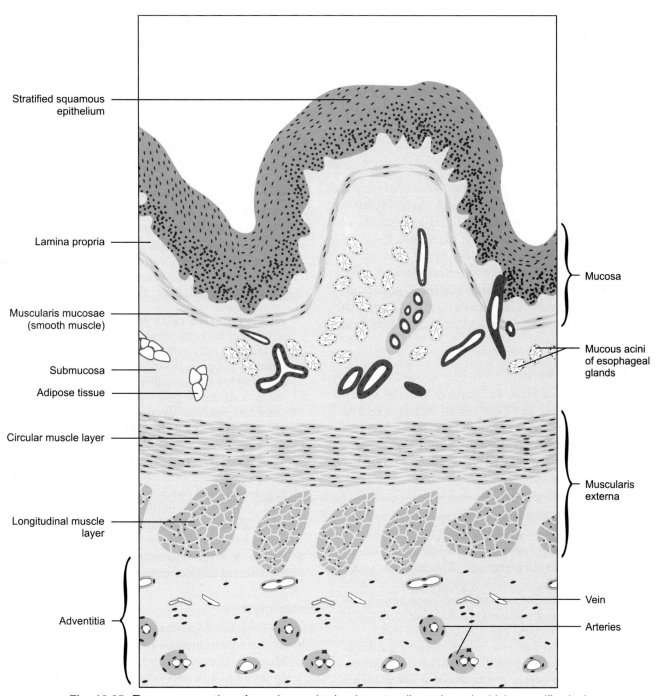

Fig. 16.35: Transverse section of esophagus (stain—hematoxylin-eosin under high magnification)

CHAPTER-16

2. **Lamina propria:** It is the layer of connective tissue that supports the epithelium. It consists of collagen fibers, elastic and reticular fibers with fibroblasts with capillaries of blood and lymph vessels and sensory nerve endings.

3. **Muscularis mucosa:** It is a thin layer of smooth muscle fibers that is arranged is an inner circular layer and an outer longitudinal layer. The contractions of these fibers allow the mixing of intraluminal food content and the ejection of secretions of various intestinal glands.

Submucosa

It primarily consists of loose areolar tissue with blood vessels and lymphatics. A submucous plexus of nerves known as **Meissener's plexus** is present circumferentially in this layer.

Muscularis Externa

It is the definitive muscular layer of the tract and causes the peristaltic movements. It primarily consists of spirally arranged smooth muscle fibers which can be identified as an inner circular layer and outer longitudinal layer. It is modified at sites to form sphincters and taeniae in large intestine. A circumferential plexus of nerves, **myenteric plexus of Auerbach** is present between the circular and longitudinal fasciculi of muscles.

Adventitia or Serosa

It is the outermost layer of connective tissue which carries the branches of blood vessels, lymphatics and nerves to the organ. It consists of visceral layer of peritoneum in parts which are peritoneal, that is, have a mesentery while it is termed adventitia in retroperitoneal parts of the tract.

Esophagus (Fig. 16.35)

It consists of the following layers:
1. **Mucosa:** Lining epithelium is stratified squamous non keratinized epithelium. The mucous membrane is thrown into folds or papillae with a core of lamina propria. Muscularis mucosa is not clearly defined except its lower end. It mainly consists of longitudinal muscle fibers of the lower end.
2. **Submucosa:** It has few mucus secreting tubuloalveolar glands and small lymphoid aggregations.
3. **Muscularis externa:** It consists of striated muscle fibers in upper 1/3rd, striated and smooth muscle fibers in middle 1/3rd and smooth muscle fibers in lower 1/3rd.
4. **Adventitia:** Is the outermost layer of connective tissue with blood vessels and nerves.

Stomach (Fig. 16.36)

It has the following four layers:
1. **Mucosa:** Mucosa is thrown into numerous gentle folds or rugae which disappear when stomach is distended. Lining epithelium is tall columar epithelium with a basal oval nucleus. The apical parts of columnar cells are filled with mucin granules. The lining epithelium invaginates into lamina propria at places to form pits called gastric pits. These are lined by same tall columnar cells and receive openings of gastric glands. Gastric glands are tubular glands lined by three types of cells:
   a. **Chief cells or zymogen cells:** These are cuboidal or low columnar cells with granular, basophilic cytoplasm and a central nucleus. They secrete enzymes like pepsin.
   b. **Oxyntic or parietal cells:** These are large ovoid cells with bright eosinophilic cytoplasm and a central nucleus, scattered between chief cells. They secrete hydrochloric acid.
   c. **Mucus secretory cells:** They are seen near the opening of the gland and consists of tall columnar cells with clear cytoplasm and basal nucleus.
   d. **Argentaffin cells:** They are few flattened endocrine cells present at base of glands that are seen only when stained with silver stain.
   Lamina propria is full of these gastric glands interspersed in connective tissue. Muscularis mucosae is well developed with an inner circular and outer longitudinal layer of smooth muscle fibers.
2. **Submucosa** has connective tissue, blood vessels and nerves.
3. **Muscularis externa:** It has three layers of fibers inner most consists of oblique fibres, middle layer has circular and outer most layer has longitudinal muscle fibres. The circular fibers are thickened and most abundant at the pyloric end forming a sphincter.
4. **Serosa:** It is the outermost covering consisting of the visceral layer of peritoneum.

Small Intestine

The inner surface of intestine has numerous circular folds which has a core of mucosa and submucosa (Fig. 16.37).
1. **Mucosa:** The lining epithelium is tall columnar epithelium. The cells have cytoplasmic extensions in the luminal side forming microvilli giving

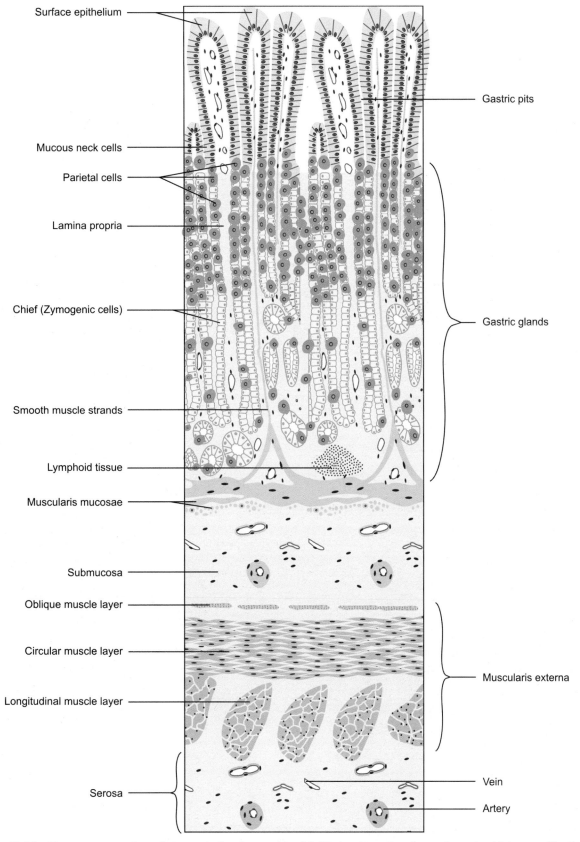

Fig. 16.36: Transverse section of stomach (fundus and body) (Stain—hematoxylin-eosin under high magnification)

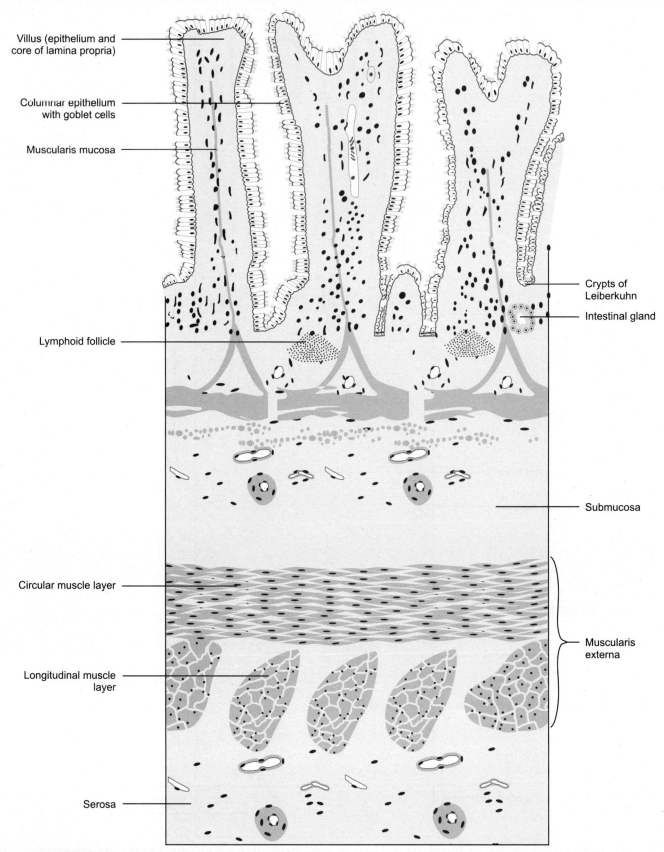

Villus (epithelium and core of lamina propria)

Columnar epithelium with goblet cells

Muscularis mucosa

Lymphoid follicle

Circular muscle layer

Longitudinal muscle layer

Serosa

Crypts of Leiberkuhn

Intestinal gland

Submucosa

Muscularis externa

Fig. 16.37: Transverse section of small intestine (Stain—hematoxylin-eosin under high magnification)

appearance of brush border (seen only on electron microscope magnification). In between columnar cells are present mucus secreting goblet cells these appear flask shaped, with an expanded upper end containing mucinous granules and a flat basal nucleus. The epithelium forms finger like projections on the surface, called villi, which consist of a core of lamina propria with few fibers of muscularis mucosae. Villi are maximally seen in duodenum. The lining epithelium invaginates into lamina propria to form crypts named as **crypts of Leiberkuhn.** The walls of crypts are lined by simple columnar cells. Lamina propria extends into villi and consists of loops of lymphatic and blood vessels. Aggregates of lymphoid follicles called Peyer's patches are seen in lamina propria, most common in ileum. Muscularis mucosae is a thin layer of inner circular and outer longitudinal muscle fibers.

2. **Submucosa:** It consists of loose areolar tissue. In duodenum, it presents with numerous acini of tubulo-alveolar glands known as Brunner's glands. The cells lining the acini are columnar cells with a flat basal nucleus and cytoplasm filled with mucus.

3. **Muscularis externa:** It consists of well developed inner circular and outer longitudinal smooth muscle fibers with intervening myenteric plexus.

4. **Serosa:** It is outermost layer and consists of the visceral peritoneum.

Large Intestine

There is marked variation in structure of various parts of intestine and is described below:

Colon

1. **Mucosa:** The lining epithelium consists of tall columnar cells with brush border. A number of goblet cells are interspersed in between columnar cells. The epithelium invaginats into lamina propria to form crypts of Leiberkuhn. Lamina propria has connective tissue, blood vessels and scattered lymphatic follicles. Muscularis mucosae is a thin layer of inner circular and outer longitudinal smooth muscle fibers

2. **Submucosa** has loose areolar tissue with blood vessels and nerve fibers.

3. **Muscularis externa** has an inner circular and outer longitudinal layer. The longitudinal muscle is thicked at regular intervals in the circumference to form three longitudinal bands called taenia coli.

4. **Serosa:** The outermost lining consists of visceral peritoneum in most parts except the posterior

aspects of ascending and descending colon which are covered with adventitia.

Appendix

1. **Mucosa:** Lining epithelium consists of tall columnar cells with few small crypts of Leiberkuhn. Lamina propria has numerous scattered lymphoid follicles. Muscularis mucosae is poorly defined.

2. **Submucosa:** It is made of loose aereolar tissue and is characterized by presence of numerous lymphoid aggregates which may bulge into the lumen.

3. **Muscularis externa** consists of inner circular and outer longitudinal layer of smooth muscles with intervening connective tissue layer. There are no teniae.

4. **Serosa:** Is the outer lining consisting of visceral peritoneal layer.

Rectum

1. **Mucus membrane:** It presents with a number of folds. Lining epithelium has tall columnar cells with scattered goblet cells. It forms crypts that dips into lamina propria, crypts of Leiberkuhn. Lamina propria has connective tissue, lymphatics, blood vessels and nerves. Muscularis mucosae is a thin layer of inner circular and outer longitudinal smooth muscle fibers.

2. **Submucosa:** It has connective tissue, lymphatics, blood vessels and nerve fibers.

3. **Muscularis externa:** It has a well defined layer of inner circular and outer longitudinal layer. There are no taeniae.

4. **Adventitia** is the outer most connective tissue covering except at upper anterior part of rectum where there is serosa.

Anal Canal

1. **Mucus membrane:** Lining epithelium varies from above downwards:
   a. It is simple columnar epithelium with crypts of Leiberkuhn in upper 1/3rd.
   b. In middle 1/3rd it is made of stratified squamous non keratinized epithelium.
   c. The lower 1/3rd it is made up of keratinized stratified squamous epithelium.
   Lamina propria and muscularis mucosae are thin layers.

2. **Submucosa:** It has areolar tissue with mucus secreting glands. It presents with venous plexuses in lower ½.

3. **Muscularis externa:** In upper 3/4th, it consists of inner well defined circular layer of smooth muscle

fibers forming internal sphincter and an outer longitudinal layer. In lower 1/4th it consists of striated muscle fibers forming external anal sphincter.

4. **Adventitia** is the outermost connective tissue covering with blood vessels and nerve.

Nerve Supply of Gastrointestinal Tract

It is made up of intrinsic and extrinsic innervations:

Intrinsic Innervation

It consists of two networks.

1. **Myenteric plexus or Auerbach's plexus:** It is present between the outer longitudinal and inner circular muscle layers and supplies them. It acts to increase the tone and rate of contraction of muscle layer and helps in peristalsis.

   Peristalsis: The stretching of gut wall by the contents, food or water, in intestinal lumen leads to a local reflex response by the myenteric plexus. This leads to a wave of contraction proximal to the stretch and an area of relaxation distal to it. Contraction and relaxation in this orderly fashion is known as peristalsis and it helps in propulsion of food from esophagus to rectum.

2. **Meissner's plexus:** This plexus is present in submucosa, inner to circular muscle layer. It supplies the glandular epithelium, endocrine cells of intestine and blood vessels and **controls intestinal secretions.**

Extrinsic Innervation

1. **Parasympathetic supply:** Preganglionic fibers are derived from vagal efferents and sacral outflow and end on myenteric and meissner's plexus. Stimulation releases acetylcholine which increases contractions of the musculature and relaxation of sphincters. It also increases gastric and intestinal secretions.

2. **Sympathetic supply:** Postganglionic fibers are derived from mesenteric (T_6 to L_2) and hypogastric ganglia (L_1, L_2) and enter the gut wall along the blood vessels. Stimulation leads to contraction of sphincters and decrease motility and tone of gut wall.

PHYSIOLOGICAL FUNCTIONS OF VARIOUS PARTS OF GASTROINTESTINAL TRACT

Oral Cavity

- The food is mixed in the mouth with saliva, rotated by tongue and chewed by teeth aided by movement of jaws.

- The bolus of food is propelled backwards by the tongue towards the pharynx and swallowed.

Deglutition (Swallowing reflex)

Deglutition is characterised by inhibition of respiration, closure of laryngeal inlet and propulsion of food to oropharynx leading to contraction of pharyngeal muscles and relaxation of upper esophageal sphincter. This allows food to enter esophagus.

Salivary Glands and Saliva

The three pairs of salivary glands namely; parotid, submandibular and sublingual secrete saliva. 1500 ml saliva is secreted per day, 70% is derived from submandibular gland while 25% from parotid and 5% from sublingual glands. Each gland consists of serous and mucous cells, except parotid which is purely serous. Serous cells secrete a thin, watery secretion with α-amylase and mucous cells secrete viscous secretion of mucins and glycoproteins which help to lubricate food.

Functions of Saliva

1. α-amylase in saliva starts digestion of starch.
2. Lubricates food, allows proper mixing to form bolus that can be easily swallowed.
3. Acts as solvent for substances to stimulate taste buds.
4. Keeps oral cavity moist, which helps clean mouth and teeth.
5. Aids in speech by facilitating movement of tongue and lips.
6. Has buffers and proline rich proteins which keep oral pH 7.0 and prevents enamel loss. Thus it prevents tooth decay.
7. Contains local immunological agents like IgA, lysosymes, lactoferrin which provide defence against bacteria and viruses.

Secretion of saliva occurs in response to

a. Parasympathetic stimulation.
b. Food in mouth, taste, smell and sight of food also augment secretion.

Esophagus

- It primarily serves as a passage for food to stomach.
- At the pharyngo-esophageal junction, the upper 3 cm acts like a sphincter with a high resting tone. This area is controlled by vagal tone. It is normally closed and relaxes only briefly during swallowing. It is named as upper esophageal sphincter.
- Food is propelled distally by peristalsis.
- 2.5 cm above gastroesophageal junction, the musculature acts like a **lower esophageal sphincter.**

It is normally closed and is under the influence of vagus nerve. It relaxes in response to peristaltic waves from above to allow passage food into stomach. It helps to prevent reflux of stomach contents into esophagus.

- **Mechanisms that prevent gastro esophageal reflux**
  a. Tone of lower esophageal sphincter.
  b. Contraction of crural fibres of diaphragm: The esophageal opening in diaphragm is encircled by circular fibers of right crura of diaphragm which contract when intraabdominal pressure is increased. Thus, they prevent reflux of stomach contents upwards.

Stomach

Stomach stores food and produces acid and pepsin to act on proteins. Gastric mucosa presents two types of glands (Fig. 16.36):

1. **Glands at pyloric and cardiac ends:** These produce mucus. Deeper portion of pyloric glands have **G-cells** which secrete gastrin.
2. **Glands in the fundus and body:** These have **parietal (oxyntic) cells** which secrete hydrochloric acid and intrinsic factor and **chief (zymogen) cells** which secrete pepsinogens.

Gastric secretions are about 2500 ml per day. The secretion and motility of stomach is regulated by vagal stimulation and by gastrin hormone.

Functions of Stomach

1. Stores food, acts as reservoir for food and converts food to uniform consistency of chyme.
2. **Functions of hydrochloric acid:**
   a. Activates pepsinogen to pepsin.
   b. Kills any ingested bacteria.
   c. Stimulates flow of bile and pancreatic juices.
   d. Helps to convert Fe^{3+} to Fe^{2+}.
3. Pepsins digest proteins.
4. Mucus protects the gastric mucosa from acid.
5. Intrinsic factor produced by parietal cells binds to vit B_{12} and facilitates its absorption in the ileum.

Small Intestine

- It is the primary site of completion of digestion and absorption of various nutrients.
- The mucosal lining consists of villi and crypts lined with enterocytes. The lining presents with simple tubular intestine glands called crypts of Leiberkuhn in entire length. Coiled acinotubular glands are seen in duodenum (Brunner glands) and lymphatic nodules are mostly seen in region of ileum.
- **Intestinal secretions consists of**
  1. Mucus by surface epithelial cells and Brunner glands.
  2. Intestinal juices produced by intestinal glands.
- About 3000 ml of isotonic intestinal fluid is produced per day.
- Various enzymes are present on the brush border of enterocytes and consist of disacharridases, peptidases, neucleases, nucleotidases, lipase and cholesterol esterase. These eneymes are responsible for complete digestion of molecules of proteins, fats and carbohydrates into simple absorbable units.
- Intestinal secretion is controlled by local mechanical and chemical stimuli. VIP (vaso instestinal peptide) increases secretion of intestinal juices while vagal stimulation increases Brunner gland secretions.
- **Intestinal motility:** It consists of three types of smooth muscle contractions:
  1. **Peristalsis:** It is the contraction and relaxation of intestinal wall in an orderly fashion which allows propulsion of food from proximal to distal part.
  2. **Segmentation contractions:** These are ring like contractions which appear at regular intervals along the gut. They help to move the chyme to and fro for absorption.
  3. **Tonic contractions:** These are prolonged contractions seen in isolated segments of instestine.
- The motility of small instestine has a basic electrical rhythm which is increased by presence of food and action of local hormones like gastrin and CCK (Cholecystokinin).

Large Intestine

- It is primarily concerned with absorption of water and Na^+.
- Mucosa of colon has mucus secreting glands. There are no villi or microvilli.
- About 1000 to 2000 ml of chyme reaches colon and 90% absorption of water takes place in colon resulting in the formation of semisolid faeces.
- Colon also houses bacteria like E.coli, Enterobacter, bacteroides and other cocci and bacilli.
- **The various effects of bacteria in colon**
  1. Help in synthesis of vitamin K and B complex.
  2. Action of bacteria on bile pigments causes formation of brown color of stools.
  3. Responsible for producing gases like CO_2 and H_2S. When it is in excess, it leads to flatus.
- Movements of colon consists of
  1. **Segmentation contractions** which help to mix contents of colon and aid absorption.
  2. **Peristalsis** to propel contents.
  3. **Mass action contractions** which help to empty colon.
- **Defecation:** Faeces is made of undigested food and intestinal secretions. Distension of rectum with feces initiates reflex contractions and relaxation of anal sphincter allowing the contents to be expelled. This is called **defecation reflex.**

Functions of Large Intestine
1. Storage of matter
2. Absorption of fluids and solutes
3. Lubrication of undigested matter to facilitate its passage
4. Protection against bacterial invasion due to presence of numerous lymphatic follicles
5. Synthesis of vitamin B from colonic flora

LIVER

It is the largest gland of the body lies in the upper part of the abdominal cavity. It lies in the right hypochondrium, epigastrium and part of left hypochondrium. It is wedge shaped. It weighs about 1.5 to 2 kg which is 1/36th of the body weight in adults while it is 1/18th of the body weight in infants (Figs 16.38, 16.39).

Anatomical Features

Liver has five surfaces, three borders, right, left, caudate and quadrate lobes, fissure for ligamentum teres, ligamentum venosum and porta hepatis.

Surfaces of Liver
Liver presents with a right surface, an anterior and a posterior surface, a superior and a inferior surface.
1. **Right surface:** It lies in relation to the undersurface of diaphragm and is convex all around. It is covered by peritoneum.
2. **Superior surface:** It is quadrilateral and shows a concavity in the middle.
3. **Anterior surface:** It is triangular and slightly convex.
4. **Posterior surface:** This surface lies between posterosuperior and posteroinferior borders which are not very well defined. In the middle it shows a deep concavity for the vertebral column. This surface has following features and relations.
   a. **Bare area (Fig. 16.39):** It is triangular in shape, has following boundaries.
   Apex: Right triangular ligament
   Base: Groove for inferior vena cava

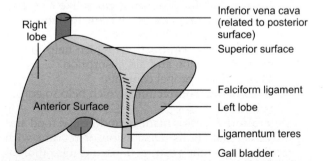

Right lobe
Inferior vena cava (related to posterior surface)
Superior surface
Falciform ligament
Anterior Surface
Left lobe
Ligamentum teres
Gall bladder

Fig. 16.38: Superior and anterior surface of liver

Upper boundary: Superior layer of coronary ligament
Lower boundary: Inferior layer of coronary ligament
It is non peritoneal and is covered by Glisson's capsule. This area is related to diaphragm, right suprarenal and upper end of right kidney.
   b. **Groove for inferior vena cava:** It is a vertical groove which lodges the inferior vena cava. It is non peritoneal and is pierced by hepatic veins.
   c. **Caudate lobe:** It is covered by the peritoneum of lesser sac. It is related to crura of diaphragm, coeliac trunk and right inferior phrenic artery.
   d. **Fissure for ligamentum venosum:** It is deep and extends to the front of caudate lobe. It contains two layers of lesser omentum. The floor of the fissure lodges the ligamentum venosum which is the remnant of ductus venosus.
   e. **Groove for esophagus:** It is the shallow vertical groove on the posterior surface of left lobe. It is covered with peritoneum.

5. **Inferior or visceral surface (Fig. 16.39):** It has following features and relations from left to right.
   a. **Gastric impression:** Concave fossa on the under surface of left lobe of liver.
   b. **Omental tuberosity or tuberomental:** It is a rounded elevation between gastric impression and lower end of fissure for ligamentum venosum.
   c. **Fissure for ligamentum teres:** A deep cleft extends from inferior border of liver to left end of porta hepatis. This lodges ligamentum teres which represents the obliterated left umbilical vein.
   d. **Quadrate lobe:** It is quadrangular in shape, bounded by inferior border of liver, porta hepatis, fossa for gall bladder and fissure for ligamentum teres. This surface is related to Ist part of duodenum, transverse colon in lower part.
   e. **Porta hepatis:** It is a transverse, non peritoneal fissure. It is the gateway to liver. The lips of porta hepatis give attachment to anterior and posterior layer of lesser omentum. The structures passing through porta hepatis are from before backward are
      — Right and left hepatic duct
      — Right and left hepatic artery
      — Right and left division of portal vein.
   f. **Caudate and papillary processes of caudate lobe**
   g. **Fossa for gall bladder:** It extends from a notch on the inferior border of liver to right end of

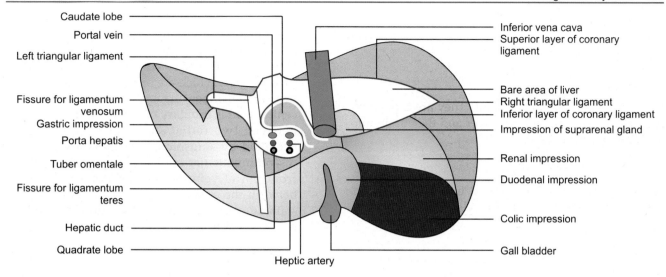

Fig. 16.39: Relations of inferior and posterior surface of liver

porta hepatis. It is not covered by peritoneum and lodges the gall bladder.

h. **Duodenal impression:** It is a gentle depression seen to the right of gall bladder.

i. **Colic impression:** It is seen further on the right side of body of gall bladder

j. **Renal impression:** It is present above and behind the colic impression.

Borders

Inferior border: It is well defined and separates the inferior surface from right and anterior surface.

Posterosuperior border: It is demarcated by superior layer of coronary ligament, upper end of groove for inferior vena cava and left triangular ligament.

Posteroinferior border: It separates the inferior and posterior surfaces. It is indicated by inferior layer of coronary ligament and groove for inferior vena cava.

Lobes of Liver

Liver is divided into two lobes right and left.

1. **Right lobe:** It is the largest lobe of liver and forms 5/6th of the liver. It presents **caudate** and **quadrate** lobes.

2. **Left lobe:** Forms 1/6th of the liver. It is flattened from above downward.

Non-peritoneal areas: These are sites where liver is not covered by the peritoneum.

1. Bare area
2. Attachment of falciform ligament
3. Groove for vena cava

4. Fossa for gall bladder
5. Porta hepatis
6. Fissure for ligamentum teres and venosum

Peritoneal Recesses of liver

1. Right and left supra hepatic recesses
2. Right and left subhepatic recesses

Right subhepatic recess is also known as **Morrison's pouch.**

Peritoneal Ligaments of Liver

1. **Falciform ligament:** It is sickle shaped, made up of two layers. It connects the undersurface of diaphragm and anterior abdominal wall to liver.
   Contents: Ligamentum teres, Paraumbilical vein, Accessory portal system of Sappey

2. **Coronary ligament:** Connects bare area of liver to diaphragm.

3. **Right triangular ligament:** Connects right surface of the liver to diaphragm.

4. **Left triangular ligament:** Connects upper left surface of liver to diaphragm.

5. **Lesser omentum:** It connects liver to lesser curvature of stomach and proximal 1.5 cm of duodenum.

Other Ligaments

1. **Ligamentum teres:** It is obliterated left umbilical vein.

2. **Ligamentum venosum:** It is remnant of obliterated ductus venosus.

CHAPTER-16

Blood Supply of Liver

80% is derived from portal vein while 20% is derived from hepatic artery.

Venous Drainage of Liver

Liver is drained by hepatic veins. They are formed by two sets of veins, upper and lower and they drain into the inferior vena cava.

Lymphatic Drainage of Liver

The lymphatics from liver drain into caval, hepatic, paracardiac and coeliac lymph nodes.

Nerve Supply of Liver

Liver is supplied by hepatic plexus which contains sympathetic and parasympathetic nerves.

Structure of Liver (Fig. 16.40)

- Liver is made up of parenchymal cells, connective tissue stroma, sinusoids, bile canaliculi, portal triads and tributaries of veins.

- On microscopic examination liver presents with polygonal (usually hexagonal) shaped hepatic lobules seperated by thin connective tissue septae.
- **Hepatic lobule:** Each lobule consist of mass of cells (hepatocytes) which are arranged in single sheets in a radial manner surrounding a central vein. The central vein is tributary of hepatic vein. The space between two radial sheets of hepatic cells is occupied by sinusoids. **Sinusoids** are lined by discontinuous flat epithelium and receive blood from portal venules and hepatic arterioles. In between the epithelium are present large deeply staining cells, **Kupffer's cells.** Kupffer's cells are part of the reticulo-endothelial system.
- Hepatocytes are hexagonal in shape and contain a large vescicular nucleus. Small intercellular channels are present between two adjacent hepatocytes. These are **bile canalculi** and are not seen on H and E staining (stained by osmic acid stain).
- At the corners of the polygonal lobule, are present portal triads.

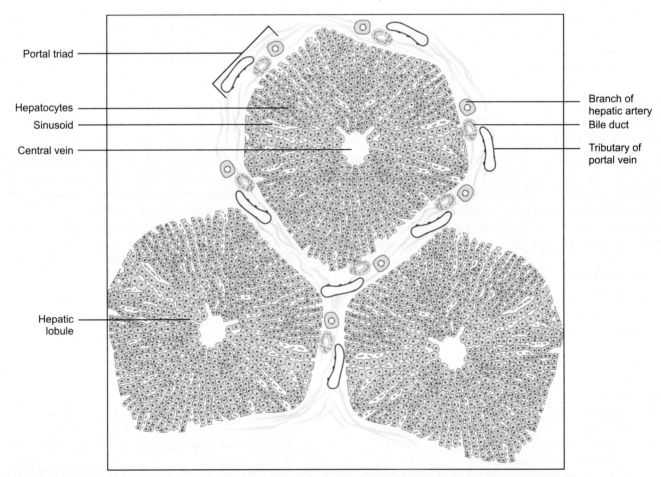

Fig. 16.40: Transverse section of Liver (Stain-hematoxylin-eosin under high magnification)

- **Portal triads (canals)** are interlobular. Each triad consists of a tributary of portal vein, hepatic artery and bile duct.
- **Portal lobule** is the term given to the polygonal territory of the liver cells centered around a portal triad. Three adjacent hepatic lobules meet at the portal triad. Hence, the corners of this polygonal portal lobule will contain three neighbouring central veins. The portal lobule becomes clearly demarcated in conditions with high hepatic pressure.
- **Liver acini (of Rappaport):** This term is given to the diamond or oval shape arrangement of hepatocytes around a terminal branch of hepatic arteriole and portal venule.

EXTRA HEPATIC BILIARY SYSTEM

It includes **right and left hepatic ducts, common hepatic duct, gall bladder, cystic duct** and **bile duct (Fig 16.41).**

Intra Hepatic Circulation of Bile

Bile is secreted by hepatocytes into the bile canaliculi which join to form canal of Herings. It then drains into ductules which join to form right and left hepatic ducts. The two hepatic ducts join at porta hepatis to form the common hepatic duct.

Bile canaliculi → Canal of Herings → Ductule → Right and left hepatic ducts

Extra Hepatic Circulation

Common hepatic duct is 3 cm long and is 4 mm in diameter. It joins with the cystic duct from gall bladder to form the common bile duct. The bile flows from liver to gall bladder and via common bile duct to the duodenum.

Gall Bladder (Fig. 16.41)

It is related to the inferior surface of the liver where it lies in the gall bladder fossa. It is pear shaped. It is 7 to 10 cm long and 3 cm wide. It has a capacity of 30 to 50 ml. It can be divided into fundus, body and neck. A small diverticulum extends in the downward and backward direction from the postero-medial wall of neck of gall bladder. This forms **Hartmann's pouch.**

Arterial supply: It is supplied by cystic artery a branch of right hepatic artery.

Nerve supply: It receives sympathetic supply through coeliac plexus and hepatic plexus. It also receives a few twigs via phrenic nerve.

Cystic Duct (Fig. 16.41)

It extends from neck of gall bladder to bile duct. It is 3 to 4 cm in length and 2 mm in diameter. The spiral valves of Heister are present in cystic duct.

Blood Supply of Gall Bladder

1. Cystic artery
2. Right hepatic artery
3. Superior pancreatico-duodenal artery and inferior pancreatico-duodenal artery

Bile Duct (Fig. 16.41)

It is formed close to porta hepatis by the union of common hepatic and cystic ducts. Usually cystic duct joins the right side of common hepatic duct at an acute angle. It is 7.5 cm in length and 6 mm in diameter. Bile duct is divided into four parts

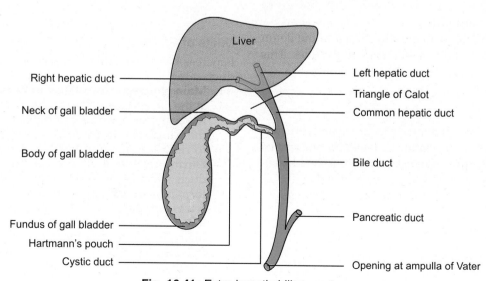

Fig. 16.41: Extra hepatic biliary system

1. Supraduodenal part
2. Retroduodenal part
3. Infraduodenal part
4. Intraduodenal part

The bile duct opens into the second part of duodenum along with pancreatic duct at the summit of ampulla of Vater. This opening is guarded by smooth muscle fibres forming a sphincter known as sphincter of Oddi.

Sphincter of Oddi: It is made up three sphincters:

1. **Sphinter of Boyden:** Choledochus sphincter (strongest), sphincter of bile duct.
2. **Sphincter Pancreaticus:** Sphincter of pancreatic duct.
3. **Sphincter of oddi proper**

Physiological Functions of Liver and Gall Bladder

- Liver performs important functions of the body:
  1. Synthesis of plasma proteins, clotting factors.
  2. Metabolism of glucose, aminoacids and lipids
  3. Inactivation of toxic substances
  4. Formation and secretion of bile.
- Bile is made up of bile salts, bile pigments and other substances in an alkaline electrolyte solution. It is secreted by hepatocytes into bile canaliculi and collected by ducts which join to form hepatic ducts.
- About 500 ml of bile is produced per day.
- Bile passes through cystic duct to gall bladder for storage between meals. It is released into 2nd part of duodenum by common bile duct following contraction of gall bladder as food enters intestine.
- Bile salts reduce surface tension and emulsify fats in food, facilitating action of lipases and diffusion of lipids in soluble form to the brush border of intestine for absorption.
- 90 to 95% of bile salts are reabsorbed in the ileum and enter portal circulation back to the liver. This is called entero-hepatic circulation of bile.

PANCREAS

It is an exocrine as well as an endocrine gland. It lies in the C of duodenum in relation to posterior abdominal wall. It extends from epigastrium to the left hypochondrium at the level of L_1 and L_2 vertebrae (Fig. 16.42).

Dimensions

Length	:	15 to 20 cm
Breadth	:	3 cm
Thickness	:	0.5 to 2 cm
Weight	:	85 to 90 gm

Anatomical Features

Pancreas can be divided into the following parts:

1. **Head:** It is the enlarged part. It lies in the C of duodenum. It consists of a superior, Inferior and a right border. It presents with an anterior and a posterior surface.

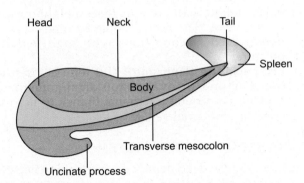

Fig. 16.42: Parts of pancreas with relations

Uncinate process: It is a triangular projection which arises from the lower and left part of the head. Anteriorly it is related to the superior mesenteric vessels and posteriorly to the aorta.

2. **Neck of pancreas:** It is a slightly constricted part which is directed **forwards, upwards and to the left.** It connects the head to the body.
3. **Body of pancreas:** The body extends from front of aorta till the left kidney and is triangular on cross section. It has three surfaces and three borders. Anterior border provides attachment to root of transverse mesocolon. Superior border presents with a conical projection called tuberomentale on right side. At the right end of inferior border emerge the superior mesenteric vessels.
4. **Tail of pancreas:** This is the narrow left end of pancreas. It lies in the lienorenal ligament together with splenic artery. It is the most mobile part of pancreas.

Ducts of Pancreas

Pancreas has an exocrine part which is drained by two ducts.

1. **Main pancreatic duct (Duct of Wirsung):** It begins at the tail and runs close to the posterior surface of the pancreas towards the right. Near the neck of the pancreas it turns downwards, backwards and to right to open into the 2nd part of duodenum. During its course it receives numerous smaller ducts which open at regular intervals at right angle forming a **herring bone pattern.**
2. **Accessory duct (duct of Santorini):** It begins in the lower part of the head and crosses in front of the main duct passing upwards and to the right. It opens into the 2nd part of duodenum at the minor papilla.

Arterial Supply of Pancreas

1. Pancreatic branches of splenic artery.
2. Superior pancreaticoduodenal artery.
3. Inferior pancreaticoduodenal artery.

Venous Drainage of Pancreas

Corresponding veins drain into superior mesenteric, splenic and portal veins.

Lymphatic Drainage of Pancreas

1. Head and neck of pancreas drain into pancreatico duodenal lymph nodes.
2. Tail and body of pancreas drain into pancreatico-splenic lymph nodes.

Nerve Supply of Pancreas

Sympathetic: It is derived from superior mesenteric and coeliac plexus. It is vasomotor.
Parasympathetic: It is derived from bilateral vagi. These stimulate pancreatic secretion.

Structure of Pancreas (Fig. 16.43)

It is made up of an exocrine and an endocrine part.

1. Exocrine part is made up of racemose glands and is devoid of definite fibrous capsule. It consists of lobules which are separated by interlobular septae. Each septa is made up of connective tissue and has blood capillaries, nerves and ducts of the gland. Each lobule is made up of ductules and serous acini. Ducts are lined by cuboidal epithelium. Junction between duct and acini is lined by cuboidal cells which are known as centro-acinar cells. The acini are lined by tall columnar cells and have a small lumen. The nucleus of acinar cells is situated at the base and the apical zone of the cells is eosinophilic due to presence of zymogen granules.

2. Endocrine part consists of islets of Langerhans. These are collections of cells scattered throughout the organ in between the exocrine acini but are more numerous in the tail. About 1 to 2 million islets are found in the human pancreas. Islet cells are polyhedral. These are divided into α and β cells according to the presence of granules stained by Mallory-Azan dye. α cells are further divided into α_1 and α_2 subtypes.

Physiological Functions of Pancreas

- Pancreas produces 1200 to 1500 ml of pancreatic juice per day.
- The exocrine portion is a compound alveolar gland and secretions are carried from small ductules to ducts and finally the duct of pancreas opens into 2nd part of duodenum.
- Pancreatic juice is alkaline (has high HCO_3^- content) and consists of various enzymes as given below:
  1. **Alpha amylase:** It digests starch
  2. **Pancreatic lipase:** It hydrolyses fat
  3. **Cholesteryl ester hydrolase:** It acts on cholesterol ester
  4. **Phospholipase A$_2$:** It acts on phospholipids.
  5. **Proteolytic enzymes:** These are secreted as inactivated proenzymes namely trypsinogen, chymotrypsinogen, proelastase and procarbo-xypeptidases. Other enzymes are nucleotidases like ribonucleases etc. Trypsinogen is activated to trypsin by enterokinases present at the brush border of intestinal mucosa. Trypsin further activates the other proenzymes. These together hydrolyse proteins.
- **Secretions of exocrine part of pancreas is controlled by**
  1. **Vagus nerve:** It stimulates secretion of enzyme rich pancreatic juice. Vagal stimulation occurs

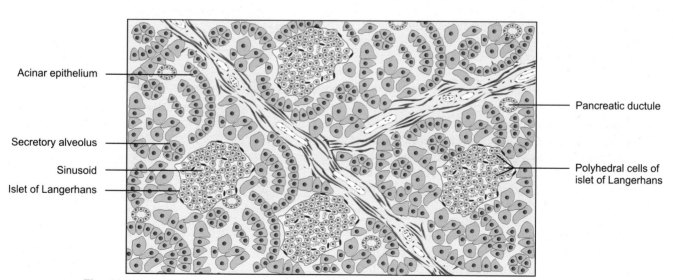

Fig. 16.43: Transverse section of pancreas (Stain-hematoxylin-eosin under high magnification)

Acinar epithelium

Secretory alveolus

Sinusoid

Islet of Langerhans

Pancreatic ductule

Polyhedral cells of islet of Langerhans

due to presence of food in upper GIT and by the sight and smell of food.

2. Hormonal regulation
   a. Secretin: It acts to increase secretion of alkaline juice rich in HCO_3^- and poor in enzymes.
   b. Cholecystokinin (CCK): It acts to increase production of pancreatic juice rich in enzymes.

DIGESTION AND ABSORPTION OF VARIOUS FOOD AND NUTRITIVE COMPONENTS IN GIT
Carbohydrates

- Carbohydrate content of diet averages 50 to 60% and consists of polysaccharides like starches (amylopectin), glycogen, disaccharides like sucrose, lactose (milk) and maltose and monosaccharides like glucose, fructose etc.
- There is no digestion of carbohydrates in stomach.
- Digestion begins in mouth by action of salivary a amylase and in small instestine by action of pancreatic a amylase. This results in the formation of small chain polymers, oligosaccharides and disaccharides. The enzymes in brush border of small intestine namely alpha-dextrinase, maltase, sucrase, lactase and trehalase complete the breakdown, convert oligosaccharides finally to glucose (mainly), fructose and galactose.
- Glucose is rapidly absorbed from jejunum and ileum. Mode of absorption is by simple diffusion and by secondary active transport via the sodium dependent glucose transporter (SGLT). (Fig. 16.44) Absorption of glucose is sodium (Na^+) dependent, high Na^+ concentration in lumen favours higher absorption.
- Galactose absorption is also via Na^+ dependent transporter while fructose is absorbed by facilitated diffusion.
- Insulin does not affect absorption in intestine.
- Maximal rate of absorption of glucose from intestine is 120 gm/hr.

Proteins

- Digestion of protein begins in stomach by action of enzyme pepsin. Pepsin is secreted from the chief cells of mucosa as a precursor, pepsinogen which gets activated by hydrochloric acid. Pepsin acts best at pH of 1.6 to 3.2 and its action ceases as the food is passed to small intestine.
- Further digestion occurs in duodenum by proteo-lytic enzymes of pancreas namely trypsins, chymotrypsins, elastases and carboxypeptidases.
- In the intestine complete digestion of polypeptides to aminoacids occurs at 3 sites, intraluminal by

pancreatic enzymes, at brush border by surface peptidases and also intracellularly by cytoplasmic peptidases. 50% of digested protein is from food while 25% is from contents of digestive juices and 25% from desquamated mucosal cells.

- Absorption of amino acids is rapid in duodenum and jejunum while slow in ileum.
- Aminoacids are absorbed by simple diffusion and by seven transport systems into enterocytes which are mostly Na^+, dependant. In 2 systems transport is independent of Na^+. H^+ dependent transport system helps absorption of di and tripeptides into the cells.
- Amino acids are further transported out into circulation by 5 basolateral transport systems, two are Na^+ dependent and three are Na^+ independent.

Lipids

- Dietary fat consists of simple fats consisting of triglycerides, compound fats like phospholipids, sphingomyelins and galacto-lipids and sterols like cholesterol.
- Digestion of fat starts in stomach by action of lingual lipase and gastric lipase. Though lingual lipase is secreted in mouth, it is active only in the stomach.
- It is in the duodenum where most of fat digestion occurs by the action of pancreatic lipases and cholesterol ester hydrolases.
- Presence of bile salts is important as it activates lipases and helps in emulsification of fats to facilitate action of lipases. Bile salts along with lipids form cylindrical molecular aggregates called **micelles** which are water soluble and allow absorption of fats. **(Fig. 16.45)**

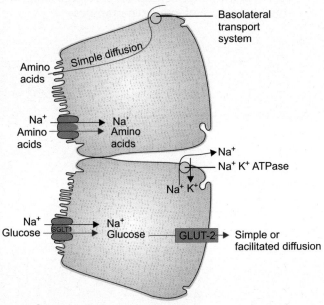

Fig. 16.44: Diagrammatic representation of absorption of glucose and amino acids in jejunum

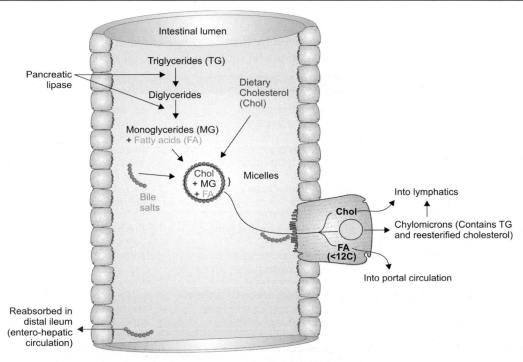

Fig. 16.45: Diagrammatic representation of absorption of fat in jejunum

- Micelles are transported to brush border along their gradient where the bile salts detach and allow the lipid content to pass by passive diffusion into the enterocytes.
- The bile salts are taken up actively back into the circulation at terminal ileum. **This enterohepatic circulation of bile salts** is an important mode of maintaining pool of bile salts.
- The monoglycerides, fatty acids and cholesterol are reesterified to triglycerides and cholesterol esters and coated with phospholipids to form chylomicrons that pass into lymphatics.
- Fatty acids pass directly into circulation. They get bound to albumin and other plasma proteins forming lipoprotein complexes for transport.

Water and Electrolytes

- Water is mostly absorbed from jejunum, and partly from ileum and colon.
- 98% of fluid reaching the intestine is reabsorbed. Ingested liquid is approximately 1.5 to 2.5 litres while 7000 ml is derived from secretions of mucosa of GIT.
- Na^+ is actively absorbed along with glucose and aminoacids in small intestines. It also diffuses passively into small and large intestines.
- Potassium (K^+) is absorbed by passive diffusion in small intestine.
- Chloride (Cl^-) is secreted into intestinal lumen by Cl^- channels and is reabsorbed in exchange for bicarbonate (HCO_3^-) ions to keep the intestinal contents alkaline.

Vitamins and Minerals

- Water soluble vitamins, B and C are absorbed rapidly in upper part of small intestine by Na^+ dependent cotransporters.
- Vitamin B_{12} is absorbed in terminal part of ileum. It first binds to an intrinsic factor secreted by the stomach and the entire IF-B_{12} complex is absorbed in ileum.
- Fat soluble vitamins are absorbed along with emulsified fat molecules, micelles.
- Calcium is absorbed in upper part of small intestine by active transport. The rate of absorption is dependent on presence of 1,25 dihydroxy cholecalciferol, a vitamin D derivative obtained from kidney. Ca^+ absorption is aided by presence of proteins and inhibited by dietary oxalates and phosphates. About 30 to 80% of ingested calcium is absorbed.
- Iron is absorbed in the ferrous form (Fe^{2+}) but most of dietary iron is in ferric form (Fe^{3+}). Hence, iron absorption is only 3 to 6% of the total ingested iron. It is absorbed in duodenum and jejunum and is actively transported out of enterocytes into circulation. In circulation it changes to Fe^{3+} form and binds to apotransferin to form transferrin, the circulating form of iron. Iron absorption is decreased by presence of dietary phytates, oxalates, and phosphates. It is increased in iron deficiency conditions.

Gastrointestinal Hormones

These are biologically active peptides that are secreted by nerve endings and mucosal cells and act in a paracrine manner to exert influence on gastro intestinal secretion and motility. They are tabulated below:

Hormone	Site of production	Action	Regulation of secretion
1. Gastrin	G-cells in antral glands of stomach	1. Stimulates gastric acid and pepsin secretion 2. Stimulates growth of gastrointestinal mucosa 3. Stimulates gastric motility	1. Increased by presence of peptides and aminoacid in stomach especially, tryptophan and phenylalanine 2. Increased by vagal stimulation 3. Inhibited by acid in antrum 4. Somatostatin inhibits gastric secretion 5. Increase in secretin, GIP, VIP in circulation inhibit gastrin secretion
2. Cholecystokinin CCK	Cells in mucosa of upper part of small intestine	1. Stimulates contraction of gall bladder 2. Stimulates secretion of pancreatic juice rich in enzymes 3. Augments action of secretin 4. Inhibits gastric emptying 5. Stimulates growth of pancreas 6. Increases production of enterokinase 7. Increases motility of small intestine 8. Stimulates secretion of glucagon hormone	1. Products of digestion especially peptides, aminocids and fatty acids stimulate its secretions 2. Enzymatic action by pancreatic juices on protein and fat and the resultant products further stimulate CCK (positive feed back) 3. Action is terminated as digested particles pass down further
3. Secretin	S-cells located in glands of upper part of small intestine	1. Induces secretion of watery alkaline rich pancreatic juice 2. Augments action of CCK 3. Increases gastric acid secretion and contraction of pyloric sphincter	1. Secretion is increased by presence of: a. Products of protein digestion b. Acid in duodenum 2. Secretion is terminated as the chyme becomes more alkaline by pancreatic juices and passes down
4. Gastric inhibitory polypeptide GIP	K-cells of mucosa of duodenum and jejunum	1. Inhibits gastric juice secretion and gastric motility 2. Stimulates insulin secretion	Secreted in response to glucose and fat in duodenum
5. VIP Vaso-intestinal peptide	Found in nerve endings of GIT	1. Inhibits gastric acid secretion 2. Increases intestinal secretion of water and electrolytes 3. Relaxes intestinal smooth muscles and sphincters	Stimulated by presence of fat in food
6. Motilin	Secreted by enterochromaffin cells and Mo cells in stomach, small and large intestine	May control gastrointestinal motility in between meals	
7. Somatostatin	Produced by D-cells of islets in pancreas and gastrointestinal mucosa.	It inhibits 1. Secretion of gastrin due to acid, VIP, GIP and secretin 3. Gastric acid secretion and motility 4. Gall bladder contraction 5. Absorption of glucose and amino acids	Secreted in response to acid in intestine

NUTRITION AND METABOLISM

Metabolism denotes 'change'. It is the continuous chemical and energy changes brought about by the body.

Anabolism: It is the process involving storage of energy either as energy rich phosphate compounds or building of protein, fat and carbohydrate molecules from basic molecules.

Catabolism: It is the process of breakdown of nutritive substances like fat, protein and carbohydrate to form smaller molecules. These molecules are further broken down to release energy. It is a complex process involving oxidation which results in 3 principle end products CO_2, H_2O and energy in the form of heat or energy rich phosphate compounds, ATP.

Energy metabolism: Catabolism of various food stuffs liberates energy. This energy is used for maintaining various functions of various parts of body, physical activity, temperature regulation, metabolism of food etc. Metabolic rate is defined as the amount of energy liberated per unit time.

Basal metabolic rate (BMR): It is the metabolic rate of an individual at rest in a room with comfortable temperature, 12 to 14 hours after last meal.

Metabolic rate is increased in:
  a. Children
  b. Pregnancy
  c. Exercise
  d. Recent intake of food
  e. Increase temperature
  f. Anxiety and stress
  g. Sympathetic stimulation

Metabolic rate is lowered in:
  a. Low temperatures
  b. Increasing age
  c. Starvation
  d. Hypothyroidism

Energy Balance

The standard unit of heat energy is calorie. It is the amount of heat required to raise the temperature of 1 gm of water by 1°C, from 15°C to 16°C. The unit used in physiology is Kcal or kilo calories which is equal to 1000 calories.

- The energy produced by burning of food stuffs is as follows:
  1 gm of carbohydrate produces 4.1 Kcal
  1 gm of protein produces 4.1 Kcal (5.3 in vitro)
  1 gm of fat produces 9.3 Kcal
- When the calorie value of the food ingested equals the energy output, the weight of an individual is maintained. If calorie intake is less, there is breakdown of endogenous stores and over a long period of time leads to weight loss. However, if calorie intake is higher then weight gain is seen.

Energy Transfer

- The food is digested as described earlier in the chapter and the nutrient components are absorbed.
- Catabolism of the absorbed compounds liberates energy which is stored by cells in the form of high energy phosphate compounds. The most important and abundant energy rich compound in our body is ATP, adenosine triphosphate. Other energy rich phosphate compounds are creatinine phosphate (mostly in muscles), triphosphates of purine or pyridone derivatives like guanosine triphosphate (GTP), uridine triphophate (UTP) etc.
- The catabolism of glucose, aminoacids and fatty acids by enzymes is primarily by oxidation reactions that utilizes a number of coenzymes that serve as hydrogen acceptors like NAD (nicotin-amide adenine dinucleotide) and NADP (nicotina-mide adenine dinucleotide phosphate) which respectively form NADH and NADPH.

Oxidative phosphorylation: It is brought about by the flaroprotein—cytochrome system, present in the inner membrane of mitochondria. It involves regeneration of coenzymes NAD and NADP from their reduced forms by a successive transfer of H^+ (protons) along the chain of flaroprotein—cytochrome system. This oxidation process is coupled with release of energy and formation of ATP, hence it is called oxidative phosphorylation. The H^+ is finally transferred O_2 forming H_2O. This process thus depends on adequate supply of O_2 and ADP. Hence, 90% of O_2 taken up by cell is used in mitochondria. ATP is used in functions required energy for example, protein synthesis, Na^+K^+ ATPase pump to maintain membrane polarity, gluconeogenesis, actin-myosin coupling etc.

Metabolism of Carbohydrates

- Carbohydrates are compounds of carbon (C), hydrogen (H) and oxygen (O) and their metabolism yields CO_2 and H_2O.
- The principal product of carbohydrate digestion is glucose. Blood glucose levels vary from 80-140 mg%. Glucose is taken up by various cells of the body and is mostly converted to glucose-6-phosphate.
- Glucose-6-phosphate is either converted to glyco-gen for storage in liver and muscle or undergoes catabolism for energy production.
- Glucose undergoes oxidation to form pyruvic acid. Pyruvic acid is converted to acetyl CoA in presence of O_2 while in the absence of O_2 it is converted to lactic acid.

- Acetyl CoA is completely oxidized to CO_2 and H_2O via citric acid cycle or Kreb's cycle.
- The oxidation of glucose to pyruvic acid yields 8 ATP. In presence of O_2 pyruvic acid gets converted to acetyl CoA and produces 6 ATP. Acetyl CoA further undergoes respiratory chain oxidation to yield 24 ATP. Thus, 36 ATP are generated in aerobic oxidation of one molecule of glucose.
- In absence of O_2 (anaerobic conditions) one glucose molecule yields only 2 ATP.
- Glucose levels and metabolism are regulated by insulin hormone.
- Glucose is filtered by kidney and mostly reabsorbed (see page no. 542).

Physiological Functions of Carbohydrates

1. They are the primary source of energy for the body. Brain and RBCs are totally dependant on glucose metabolism for their energy.
2. Adequate presence of carbohydrates in body ensures proper protein utilization as proteins are not broken down to provide for energy.
3. Excess glucose is stored as glycogen especially in liver and muscles for use in conditions which demand more energy.
4. Components of carbohydrates are present in various parts of body for example:
   a. Mucopolysaccharides (carbohydrates with uronic acid and amino sugars) are present in bones, cartilage, collagen etc.
   b. Glycoproteins: These are complexes of carbohydrate with polypeptides. They are present as structural components of cell membranes, they form hormones.
   c. Nucleotides precursors of DNA and RNA consists of sugar moiety in their structure.

Metabolism of Fat

- Fatty acids are compounds of carbon (C), hydrogen (H) and oxygen (O) and their metabolism yields CO_2 and H_2O.
- The products of lipid digestion consist mostly of fatty acids, triglycerides, phospholipids and cholesterol. Triglycerides are made up of three fatty acids bound to one molecule of glycerol.
- Fatty acids undergo β oxidation in mitochondria to produce acetyl CoA which enters citric acid cycle. 44 ATP are produced by complete oxidation of one molecule of free fatty acids.
- Acetyl CoA thus produced, can be utilized to form one of the following:
   1. Ketone bodies: These are produced in liver and consist of acetoacetate, a hydroxybutyrate and

acetone. Normal blood ketone level is 1 mg/dl. Ketone bodies metabolized in periphery. In conditions where there is increase mobilization of free fatty acids like diabetes mellitus starvation there is increased production of ketone bodies. Excess circulating ketone bodies lead to condition called ketosis which is associated with metabolic acidosis.
   2. Fatty acids: Acetyl CoA can be reutilized to produced fatty acids.
   3. C-atoms Acetyl CoA is used in synthesis of cholesterol, haem porphyrin etc.
   4. Acetyl CoA is precursor for synthesis of neurotransmitter acetylcholine.

Essential fatty acids: These consist of linoleic, linolenic and arachidonic acids which are polyunsaturated fatty acid. They can not be synthesized in the body and hence are an essential part of diet.

Physiological Functions of Fat (Lipids)

1. Lipids (phospholipids and cholesterol) are present as structural components of all cell membranes.
2. Provide for an alternative source of energy to body.
3. Deposits of fat in subcutaneous regions provides insulation against temperature, while fat around internal viscera provides cushion effect preventing injury.
4. Cholesterol is the precursor for formation of steroid hormones, bile salts, prostaglandins. It forms a structural component of cell membranes.
5. Fat acts as carrier for lipid soluble vitamins.
6. Extra fat is stored in adipose tissue.

Metabolism of Proteins

- The basic building block of proteins are amino acids.
- Amino acids are compounds of carbon (C), hydrogen (H), oxygen (O) with nitrogen (N) and their metabolism yields CO_2, H_2O and NH_3 (ammonia).
- Amino acids are obtained from digestion of dietary proteins and also from metabolism of body proteins. This forms the amino acid pool of the body. Amino acids in body are used up in following ways:
   a. Synthesis of proteins: Structural body proteins or hormones, enzymes, purine and pyrimidine.
   b. Amino acids are transported in circulation for uptake by various organs.
   c. Degradation to urea.
   d. Carbon atoms of amino acids are used in synthesis of glucose (gluconeogenesis).

Physiological Functions of Proteins

1. Proteins are an essential structural components of all cells.
2. They are required for synthesis of various structural and cellular components and thus are responsible for repair and maintenance of cells and tissues.
3. Proteins are the raw material for synthesis of various enzymes, hormones, antibodies, plasma proteins, haemoglobin etc.
4. Proteins act as alternative energy source during conditions of starvation that is lack of adequate carbohydrates and fats.

As proteins are not stored, starvation over long periods leads to loss of protein mass of body mainly muscle leading to decrease body weight and weakness.

Nitrogen Balance

Proteins in the body are in a state of dynamic equilibrium, a balance is maintained between protein breakdown (eg. aging, menstruation etc.) and protein synthesis from amino acid pool. Adequate intake of protein in diet is essential to maintain the amino acid pool in body. The primary source of nitrogen in body is protein. Hence, when the nitrogen content of diet equals nitrogen loss in urine and feces (nitrogen equilibrium), the individual is said to be in nitrogen balance. If protein intake is increased in a normal individual, the extra amino acids are deaminated and urea excretion increases, maintaining nitrogen balance. However, in conditions like diabetes mellitus and during starvation and forced immobilization, nitrogen losses exceed intake and the nitrogen balance is negative. During growth or recovery from severe illness, or following administration of anabolic steroids such as testosterone, nitrogen intake exceeds excretion and nitrogen balance is positive.

- The first step in metabolism of amino acids is the oxidative deamination, that is removal of molecule of ammonia (NH_3) to produce corresponding ketoacid. Most of these reactions are coupled with interconversion of another ketoacid (usually a ketoglutarate) to amino acid (glutamic acid). This is known as transamination.

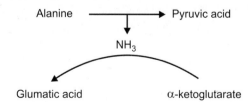

- The non-nitrogenous residues remaining after deamination enter the common metabolic pool and are either completely catabolised to CO_2 or are built up into other body constituents.

- In general the essential amino acids are glucogenic, they give rise to compounds that can readily be converted to glucose. All the non-essential amino acids are ketogenic, they give rise to ketone bodies.

Essential Amino Acids

Essential amino acids are those which cannot be synthesized by the body in amounts sufficient to fulfill its normal requirements. These consist of the following: valine, leucine, isoleucine, threonine, methionine, phenylalanine, tryptophan, lysine, hitidine and arginine.

Urea Formation

NH_3 formed by deamination of amino acids is toxic and is converted to a non toxic compound called urea in the liver. Normal blood urea levels vary from 20 to 40 mg/dl. Urea is filtered by the kidneys and excreted in the urine. It accounts for more than 80% of total urinary nitrogen.

Nitrogen Containing Constituents in Urine

The chief nitrogen containing waste products in urine are: Urea, creatinine, creatine, ammonium ions and uric acid.

1. **Urea:** Urea is formed in the liver from ammonia derived from metabolism of amino acids. On a normal protein diet, urinary urea is derived from proteins in diet. In protein deficient diet which is otherwise adequate in energy content, amino acids and hence urea is derived from breakdown of tissue proteins. In starvation, tissue protein, specially muscle protein is broken down into amino acids on a much larger scale. Most of this is deaminated and the residues are utilized for energy purposes and to maintain the blood sugar levels. Hence, in starvation urea excretion is on a much larger scale.

2. **Creatine and creatinine:** Creatine is synthesized in the liver from arginine, glycine and methionine. Creatine occurs in greatest concentration in skeletal muscle, with lesser amounts in heart muscle, brain and uterus. In skeletal muscle, it is phosphorylated to form phosphorylcreatine, which is an important energy store for ATP synthesis. Creatine is not a normal constituent of the urine but may appear in children, pregnancy and myopathies. Creatinine in urine is formed from phosphorylcreatine. The rate of creatinine excretion is relatively constant.

Nucleic Acid Metabolism

- Cells synthesize nucleic acids, ribonucleic acid (RNA) and deoxyribonucleic acid (DNA). Nucleic

acids are made up of polymers of nucleotides. Nucleotides are made up of:
  a. Nitrogenous base: Purine or Pyrimidine
  b. Pentose sugar: Ribose or Deoxyribose
  c. Phosphate group
- Purine bases are adenine and guanine. Pyrimidine bases are cytosine, thymine and uracil. Combination of a purine or promidine base with pentosugar is called nucleoside. Nucleosides are components of various co-enzymes in the cell namely NAD, NADP, ATP etc. Addition of phosphate group to nucleoside forms nucleotide.
- The nucleic acid content of food is digested in the duodenum and small intestine, with liberation of nucleotides, nucleosides and free purines and pyrimidines. RNA is continuously being broken down by enzyme systems within the cell.
- Metabolism of purines : Purine nucleotides are released during the breakdown of tissue nucleic acids, food nucleic acids. These bases can either be reconverted to their respective nucleotides or are oxidized to uric acid.
- Pyramidines are catabolized to form CO_2 and NH_3.

Uric Acid

Uric acid is the end product of breakdown of purines. Normal blood uric acid levels range from 2 to 4 mg/dL. Uric acid is filtered by the kidney. 98% of the filtered uric acid is reabsorbed and most of the urinary uric acid comes from tubular secretion. The uric acid excretion on a purine-free diet is about 0.5 g/24 hours on a regular diet is about 1 g/24 hours.

Nutrition

Nutrition is a dynamic process in which the food that is consumed is digested, its nutrients are absorbed and finally distributed to all body tissues for proper utilization.

The dietary consituents of food are : proteins, fats, carbohydrates, vitamins, minerals, dietary fibre and water.

Energy Requirement of Body

- Average calorie requirement of a sedentary individual is 1900 to 2200 Kcal / day.
- Additional calories are required for working or exercising. Pregnancy puts an additional demand of 300 Kcal / day while lactation increases demand by 550 Kcal / day.

Carbohydrates

Carbohydrates form the main bulk of diet and provide 50% of calorie intake of food. Their daily requirement varies from 300 to 500gm. The common sources are starches (present in cereals, millets, roots and tubers), sugars, cellulose (dietary fibre).

Fats

Dietary fat provides for about 20 to 25% of daily calorie requirement of body. Daily requirement for fat varies from 10 to 20 grams. The common sources are animal sources like ghee, butter, fish and plant sources like groundnut, mustard and coconut oil.

Proteins

Daily protein requirement is about 0.8 to 1 gram per kg body weight. Dietary sources of protein are animal sources like milk and milk products, eggs, meat, fish etc., plant sources like pulses, cereals, dry fruits, nuts, beans, etc,

Vitamins

Vitamins are essential organic compounds obtained from diet. They are required in small quantities and act as important co-factors and catalysts of various reactions in the body. They are divided into two groups namely fat soluble vitamins and water soluble vitamins. These are described below :

1. **Fat soluble vitamins:** These vitamins are absorbed in the small intestine along with dietary fats. Presence of adequate bile salts is necessary for their absorption. They are stored in liver and are not excreted by urine. Deficiency of these vitamins is rare but excess intake can cause hypervitaminosis and toxicity.
   Fat soluble vitamins are:
   a. Vitamin A
   b. Vitamin D
   c. Vitamin E
   d. Vitamin K
2. **Water soluble vitamins:** These vitamins are absorbed in the small intestine by simple diffusion. They are not stored in the body and excess is excreted via urine. Deficiency of these vitamins occurs sooner while excess intake is harmless.
   Water soluble vitamins are :
   a. Vitamin B complex
   b. Vitamin C

Minerals

The body contains some 50 minerals which serve specific functions in the body. The important minerals include:

Sodium is the primary mineral component of extracellular fluid. It helps to maintain ECF volume. It is also responsible for functioning of various cells, muscle fibers and nerves.

Calcium is the most abundant mineral in the body. It is responsible for maintainance of bones and teeth, helps in contraction of muscles, responsible for clotting of blood.

Phosphorus is primarily present in bones and teeth and is responsible for maintainance of bones and teeth. It is also a component of energy compounds like ATP, ADP, DNA and RNA.

Iron is mostly a component of haemoglobin (see page no. 454).

Iodine is required for synthesis of thyroid hormones.

Potassium is mostly present intracellularly. It is responsible for maintaining cell membrane polarity specially in the nerve and muscle fibre cells.

Sulphur is a component various proteins, hormones and vitamins.

Chloride is mostly present in ECF and plays a role in acid base and water balance. It is also a part of the hydrochloric acid secreted by stomach.

Dietary Fibre

Dietary fibres are made up of carbohydrate derivatives like pectin, cellulose, hemicellulose and non-carbohydrate substances like lignin. They cannot be digested and pass as such to the colon where they absorb water and increase the bulk of the intestinal contents which facilitates intestinal movements and defecation. Deficiency of dietary fibre is associated with constipation, cancer of colon, colonic diverticulosis, heart disease and gall bladder stones.

Water

Water is an essential requirement for life. It is the medium in which most of the chemical activities in the body take place.

CLINICAL AND APPLIED ASPECT

ORAL CAVITY

- General features of teeth
  — The first premolars are usually the largest teeth
  — The third molar is often known as the 'wisdom tooth'. Now a days the 3rd molars may appear very late or become impacted in the jaw. This is because there has been a gradual decrease in size of the jaw of humans over a period a time.
  — The permanent molars have no deciduous predecessors.

- Osteomyelites of the jaw after tooth extraction, though rare, is more commonly seen in lower jaw than upper jaw. This is because, the lower jaw is supplied by a single inferior alveolar artery. Therefore, damage to this artery during extraction produces bone necrosis. The upper jaw on the other hand receives segmental supply by three arteries namely, posterior superior, middle superior and anterior superior alveolar arteries. Therefore ischaemia does not occur following injury to an individual artery.
- **Dental caries** is the disintegration of one of the calcified structures covering the pulp cavity. The most important cause is inadequate oral hygeine. It leads to inflammation and pain in the involved tooth due to exposure of the pulp cavity.
- Congenital anomalies of the tongue can be:
  — **Aglossia,** complete absence of the tongue, due to total developmental failure.
  — **Bifid tongue,** due to non fusion of lingual swellings.
  — **Lingual thyroid,** the median thyroid rudiment fails to grow caudally and thyroid tissue persists within the substance of the tongue.
  — **Tongue tie:** This occurs due to shortening of the frenulum linguae and can interfere in speech. It can be easily excised.
- Paralysis of muscles of soft palate due to lesion of vagus nerve produces
  — Nasal regurgitation of liquids
  — Nasal twang in voice
  — Flattening of the palatal arch on the side of lesion
  — Deviation of uvula, opposite to the side of lesion.
- **Congenital anomalies of face:** These occur due to failure or incomplete fusion of the various processes that form the external part of face during development. They are of the following types:
  — **Cleft upper lip:** Median cleft lip is rare and occurs if the philtrum fails to develop from the frontonasal process. Lateral cleft is more common it may be on one or both sides of the philtrum. Unilateral cleft lip occurs if maxillary process of one side fails to fuse with the corresponding frontonasal process. Bilateral cleft lip occurs if both the maxillary processes fail to fuse with the frontonasal process. The cleft may be a small defect in the upper lip or may extend into the nostril splitting the upper jaw. It may rarely extend to the side of nose along the nasolacrimal groove as far as the orbit (medial angle of the eye). The later is called as oblique facial cleft. The nasolacrimal duct is not formed in these cases.

— **Cleft lower lip:** It is always median and rare. It occurs when the two mandibular processes do not fuse with each other. The defect usually extends into the lower jaw.

— **Cleft palate:** The defective fusion of various segments of the palate gives rise to clefts in the palate. These vary considerably in degree, leading to the following varieties of cleft palate.

i. **Complete cleft palate:** It can be unilateral or bilateral.

ii. **Incomplete or partial cleft:** It can be in form of bifid uvula, cleft of soft palate or cleft of soft palate extending into the hard palate.

Cleft lip leads to facial deformity while cleft palate is also associated with regurgitation of milk into the nose of new borns and can lead to aspiration pneumonitis. There is defective development of speech in cleft palate involving hard palate.

SALIVARY GLANDS

- **Xerostomia** is dry moutlh: This occurs due to lack of secretion of salivary glands. It can occur in anxiety, dehydration or pathologies like auto-immune diseases of salivary glands or radiation injuries.
- **Sialorrhea** is hypersecretion of saliva.
- **Mumps:** It is an infection caused by a virus which has special affinity for the parotid glands and results in swollen and painful glands. Pain is severe as the gland is surrounded by a tough capsule. Mastica-tion is also painful due to inflammation of the glenoid process of gland which is closely related to the tempromandibular joint. Mumps is self limiting and requires only supportive care. Rarely it can lead to complications like bronchitis, orchitis (infection of testis) and pancreatitis.
- Infection of parotid gland usually occurs as a conse-quence of retrograde bacterial infection from mouth through the parotid duct. Severe infection leading to an abscess is drained by giving a horizontal incision over it. A vertical incision is avoided as it can lead to injury to branches of the facial nerve.

ESOPHAGUS

- **Aerophagia:** It is the swallowing of air during eating and drinking. It leads to belching.
- **Gastro esophagial reflux disease (GERD):** It is the reflux of the acidic contents of stomach retrograde into the esophagus. It usually occurs due to:
  — Loss of LES tone—as seen in pregnancy, anxious individuals.
  — Hiatus hernia—due to widening of esophageal opening in diaphragm.

GERD leads to chronic inflammation and occasionally formation of ulcer in lower end of esophagus.
- **Dysphagia:** It is defined as difficulty in swallowing. It can be to liquids or solids. In the elderly, it is an important symptom of esophageal cancer.
- The lower end of oesophagus is drained by two venous channels. The left gastric vein drains into the portal vein of liver and the hemiazygous vein drains into the inferior vena. Thus, it is a site of **portocaval anastomosis**. In cirrhosis of liver associated with portal hypertension there is back pressure in the portal circulation. This leads to opening of the anastomotic channels in the lower end of esophagus. These engorged veins (esophageal varices) are friable and can burst at any time causing hematemesis (vomitting of blood).
- **Achalasia cardia:** It is the congenital absence of ganglionic cells or myenteric plexus of nerves in the esophageal wall. This leads to neuromuscular incoordination and accumulation of food in the esophagus, as the lower end fails to dilate in response to bolus of food.
- The constrictions of esophagus have to be borne in mind to avoid injury during endoscopy.

STOMACH

- **Peptic ulcer:** It is the break in the mucosal lining of stomach or first part of duodenum. It occurs due to:
  — Disruption of mucosal barrier: This can be caused by excess or prolonged use of pain killers, infection with helicobacter pylori, damage by bile salts etc.
  — Excess secretion of gastric acids: It is usually caused by abnormal response to gastrin, may also occur in gastric tumors. The patient presents with complaints of epigastric pain especially after meals.
- **Vomiting:** It is the forceful expulsion of contents of stomach and small intestine (usually food, gastric secretions along with bile and intestinal secretions) from the mouth to exterior. Vomiting centre is present in the medulla and can be stimulated by afferents from GIT (irritation of mucosa), vestibular apparatus of ear, limbic system (emotional stimuli) etc. or diretly by drugs like digitalis etc.
- Patient with carcinoma stomach usually develop left side supraclavicular lymphadenopathy (lymph nodes enlargement) in late stages. This is because stomach, pancreas, testis etc. drain lymph into the thoracic duct which opens at the juction of left internal jugular vein with subclavian vein on the left side.

SMALL INTESTINE

- Ist part of duodenum has highest risk of peptic ulcer because it is directly exposed to gastric juices containing acid.
- In malignancy of neck of pancreas a part of duodenum is also removed because the head of pancreas and duodenum have a common blood supply. Head of pancreas cannot be removed without damaging blood supply to the duodenum. Hence, both are removed.

LARGE INTESTINE

- Taenia coli, converge at the base of appendix as they do not extend to appendix. This is the identifying feature for appendix.
- Sympathetic preganglionic supply to appendix is from T_{10} spinal segment and the skin over umbilicus is also supplied by T_{10} spinal segment. Hence, pain of appendicitis is felt at the umbilicus (referred pain).
- McBurney's point (Fig. 23.9): It is the point of junction of medial 2/3rd and lateral 1/3rd of a line extending from right anterior superior iliac spine to umbilicus. The initial pain of appendicitis is refered to umbilicus but later on, with involvement of parietal peritoneum, pain is felt at McBurney's point. Maximum tenderness on palpation is also felt at this point.
- Anal column contain radicles of superior mesenteric vein. In case of portal obstruction or in patients with chronic constipation these veins get dilated and become tortuous. This is known as **internal haemorrhoids** or **piles.** On internal examination the position of piles is 3, 7 and 11'o clock.
- **Diarrhea:** It is defined as passage of poorly formed stools usually liquid in consistency at increased frequency. It can be due to following reasons:
  — Acute diarrhea is usually due to bacterial or viral infections.
  — Ingestion of toxic or poisonous substance.
  — Drug induced, e.g., Ampicillin, Cephalosporin etc.
  — Chronic diarrhea is diarrhea occurring for more than four weeks. It is due to instestinal diseases leading to malabsorption.
- **Constipation:** It is a clinical condition characterized by persistent infrequent defecation usually associated with hard stools, difficulty in defecation and feeling of incomplete defecation.

LIVER AND GALL BLADDER

- **Cholecystectomy** is the surgical removal of gall bladder.

- Most common pathology for which cholecystectomy is performed is cholelithiasis or gall stones. Gall stones can cause chronic inflammation of gall bladder, obstruction of bile duct leading to jaundice and occasionally are associated with gall bladder cancer.
- Kocher's incision is used for cholecystectomy. The incision commences at the tip of the xiphoid process and passes down and to the right, parallel to the costal margin and two finger-breaths below it. 9th thoracic spinal nerve is prone to injury with this incision. However, these days laparoscopic cholecystectomy is mostly performed. The post operative morbidity is very low with laparoscopic procedure than with open laparotomy (Kocher's incision).
- Cystic artery is ligated in Calot's triangle in cholecystectomy. The triangle of Calot is formed by the common hepatic duct on the left, the cystic duct on the right and liver above.

PANCREAS

- Malignant growth of head of pancreas may obstruct the bile duct leading to obstructive type of jaundice.
- Steatorrhea: It is the passage of large, bulky, clay coloured stools due to presence of increased amount of undigested lipid content of food. It most commonly occurs due to deficiency of pancreatic lipase enzyme. It may also occur in patients with malabsorption syndrome due to damage or removal of ileum.

NUTRITION

- **Protein energy malnutrition (PEM):** It is a clinical condition which results due to deficient intake of diet specially in energy (carbohydrates) with or without protein deficiency. It is the major cause of morbidity and mortality in children specially under the age of 5 years in our country. PEM is assessed in school children by measuring weight, height and midarm circumference. The most common causes of PEM are:
  — Poverty
  — Ignorance regarding diet
  — Repeated worm infestation
  — Poor hygiene
  The two clinical conditions associated with PEM are kwashiorkor and marasmus.

Recommended intake of nutrients

Item	Requirement (recommended in adults)
Calories	Male: 2200 to 2800 calories Female: 1900 to 2200 calories (pregnancy + 300 calories, lactation + 550 calories)
Protein	0.9 to 1 g/kg (in children 1.2 to 1.5 gm/kg) (pregnancy + 15 gm/day, lactation + 25 gm/day)
Carbohydrate	50 to 60% of total calories
Fat	15 to 20% of total calories
Vitamin A	600 µg
Vitamin D	100 IU
Vitamin K	0.03 mg/kg
Vitamin B1 (Thiamin)	0.5 mg/1000 calories
Vitamin B2 (Riboflavin)	0.6 mg/1000 calories
Niacin	6.6 mg/1000 calories
Folic acid	100 µg
Vitamin B12	1 µg
Vitamin C	60 mg
Calcium	500 mg (1000 mg in pregnancy and lactation)
Iron	28 mg (30 to 60 mg in pregnancy and lactation)
Iodine	150 µg

Sources of vitamins and disorders associated with their deficiency

Vitamin	Source	Deficiency disorder
Vitamin A	Yellow and green vegetables, milk, ghee, cream Liver	Night blindness. Dry skin and hair. Increase respiratory, urinary and digestive tract infections. Drying and finally destruction of cornea known as keratomalacia.
Vitamin D	Produced in the body in skin following sunlight exposure and then finally by liver and kidney. Fish oil, Egg yolk.	Defective mineralization of bones leading to rickets in children and osteomalacia in adults.
Vitamin E	Nuts, liver, seed oils, fish oil, green leafy vegetables.	Nil of significance.
Vitamin K	Synthesized by intestinal bacteria. Green leafy vegetables, cauliflower, cabbage, liver, pork.	Bleeding disorder due to defective synthesis of coagulation factors.
Vitamin B1 (Thiamine)	Whole grains, nuts, potato, yeast, liver and eggs.	Beri-beri, polyneuritis.
Vitamin B2 (Riboflavin)	Whole grains peanuts, peas, egg and non-vegetarian food.	Dermatitis, angular stomatis, glossitis, cataract and corneal defects.
Niacin	Whole grain, beans, mushrooms, nuts, meat and fish.	Dermatitis, diarrhea and psychological defects. Condition is known as pellagra.
Vitamin B6 (Pyridoxine)	Yeast, tomatoes, potatoes, corn, spinach, whole grains, legumes, liver, fish.	Dermatitis of eyes and mouth, peripheral neuritis.
Vitamin B12 (Cyanocobalamin)	Cheese, milk, egg, meat.	Megaloblastic anemia.
Pantothenic acid	Yeast, green vegetables, cereals, liver, kidney and egg.	Fatigue, muscle cramps.
Folic acid	Green leafy vegetables, broccoli, bread, fruits.	Megaloblastic anemia.
Biotin	Egg yolk, liver, milk, mushroom.	Skin and hair dryness, fatigue, depression.
Vitamin C	Tomatoes, green vegetables, citrus fruits.	Scurvy due to poor collagen formation leading to swollen gums, poor wound healing and fragile blood vessels. Anemia.

Chapter 17

Urinary System

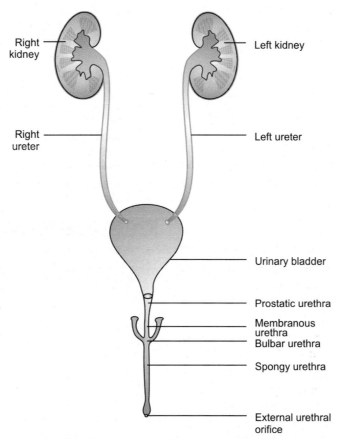

Fig. 17.1: Parts of urinary system in male

INTRODUCTION

The excretory function of the body is primarily carried out by a pair of kidneys. The other excretory organs of the body are skin (produces sweat), GIT (excretes faeces), respiratory tract (excretes CO_2). Kidneys are responsible for the filtration of blood and removal of waste substances like urea, creatinine, uric acid and others from the body. The filtrate under goes a process of reabsorption and secretion which results in the formation of urine. The urine is carried from the kidneys to the urinary bladder by the ureters and is expelled to exterior during micturition through urethra. Kidneys, ureters, urinary bladder and urethra form the urinary system. This system helps in regulating the solute and water content of the body there by, regulating the composition and volume of extracellular fluid.

KIDNEYS

Kidneys are a pair of excretory organs lying in relation to the posterior abdominal wall, on each side of vertebral column (Figs 17.1 to 17.4).

The kidneys are bean shaped and reddish brown in colour. Each kidney extends from T_{12} to L_3 vertebrae. Right kidney is lower than the left, due to presence of liver. Long axis of each kidney is directed downwards and laterally while the transverse axis is directed backwards and laterally. Hence, upper pole is nearer to the vertebral column than lower pole.

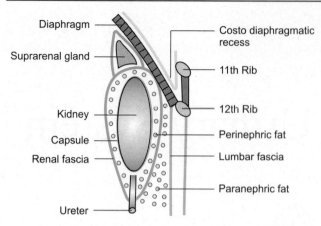

Fig. 17.2: Relations and coverings of kidney

Dimensions (in adults)

Length   :   11 cm
Breadth   :   6 cm
Thickness :   3 cm
Weight   :   130 to 170 gm.

Coverings of Kidney

From within outward (Fig. 17.2)

1. **Fibrous capsule:** It is a fibrous condensation of stroma of kidney. It covers the kidney entirely and lines the wall of renal sinus. It also covers major and minor calyces and pelvis of ureter. It can be stripped off in a healthy kidney.
2. **Perinephric fat:** It lies next to fibrous capsule fills the renal sinus and is abundant along the borders.
3. **Renal fascia (fascia of Gerota):** Renal fascia is the condensation of extra peritoneal tissue. It consists of an anterior layer **(fascia of Toldt's)** and a posterior layer **(fascia of Zuckerkendl).**

4. **Paranephric fat:** It lies between renal fascia and thoraco-lumbar fascia. It is abundant on the posterior surface of lower part of the kidney. It provides a cushion for the kidney.

Presenting Parts

Each kidney presents the following parts

1. **Upper end:** It lies 2.5 cm from median plane. It is more rounded and is related to suprarenal gland.
2. **Lower end:** It lies 7.5cm from the median plane and is broader. It lies about an inch above iliac crest.
3. **Medial border:** It is convex and presents with a central concavity for the hilum. Hilum is a vertical cleft through which the following structures enter or leave the kidney (anterior to posterior):
   — Renal vein
   — Renal artery
   — Pelvis of ureter
   Other structures present in hilum are renal lymphatics, nerves and perinephric fat.
4. **Lateral border:** It is convex, thick and lies on a more posterior plane.
5. **Anterior surface:** It is convex, irregular and directed forwards and laterally.
   Relations: from above downward (Fig. 17.3).

Right kidney	Left kidney
a. Right suprarenal	a. Left suprarenal
b. 2nd part of duodenum	b. Spleen
c. Right lobe of liver	c. Postero-inferior surface of stomach, body of pancreas and splenic artery
d. Right colic flexure	d. Left colic flexure
e. Coils of jejunum	e. Coils of jejunum

6. **Posterior surface:** It is flat and is directed backwards and medially. It is completely non peritoneal. The posterior surface of both the kidneys are related to similar structures as tabulated below (Fig. 17.4):

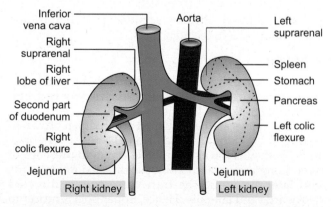

Fig. 17.3: Anterior relations of right and left kidney

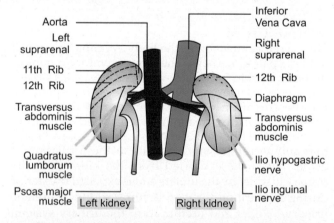

Fig. 17.4: Posterior relations of right and left kidney

Upper part of kidney (within outward)	Lower part of kidney
a. Diaphragm	a. Psoas major muscle
b. Costo-diaphragmatic recess of pleura	b. Quadratus lumborum muscle
c. 12th rib on right side and 11th, 12th ribs on left side	c. Anterior layer of thoraco-lumbar fascia
	d. Transversus abdominis with fascia transversalis
	e. Paranephric fat
	f. Subcostal nerve and vessels
	g. Iliohypogastric nerve
	h. Ilioinguinal nerve
	i. 4th lumbar artery on the right side

Arterial Supply of Kidney

Each kidney is supplied by the **renal artery** which is a branch of abdominal aorta

- Each renal artery divides into anterior and posterior trunks which enter the kidney via the hilum.
- Anterior trunk further divides into 4 segmental arteries and posterior trunk continues as posterior segmental artery.
- Each segmental or lobar artery divides successively into interlobar arteries, arcuate arteries and interlobular arteries.
- The interlobular arteries give rise to afferent arterioles which further divide to form a tuft of capillaries called the glomerulus.
- The glomerular capillaries rejoin at the other end and form the efferents arterioles.
- Each efferent artriole further divides into peritubular capillaries which surround the renal tubules. The efferent arterioles of juxta-medullary nephrons give rise to vasa recta which run along the loop of Henle in the medulla.
- The peritubular capillaries and vasa recta finally drain into the interlobular veins.

Venous Drainage of Kidney

Each kidney is drained by a renal vein which further drains into the inferior vena cava. The left renal vein is longer than the right vein.

Lymphatic Drainage of Kidney

Lymphatics from kidney run along the renal vessels and drain into lateral aortic lymph nodes.

Nerve Supply of Kidney

1. **Sympathetic supply:** Preganglionic fibres are derived from T_{10} to L_1 spinal segments. They form a renal plexus around the renal vessels. The sympathetic supply is vasomotor. It also supplies the JG cells.
2. **Parasympathetic supply:** It is derived from vagus nerve.

Structure of Kidney

On a coronal section, kidney presents with two regions, an inner pale appearing medulla, and an outer brownish red cortex (Fig. 17.5).

Medulla

It is made up of renal pyramids. They are 8–18 in number. Pyramids are striated, pale and conical masses. Base of a pyramid is directed externally towards the cortex. Apex forms the **renal papilla** which opens into a minor calyx in the renal sinus. Renal papilla is perforated by numerous openings of ducts of Bellini. Urine passes from these ducts into the minor calyces.

Cortex

It has a granular appearance and is surrounded by the fibrous capsule. It consists of two parts

1. **Renal columns:** These consist of cortical tissue which extends from the surface to the renal sinus, between renal pyramids.
2. **Cortical arches:** These are arches of cortical matter present between base of pyramid and surface of kidney.

Renal Sinus

Cavity within the kidney at the level of hilum is the renal sinus. It is lined by the renal capsule.

Contents of Renal Sinus
1. Renal artery
2. Renal vein
3. Lymph vessels
4. Nerves

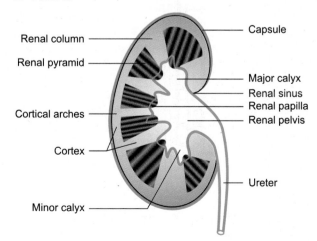

Fig. 17.5: Coronal section of kidney

5. Perinephric fat
6. Minor calyces, 7 to 13
7. Major calyces, 2 to 3
8. Pelvis of ureter

Microscopic Structure of Kidney

Kidney is made up of numerous uriniferous tubules. A uriniferous tubule consists of two parts namely:
a. Excretory part: Nephron
b. Collecting part: Collecting tubule

It is supported by fine connective tissue containing blood vessels, lymphatics and nerves.

Nephron

Nephron is the functional unit of kidney (Fig. 17.6). There are about 1.3 million nephrons in each kidney. Each nephron consists of two parts namely: renal corpuscle and renal tubule.

1. **Renal corpuscle:** It is made up of glomerulus and Bowman's capsule. Filtration of blood occurs at glomerulus which is formed by the invagination of tuft of capillaries into the proximal dilated end of nephron known as Bowman's capsule. The capillaries originate from an afferent arteriole and drain into an efferent arteriole. Filtration occurs across the **glomerular membrane** which is made up of:

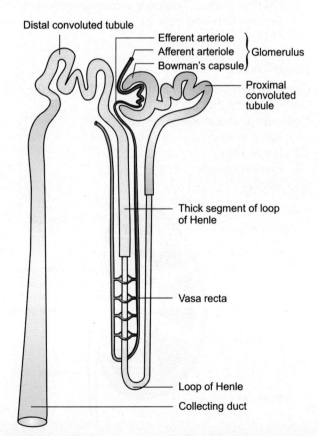

Distal convoluted tubule

Efferent arteriole
Afferent arteriole } Glomerulus
Bowman's capsule

Proximal convoluted tubule

Thick segment of loop of Henle

Vasa recta

Loop of Henle

Collecting duct

Fig. 17.6: Diagrammatic representation of parts of a nephron

a. **Endothelium of capillaries:** it is fenestrated with pores having a diameter of 70 to 90 nm.
b. **Stellate cells or mesangial cells:** These are present between the endothelial cells and their basement membrane.
c. **Basement membrane of endothelium.**
d. **Basement membrane of epithelial layer of Bowman's capsule.**
e. **Epithelium of capsule:** It consists of simple squamous cells with intersperced specialized cells called podocytes.

The passage of substances across this membrane depends upon their size and electrical charges. It allows free passage of neutral substances less than 4 nm while inhibits passage of substances above 8 nm.

2. **Renal tubule:** The composition and volume of the fluid filtered at glomerulus is altered as it passes through the renal tubules. Renal tubules are responsible for selective reabsorption of the filtrate and secretion of substances not filtered at glomerulus resulting in formation of urine. Each renal tubule consists of the following parts:
   a. **Proximal convoluted tubule (PCT):** It is 15 mm long and 55 µm in diameter. It is lined by single layer of cuboidal cells which are rich in mitochondria.
   b. **Loop of Henle:** This part decides the length of a nephron. Nephrons with smaller length are more numerous and nephrons with larger loops constitute only 15%. The longer nephrons are located in the juxtamedullary portion of renal cortex. Loop of Henle consists of two parts:
      — **Descending limb:** It is the thin tubular part lined by flat cells and continues from proximal convoluted tubule. The length varies from 2 to 11mm.
      — **Ascending limb:** It is thin in lower half and thick in upper part. The thick tubular segment is about 12 mm length and is lined by cuboidal cells.
   c. **Distal convoluted tubule (DCT):** It is 5 mm long and continues from distal end of ascending limb. It is lined by a layer of low cuboidal cells.

Juxta Glomerular Apparatus

It is the term given to the collection of specialised cells of renal tubule and the associated afferent arteriole of a nephron. It consists of the following parts:

1. **Juxta glomerular cells (JG cells):** These are modified endothelial cells of afferent arterioles. They are seen in the anteriole just before they enter the glomerulus. These cells are rich in endoplasmic reticulum, mitochondria and ribosomes. These cells

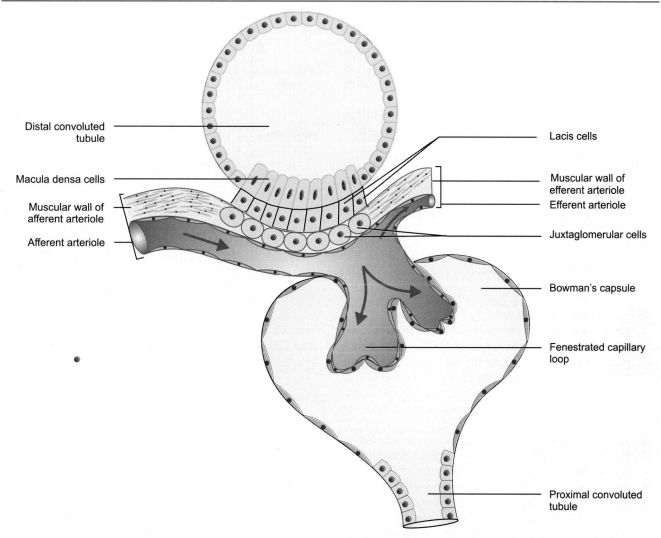

Fig. 17.7: Juxta glomerular apparatus

synthesize and store the enzyme **Renin**. They are innervated by the sympathetic nerves and respond to pressure changes between the afferent arterioles and interstitium of kidney. Hence, they act as **baroreceptors** (Fig. 17.7).

2. **Macula densa cells:** These are specialized tubular cells located at the junction of thick ascending limb of loop of Henle and distal convoluted tubule, lying in close apposition to the afferent arteriole. They act as **chemoceptors.** They respond to the changes in Na^+ load reaching them.

3. **Mesangial cells or Lacis cells:** These cells lie between the capillary loops in relation to both JG cells and macula densa cells.

Collecting Tubules (CT)

The distal convoluted tubules coalesce to form collecting ducts. Each duct is about 20 mm long and passes from cortex to medulla. It ends into the pelvic calyces of kidneys. It is lined by cuboidal cells consisting of principal (P) cells and intercalated (I) cells. P cells are involved in Na^+ reabsorption while I cells are concerned with HCO_3^- transport.

Functions of Kidneys

- Kidneys are the main excretory organs of our body that eliminate metabolic waste products like ammonia, urea, uric acid, creatinine etc. by the formation of urine.
- They play an important role in the regulation of extra cellular fluid volume by controlling the water and electrolyte balance
- Kidneys are responsible for control of the acid base balance of body.
- Kidneys also have an endocrine function and secrete the following hormones:

1. Erythropoetin: It is secreted from the endo-thelium of peritubular capillaries in response to hypoxia. Erythropoetin stimulates hemopoeisis.
2. 1, 25-dihydroxycholecalciferol (calcitriol): It is produced by the cells of PCT and it regulates calcium metabolism.
3. Renin: It is secreted by JG cells and regulates extracellular fluid volume and blood pressure.

URETERS

Ureters are thick walled tubes extending from the corres-ponding kidney to the urinary bladder. They are two in number and lie in relation to the posterior abdominal wall (Fig. 17.8).

Length : 25 cm
Diameter : 3 mm

Parts of Ureter

There are three parts of ureter

1. **Pelvis of ureter:** The urine flows from minor calyces which join to form major calyces. There are 2 to 3 major calyces in each kidney. The major calyces join to form the pelvis of ureter also called renal pelvis at the hilum of kidney. It is funnel shaped and continues with abdominal part of ureter at the level of lower end of the kidney.
2. **Abdominal part of ureter:** This part is related to the posterior abdominal wall. It extends from lower end of the kidney to bifurcation of common iliac artery. **It lies in relation to the tip of transverse processes of lumbar vertebrae.** It passes downward and slightly medially. It is covered by parietal peritoneum of posterior abdominal wall anteriorly. It is plastered to the parietal peritoneum.
3. **Pelvic part of ureter:** It extends from the bifurcation of common iliac artery to the entry of ureter in urinary bladder. It is divided into three parts.
   a. **Vertical part or 1st part:** It extends from the bifurcation of common iliac artery to the ischial spine. Here, it runs along the lateral pelvic wall beneath the peritoneum.
   b. **Oblique part of ureter or 2nd part:** It extends from the ischial spine to the superolateral angle of base of bladder, passing forwards and medially. In female it lies at the level of internal os of uterus, 1.5 cm lateral to it. The uterine artery crosses over it at this point.
   c. **Intravesical part or 3rd part:** It lies inside the musculature of urinary bladder. It is 2 cm in length and runs obliquely.

Arterial Supply of Ureter

Ureter is supplied by branches of various arteries along its course. These are renal artery, gonadal artery, lumbar

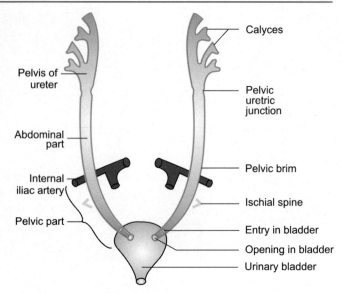

Fig. 17.8: Parts of ureter

arteries, peritoneal arteries, common iliac artery, internal iliac artery, inferior vesical artery, uterine and vaginal arteries in female.

Venous Drainage of Ureter

Corresponding veins drain into inferior vena cava.

Lymphatic Drainage of Ureter

Lymphatics of ureter drain into
1. Para-aortic lymph nodes, from upper part.
2. Common iliac lymph nodes, from intermediate part.
3. Internal iliac and external iliac lymph nodes, from lower part.

Nerve Supply of Ureter

1. **Sympathetic supply:** Preganglionic fibres are derived from T_{10}, T_{11}, T_{12} and L_1 spinal segments. Post ganglionic fibres are distributed via renal, gonadal and hypogastric plexuses.
2. **Parasympathetic supply:** It is derived from bran-ches of vagus and pelvic splanchnic nerves.

Structure of Ureter

It is made up of three coats (Fig. 17.9). From without inwards these are:
1. **Outer fibrous coat:** It is made up of loose connective tissue. It contains numerous blood vessels and fat cells.
2. **Middle smooth muscle coat:** It is a well developed layer consisting of an inner longitudinal and an outer circular muscle layer. A third layer of long-

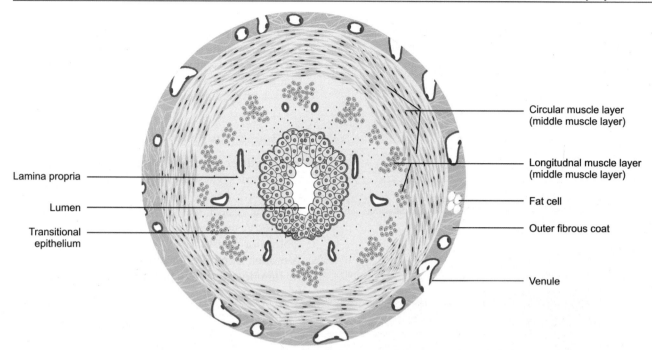

Lamina propria

Lumen

Transitional epithelium

Circular muscle layer (middle muscle layer)

Longitudnal muscle layer (middle muscle layer)

Fat cell

Outer fibrous coat

Venule

Fig. 17.9: Transverse section of Ureter (Stain-hematoxylin-eosin under high magnification)

itudinal fibres is present outside the circular coat in the lower 1/3rd of the ureter.

3. **Inner mucous membrane:** It is lined by transitional epithelium which is 4 to 5 cell thick. The epithelium rests on fibrous tissue containing many elastic fibres known as lamina propria. The lamina propria has diffuse connective tissue with scattered lymphoid tissue. The mucosa shows a star shape appearance as it is thrown into many folds.

Functions of Ureters

Ureters primarily conduct urine from the corresponding kidney to the bladder.

Following are the factors responsible in preventing reflux from urinary bladder to ureter.

a. Obliquity of ureters when they enter the bladder wall.

b. Peristalsis of ureteric muscles helps in draining urine in the form of a jet not as continuous drops.

c. Anterior wall of intravesical part of ureter acts as a flap valve.

URINARY BLADDER

It is a muscular bag which acts as a reservoir of urine (Figs 17.10, 17.11).

Position: It lies in pelvis in adult while in children it is an abdomino-pelvic organ.

Shape: Ovoid when distended, tetrahedral when empty.

Capacity

Anatomical capacity : 1000 ml
Physiological capacity : 450 ml

Presenting Parts

It presents the following parts when empty

1. **Apex:** It is directed forwards and upwards. The urachus or median umbilical ligament is attached to it.

2. **Base:** It is also called the postero-inferior surface. It is directed backward and downwards. It is non peritoneal except at a small part in respect of upper part of seminal vesicles in male.

3. **Superior surface:** It is triangular in shape and covered with peritoneum.

4. **Infero-lateral surfaces:** There are two inferolateral surfaces.

5. **Anterior border:** It separates the inferolateral surfaces, and extends from the apex to the neck of bladder.

6. **Posterior border:** It separates the superior surface from base of bladder.

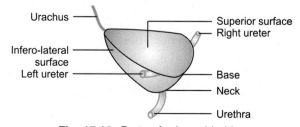

Urachus

Infero-lateral surface

Left ureter

Superior surface

Right ureter

Base

Neck

Urethra

Fig. 17.10: Parts of urinary bladder

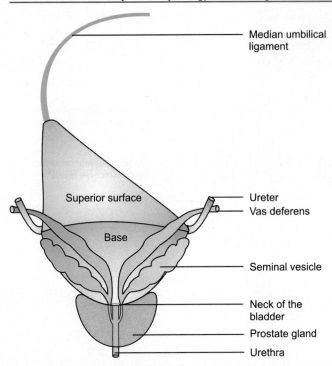

Fig. 17.11: Relations of urinary bladder

7. **Lateral border:** Each lateral border separates the inferolateral surface from superior surface.
8. **Neck:** Lowest point of the bladder from where urethra begins is the neck of bladder. In case of male, the neck is surrounded by prostate gland.

In distended bladder: Inferolateral surfaces become anteroinferior surfaces. The anteroinferior surfaces are nonperitoneal.

Ligaments of Bladder

They are classified as true and false ligaments.

True ligaments: These are fibrous bands formed by condensation of pelvic fascia containing few smooth muscle fibres. These ligaments help to support the bladder. They are 9 in number

1. Median umbilical ligament: It is the remnant of urachus. It extends from apex of bladder to umbilicus.
2. Four pubo-prostatic ligaments: These are also called pubovesical ligaments. They extend from the bladder neck to the symphysis pubis and to the tendinous arch of pelvic fascia.
3. Two lateral ligaments: These extend from each of the infero-lateral surfaces of bladder to pelvic fascia.
4. Two posterior true ligaments: These extend from the base of bladder to lateral pelvic wall. Each contains a plexus of vesical veins.

False ligaments: These are just peritoneal folds. They are seven in number.

1. Three anterior peritoneal folds: These peritoneal folds are present over the median umbilical ligament and the two obliterated umbilical arteries.
2. Two lateral false ligaments: These extend from the bladder to lateral pelvic wall.
3. Two sacro genital folds posteriorly.

Arterial Supply of Urinary Bladder

Urinary bladder receives arterial supply through following arteries. These are the branches of internal iliac artery.

1. Superior vesical artery
2. Inferior vesical artery
3. Obturator artery
4. A branch from inferior gluteal artery
5. In female–uterine artery also supplies urinary bladder

Venous Drainage of Urinary Bladder

Venous drainage is through vesical plexus of veins which is situated along the inferolateral surface of bladder. It drains into internal iliac vein along the posterior ligament of bladder.

Lymphatic Drainage of Urinary Bladder

Lymphatics from bladder drain into external iliac group of lymph nodes.

Nerve Supply of Urinary Bladder

Urinary bladder is supplied by sympathetic and para-sympathetic divisions of autonomic nervous system (Fig. 17.12).

1. **Sympathetic supply:** Preganglionic fibres are derived from T_{11}, T_{12}, L_1 and L_2 segments of spinal cord and relay in superior hypogastric plexus. Post ganglionic fibres supply the body and neck of urinary bladder. Sympathetic neurons stimulate the sphincter vesicae and inhibit the detrusor muscle. This is responsible for retention of urine. Painful sensation is also carried by the sympathetic fibres.
2. **Parasympathetic supply:** Preganglionic fibres are derived from lateral horn of S_2, S_3, S_4 spinal segments and form nervi erigentes. Post ganglionic fibres arise form the bladder wall or parasympathetic ganglia near the bladder. Parasympathetic is stimulator to detrusor muscle and is responsible for micturition (passing of urine). Sense of distension is carried by parasympathetic fibres.

Inner Aspect of Bladder

- On naked eye examination, the mucosa presents with irregular folds, in an empty bladder, as it is loosely attached to underlying muscular coat. These folds flatten out as the bladder starts filling with urine (Fig. 17.13).
- **Trigone:** It is seen as a triangular area in the lower part of base of bladder where the mucosa is adherent to underlying muscular coat. Hence, it is smooth. Base of trigone is formed by the interureteric ridge which extends between the two openings of ureters while the apex is directed downwards and leads to the internal urethral meatus.
- Bladder mucosa is derived from endoderm except trigone of the bladder which developes from mesoderm.

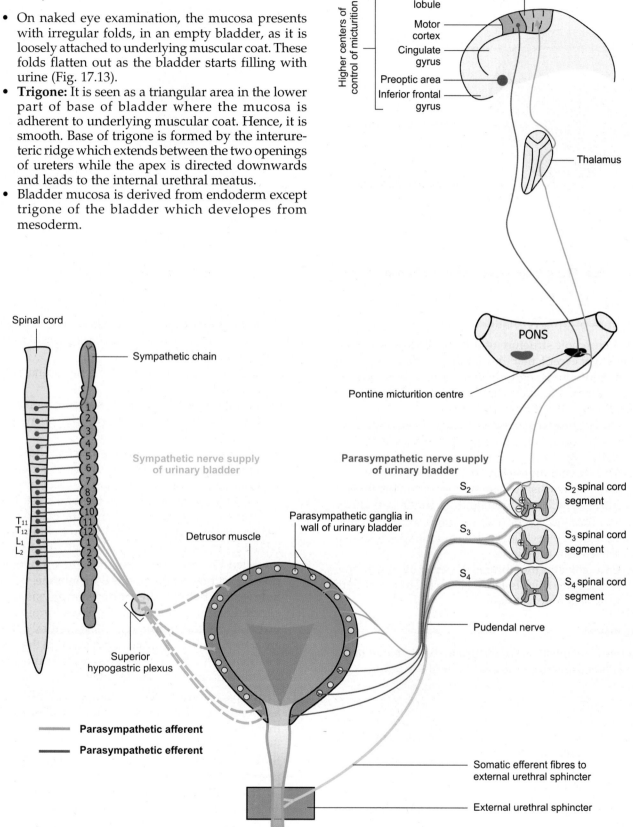

Fig. 17.12: Nerve supply of urinary bladder

CHAPTER-17

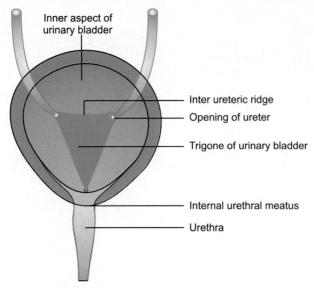

Fig. 17.13: Inner aspect of urinary bladder

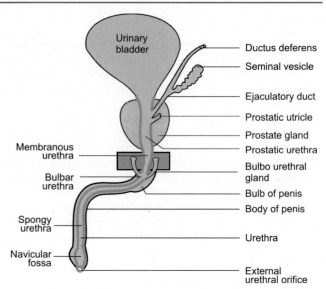

Fig. 17.14: Male urethra

Structure of Urinary Bladder

The microscopic structure of urinary bladder is similar to the ureter except, that the middle smooth muscle coat has an additional longitudinal layer of muscle outside the circular muscle layer. The bladder is made up of three coats. From without inwards these are:

1. **Outer fibrous coat:** It is made up of loose connective tissue. It contains numerous blood vessels and fat cells.
2. **Middle smooth muscle coat:** It is a well developed layer and consists of a meshwork of smooth muscle fibres which are arrnaged as inner and outer longitudinal layers with an intermediate circular or oblique muscle layer. This muscle coat is known as Detrusor muscle.
3. **Inner mucous membrane:** It is lined by transitional epithelium which is 4 to 5 cell thick. The epithelium rests on a fibrous tissue.

URETHRA

It is the distal most part of the urinary system that helps to conduct urine from the bladder to the exterior.

Male Urethra

In males it is 18 to 20 cm long and extends from bladder neck to tip of penis. It is S-shaped in flaccid penis while J-shaped in erected penis (Fig. 17.14).

Parts of Male Urethra

1. **Prostatic part of urethra (3 cm long):** It is the widest and most dilatable part. It extends from neck of urinary bladder to prostatic utricle and passes through anterior part of prostate. Inner aspect of posterior wall of prostatic urethra presents with following features:
   a. **Urethral crest:** It is a median longitudinal ridge of mucus membrane.
   b. **Colliculus seminalis:** This is an elevation in the middle of urethral crest with the opening of prostatic utricle at its summit.
   c. **Openings of ejaculatory ducts:** These are present on each side of the orifice of utricle
   d. **Prostatic sinuses:** These are vertical grooves present one on each side of urethral crest. They present with openings of prostatic glands.
2. **Membranous part of urethra (1.5 to 2 cm long):** It is the narrowest and least dilatable part. It runs from lower end of prostate through the deep perineal pouch and pierces the perineal membrane, 2.5 cm below and behind the pubic symphysis. It is surrounded by striated muscle fibres forming the **external urethral sphincter.** Bulbo-urethral glands are present one on each side of this part in the deep perineal pouch. It presents with numerous openings of urethral glands, internally.
3. **Penile part of urethra (15 cm long):** It is also known as spongy part. It first runs forwards and upwards in the bulb of penis. Then it bends downwards and lies in the corpus spongiosum of penis. It ends at the external urethral meatus at tip of glans penis. It presents with two dilatations
   a. **Intrabulbar fossa, at its commencement**
   b. **Navicular fossa, within glans penis:** The ducts of bulbourethral glands open into penile urethra, 2.5 cm below its origin.

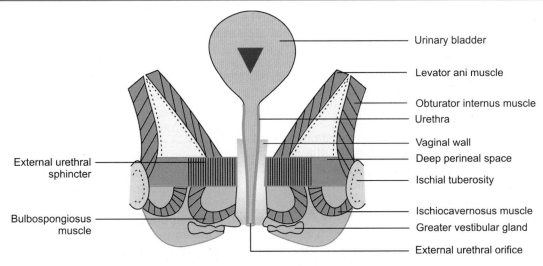

Fig. 17.15: Female urethra

The external urethral meatus is the narrowest part of urethra and is in the form of a sagittal slit about 6 mm long.

Blood Supply of Urethra

It is obtained from vessels supplying prostate and penis.

Lymphatic Drainage of Urethra

Lymphatics from urethra drain into internal and external iliac lymph nodes, deep and superficial inguinal lymph nodes.

Female Urethra

- In female, urethra is only 3.8 to 4 cm long (Fig. 17.15).
- It extends from neck of bladder to the external urethral orifice which lies in the vestibule.
- It is embedded in anterior wall of vagina.
- Internally, the mucosa of urethra is folded extensively and contains numerous mucus glands.
- On each side, in the upper part, are present paraurethral glands of Skene (homologus to prostate in male).
- It is easily dilatable.

Urethral Sphincters

These consist of muscle fibres which enclose the urethra at two sites and control the flow of urine.

1. **Internal urethral sphincter/shpincter vescicae:** It is made up of involuntary smooth muscle fibres interspersed with elastic and collagen fibres. It lies subjacent to the neck of bladder (around prostatic urethra, above the opening of ejaculatory ducts in males). It is supplied by sympathetic nerves. Sympathetic supply maintains the tone of internal sphincter which allows for the filling of bladder.

2. **External urethral sphincter/sphincter urethrae:** It is made of voluntary, striated muscle fibres present just above external meatus in deep perineal space. It is supplied by pudendal nerve (S_2, S_3, S_4). Pudendal nerve is responsible for contraction of the external sphincter which helps in voluntary control of micturition.

FORMATION OF URINE

- Kidneys receive 1.2 to 1.3 litres of blood per minute and produce urine at the rate of 1 ml per minute.
- There are three processes involved in urine formation
  - **Filtration:** This occurs in glomerulus.
  - **Reabsorption:** It is the active transport of various solutes like Na^+, K^+, Cl^-, Ca^{2+}, HPO^{2-}_4, uric acid, amino acid and glucose with passive movement of water from the lumen of tubules into the peritubular capillaries. Creatinine is the important solute which is filtered but is not reabsorbed at all.
  - **Secretion:** It is the transport of solutes like K^+, H^+ and uric acid from peritubular capillaries into the lumen of the tubules.
- The plasma is filtered at the glomerulus and passes into the Bowman's capsule.
- The glomerular filtrate is known as ultrafiltrate. It has similar osmolality and electrolyte content as plasma but has no proteins or cells.
- The normal **glomerular filtration rate (GFR)** is 125 ml/minute. This equals 170 to 180 litres/day. However, daily urine output is 1.5 to 2 liters. 99% of the filtrate is therefore reabsorbed in normal conditions.

Factors Affecting GFR

1. **Hydrostatic pressure gradient:** Increase pressure in capillaries leads to increase GFR while increase pressure in Bowman's capsule decreases GFR.
   a. **Factors affecting capillary pressure**
      — **Renal blood flow:** Decreases with age. Hence, GFR also decreases with age.
      — **Systemic blood pressure:** GFR is maintained at systemic BP of 90 to 220 mmHg due to autoregulation in kidney. Fall of systolic BP below 90 mmHg reduces GFR sharply.
      — **Contraction of afferent arteriole:** This reduces renal plasma flow and hence GFR while efferent arteriolar contraction increases capillary pressure and GFR.
   b. **Factors affecting hydrostatic pressure in Bowman's capsule:** Ureteral obstruction associated with hydronephrosis or edema of kidneys increases pressure in Bowman's capsule leading to fall in GFR.
2. **Osmotic pressure gradient between capillaries and Bowman's capsule:** A decrease in concentration of plasma proteins, as in hypoprotenemia, leads to increase in GFR. In dehydration however, due to the altered plasma osmolality GFR decreases.
3. **Size of capillary bed:** Contraction of mesangial cells cause reduction in total area available for filtration by encroaching on capillary bed. This leads to decrease in GFR. Angiotensin II is an important regulator of contraction of mesangial cells.
4. **Permeability of capillaries:** Increase permeability of glomerular membrane due to damage by various diseases like glomerulornephritis results in increase GFR with increase filtration of plasma proteins (known as proteinuria).

Auto Regulation of Renal Blood Flow

The vascular bed of renal cortex has an intrinsic capacity to maintain a constant rate of blood flow by altering local vascular resistance to variations in perfusion pressures (90-220 mmHg). This is achieved by changes in the intrinsic tone of musculature of the afferent arterioles. It is also regulated by the macula densa cells. Any decrease in renal blood flow leads to decrease in GFR and subsequently a decrease in load of solute (Na^+, Cl^-) to the DCT. This is sensed by macula densa cells and they regulate local renin-angiotensin response via juxta-glomerular cells which increases local blood flow.

Tubular Function

The tubules of nephrons reabsorb most of the filtrate. Some molecules are secreted by the tubules which adds to the filtrate and ultimately leads to formation of urine.

The chapter describes reabsorption and secretion of important substances like glucose, Na^+, K^+, Cl^-, HCO_3^-, H^+ and water (Figs 17.16 to 17.19).

Glucose Reabsorption

- Glucose is filtered across glomerulus at 100mg/mt.
- 100% glucose is reabsorbed at the proximal part of proximal convoluted tubules (amino-acids are also reabsorbed completely at PCT).
- Glucose is transported by the sodium (Na^+) dependant glucose transporter (SGLT-2) into the tubular epithelium. This is an example of **secondary active transport** similar to that in intestines.
- It is transported out of cell into interstitium by glucose transporter (GLUT-2) along its gradient and enters the peritubular capillaries by diffusion.
- Renal threshold for glucose is the plasma level of glucose beyond which significant amount of glucose starts appearing in urine. This is called **glycosuria.** Glycosuria is seen when plasma glucose level rises above 180 mg/dl. This is the T_m or transport maximum of glucose. All the transport sites are occupied and no more glucose can be reabsorbed.

Na^+ Reabsorption

- About 98-99% of Na^+ gets reabsorbed by nephrons at PCT, loop of Henle, DCT and collecting tubule. **This is an active transport.**
- **In PCT:** 80% Na^+ is reabsorbed in PCT. It is mostly transported by Na^+ glucose cotransporter into the cell. It also directly enters interstitium by Na^+ Cl^- channels. From cells, it is actively pumped out by Na^+ K^+ ATPase pump which maintains the chemical and electrical gradient for uptake of Na^+. Increase in osmolality of interstitium results in diffusion of water passively into tubular cells and then into peritubular capillaries.
- **In loop of Henle:** Na^+ is absorbed with Cl^- in thin ascending segment of loop of Henle by passive diffusion across the channels. In the thick ascending segment however it is actively transported by Na^+-K^+-Cl^- symporter.
- **In DCT and CT:** Na^+ is mostly absorbed coupled with Cl^-. The rest is absorbed in exchange with H^+ or K^+ ions which are secreted into the lumen.

Regulation of Na^+ Excretion

Na^+ is the most abundant and hence an important osmotically active ion in the extracellular fluid **(ECF).** Thus, regulation of Na^+ balance is important to maintain the homeostasis of the body. Factors regulating Na^+ secretion are:
1. **Hydrostatic and osmotic pressures**
   a. Increase in GFR results in increase reabsorption of Na^+.

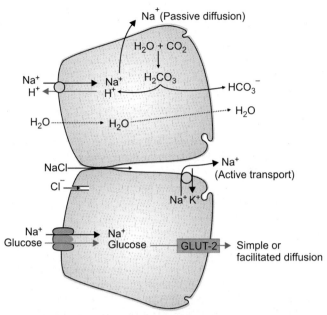

Fig. 17.16: Diagrammatic representation of absorption of various solutes and water in PCT

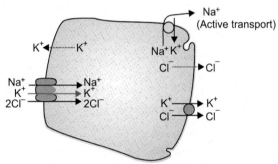

Fig. 17.17: Diagrammatic representation of absorption of various solutes in thick ascending loop of Henle

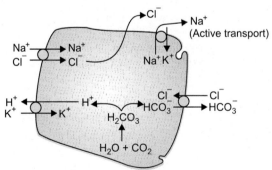

Fig. 17.18: Diagrammatic representation of secretion of H+ in DCT

b. Decrease in extracellular fluid volume results in reduced hydrostatic pressure in peritubular capillaries leading to increase Na+ reabsorption in PCT. Water moves in with Na+ and helps to correct the ECF volume.

c. Increase Na+ load results in increase excretion. This is because the excess load overcomes the maximum reabsorptive capacity. This is called Natriuresis.

2. **Effect of hormones—Aldosterone:** It increases activity of Na+ K+ ATPase pump and thus increases the gradient for Na+ in DCT and CT resulting in increased Na+ reabsorption. It is produced in response to low extra cellular fluid volume (ECFV) and low Na+ intake.

Water Excretion

- Water is reabsorbed mostly by **passive diffusion** by the osmotic gradient caused by Na+ and Cl– absorption.
- 60 to 70% gets absorbed in PCT, about 15% is removed by the thin descending limb of loop of Henle. The ascending limb of loop of Henle is impermeable to water. DCT is minimally permeable to water. Rest of the water is absorbed in collecting tubules. Thus 99.7% water is reabsorbed.
- Water reabsorption in CT is controlled by **antidiuretic hormone (ADH).** ADH helps in water reabsorption. Decrease ADH levels limit the reabsorption in collecting tubules and causes diuresis, there is increase urine output which is hypotonic.
- **Water diuresis:** It is produced by drinking large amounts of water. Excess water results in reduced plasma osmolality which inhibits ADH secretion leading to diuresis. The maximal urine flow in this condition is 16ml/mt as it affects absorption in CT only.
- **Osmotic diuresis:** Administration of substances like mannitol, which are freely filtered at glomerulus but are not reabsorbed creates an osmotic gradient in the lumen of tubules and prevents water from leaving the lumen. Increase osmolality also decreases Na+, Cl-, K+ reabsorption leading to marked increase in urine volume with loss of electrolytes.

K+ Excretion

- Most of the K+ (upto 90%) filtered is reabsorbed in PCT. **This is an active transport.**
- **In DCT:** K+ is secreted in exchange for Na+. Tubular secretion of K+ is decreased if Na+ or K+ are depleted. Aldosterone activates Na+ K+ ATPase pump in the basolateral membrane of cell of DCT and increases intracellular K+ levels. This leads to increase secretion of K+.
- Excess H+ (acidosis) leads to inhibition of secretion of K+ at DCT.
- Loop diuretics like Frusemide (Lasix) inhibit action of Na+ Cl- transporter in thick ascending loop of Henle. This leads to increase excretion of Na+ and water. The increase Na+ load to DCT also increases the Na+ K+ exchange resulting in increase secretion

of K^+. Hypokalemia can occur in patients receiving high doses of lasix for long time.

- Spironolactone (Aldactone) acts by inhibiting Na^+ K^+ exchange at CT by inhibiting aldosterone. This results in excess excretion of Na^+ and water and causes diuresis with minimal secretion of K^+.

H^+ Secretion

- For each Na^+ reabsorbed, one H^+ ion is secreted in exchange into the lumen. **This is an example of active transport.**
- **In PCT:** H^+ combines with the HCO_3^- in filtrate and forms H_2CO_3 in the presence of carbonic anhydrase which again dissociates to H_2O and CO_2. These diffuse into the cell and reform H_2CO_3 within the cell which dissociates to H^+ and HCO_3^-. HCO_3^- enters the interstitium along the electrical gradient created by Na^+ K^+ ATPase pump. H^+ is secreted back into lumen. More than 3/4th of H^+ is secreted in PCT.

- **In DCT and CT:** About 15% of H^+ secretion occurs here. This is brought about by maintaining a constant gradient for secretion of H^+ into the lumen by the following methods:
  a. H^+ combines with HPO_4^{2-} to form $H_2PO_4^-$
  b. H^+ also combines with NH_3 (ammonia) in PCT and DCT to form NH_4^+ which cannot be absorbed
- The buffering of H^+ by the above 3 methods (HPO_4^{2-}, NH_3, HCO_3^-) maintains the pH of tubular fluids.
- Acidification of urine upto pH 4.5 is attained in collecting tubules.

Factors Affecting H^+ Secretion

1. **Intracellular pCO_2:** pCO_2 rises in respiratory acidosis due to hypoventilation as in emphysema. There is increase intracellular formation of H_2CO_3 and increase production of H^+ ions leading to increase H^+ secretion. (It is reversed in hyperventilation)

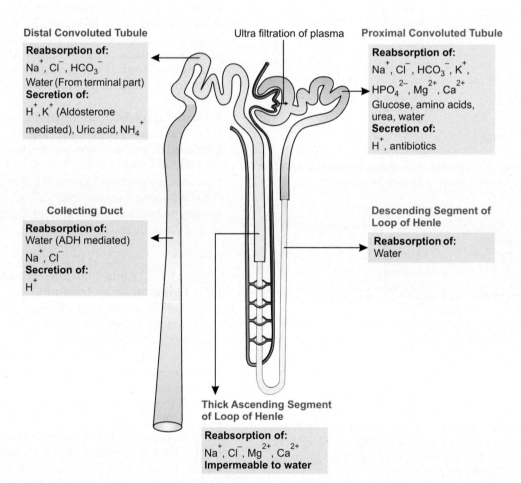

Distal Convoluted Tubule

Reabsorption of:
Na^+, Cl^-, HCO_3^-
Water (From terminal part)
Secretion of:
H^+, K^+ (Aldosterone mediated), Uric acid, NH_4^+

Ultra filtration of plasma

Proximal Convoluted Tubule

Reabsorption of:
Na^+, Cl^-, HCO_3^-, K^+,
HPO_4^{2-}, Mg^{2+}, Ca^{2+}
Glucose, amino acids, urea, water
Secretion of:
H^+, antibiotics

Collecting Duct

Reabsorption of:
Water (ADH mediated)
Na^+, Cl^-
Secretion of:
H^+

Descending Segment of Loop of Henle

Reabsorption of:
Water

Thick Ascending Segment of Loop of Henle

Reabsorption of:
Na^+, Cl^-, Mg^{2+}, Ca^{2+}
Impermeable to water

Fig. 17.19: Diagrammatic representation of reabsorption and secretion of important ions and water in various part of a nephron and its collecting duct

2. **K⁺ concentration:** In hypokalemia, there is intracellular acidosis leading to excess H⁺ secretion.
3. **Carbonic anhydrase inhibitors,** e.g., Acetazolamide—Inhibits formation of H_2CO_3 in the cells and hence there is low intracellular levels of H⁺ resulting in decrease secretion of H⁺, while increase secretion of K⁺
4. **Aldosterone:** Increase aldosterone increases Na⁺ reabsorption, increasing H⁺ and K⁺ secretion and increasing HCO_3^- reabsorption.

Bicarbonate Ion (HCO_3^-) Excretion

- Most of filtered HCO_3^- combines with H⁺ in luminal aspect of cells and forms H_2CO_3 which dissociates to H_2O and CO_2 that enters the cells.
- Within the cells it again forms H_2CO_3 along with cellular CO_2 and dissociates to H⁺ and HCO_3^-.
- HCO_3^- enters the interstitium along the electrical gradient created by Na⁺ reabsorption.

Chloride Ion (Cl⁻) Transport

- 99% of Cl⁻ is reabsorbed. In PCT and DCT Cl⁻ is transported along with Na⁺ along the electrical gradient passively. In loop of Henle it is transported by the Na⁺ 2Cl⁻ K⁺ sympoter.
- Cl⁻ passes into interstitium along the electrical gradient created by transport of Na⁺ by Na⁺ K⁺ ATPase pump.

- Cl⁻ transport varies inversely with HCO_3^- transport. Reabsorption of Cl⁻ is increased when HCO_3^- reabsorption is decreased.

Counter Current Mechanism

The reabsorption of water and various solutes from the nephrons depends on the osmolality of the interstitial fluid in the cortex and medulla. The osmolality of interstitial fluid of cortex is similar to the plasma while it increases progressively from outer to inner medulla. The counter–current mechanism helps to maintain high osmolality levels in the interstitium of medulla of kidneys allowing for maximal urine concentration. It has two parts (Fig. 17.20):

1. **Counter current multiplier system**
   - This is the function of loop of Henle and is especially seen in juxta medullary nephrons which have long loops.
   - The thin descending limb is permeable to water while it is not permeable to NaCl resulting in formation of hypertonic tubular fluid.
   - The thin segment of ascending limb on other hand is freely permeable to NaCl. The thick segment of ascending limb also actively transports Na⁺ K⁺ and Cl⁻ out of tubules. However, the ascending limb is practically

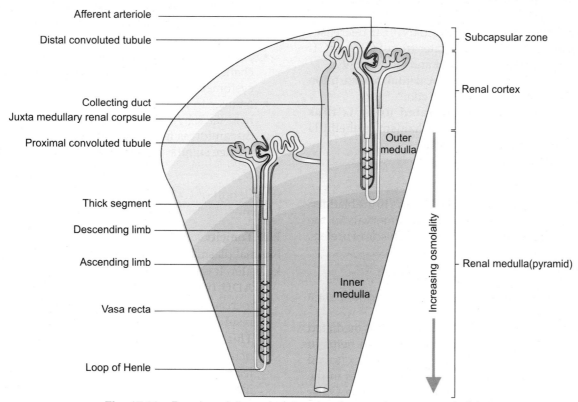

Fig. 17.20: Renal medulla and cortex showing counter current principle

impermeable to water. This results in formation of hypotonic fluid in the lumen.
— The continuous inflow of isotonic fluid from PCT, and active pumping out of NaCl from thick ascending limb increases the osmolality of interstitium.
— The hypotonic solution is passed to DCT.
— Urea is also absorbed from the collecting ducts in the medulla and contributes to interstitial osmolality

2. **Counter current exchange system**
— This is the function of vasa recta. Vasa recta are loops of peritubular capillaries derived from efferent arterioles which accompany juxta medullary nephrons in the form of hair pin loops.
— The solutes diffusing out from the ascending limb enter the vasa recta and water moves passively from descending limb at the other end. Thus the intra vascular tonicity is maintained. This ensures that no solute is removed from interstitum, thus maintaining the osmolality.

Hormones Affecting Renal Tubular Function

1. **ADH:** It increases permeability of DCT and CT to water.
2. **Aldosterone:** It increases action of $Na^+ K^+$ ATP ase pump resulting in increase reabsorption of Na^+ and increase secretion of K^+.
3. **Atrial Natriuretic Peptide (ANP):** It decreases reabsorption of Na^+ and water from PCT and CT. Decreases secretion of ADH and aldosterone.
4. **Parathormone:** It increases calcium reabsorption and increases phosphate secretion.

The formation of concentrated urine is thus contolled by counter current mechanism in medulla of kidney and serum ADH levels.

Physiology of Ureteres

The ureters propel urine from the kidneys to the bladder. Peristaltic waves are seen at regular intervals in the ureters and are the intrinsic property of muscle of ureters.

Physiology of Urinary Bladder Function

Urinary bladder receives urine from the kidneys via a pair of ureters.
Micturition: It is the act of passing urine. It is mediated by the contraction of detrusor muscle which helps in emptying urine from bladder. It is a spinal reflex (sacral reflex), facilitated or inhibited by higher centres in the brain and has an element of voluntary control also. Other factors that aid emptying of bladder are, increased intra-abdominal pressure brought about by contraction of abdominal wall muscles and diaphragm and relaxation of pelvic diaphragm and perineal muscles.

Physiological Capacity of Bladder

In new born : 30 to 50 ml
In infants : 200 ml
In adults : 450 to 600 ml (Anatomical capacity is 1 litre)

Urine stored in the bladder does not show any change in the chemical composition.

Micturition Reflex

- It is the reflex that helps to empty the bladder and pass urine to the exterior.
- As urine starts filling, the strech receptors in the bladder wall are stimulated and impulses travel along pelvic nerves to sacral dorsal nerve roots.
- The efferent path of this reflex is along the same parasympathetic outflow that is, the pelvic nerves or nervi arigentes. It leads to contraction of detrusor muscle, relaxation of perineal muscles and external urethral sphincter.
- The reflex is under the control of facilitatory and inhibitory impulses from CNS (pontine centers). These higher centers are responsible for voluntary control of micturition which is gradually learnt during early period of life (toilet training).
- Study of changes in intravesical pressure with the changes in the fluid volume in bladder is known as cystometrogram.
- Ist urge to pass urine is felt at 150 ml. This can be held back by voluntary control. Marked sense of discomfort is felt at 450 ml The pressure does not change significantly till the organ is relatively full.

Regulation of Extracellular Fluid Composition and Volume

ECF Tonicity
Normal plasma osmolality is 280 to 295 milli-osmoles/kg water. It is regulated by:
1. **ADH (vasopressin) actively:** Increase osmolality increases ADH secretion from hypothalamus. This results in increase water reabsorption in CT.
2. **Thirst mechanism:** Stimulation of osmoreceptors of hypothalamus due to increase osmolality of ECF leads to increase thirst and hence water intake is increased.

ECF Volume

It is determined by:

1. **Plasma osmolality:** Na^+ is the most important and abundant osmotically active solute in ECF. Regulatory mechanisms of Na^+ levels control the ECFV. These have been discussed.
2. **Control of water excretion:** It occurs via following ways:
   a. **ADH secretion:** Increase plasma osmolality and decrease ECFV increases ADH secretion leading to increase solute free water absorption from DCT and CT.
   b. **Angiotension II activity:** Decrease in effective circulating blood volume as seen in haemorrhage, acute hypotension, heart failure and other causes of edema and ascites, leads to secretion of renin from J.G. apparatus. There is increase angiotensin II formation which leads to :
      i. Vaso constriction.
      ii. Production of aldosterone. This stimulates Na^+ and associated water reabsorption from DCT and CT.
      iii. Stimulates secretion of ADH which cause increase water reabsorption.
      iv. Stimulates thirst mechanism increasing water intake.
   c. **Atrial natriuretic peptide (ANP) activity:** Increase in ECFV stimulates production of ANP from atrial tissue which leads to:
      i. Efferent arteriolar constriction. This results in increase capillary pressure, increase GFR resulting in natriuresis.
      ii. Afferent arteriolar relaxation causing increase capillary pressure and natriuresis.
      iii. Decreases secretion of ADH and aldosterone.

Control of pH or H$^+$ concentration in ECF

- Body pH, both intracellular and extracellular, is usually maintained at 7.4 ± 0.05 units.
- pH is stabilized by presence of various buffers named below :
  1. Blood buffers
     a. Haemoglobin: provides 90% of buffering capacity of blood
     b. Plasma proteins
     c. Carbonic acid-bicarbonate system
  2. Interstitium buffer: Carbonic acid-bicarbonate system
  3. Intracellular buffer
     a. Protein system
     b. Phosphate system

CLINICAL AND APPLIED ASPECT

KIDNEY AND URETER

- Kidneys move with respiration. The extent of movement varies from 1.5 to 2.5 cm.
- **Renal angle:** It is the angle between lateral border of erector spinae muscle in the back and the 12th rib. It is so named as the posterior surface of kidney is related here. Retroperitoneal approach to kidney in surgeries is via an incision from the renal angle.
- **Pain of renal colic:** It is a spasmodic pain, arising in kidneys, usually due to presence of a stone (calculus) in the pelvi-calyceal system.
  The pain is referred from renal angle or the lumbar region to the umbilicus and groin. This is because of same segmental supply of kidney (via T_{10}, T_{11}, T_{12}, L_1) and umbilicus (T_{10}) and groin (L_1) .
- **Polycystic kidney:** It is a developmental defect which may be secondary to a genetic defect. In this condition the excretory system of kidney fails to unite with the collecting system during development of fetus. This results in multiple cyst formation due to accumulation of urine. The kidneys are enlarged with multiple cysts of varying size and this condition can be picked up on ultrasound during pregnancy.
- **Pain of ureteric colic:** This occurs due to spasm of ureteric muscles, usually secondary to presence of a calculus in ureter. Due to same segmental supply. the pain is referred to groin and tip of penis in males.
- The uterine arteries are ligated during hysterectomy (that is surgical removal of uterus) as they approach the uterus at level of interval os. Injury to ureter, may take place if care is not taken. This is because, at this point the uterine arteries cross over the ureters from lateral to medial side.

URINARY BLADDER

- Cystoscopy is the examination of interior of bladder by a fiberoptic scope called cystoscope. The interureteric ridge is seen as a pale band and acts as a guide to ureteric orifices on each side, so that a catheter can be introduced into the ureter. Catheterization of ureters is done during retrograde pyelography to evaluate and repair ureteric injuries.
- Highest centre of control of micturition is paracentral lobule of cerebral hemisphere. Other centres are:
  — Detrusor centre in pons
  — Sacral micturition centre (S_1 S_2 S_3): It is responsible for micturition reflex.

CHAPTER-17

- Incontinence of urine is the involuntary passage of urine. It can be due to
  - Injury of bladder/urethral wall, e.g., in the formation of fistula, leading to continuous dribling of urine.
  - Stress incontinence: It occurs due to weakness of the fascial support to bladder neck. Any increased in intra-abdominal pressure like during laughing or coughing results in increase pressure in the bladder and incontinence.
  - Bladder muscle dysfunction. There is over activity of detrusor muscle fibres leading to urgency and urge incontinence.
- Interruption of afferent pathway at the level of S_2, S_3, S_4 is seen in lesions of dorsal roots of spinal cord like tabes dorsalis. Reflex micturition is abolished. Patient is unaware of distension and bladder becomes distended, thin walled and hypotonic. Overdistension leads to evacuation which is in the form of overflow incontinence. This is called automatic bladder.
- Interruption of afferent and efferent nerves of arc of micturition reflex, as seen in injuries to cauda equina, leads to complete loss of voluntary micturition. Bladder initially is flaccid but regains contractions which are irregular, ill sustained. Initiation of micturition is difficult and there is constant irregular dribbling of urine. This is decentralized bladder.
- In transection of spinal cord above S_2 level: There is initially a stage of **spinal shock** and bladder becomes atonic. There is difficulty to initiate micturition on one's own due to loss of voluntary function. There is overflow incontinence when the intravesical pressure exceeds sphincter tone.
  Late stage: Local spinal reflex develops and bladder contracts at regular intervals without any control of higher centres. There is also loss of voluntary control. This results in automatic bladder which starts to empty every time it is filled.
- **Urinary Tract Infection (UTI):** It can be upper urinary tract or lower urinary tract infection.
  - **Cystitis:** It is infection of urinary bladder. Most common site of UTI is the bladder. It is more common in sexually active females. The symptoms are due to inflamation of mucosa of bladder. There is sensation of frequency and urgency to pass urine, burning sensation while passing urine, pain in lower abdomen after passing urine and occasionally haematuria.
  - **Pyelonephritis** is infection of kidney which is usually due to repeated lower urinary tract infections.
  - **Urethritis** or infection of urethra is usually a sexually transmitted condition due to infection by Neisseria gonorrhea bacteria.

NORMAL AND ABNORMAL RENAL FUNCTION

Functional capacity of kidneys is mostly evaluated using urine and blood tests.

Urine Examination

- Urine output:
  - **Normal** urine output is 1 to 1.25 litres/day
  - **Oliguria** is defined as urine output < 400 ml/day. 400 ml is the minimal volume of urine required to remove the various toxic wastes from body. Oliguria is seen in diseases of kidney affecting the nephrons or in acute renal failure secondary to sudden fall in intravascular pressure as in hypovolemia due to excess bleeding.
  - **Anuria** is the complete absence of urine output.
  - **Polyuria** is defined as urine output > 2.5 lt / day. It is seen in certain chronic renal diseases in which the concentrating ability of kidney is lost or in conditions with excess solute load like diabetes mellitus.
- **Color and appearance:** Normal color of urine is pale yellow due to presence of urobilin. High colored urine is seen in
  a. Dehydration
  b. Jaundice due to presence of excess urobilin.
  c. Certain dyes like pyridium and drugs like rifampicin produce orange color urine.
  The urine normally appears as a clear liquid. It becomes slightly turbid on standing after exposure to air. Increased turbidity is seen in conditions associated with excess shedding of epithelial or pus cells as in infections or in conditions associated with increase secretion of crystals and proteins in urine
- **Specific gravity:** It is determined by the presence of electrolytes like Na^+, K^+, Cl^- and urea. Normal specific gravity of urine varies from 1010 to 1025 (in dehydration). Specific gravity is increased in dehydration, diabetes mellitus, albuminuria. Specific gravity is reduced in cases of deficiency of ADH and in tubular diseases in which there is loss of concentrating power of urine.
- **Urine pH** is usually 4.5 to 6.5. It is slightly acidic. On exposure to air, urea splits to release NH^{4+} and gives alkaline reaction.
- **Biochemical analysis:** The various biochemical products most commonly checked in urine are:

— **Glucose:** Normally absent. Glycosuria, that is, presence of glucose in urine is seen in diabetes mellitus.
— **Proteins:** Total protein excreted in urine in 24 hours is less than 150 mg. Protein in urine is derived from the cellular contents of shedding epithelial cells from the urinary tract. Plasma proteins are not present in urine normally as they cannot be filtered. **Proteinuria** is excretion of > 150 mg/day of protein. Albumin is the smallest plasma protein and is the most common plasma protein found in urine as it readily crosses damaged and diseased glomerular membranes. The various conditions associated with proteinuria are
  i. Diseases involving the nephrons, glumerulonephritis, nephrotic syndrome.
  ii. Excess formation of protein molecules as in multiple myeloma.
  iii. Increased shedding of epithelial cells as in urinary tract infections.
— **Ketone bodies:** Normally not detected. Ketonuria is seen in patients with diabetes mellitus or with history of prolonged starvation or protracted vomitings.
— **Bilirubin:** Small amount of urobilirubilinogen is excreted in urine (most is reabsorbed) that gives it the pale yellow color. Excess excretion of urobilirubin is called bilirubinuria and occurs in jaundice. Presence of bile salts and bile pigments along with bilirubinuria is seen in obstructive type of jaundice.
— **Blood and Haemoglobin:** Is normally absent in urine. Haematuria (blood in urine) occurs in inflammatory diseases of nephrons, e.g., acute glomerular nephritis. Haemoglobinuria occurs due to excess breakdown of RBCs and is seen in conditions associated with acute haemolysis.
• **Microscopy of urine:** The urine is centrifuged and the sediment obtained is studied under microscope.
Normal microscopy
— Pus cells or empty WBCs 1 to 2 / HPF, upto 6 is normal.
— Epithelial cells – may be seen.
— RBCs – Nil.
Abnormal microscopy is presence of
— Bacteria.
— RBCs as in hematuria.
— Granular casts: Large hyaline casts are suggestive of tubular / glomerular destruction.
— Presence of albumin, glucose, ketones.

Blood Tests to Assess Renal Function

These include measurement of the levels of following metabolites in blood
• **Blood urea:** It is the earliest metabolite that rises in blood in various diseases of kidney.
• **Serum creatinine:** It is the most sensitive indicator of kidney function.
• Serum uric acid.
• Serum electrolytes: Na^+, K^+, Cl^-.

Renal Clearance Tests

These are slightly advanced tests for assessing glomerular function. This tests the rate of clearing of inulin(most common substance used) after giving an injection of inulin in a specific dose.

Other Tests

Ultrasound, CT scan, MRI, Intravenous pyelography are the other tests used to evaluate the various diseases of kidney.

UREMIA

It is the accumulation of break down products of protein metabolism due to chronic renal failure. There are elevated levels of blood urea nitrogen (BUN), and creatinine. It leads to lethargy, anorexia and vomiting and in late stages cause drowsiness, confusion, disorientation, headache and convulsions. Treatment is haemodialysis or renal transplant.

ACID-BASE ABNORMALITIES

• **Respiratory acidosis:** Reduced or poor ventilation results in a rise in arterial pCO_2 which increases the formation of H_2CO_3 and hence HCO_3^- and H^+. Increase in H^+ causes lowering of pH. Renal compensation occurs in two ways:
  — Increase load of HCO_3^- in glomerular filterate is associated with increased reabsorption.
  — Increase in pCO_2 leads to increase in intracellular H^+ and HCO_3^- resulting in increased secretion of H^+.
Both these mechanisms correct the pH.
• **Respiratory alkalosis:** Increased ventilation (hyper ventilation) leads to fall in pCO_2. Renal compensation occurs by reducing H^+ secretion and decreasing HCO_3^- reabsorption leading to lowering of pH.
• **Metabolic acidosis:** It is due to accumulation of acid substances, e.g., ketoacids in diabetes mellitus, ingestion of alcohol or salicylates or due to loss of HCO_3^- as in diarrhea. Increase H^+ is buffered by

HCO_3^- and plasma proteins. The following compensatory mechanisms start operating:

— **Respiratory compensation**
   a. Extra H_2CO_3 formed increases pCO_2 levels.
   b. Increase H^+ stimulates respiration.
   c. Both lead to rapid expulsion of CO_2 which corrects excess pCO_2 levels and normalizes the pH.

— **Renal compensation**
   a. There is increase in formation of H_2CO_3 intracellularly. This leads to increase H^+ and HCO_3^- in the cells which results in increase tubular secretion of H^+.
   b. H^+ are secreted in exchange for Na^+ and along with the Na^+ one HCO_3^- passes out of the cell into interstitium.

   c. Gradient for secretion of H^+ is maintained by the removal of H^+ ions in the tubular lumen by urine buffers like HPO_3^{2-} and NH_3.

- **Metabolic Alkalosis:** Plasma HCO_3^- levels and pH increase in cases of excess vomiting resulting in loss of HCl and in patients giving history of excess ingestion of HCO_3^- or lactate. The following compensatory mechanisms start operating:
— **Respiratory compensation**
   a. Increase HCO_3^- leads to increase binding with H^+.
   b. Lowering of H^+ leads to decrease respiratory drive. The pCO_2 level increase. CO_2 binds to H_2O and regenerates H^+.
— **Renal compensation:** Is slight by increasing HCO_3^- excretion. **1st stage is spinal shock:** Bladder is flaccid, with retention of urine and over distension.

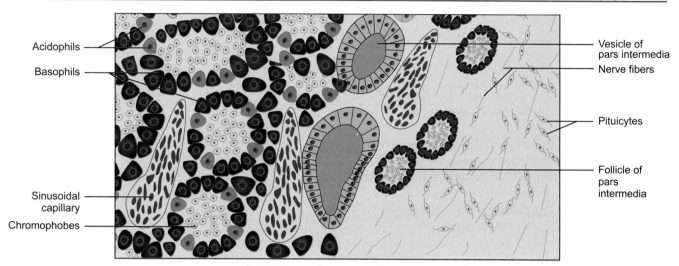

Fig. 18.3: Histology of pituitary gland

Venous Drainage of Pituitary Gland

Short veins from pituitary gland drain into neighbouring dural venous sinuses. The hormones produced in the gland pass out of it through the venous blood to the target sites.

Endocrine Function of Pituitary Gland (Fig. 18.3)

- Pituitary gland consists of an anterior lobe and a posterior lobe connected by a small pars intermedia (intermediary lobe).
- The anterior lobe has two types of cells namely, chromophobes and chromophils. The exact function of chromophobes (non staining cells) is not known. Chromophils are the cells which produce hormones.
  Chromophils are granular secretory cells and are further divided into:
  a. **Basophils:** These consists of:
    1. **Gonadotropes:** They secrete FSH (Follicular stimulating hormone) and LH (Leuteinising hormone).
    2. **Thyrotropes:** They secrete thyroid stimulating hormone (TSH). TSH stimulates growth and vascular supply of thyroid gland. It increases rate of thyroid hormone production.
    3. **Corticotropes:** They secrete adreno corticotropic hormone (ACTH). ACTH controls the growth and secretion of zona fasciculata and zona reticularis of adrenal gland.
  b. **Acidophils:** These consists of:
    1. **Mammotropes:** They secrete prolactin.
    2. **Somatotropes:** Secrete growth hormone (GH).

- The posterior lobe primarily has endings of axons from supra-optic and paraventricular nuclei of hypothalamus and secretes hormones conducted from hypothalamus. These are:
  1. Vasopressin (ADH)
  2. Oxytocin
- The intermediate lobe is primarily rudimentary and produces melanocyte stimulating hormone (MSH).

FSH (Follicle Stimulating Hormone)

It is a glycoprotein hormone.

Actions of FSH
  1. **In males:** It maintains the spermatogenic epithelium and sertoli cells. It facilitates spermatogenesis.
  2. **In females:** It stimulates growth of ovarian follicles, recruiting new follicles in each menstrual cycle and facilitates secretion of estrogen hormone. It also maintains ovarian growth.

Control of secretion of FSH is via the following:
  1. **GnRH (Gonadotrophin releasing hormone):** This is produced by hypothalamus in a regular pulse like fashion and stimulates secretion of FSH. GnRH secretion is reduced by negative feedback of high estrogen and progesterone level in females and high testosterone levels in male.
  2. **Estrogen and progesterone:** These hormones are produced by ovary. Increasing levels of estrogen and progesterone inhibit secretion of FSH from anterior pituitary.
  3. **Inhibin B:** It is produced by ovary and inhibits secretion of FSH. Low levels of inhibin B during onset of menstruation results in increase in level of FSH.

LH (Leuteinizing hormone)

It is a glycoprotein hormone.

Actions of LH

1. In males, it maintains the levels of Leydig cells in testes and stimulates production of testosterone from them.
2. In females, it stimulates ovulation and secretion of estrogen and progesterone hormone from corpus leuteum. It is responsible for maintaining corpus luteum.

Control of secretion of LH is via the following:

1. GnRH, it is similar to FSH control.
2. Estrogen and progesterone in females and testosterone in male exert negative feedback on anterior pituitary and inhibit secretion of LH.
3. Estrogen also exerts a positive feedback in midcycle of menstrual cycle that causes sudden increase in secretion of LH. This is by positive feedback on pituitary. The LH surge causes ovulation.

TSH

It is a glycoprotein hormone. Average plasma level is 2 μgm/ml (0.2 to 5 μgm/ml).

Action of TSH

Effects of TSH on thyroid gland are:
1. Increase iodide trapping.
2. Increase binding of iodine to thyrosine.
3. Increase synthesis of T_3 and T_4.
4. Increase secretion of thyroglobulin and increase in endocytosis of the colloid with thyroid hormones, resulting in increased release of T_3 and T_4 into circulation.
5. Increase blood flow and growth of thyroid gland.

Control of Secretion of TSH

Plasma levels of TSH are regulated by the following mechanisms:
1. Negative feedback mechanism: increase in plasma T_3 and T_4 levels act on the pituitary and decrease the secretion of TSH.
2. Thyrotropin releasing hormone (TRH): It is secreted by hypothalamus and stimulates secretion of TSH from pituitary. Release of TRH is partly inhibited by T_3, T_4.

ACTH

It is a polypeptide hormone. Secretion of ACTH shows normal diurnal variation, with maximum secretion occurring in early hours of morning. It is also stimulated by stress. Cortisol levels are higher in early morning and after any stress.

Functions of ACTH

1. It regulates the basal and stress induced secretion of glucocorticoids from adrenal cortex.
2. It also regulates secretion of mineralocorticoids to some extent.
3. It controls the growth of adrenal cortex.

Control of Secretion of ACTH:

1. It is inhibited by plasma glucocorticoid levels.
2. Corticotrophin releasing hormone (CRH): It is secreted by hypothalamus and stimulates secretion of ACTH from pituitary.

Prolactin

It is polypeptide hormone.

Action of Prolactin

1. Prolactin helps in the growth of alveolar glandular tissue of mammary gland and stimulates milk secretion during pregnancy.
2. It inhibits the effects of gonadotrophins especially LH leading to anovulation. This is the basis for natural contraception in females who are exclusively breast feeding their new borns after delivery.

Control of Secretion of Prolactin

1. Prolactin secretion is increased by sleep, exercise, stress, lactation and pregnancy. It is also increased by the release of prolactin releasing factors (PRF) from hypothalamus.
2. Prolactin secretion is inhibited by prolactin inhibitory factor (dopamine) which is secreted from hypothalamus and by negative feedback on pituitary by high levels of prolactin in circulation.

Growth Hormone

Growth hormone is a polypeptide. It is produced at the rate of 0.2 to 1.0 mg/day in adults and has a plasma half life of 6 to 20 minutes.

Actions of Growth Hormone

1. It stimulates growth of cartilage and epiphyseal plates, thus increasing bone growth. GH acts via somatomedins. These are polypeptide growth factors secreted by the liver. The primary somatomedins are IGF-I (insulin like growth factors) and IGF-II. GH itself increases the levels of IGF-I.
2. **Effect on protein metabolism:** GH increases protein synthesis and synthesis of soluble collagen.
3. **Effect on carbohydrate metabolism:** GH increases blood glucose by increasing hepatic glycogenolysis and glucose output. It also has an anti-insulin action on glucose uptake in muscles.

4. **Effect on fat metabolism:** GH increases free fatty acid levels and ketone bodies and hence facilitates gluconeogenesis.

5. **Effect on electrolytes:** It increases Ca^{2+} absorption from intestine and decreases Ca^{2+}, Na^+, K^+ and PO_4^{3-} excretion by kidneys to increase availability for growth.

Regulation of Secretion of Growth Hormone

- Hypothalamus produces GHRH (Growth hormone releasing hormone) and GHIH (Growth hormone inhibiting hormone) or somatostatin.
- GHRH is stimulated by exercise, low blood glucose levels, fasting, increase aminoacid levels, stress and by glucagon. These factors hence increase GH secretion.
- GHIH is stimulated by high blood glucose and free fatty acid levels, cortisol, growth hormone. These stimuli hence decrease GH levels.

Physiology of Growth

Growth is an orderly sequence of increase in size and number of cells, increase in length, size and weight of body accompanied with maturation of functions. In humans growth is rapid after birth, in infancy and continues gradually till puberty. A marked increase in growth known as **growth spurt,** occurs during puberty after which there is cessation of growth due to closure of epiphyses. Growth spurt occurs earlier in girls than boys. The pattern of growth is affected by following factors:

1. **Genetic factors**
2. **Nutritional factors:** Diet adequate in energy, protein and minerals is important to ensure proper growth. The rate of growth is slightly increased in children specially after starvation or illness which is called 'catch up growth' provided the nutrition in restored.
3. **Age:** Growth is rapid in children. In old age there is negative growth due to increase cellular degeneration.
4. **Hormonal factors:**
   a. **Growth hormone**
   b. **Thyroid hormones:** These hormones are responsible for rapid growth in infancy and for the pubertal spurt.
   c. **Androgens:** Increase growth hormone and IGF-1 activity and are anabolic.
   d. **Glucocorticoids:** Regulate growth. However, in high doses inhibit rate of growth.
   e. **Insulin:** It is important for uptake of glucose, amino acids which are required for growth. Deficiency of insulin leading to diabetes in children results in decreased rate of growth due to increase breakdown of fat and protein.

POSTERIOR PITUITARY HORMONES

The hormones secreted from posterior pituitary are actually synthesized in the hypothalamus and transported down the hypothalamo-hypophyseal tract of nerves to posterior lobe of pituitary. They are stored in posterior pituitary and secreted in response to the appropriate stimuli.

ADH (Antidiuretic Hormone)

It is also called **vasopressin.** It is a polypeptide hormone with a biological half like of 16 to 20 minutes.

Actions of ADH

1. **Main function:** It acts on the collecting ducts of the kidneys and increases the permeability to water. This increases water reabsorption, thereby decreasing urine volume and making it more concentrated.
2. Accessory functions:
   — Increases glycogenolysis in liver.
   — Stimulates secretion of ACTH from anterior pituitary to regulate aldosterone secretion.
3. In high doses that is, in pharmacological doses it acts as a vasoconstrictor.

Control of Secretion of ADH

1. Osmolality of plasma: Any increase in plasma osmolality stimulates the osmoreceptors in anterior hypothalamus and increases secretion of ADH. The potent stimulus is Na+ levels followed by high blood glucose levels.
2. **ECF volume:** Hypovolemia stimulates ADH secretion and vice versa.
3. Miscellaneous stimuli for ADH secretion are pain, emotional excitement, nausea, surgical stress.
4. Alcohol intake decreases secretion of ADH.
   — The net effect of ADH hormone is in the maintainance of ECF volume and plasma osmolality.

Oxytocin

It is an octapeptide hormone.

Actions of Oxytocin

1. **On female breast:** It stimulates contraction of myoepithelial cells resulting in ejection of milk from primed breasts (that is in pregnant and lactating women).
2. On uterus:
   a. It increases sensitivity of pregnant uterus to self by increasing oxytocin receptors in the uterine muscle. It stimulates contraction of uterine muscles during labor.

b. It also causes uterine contractions in non pregnant uterus during sexual excitation which help in sperm transport.

3. In males, it may help to propel sperm in the duct forwards during ejaculation.

Control of Secretion of Oxytocin

1. Oxytocin release is primarily increased by stimulation of touch receptors in the breast especially at nipples. This is called suckling reflex. As the baby sucks on the nipple of breast milk is ejected in lactating mothers.
2. It is also stimulated by sexual excitement.
3. Its secretion is decreased by stress and sympathetic overactivity.

HYPOTHALAMUS

Anatomy of Hypothalamus is described in chapter no. 8 (page no. 222).

Endocrine Function of Hypothalamus

- Hypothalamus controls the secretion of various hormones from the pituitary by secreting the following hormones.
  1. TRH (Thyrotrophin releasing hormone): It acts on anterior pituitary and stimulates release of TSH.
  2. CRH (Corticotrophin releasing hormone): It acts on anterior pituitary and stimulates release of ACTH.
  3. GHRH (Growth hormone release hormone) GHIH (Growth hormone inhibiting hormone):

GHRH stimulates while GHIH inhibits release of growth hormone from anterior pituitary.

4. Prolactin Inhibiting Factor (PIF): It is released in pulses by hypothalamus and inhibit secretion of prolactin from anterior pituitary. This helps to control levels of prolactin in circulation.
5. GnRH (Gonadotrophin releasing hormone): This controls secretion of FSH and LH from anterior pituitary.

- It synthesizes posterior pituitary hormones namely, ADH and oxytocin which are transported via the hypothalamo-hypophyseal system to the pituitary.

PINEAL GLAND

It is a small gland arising from roof of third ventricle, at posterior end of corpus callosum in brain. It secretes the hormone melatonin into CSF and blood. The levels of melatonin are controlled by sympathetic nerve activity and is maximal at night (darkness). The physiological function is not clear but it has a role in inhibiting gonadotrophin releasing hormones (GnRH) and may regulate puberty.

THYROID GLAND

Thyroid gland is a brownish red endocrine gland situated in lower part of neck, in front and sides of lower end of larynx and upper part of trachea. It lies opposite the level of C_5 to T_1 vertebrae.

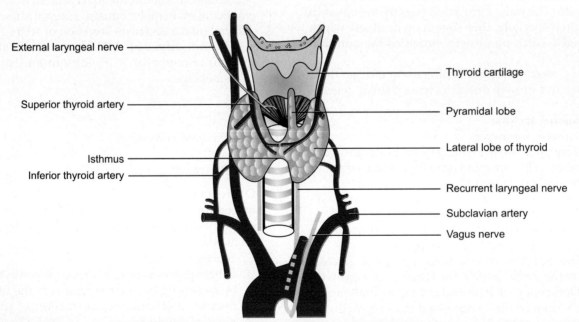

External laryngeal nerve
Superior thyroid artery
Isthmus
Inferior thyroid artery

Thyroid cartilage
Pyramidal lobe
Lateral lobe of thyroid
Recurrent laryngeal nerve
Subclavian artery
Vagus nerve

Fig. 18.4: Thyroid gland, its arterial supply and relations

Anatomical Features

The gland consists of two lobes connected by an isthmus (Fig. 18.4). Each lobe extends from the middle of thyroid cartilage above to the 6th tracheal ring below. It is enclosed by the pretracheal layer of deep cervical fascia.

Each lobe is pyramidal in shape and measures 5 cm in length, 3 cm in breadth and 2 cm in thickness. It presents with following features:

a. **Apex:** Is directed upwards, towards the oblique line of thyroid cartilage.

b. **Base:** Extends to the 5th or 6th ring of trachea.

c. **Two borders:** Anterior border is thin while the posterior border is rounded and poorly defined.

d. **Superficial or lateral surface and medial surface:** Lateral surface is covered by the strap muscles of neck, fascia and skin. Posterolateral part overlaps the carotid sheath and its contents. Medial surface overlaps the larynx and trachea.

Isthmus overlies the 2nd, 3rd and 4th tracheal rings and joins the two lateral lobes together. It is 1.25 cm in both vertical and transverse diameters. It has an anterior and posterior surface and upper and lower border.

Pyramidal lobe is occasionally presents and projects upwards from the isthmus usually on the left side.

Capsules of the Thyroid Gland

The gland is enclosed in:

a. **True capsule:** It is the peripheral condensation of connective tissue of the gland forms its true capsule. A dense network of capillary plexus lies deep to it.

b. **False capsule:** It is derived from the pretracheal fascia which splits to enclose the gland. It is much denser in front than behind. On the medial surface of thyroid lobe it thickens to form the suspensory ligament of Berry which connects the lobe to the cricoid cartilage.

In between the two capsules are present parathyroid glands and trunks of blood vessels.

Arterial Supply of Thyroid Gland (Fig. 18.4)

The gland is supplied by following arteries on each side

1. **Superior thyroid artery,** a branch from external carotid artery.
2. **Inferior thyroid artery,** a branch of thyrocervical trunk from the first part of subclavian artery.
3. **Thyroidea ima artery** (present in 30% cases), a branch of brachiocephalic trunk.
4. **Accessory thyroid arteries:** Branches from tracheal and oesophageal arteries also supply the gland.

Venous Drainage of Thyroid Gland

Thyroid gland is drained by three sets of veins. These are

1. Superior thyroid vein
2. Middle thyroid vein
3. Inferior thyroid vein/veins

Lymphatic Drainage of Thyroid Gland

1. The upper part drains into prelaryngeal and jugulo-digastric lymph nodes.
2. The lower part drains into pretracheal lymph nodes

Nerve Supply of Thyroid Gland

1. **Parasympathetic supply:** Vagus nerve.
2. **Sympathetic supply:** It is derived from the periarterial plexus of nerves. These are derived from postganglionic sympathetic fibres from the superior, middle and inferior cervical ganglia. They are vasomotor to blood vessels.

Functions of Thyroid Gland

1. It produces two thyroid hormones T_3 and T_4 which are required for the normal growth and development of the body. They also maintain the metabolic rate of body.
2. It also produces calcitonin. This hormone has a role in calcium metabolism.

Structure of Thyroid Gland (Fig. 18.5)

- Thyroid gland is enclosed in a fibrous capsule. The capsule sends numerous septae inside the gland and divides it into lobules.
- Each lobule is made up of acini or follicles lined by follicular cells. These cells may be cuboidal to columnar in shape depending upon the secretory activity of the gland. Nucleus is rounded and centrally placed. The follicular cells rest on a basement membrane. A rich network of capillaries is present in relation to this basement membrane.
- In the centre of each follicle a homogenous eosinophilic material known as colloid is present in varying amounts depending upon the secretory activity of the gland.
- The parafollicular cells or C-cells are present between the follicular cells and their basement membrane.
- Follicular cells secrete T_3 and T_4 hormones.
- Calcitonin is secreted by parafollicular cells.

Formation and Secretion of Thyroid Hormones

Thyroid gland primarily produces and secretes thyroxine (T_4) and tri-iodo-thyronine (T_3). The parafollicular cells produce calcitonin.

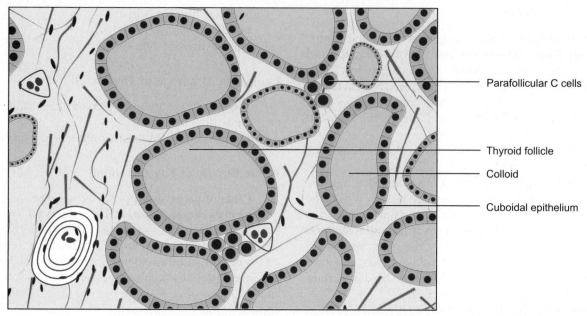

Fig. 18.5: Histology of thyroid gland

Synthesis of T_3 and T_4

- The cells of thyroid gland synthesize thyroglobulin, a glycoprotein, which is secreted into the lumen of acini and forms the colloid. It consists of tyrosine molecules and the enzyme thyroid peroxidase.
- Iodine (I_2) ingested in the food is converted to iodides (I^-) and absorbed. The minimal dietary requirement of iodine to maintain thyroid function is 150 micrograms in adults.
- The thyroid gland actively takes up iodide from circulation. Na^+ and I^- are cotransported into thyroid. This is called iodine trapping.
- Iodide is oxidized to iodine which enters the lumen of acini and binds to the tyrosine residues in the colloid. The oxidation of iodide and binding of iodine is facilitated by the enzyme, thyroid peroxidase. It forms mono-iodotyrosine (MIT) then di-iodotyrosine (DIT) and 2 molecules of DIT combine to form thyroxine (T_4). T_3 is formed by combination of MIT and DIT. This is called **coupling reaction.**

Note: Thyroid gland contains 95% of total I_2 content of body. Besides thyroid gland, kidneys also take up I^- for excretion. Other organs that transport I^- are salivary glands, gastric mucosa, ciliary body of eye, choroid plexus, mammary gland, pituitary and placenta.

- The colloid can be stored for a couple of months. When required it is ingested by acinar cells and merges with intracellular lysosomes to release T_3, T_4, DIT and MIT. MIT and DIT are deiodinized and iodine is utilized while T_3 and T_4 are released into circulation.
- T_3 and T_4 circulate in the body bound to plasma proteins, mostly to thyroid binding globulin and rest to albumin and transthyretin. They are present in free on unbound form in negligible quantity. However, it is this free, unbound form which is biologically active.
- T_3 and T_4 are deiodinated in liver and kidneys, and excreted in stool and urine.

Distinguishing features of T_3 and T_4

Feature type	T_4 is the prohormone and is converted to T_3 in tissues	T_3 is the active hormone
Secretion by thyroid gland	80 microgram / day	4 microgram / day
Plasma levels	8 microgram / dl	0.15 microgram / dl
Plasma protein binding	99.98% (free is 0.02%)	98.8% (free is 0.2%)
Action and t½	Slow onset of action, t½ 6-7 days	Rapid onset of action with short ½ life

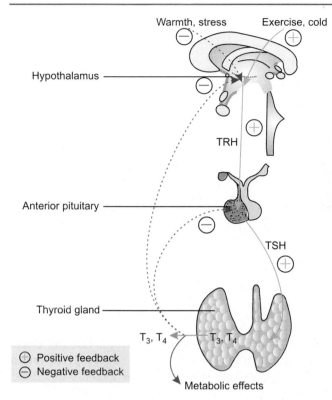

Warmth, stress   Exercise, cold

Hypothalamus

TRH

Anterior pituitary

TSH

Thyroid gland

T_3, T_4 T_3, T_4

⊕ Positive feedback
⊖ Negative feedback

Metabolic effects

Fig. 18.6: Diagrammatic representation of regulation of secretion of thyroid hormones

Regulation of Formation and Secretion of T_3 and T_4 (Fig. 18.6)

Thyroid hormone synthesis is primarily regulated by TSH, thyroid stimulating hormone.

Effects of Thyroid Hormones in the Body

1. **Calorigenic action:** Thyroid hormones increase the O_2 consumption of active tissues except in brain, testes, ovaries, uterus, lymph nodes, spleen, pituitary.
2. T_3 and T_4 increase the **basal metabolic rate (BMR)** of body and lead to heat production.
3. **Protein metabolism:** Thyroid hormones increase catabolism and protein breakdown.
4. **Carbohydrate metabolism:** Thyroid hormones increase the rate of absorption of glucose from GIT leading to transient hyperglycemia after a carbohydrate rich meal.
5. **Fat metabolism:** Thyroid hormones decrease circulatory cholesterol by increasing LDL formation. This effect is only physiological.
6. **Growth and development:** T_4 is essential for normal body growth and skeletal maturation.

7. **Nervous system:** Thyroid hormones regulate brain development. In children upto 2 years they are responsible for myelination and development of neurons and their vascular supply. In adults they regulate cerebral blood flow and O_2 consumption and are responsible for alertness responses, memory and learning ability and aid in peripheral neuromuscular coordination.
8. **Effect on CVS:** Thyroid hormones are ionotropic, they increase heart rate by increasing sensitivity of cardiac muscle to circulating catecholamines. They are chronotropic as they increase force of contraction of heart by effect on myosin. High levels of thyroid hormones cause vasodilatation.
9. **Effect on skeletal muscles:** Responsible for maintenance of neuromuscular coordination.
10. **Other effects:** Thyroid hormones are necessary for:
    a. Conversion of carotene to vitamin A in liver
    b. Proper lactation, milk production
    c. Normal menstrual cycle and fertility
    d. Increase appetite and motility of GIT.

Calcitonin

It is a polypeptide hormone produced by parafollicular, C-cells, of thyroid gland. Normal plasma calcitonin levels are 0.2 μgm/ml. It is metabolised by the kidney.

Actions of Calcitonin

It helps to lower serum calcium levels by acting on bones and kidneys in the following manner:
    a. Inhibits bone resorption by decreasing activity of osteoclasts
    b. Increases urinary excretion of calcium and phosphorus.

Regulation of Secretion of Calcitonin:

Secretion of calcitonin is stimulated by:
    a. High serum calcium levels of > 9.5 mg%
    b. Hormones like gastrin, secretin
    c. Dopamine, β-adrenergic agonists.

THYMUS (FIG. 18.7)

It is small gland, located in superior mediastinum and is made up of an inner medulla and outer cortex. It is most active in young adults and consists of lymphoid tissue which promotes development of immunologically competent T-lymphocytes. With increasing age, its function diminishes and glandular tissue is replaced by fibrous tissue and fat. It produces thymosin. which helps in proliferation of T-lymphocytes.

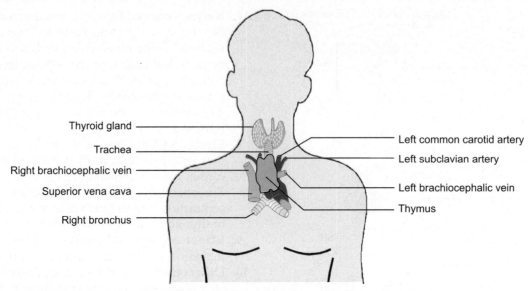

Fig. 18.7: Thymus and its relations

PANCREAS (FIG. 16.42, 18.8)

Detail of anatomy and the exocrine function of pancreas are described in chapter no. 16 (see page no. 518).

Endocrine Function of Pancreas (Fig. 18.8)

Pancreas contain ovoid collection of cells scattered throughout its substance that are known as Islet of Langerhans. There are about 1-2 million islets in pancreas and they make upto 2% of its volume. There are four distinct types of cells in the islets which secrete four hormones:

1. **α cells (A cells):** They form 20% of total cells and secrete glucagon.
2. **β cells (B cells):** They are the most abundant, 60% of cells and they secrete insulin.
3. **δ cells (D cells):** These secrete somatostatin.
4. **F cells:** These secrete pancreatic polypeptide.

The α and β cells are innervated by parasympathetic and sympathetic nerve endings. Each type of cell controls secretion of other cells by paracrine control.

Insulin

It is a polypeptide hormone synthesized in rough endoplasmic reticulum of a cells of the islets. It is produced at rate of 1 U/hour and basal plasma levels are 0 to 50 µU/ml. Its plasma half life is 5 minutes. It acts by binding to insulin receptors on the target cells. 80% insulin is metabolized by liver and kidneys.

Actions of Insulin

Insulin facilitates transport of glucose and associated aminoacids and K$^+$ into insulin sensitive cells that is primarily muscles and adipose tissues. **The net effect of the action of insulin is synthesis of glycogen, protein and fat for storage.** The various actions are described below:

a. **Adipose tissue**
   1. Increase glucose entry
   2. Increase fatty acid synthesis
   3. Increase glycerol phosphate synthesis
   4. Increase triglyceride deposition
   5. Activation of lipoprotein lipase
   6. Inhibition of hormone-sensitive lipase
   7. Increase K$^+$ uptake

b. **Muscle**
   1. Increase glucose entry
   2. Increase glycogen synthesis
   3. Increase amino acid uptake
   4. Increase protein systhesis in ribosomes
   5. Decrease protein catabolism
   6. Decrease release of gluconeogenic amino acids
   7. Increase ketone uptake
   8. Increase K$^+$ uptake

c. **Liver**
   1. Decrease ketogenesis
   2. Increase protein synthesis
   3. Increase lipid synthesis
   4. Decrease glucose output due to decreased gluconeogenesis and increased glycogen synthesis

d. **General actions of insulin**
   Insulin increases cell growth and has a role in growth of body.

Note: Glucose transport which is not dependant on insulin occurs in brain, RBCs, kidney and intestine.

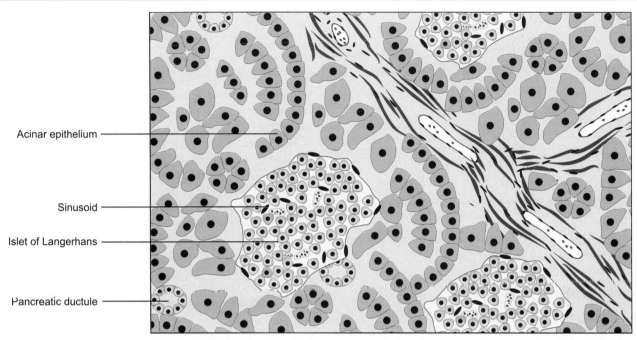

Acinar epithelium

Sinusoid

Islet of Langerhans

Pancreatic ductule

Fig. 18.8: Histology of pancreas

Regulation of Insulin Secretion

1. Insulin secretion is increased by
   a. High plasma glucose levels
   b. Amino acids especially arginine, leucine and lysine
   c. Fat derivatives especially b ketoacids
   d. Increase intracellular cAMP levels: This can be due to stimulation by:
      – β-adrenergic agonists like salbutamol
      – Glucagon
      – Drugs like theophylline
   e. **Neural control:** Parasympathetic stimulation, via right vagus nerve, stimulates insulin secretion
   f. **Hormonal control:** GIT hormones like glucagon, secretin, CCK, gastrin etc. stimulate insulin secretion. Other hormones that stimulate release of insulin are growth hormone, thyroid hormone, steroids.

2. Insulin secretion is decreased by
   a. **Decrease intracellular levels of cAMP:** Use of drugs like a adrenergics, e.g., epinephrine and β adrenergic blockers, e.g., propronolol and atenolol.
   b. **Neural control:** Sympathetic stimulation stimulates a adrenergic response decreasing secretion of insulin.
   c. **Hormonal control:** Somatostatin inhibits insulin release.
   d. **Drugs:** Diuretics like thiazides deplete K^+, decreasing insulin secretion. Other drugs like phenytoin and diazoxide directly inhibit insulin secretion.

SUPRARENAL GLANDS (ADRENAL GLANDS)

Adrenal glands are a pair of endocrine glands, one each situated in relation to the upper pole of kidney (Fig. 18.9). They lie retroperitoneally on each side of vertebral column in relation to posterior abdominal wall. They are golden yellow in colour and weigh about 5 gm.

Shape: Right gland is triangular or pyramidal in shape. Left suprarenal gland is semilunar in shape.

Dimensions:

Vertically	:	3 cm
Breadth	:	2 cm
Thickness	:	1 cm

Right Suprarenal Gland
- It is triangular or pyramidal in shape. It presents with an apex which is directed above, and a base, directed below. The base overlaps the upper pole of right kidney.
- The anterior surface is divided into medial and lateral areas by a vertical ridge, which is known as anterior border.
- The medial area is related to inferior vena cava while the lateral area is related to upper part to liver and superior duodenal flexure.
- Near the apex on the anterior surface, lies the hilum through which right suprarenal vein emerges in an upward and forward direction.

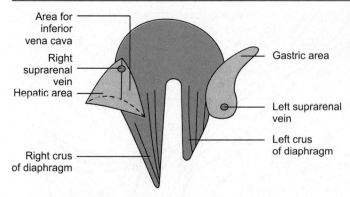

Fig. 18.9: Anterior relations of surarenals

- Posterior surface is related to diaphragm in upper part and kidney in lower part.

Left Suprarenal Gland

- It is longer and semilunar in shape. The upper end is narrow and is related to medial end of spleen. The lower end is broad and is directed downward and medially. It presents the hilum through which left suprarenal vein passes.
- Anterior surface is divided into upper and lower area. Upper area is related with the posterior surface of stomach. Lower area is non peritoneal and overlapped by body of the pancreas and crossed by splenic artery.
- Posterior surface is divided into medial and lateral area. Medial area is related to left crus of diaphragm and lateral area is related to anterior surface of left kidney.

Arterial Supply of Adrenal Gland

Each gland is supplied by the following arteries:
1. Superior suprarenal artery, branch of inferior phrenic artery
2. Middle suprarenal artery, branch of abdominal aorta
3. Inferior suprarenal artery, branch of renal artery

Venous Drainage of Adrenal Gland

Right suprarenal vein drains into inferior vena cava. Left suprarenal vein drains into left renal vein.

Lymphatic Drainage of Adrenal Gland

Lymphatic drains into lateral aortic lymph nodes.

Nerve Supply of Adrenal Gland

1. Medulla is supplied by preganglionic sympathetic fibres via coeliac plexus from T_8 to L_1.

2. Cortex is controlled by ACTH secreted by anterior pituitary.

Structure of Suprarenal Gland (Fig. 18.10)

Suprarenal gland is covered by thick fibrous capsule. Beneath capsule it presents two parts, outer cortex and inner medulla.
1. **Cortex:** It forms the main mass of gland. It consists of three cellular zones namely
    a. **Zona glomerulosa:** It consists of small polyhedral cells arranged in rounded clusters. These cells secrete mineralocorticoids.
    b. **Zona fasciculata:** It consists of large polyhedral cells with basophilic cytoplasm, arranged in straight columns. These columns have two cell width containing sinusoids between them. Cells of zona fasciculata secrete glucocorticoids.
    c. **Zona reticularis:** This is the innermost part of the cortex. It consists of branching interconnecting columns of round cells. Cells of zona reticularis secrete sex hormones.
2. **Medulla:** It consists of groups of columns of chromaffin cells separated by wide venous

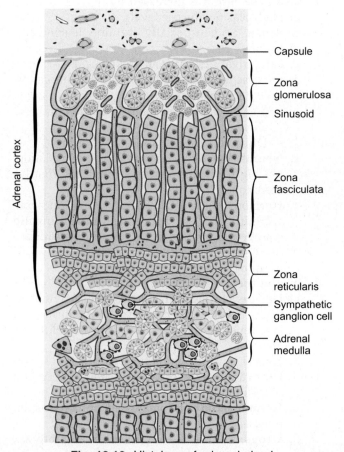

Fig. 18.10: Histology of adrenal gland

sinusoids. Single or small groups of neurons are found in medulla. They secrete adrenaline and noradrenaline.

Development of Suprarenal glands

1. **Cortex** is derived from proliferation of coelomic mesothelium on each side of the root of dorsal mesentery of primitive gut.
2. **Medulla** is derived from neural crest.

Endocrine Function of Adrenal Gland (Fig. 18.10)

Adrenal Cortex

Adrenal cortex is essential for life: It produces steroid hormones which are derivatives of cholesterol. These are:

1. **Mineralocorticoids:** Aldosterone and deoxycortico-sterone. Aldosterone has a short half life of 20 minutes. It is metabolized in liver and kidneys and excreted in urine.
   Actions of Aldosterone: It primarily helps to maintain ECF volume.
   a. It acts on the DCT and CT of kidneys and results in increase Na^+ reabsorption and K^+ excretion. This is associated with a net reabsorption of water.
   b. It also increases reabsorption of Na^+ from saliva, sweat, GIT.
   Regulation of aldosterone secretion
   a. **Renin angiotensin system control:** Lowering of ECF volume and low plasma Na^+ stimulates renin—angiotensin system which further stimu-lates secretion of aldosterone. This is seen in cases of hemorrhage and hypovolemia which occur due to surgery or trauma. Aldosterone corrects the ECF volume by Na^+ and water retention.
   b. **ACTH:** ACTH is produced by anterior pituitary and has minimal stimulatory action on aldosterone secretion.
   c. **K^+ levels:** Hyperkalemia stimulates aldosterone secretion.
2. **Glucocorticoids:** These are cortisol, and corticoste-rone. They circulate in blood by binding to corticosteroid binding globulin (CBG) which is an a-globulin present in plasma. The half life of cortisol in 60-90 mts and corticosterone is 50 minutes. They are metabolized in liver and excreted by urine. Levels of cortisol binding globulin are increased in pregnancy while they are decreased in cirrhosis of liver and renal diseases like nephrosis. Hence, there is increase in total cortisol levels in pregnancy and decrease in total cortisol levels in liver and kidney diseases.

Actions of Glucocorticoids
a. Metabolic effects: The net result of glucocorti-coid action is hyperglycemia. They increase protein and fat metabolism making amino acids, fatty acids and ketone bodies available for gluconeogenesis. They increase hepatic glyco-genolysis.
b. Permissive action: Action of glucagon to increase blood glucose levels is facilitated by glucocorticoids. Glucocorticoids help catechola-mines to maintain normal vascular reactivity and facilitate gluco-neogenesis and calorigenic action of cate-cholamines.
c. Water and electrolyte balance: They have a mild mineralocorticoid activity.
d. Bone metabolism: They have a role in remodel-ing of bone by decreasing Ca^{2+} deposition and mineralization of bone.
e. Effect on blood cells: Administration of glucocorticoids lowers basophils and eosino-phils while increasing neutrophils and platelet count.
f. Effect on nervous system: They increase brain activity. Hence, they are not recommended for use in patients with history of convulsions, e.g., epilepsy.
g. During stress: Increase in glucocorticoid levels (due to increase in ACTH secreted in response to stressful stimuli) along with catecholamines help maintain the vascular integrity and provide for energy to counter any adverse condition.
h. Antiinflammatory action: This is seen when glucocorticoids are administered as drugs and is not their normal physiological action. They decrease local and systemic response to inflammation and allergy.

Regulation of secretion of glucocorticoids (Fig. 18.11): The secretion of glucocorticoids is controlled by ACTH (Adreno-corticotropic hormone) which is secreted by anterior pituitary.

3. **Adrenal androgens:** These are dehydroepiandro-sterone and androsteredione. They have only 20% activity of testosterone. In females, they are converted to estrogen in the peripheral circulation, providing a secondary source of these hormones besides ovaries. Their levels are also controlled by ACTH.

Adrenal Medulla

It is not essential for life. Adrenal medulla secrets catecholamines namely:
1. **Epinephrine:** It is primarily produced in adrenal medulla.

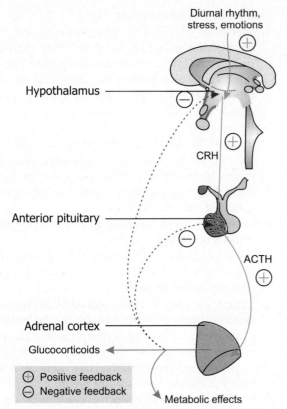

Fig. 18.11: Diagrammatic representation of regulation of secretion of glucocorticoids

2. **Norepinephrine:** Norepinephrine is also produced in peripheral and central adrenergic neurons besides adrenal medulla.
3. **Dopamine:** It is also produced in brain and by sympathetic ganglia besides adrenal medulla.

The half life of catecholamines is 2 minutes. They are methoxylated to metanephrine and normetanephrine and further oxidized to form, vanilylmandelic acid (VMP), which are excreted into urine.

Actions of Epinephrine and Norepinephrine
1. **Effects on CVS**
   a. Increase heart rate and force of contraction leading to increase in cardiac output and in systolic blood pressure.
   b. Produce vasoconstriction except in skeletal muscles and liver where their action causes vasodilatation.
2. **Metabolic effects**
   a. Increase blood sugar levels by stimulating glycogenolysis in liver and muscle. Also decrease insulin secretion.
   b. Increase free fatty acid mobilization by stimulating lipases in adipose tissue and muscle. This provides energy to kidney and cardiac muscle.

   c. Increase the basal metabolic rate.
3. **Effects on CNS**
   a. Increase anxiety, restlessness.
   b. Increase alertness response.
4. **Other actions**
   a. Decrease GIT motility, lead to constipation.
   b. Relax detrusor muscle and contract urinary sphincter, cause urinary continence.
   c. Stimulate sweating.
   d. Produce bronchodilatation.
   e. Responsible for dilatation of pupil and relaxation of accommodation (ciliary muscle) of eye for far vision.

Actions of Dopamine
Physiological actions are not well defined.
1. It produces ionotropic effect on heart, increasing cardiac output and systolic BP. High levels also cause vasoconstriction.
2. In kidneys, dopamine causes vasodilatation and natriuresis. It is an important hormone in maintaining local perfusion of the kidneys.

Regulation of Secretion of Adrenal Medulla
1. **Neural control:** Medulla is supplied by splanchnic nerves which secrete acetylcholine. This stimulates secretion of catecholamines. The splanchnic nerve activity is in turn controlled by hypothalamus.
2. **Sympatho-adrenal medullary response:** Increase secretion occurs as a generalized sympathetic response to emergency situations like fear, anxiety, injury, bleeding, asphyxia.

HORMONES REGULATING CALCIUM METABOLISM

Calcium Metabolism

The human body on an average contains 1100 gm of calcium. 99% of the calcium is in bones. Normal plasma calcium levels are 9 to 11 mg/dl. Ca^{2+} is absorbed from the small intestine by active transport. It is transported in blood partly bound to plasma proteins and partly in free ionized form (Ca^{2+}). Ca^{2+} is largely filtered by kidney and 98 to 99% is reabsorbed. The Ca^{2+} in bones is mostly (95 to 98%) integral to bone formation and 2 to 5% acts as reservoir for exchange with plasma.

Functions of Ca^{2+} (ionized form) are:
1. It is necessary for blood coagulation.
2. Ca^{2+} acts as a secondary messenger in cellular functions.
3. Ca^{2+} ions are responsible for contraction of muscles.
4. It is necessary for normal nerve function.

Phosphorous Metabolism

It is found in ADP, ATP, cAMP, 2,3DPG, many proteins and other molecules in body. Total body content is about 500-800 gm of which 85-90% is in the bones. It is absorbed from small intestine by active and passive transport. Plasma phosphorous levels are 12 mg/dl. 2/3rd of phosphorous circulates as organic compounds while 1/3rd is present in ionic form like PO_4^{3-}, HPO_4^{2-}, H_2PO. It is filtered by kidney and 85 to 90% is reabsorbed. Levels of serum Ca^{2+} vary inversely with serum PO_4^{3-} levels. The ratio of calcium to phosphorus in bone is 1.7:1.

Hormones controlling Ca^{2+} and PO_4^{3-} metabolism
1. Vitamin D
2. Parathormone
3. Calcitonin

Vitamin D

Formation of vitamin D: Cholecalciferol is produced in skin by action of U to V rays. This is converted to 25, hydroxy-cholecalciferol in liver and then to 1, 25 dihydroxy-cholcalciferol by 1α hydroxylase in the kidney. 1, 25-$(OH)_2D_3$ or calcitriol is the active form of vitaminD.

Actions of Vitamin D:
It increases serum calcium and phosphorous levels by :
1. Increasing the Ca^{2+} absorption from small intestine.
2. Increasing Ca^{2+} reabsorption from kidneys.
3. Mobilizing Ca^{2+} and PO_4^{3-} from bone.

Regulation of Vitamin D
1. Decrease in plasma Ca^{2+} and PO_4^{3-} levels stimulate formation of 1, 23, $(OH)_2 D_3$ directly via kidney and indirectly by increasing parathormone levels. Increase in Ca^{2+} and PO_4^{3-} levels inhibits formation of 1, 25 $(OH)_2D_3$ in kidneys.
2. Prolactin stimulates 1α hydroxylase and increases 1, 25$(OH)_2D_3$ levels. This action is important during lactation.
3. Estrogen also increases 1, 25 $(OH)_2 D_3$ levels. Low estrogen levels in menopause lead to low activity and low Ca^{2+} levels.
4. Growth hormone and calcitonin increase 1, 25 $(OH)_2 D_3$ levels.
5. T_4 decreases levels of 1,25 $(OH)_2D_3$ and there is osteoporosis in hyperthyroidism.

PARATHYROID GLANDS (FIG. 18.12)

These are endocrine glands situated in close relation to the thyroid gland and hence they are named as parathyroid glands. They are four in number, two superior and two inferior.

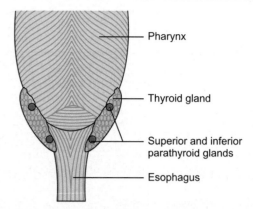

Fig. 18.12: Parathyroid glands

Size and shape: They are lentiform in shape and resemble the size of a split pea. Each measures around 6 mm × 4 mm × 2 mm.

Superior Parathyroids

One superior parathyroid gland is present on each side, near the middle of the posterior border of thyroid gland. They develop from the 4th pharyngeal pouch.

Inferior Parathyroids

One inferior parathyroid gland, lies near the lower pole along the posterior border of thyroid gland on each side. They develop from the 3rd pharyngeal pouch.

Arterial Supply of Parathyroid Gland

Superior parathyroids: From the anastamosis between superior and inferior thyroid arteries.
Inferior parathyroids: From inferior thyroid arteries.

Nerve Supply of Parathyroid Gland

It receives sympathetic (vaso-motor) supply from superior and middle cervical sympathetic ganglia.

Function of Parathyroid Glands

They secrete parathormone with maintains the calcium balance of body.

Parathyroid Hormone (Parathormone) (Fig. 18.13)

Parathormone is secreted by the 'chief cells' of parathyroid gland. **It is essential hormone for life.**

Actions of parathormone: The net effect of parathormone is increase in plasma Ca^{2+} and decrease in plasma

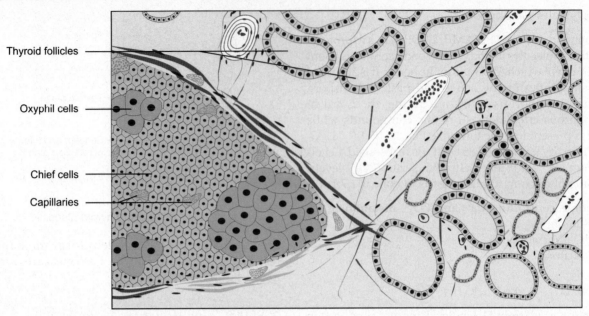

Fig. 18.13: Section of parathyroid gland (Stain—hematoxylin-eosin under high magnification)

PO_4^{3-} levels. Activity of parathormone increases bone resorption. Parathormone acts in the following manner:

1. Increases osteoclastic activity, mobilizing Ca^{2+} from bone and causing bone resorption.
2. Increases plasma Ca^{2+} levels by decreasing Ca^{2+} excretion by kidney and increasing formation of 1, 25 $(OH)_2 D_3$.
3. Decreases plasma PO_4^{3-} levels by decreasing reabsorption from kidneys (results in phosphaturia).

Regulation of secretion: Circulating Ca^{2+} levels provide negative feedback on parathyroid glands to regulate parathormone. Low Ca^{2+} levels stimulate parathormone secretion.

Calcitonin

It is produced by parafollicular C-cells of thyroid gland. **Action of calcitonin:** It helps in bone remodeling by inhibiting bone resorption. It decreases osteoclastic activity. It increases urinary excretion of Ca^{2+}, decreases renal formation of 1, 25 $(OH)_2 D_3$ and decreases Ca^{2+} absorption from GIT.

ENDOCRINE FUNCTION OF KIDNEY

Kidneys are responsible for production of two hormones:

1. **Renin: Angiotensin system**
   — The juxtaglomerullar cells (JG cells) produce and secrete renin which acts on circulating angiotensinogen in plasma and converts it to angiotensin-I.
   — Angiotensin-I gets converted to angiotensin II by angiotension converting enzyme located in the endothelial cells, especially in pulmonary circulation.
   — Angiotensin II acts as a pressor agent. It causes arteriolar vasoconstriction. It has a very short plasma t½ of 1 to 2 minutes.
   — Renin also stimulates secretion of aldosterone from adrenal cortex.
   — Renin-angiotensin system is also located in placenta.

Functions of renin angiotensin system: It primarily helps to regulate ECF volume and blood pressure. This is brought about by the following:

a. Macula densa response : When ECF volume is lowered, as in cases of haemorrhage and dehydration, the resulting low BP causes decrease in GFR. The net result is low Na^+ and Cl^- load in DCT. This stimulates macula densa cells. This stimulation causes secretion of renin from JG cells.

b. JG cells response : They are directly stimulated by changes in intra-arteriolar blood pressure. Low BP stimulates secretion of JG cells. Also increase in local prostaglandin levels stimulate JG cells directly.

Regulation of secretion of renin: Renin secretion is increased by sympathetic activity and decreased by increase level of angiotensin II and vasopressin.

2. **Erythropoietin:** It is a circulating glycoprotein that is secreted by interstitial cells of the peritubular capillary bed of kidneys. It is also produced by the

liver. It increases the number of stem cells in bone marrow that convert to red blood cells. Erythropoietin is stimulated by hypoxia and results in enhanced production of RBCs to improve O_2 carriage.

OVARY AND TESTIS

These are described in reproductive system (see page nos 577 and 586).

GIT HORMONES

These are described in digestive system (see page no. 522)

CLINICAL AND APPLIED ASPECT

PITUITARY

Tumours of pituitary gland usually produce two types of symptoms:
- **Pressure symptoms**
  — Bitemporal hemianopia, due to pressure on the optic chiasma.
  — Deepening of pituitary fossa, due to intrasellar growth. In X-ray photographs of the skull a characteristic ballooning of the hypophyseal fossa (sella turcica) may be seen. The clinoid processes may also be eroded.
- **Endocrine symptoms:** These occur due to excessive secretion of a particular hormone by the tumor cells, e.g., acromegaly (due to excess of growth hormone), Cushing's syndrome (due to excess of ACTH).

Pituitary can be approached surgically via the transfrontal or the trans-sphenoidal routes through these sinuses.

PROLACTIN HORMONE

Hyperprolactinemia: Excess prolactin levels can be caused by certain conditions other than pregnancy.
- Pituitary tumors.
- Drugs, which are dopamine antagonists, e.g., antipsychotic and antiepileptic drugs.
- Hypothyroidism: This results in increase in levels of TRH which stimulates secretion of prolactin.

In females, this leads to galactorrhea that is expression of milk from breasts and cessation of menstruation known as amenorrhea. Cessation of menstruation occurs due to inhibition of action of LH and FSH leading to anovulation. It leads to lack of libido and impotence in males and females.

GROWTH HORMONE

- **Gigantism:** This condition occurs due to excess secretion of growth hormone during childhood or growing years. It is mostly due to presence of a pituitary tumor and leads to tall stature, large hands and feet. Growth hormone has a facilitatory action like prolactin and this causes gynaecomastia and impotence in males.
- **Acromegaly:** This condition occurs due to excess secretion of growth hormone in adults (after epiphyseal closure). It leads to enlargement and widening of metacarpals, metatarsals and mandible (there is protrusion of chin known as prognathisn) with hypertrophy of soft tissues and enlargement of heart, kidney, spleen, adrenals, etc.

ADH

- ADH secretion can be stimulated by giving sucrose or mannitol which act as potent stimulators of osmoreceptors.
- Diabetes insipidus: It is a condition in which there is marked deficiency of ADH due to diseases of hypothalamus or pituitary or inability of kidneys to respond to ADH. This leads to increase volume of urine, polyuria and increase thirst, polydipsia.
- Syndrome of inappropriate hypersecretion of ADH (SIADH): It occurs due to excess circulating levels of ADH produced by pituitary tumors or lung tumors. This results in increase water retention. Increase in ECF volume results in lowering of aldosterone which causes excess secretion of Na+. The net result being dilutional hyponatremia which leads to water intoxication.

THYROID GLAND AND THYROID HORMONES

- Thyroid gland moves up and down with deglutition because it is enclosed in the pretracheal fascia which blends with the laryngeal cartilages and the hyoid bone.
- Enlargement of thyroid gland is known as goitre. It commonly occurs in India due to iodine deficiency. Rarely goitre can be due to tumors. If large it tends to push backwards pressing the sides of the trachea and esophagus.
This results in three characteristic symptoms
  — Dyspnea (difficulty in breathing), due to pressure on trachea.
  — Dysphagia (difficulty in swallowing), due to pressure on oesophagus
  — Dysphonea (hoarseness of voice), due to pressure on recurrent laryngeal nerve which lies in the tracheo-oesophageal groove.
- During thyroidectomy (surgical removal of thyroid gland) following care must be taken
  — Superior thyroid artery is ligated as near as possible to the upper pole to avoid injury to the external laryngeal nerve.
  — Inferior thyroid artery on the other hand should be ligated well away from the lower pole as the recurrent laryngeal nerve forms a close relationship with it near the gland.

— To avoid haemorrhage during thyroidectomy, the gland is removed along with the true capsule. This prevents damage to the dense capillary network that lies just below the capsule.

- The following congenital anomalies can occur during development of thyroid gland
  — Ectopic position of gland: It may be situated at base of tongue or above or below hyoid bone.
  — Absence of one of the lobe or isthumus.
  — Persistence of thyroglossal duct. This can lead to formation of thyroglossal cyst and fistula.
- **Hypothyroidism:** It is a condition which occurs due to the deficiency of thyroid hormones in body.
  Etiology
  — Iodine deficiency.
  — Destruction of thyroid tissue, e.g., Hashimoto thyroiditis.
  — Pituitary or hypothalamic dysfunction.
  — Removal of thyroid gland for tumors.

  Effects on body
  — BMR is low leading to cold intolerance, weight gain.
  — Memory is poor with slow mentation, slow speech and physical lethargy.
  — Muscular weakness and cramps are common.
  — There is accumulation of various molecules polysaccharides, hyaluronic acid, due to poor catabolism, in skin leading to dry, coarse and puffy appearance of skin. This is known as myxedema which is a non pitting type A edema often seen on face and hands.
  — Skin color becomes yellowish due to excess carotene, carotenemia.
  — Constipation occurs due to slowing of intestinal motility.
  — Altered ovarian function, anovulation is leading to common menstrual irregularities, usually periods are delayed but heavy.
  — Increase in TSH levels due to low T^3 and T^4 leads to increase growth and hyperplasia of thyroid gland which can produced **goiter.**
  — There is anaemia, normocytic normochromic type, due to lowered bone marrow metabolism.

  Treatment: Hypothyroidism is treated by administration of synthetic thyroid hormone preparations like eltroxin. Dosage needs to be titrated according to physical response and subsequent serum TSH levels.
- **Crenitism:** This condition results due to congenital deficiency of thyroid hormones.
  Etiology: It can be due to severe hypothyroidism in mother, presence of antithyroid antibodies in mother or congenital abnormalities in fetus.
  Characteristic features
  — Dwarfism, stunted growth, slow skeletal muscle growth. Characteristic appearance is short height with pot bellies

  — Gross mental retardation
  — Deafmutism
  — Coarse skin and scanty hair
  — Poor sexual development
  — Other features of hypothyroidism.

  Management: It is important to screen all newborn babies for serum TSH level as congenital hypothyroidism is the most common cause of preventable mental retardation. Institution of replacement therapy with thyroid hormones at birth can prevent abnormalities.
- **Hyperthyroidism:** This condition is due to excess circulating levels of thyroid hormones.
  Etiology
  — **Grave's disease:** It is an autoimmune disorder in which there is production of long acting stimulating antibodies to thyroid gland.
  — Tumors of pituitary or thyroid glands which are secreting hormones.

  Effect on body
  — Increase BMR, this leads to heat intolerance.
  — Increase sympathetic overactivity leads to:
    a. Increase heart rate, palpitations
    b. Anxiety, nervousness
    c. Sweating
    d. Increase cardiac output with peripheral vasodilatation, increase pulse pressure.
  — Weight loss due to increase catabolism.
  — Muscle weakness due to protein catabolism, known as thyrotoxic myopathy.
  — Increase nervous activity which is seen as:
    a. Fine tremors of outstretched hands
    b. Brisk tendon reflexes
    c. Irritability, insomnia.
  — Increase in intestinal motility associated with diarrhoea and hyperphagia (excess hunger).
  — Menstrual irregularity in the form of frequent scanty periods may occur.
  — **Exophthalmos:** Is characteristic of Grave's disease. It is the protrusion of eye balls due to swelling of extra-ocular muscles and tissues.
  — **Thyrotoxicosis:** Extreme increase in levels of thyroid hormones leads to excess activity of heart, increase O_2 consumption and can cause high output heart failure.

  Management: Treatment of hyperthyroidism is according to the underlying cause.
  — It includes symptomatic treatment with drugs to decrease heart rate, e.g., propanolol.
  — **Antithyroid drugs:** These are of three types:
    a. Thiourylenes: e.g., propylthiouracil. They inhibit iodination of MIT and block coupling reaction of MIT and DIT. They also inhibit peripheral conversion of T_4 to T_3.
    b. Drugs which inhibit iodide trapping by gland cells. These are chlorate, thiocyanate, perchlorate. These are not used clinically.

c. Iodide: Iodine is essential for normal functioning of gland. However, high doses of iodide is inhibitory to oxidation of iodine, and iodination reaction. It decreases effect of TSH, allows excess colloid accumulation thus decreasing overall release of T_3 and T_4. This action is short acting, may be for 7-10 days. Hence, this primarily used preoperatively to reduced thyroid activity at surgery.
— **Radioactive iodine:** Isotope of iodine, ^{123}I is used. In large amounts rapid uptake of radioactive iodine destroys the thyroid cells due to radiation. It is useful in treatment of cancers of thyroid gland.
— **Thyroidectomy** is surgical removal of thyroid gland. It is required in case of tumors.

INSULIN HORMONE

- **Diabetes mellitus (DM):** It is a condition caused by deficiency of insulin hormone. Causes of deficiency of insulin:

— **Genetic:** Is associated with type I diabetes mellitus. It may be autoimmune in origin.
— **Hereditary:** Family history is predisposing factor for diabetes.
— **Age:** Incidence of diabetes increases with advancing age.
— **Obesity:** Excess fat tissue becomes resistant to action of insulin leading to diabetes.
— **Damage to pancreas:** Due to surgery or pancreatitis.
— Conditions associated with raised levels of hormones which are antagonist to the actions of insulin also can cause diabetes for eg. acromegaly (growth hormone excess), Cushing syndrome (glucocorticoid excess).

Types of diabetes mellitus: It is classified into type I and type II diabetes. The features of each type is tabulated below:

	Type I	Type II
Onset	Juvenile onset DM, usually occurs at < 14 years	Maturity onset DM usually occurs above 40 years
Body weight	Thin built	Obese
Genetics	Genetic defect may be present	Family history is usually positive
Insulin level	Low	Normal
Insulin sensitivity	Present	Absent, insulin resistance is seen
Complications	Ketosis is common	Acute complications are rare, usually long term sequelae occur
Treatment	Insulin	Diet, weight control, oral hypoglycemic drugs

Clinical features: These occur due to lack of insulin activity which leads to hyperglycemia.This causes:
— Polyuria, polydipsia (increase thirst), glycosuria.
— Increase risk of skin and urinary tract infections, delayed healing of wounds.
— Long term, it leads to retinopathy, renal disease (nephropathy) and neurological abnormalities, neuropathies.
Lack of glucose uptake by cells in periphery leads to increase break down of body protein which is used for gluconeogenesis. This eventually leads to muscle wasting and weight loss.
— Increase break down of fat leading to accumulation of free fatty acids and ketone bodies. This can lead to metabolic acidosis in severe cases.

Management: This includes:
— Diet and weight managment: It is advisable for obese patients to loose weight. Patients are advised to take frequent small meals.
— Drugs
a. Insulin: It is available as injections which are given subcutaneously.

b. Oral hypoglycemic drugs: These are of two types:
i. Sulphonylureas, e.g., Glipizide, glyburide etc. increase secretion of insulin by increasing cellular Ca^{2+} influx. They require presence of some α cells.
ii. Biguanides like metformin act by reducing gluconeogenesis and improving insulin sensitivity of cells.

- **Hypoglycemia (Due to insulin excess):** It usually occurs as a result of sudden changes in dosage of insulin or missing a meal after insulin injection or after excessive excercise. Hypoglycemia results when blood glucose falls below 60 mg%. It leads to dizziness, hunger, sweating, anxiety. Severe hypoglycemia affects cerebral function leading to confusion, irritability, fatigue, convulsions and coma.

ADRENAL HORMONES

- **Phaeochromocytoma:** It is the tumor of chromaffin (epinephrine and norepinephrine secreting) cells which leads to excess hormone production. Clinical features are hypertension, headache, sweating, weakness, blurred vision due to dilated pupils of eye.

- **Hyperaldosteronism:** It is due to excess aldosterone secretion. It is of two types namely:
  - Primary hyperaldosteronism (Conn's syndrome): It is due to excess mineralocorticoid secretion, usually due to presence of an adrenal tumor. This leads to Na^+ retension causing hypertension, K^+ depletion causing muscular weakness, hypovolemic alkalosis and tetany. Renin secretion is suppressed.
  - Secondary hyperaldostenonism: It is seen in conditions that are associated with high renin activity stimulated by low intravascular volume. Examples of such conditions are congestive heart failure, liver cirrhosis, nephrosis. There is peripheral edema and hypertension. K^+ levels are normal.
- **Cushing's syndrome:** It is a clinical condition arising out of either:
  - Adrenal tumors producing glucocorticoids. It is associated with low ACTH.
  - Increase ACTH secretion due to pituitary or lung tumors.

  Clinical effects
  - Thin skin, easy bruising, thinning of hair.
  - Poor muscle development.
  - Poor wound healing.
  - Redistribution of fat: Increase fat deposition in abdominal wall, face and upper back **(buffalo hump).**
  - Salt and water retention due to minerolocorticoid action leading to generalised edema, facial edema is termed as **moon facies.**
  - Hyperglycemia, hypertension.
  - Osteoporosis due to protein metabolism, loss of matrix and decrease Ca^{2+} uptake.
- **Addison's disease:** Primary adrenocortical insufficiency. There is destruction of adrenal cortex by tumors or by infections like tuberculosis. Deficiency of hormones causes hypotension, anorexia, vomiting, diarrhea, decrease ability to stand stress. It can lead to circulatory collapse during stress.
- **Congenital adrenal hyperplasia:** The primary defect is deficiency in enzymes that convert cholesterol to cortisol. Low levels of cortisol stimulates ACTH secretion and this increases adrenal activity. The net effect is excess production of adrenal androgens. In males, excess androgens leads to precocious puberty in boys. In females, there is virilization with deepening of voice, enlarged clitoris, growth of hair in male areas and stoppage of menstruation.

VITAMIN D

- **Rickets:** Vitamin D deficiency in children causes rickets. This is characterized by hypocalcemia and low phosphate levels. This causes weakness and retarded growth of bones, malformation of weight bearing bones and dental defects.
- **Osteomalacia:** In adults, vitamin D deficiency causes osteomalacia. There is a slow and steady loss of mineral from bone. This leads to bone pain and muscular pain.

PARATHYROID GLAND AND PARATHORMONE

- The parathyroids are closely related to the thyroid gland and **during thyroidectomy they can be removed by mistake as a lymph node or fat lobules. This leads to hypoparathyroidism which causes hypocalcaemia leading to tetany.**

- **Hypoparathyroidism:** Low parathormone levels usually result from removal of parathyroid glands, parathyroidectomy, usually accidentally during removal of thyroid gland. This results in low plasma Ca^{2+} levels which leads to increased neuromuscular excitability. This is characterized by:
  - **Chvostek's sign:** Tapping at angle of jaw, site of facial nerve, leads to quick contraction of ipsilateral face muscles.
  - **Trousseau's sign:** This is characterized by spasm of muscles of upper limb leading to flexion at wrist and thumb with hyperextension of other four fingers. In mild cases, this can be precipitated by occluding blood circulation at upper arm by inflating sphygmomanometer cuff for few minutes.
  - There is tetany leading to intestinal colic, laryngeal muscle spasm leading to stridor, asphyxia and even death.
- **Hyperparathyroidism:** Excess parathormone secretion can occur in the following two ways:
  - Primary hyperparathyroidism: This is caused by tumours secreting parathormone. It is associated with high circulating plasma calcium levels.
  - Secondary hyperparathyroidism: Excess production of parathormone occurs secondary to low plasma Ca^{2+} levels which may be a result of chronic renal failure or prolonged rickets.

Clinical features of hyperparathyroidism. There is demineralization of bones leading to spontaneous fractures with irregular reformation. Due to hypercalcemia there is formation of renal stones.

Male and Female Reproductive System

INRODUCTION

Reproductive system is responsible for propogation of species for survival and existence of an organism.

FEMALE REPRODUCTIVE SYSTEM

The anatomy of female reproductive is studied under two headings.

1. **External genitalia:** Female external genitalia is also known as vulva. It includes (Fig. 19.1).
   a. Mons pubis
   b. Labia majora
   c. Labia minora
   d. Vestibule
   e. Clitoris
   f. Bulb of the vestibule

   g. Greater vestibular glands (Bartholin's gland)
   h. Vaginal orifice
2. **Internal genitalia:** The structures lie in the pelvis and perineum. During pregnancy however, uterus enlarges to become an abdominal organ. Internal genitalia consists of
   a. Uterus and cervix.
   b. A pair of fallopian tubes
   c. Vagina
   d. Two ovaries

MONS PUBIS

It is a rounded, median cutaneous elevation in front of the symphysis pubis. It is made up of fibrofatty tissue. At onset of puberty, coarse pubic hairs grow over the mons pubis.

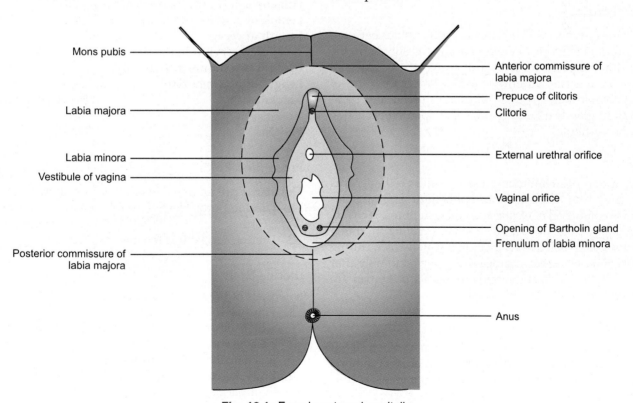

Fig. 19.1: Female external genitalia

LABIA MAJORA

Labia majora correspond to scrotum in male. They are a pair of longitudinally placed, cutaneous elevations overlying dense connective tissue and adipose tissue with scanty smooth muscle fibres. They are well developed and in apposition in young girls and nullipara while in multipara they may be wide apart and thinned out. The skin contains numerous sweat and sebaceous glands. After puberty coarse hair follicles appear over the labia. Their inner aspect however remains smooth. Anteriorly, they continue upwards as mons pubis. Posteriorly, they merge in midline to form posterior comissure and continue with perineum. The distal end of round ligament of uterus attached to subcutaneous tissue of each labia majus.

LABIA MINORA

These are a pair of thin, elongated, cutaneous folds, present one on each side, on inner aspect of labia majus. In young and nullipara they are not visible unless labia majora are separated while in multipara they usually are visible through the gap in labia majora. They converge anteriorly and split to enclose the clitoris, forming a hood over it called prepuce and a fold called frenulum of clitoris below it. Posteriorly, they join to form frenulum of vestibule or the fourchette.

VESTIBULE

It is the area enclosed by labia minora and lies between frenulum of clitoris to the frenulum of vestibule. In the midline, it presents with a opening of the external urinary meatus, anteriorly and a larger opening of vagina below it. Ducts of Bartholin's gland and para-urethral glands (Skene glands) also open on each side of the vestibule.

Hymen

It is a fold of membrane present in the vestibule. It is lined by stratified squamous epithelium on both sides and is composed of elastic and collagen fibres. It covers the vaginal opening. It has a small opening in young and sexually inactive women. It is usually torn during first coitus. However, characteristic tears occur only after child birth. The membranous remnants of hymen are called carunculae myritiformis.

CLITORIS

It corresponds to the penis of males, embryologically. It lies in the mid line, at the anterior end of labia minora. It is composed of erectile tissue and has a glans, corpus and two crurae. It is richly supplied by nerve endings and blood vessels.

BULBS OF VESTIBULE

These are a pair of elongated, erectile tissue containing a rich plexus of veins which embrace the sides of vaginal orifice. Vestibular bulbs are covered superficially by bulbo-spongiosus muscles. They correspond to the corpus spongiosum of penis in males, embryologically.

GREATER VESTIBULAR GLANDS

They are also called **Bartholin's glands.** Each gland is about 1.5 cm size and is situated behind the bulb of vestibule, in the superficial perineal pouch. The duct of each gland is 1.5 to 2 cm long and it opens on each side of vaginal orifice, below the hymen, at the junction of anterior 2/3rd with the posterior 1/3rd. These glands secrete mucus that keeps the vulva moist.

VAGINAL ORIFICE

The lower end of vagina opens in the vestibule posterior to urethral orifice forming the vaginal orifice.

UTERUS

It is a hollow, pyriform shaped, muscular organ of the female genital tract. It lies in the pelvic cavity between urinary bladder, anteriorly and rectum and sigmoid colon, posteriorly (Fig. 19.2).

Dimensions (In nulliparous adult female)

Length of fundus and body	: 5 cm
Length of cervix	: 2.5 cm
Total uterocervical length	: 7.5 cm
Breadth (maximum at fundus)	: 5 cm
Length of uterine cavity	: 6 cm
Thickness	: 2.5 cm (1.25 cm each wall)
Weight	: 50 to 80 gm

Presenting Parts

The uterus presents two main regions namely
1. Uterine body (corpus uteri): It forms the upper 2/3rd.
2. Uterine cervix: It is the lower 1/3rd.

Uterine Body

It consists of the following parts:
1. **Fundus:** It is the expanded upper end of the body which lies above an imaginary horizontal plane passing through the opening of two uterine tubes. It is usually directed forwards.
2. **Body:** It extends from fundus to isthmus, it is wider in upper part and narrow below. The lumen of the body is known as uterine cavity. The lumen is flat

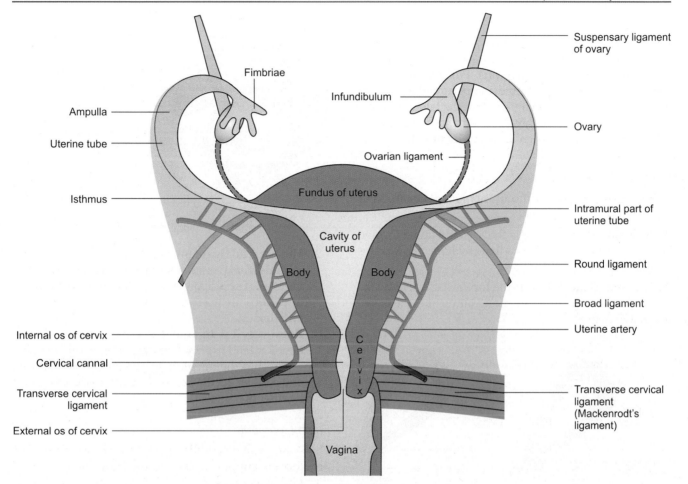

Fig. 19.2: Uterus, uterine tubes and ovaries

anteroposteriorly. Anterior surface of body is flat and is directed downwards and forwards. Posterior surface is convex and is directed upwards and backwards. Each lateral border gives attachment to the broad ligament of the uterus.

3. **Lateral angle or the cornu of the uterus:** Each angle projects outwards from the junction of fundus and the body. The cornu presents with the following attachments on each side
   a. Uterine tube
   b. Round ligament
   c. Ligament of ovary

4. **Isthmus:** It is a constricted part present between the body and uterine cervix. It is 0.5 cm in length.

Cervix

Cervix of the uterus is cylindrical in shape and extends from internal os to external os. It presents with a vaginal part that lies within the upper end of vagina and a supra vaginal part which is present above the level of vagina,

below the isthmus. It is more fixed than the body. Three pairs of ligments attach cervix to pelvic wall namely
   a. Mackenrodt's ligaments
   b. Uterosacral ligaments
   c. Pubocervical ligaments
   Cervix is twice the length of body in children whereas in adults the body is twice the length of cervix.

Important Relations of Cervix (Supravaginal part)

On each side
1. Ureter: Each ureter lies 2 cm lateral to cervix, at the level of internal os.
2. Uterine artery.
3. Mackenrodt's ligament.
4. Broad ligament.
5. Para cervical lymph nodes.

Posteriorly
1. Pouch of Douglas (with or without coils of intestine)
2. Sigmoid colon

Anteriorly: Base of urinary bladder.

Peritoneal Relations of Uterus

Fundus of uterus is fully covered by the peritoneum from all the sides. Anterior surface of the body is covered by the peritoneum upto the isthmus. Posterior surface of the body is completely covered and peritoneum extends upto posterior fornix of vagina. Both the lateral borders are non peritoneal and give attachment to the double fold of peritoneum known as **broad ligament.**

Axis of Uterus

The normal position of the uterus is anteversion and anteflexion.

Anteversion (Fig. 19.3): It is the forward angle formed between the axis of cervix and that of vagina. It measures about 90 degrees.

Anteflexion (Fig. 19.3): It is the forward angle between the body and the cervix at the isthmus and measures about 125 degrees.

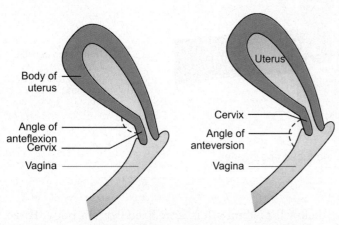

Fig. 19.3: Normal position of uterus

Ligaments of Uterus (Fig. 19.4)

Ligaments of uterus can be studied as true and false ligaments.

True Ligaments

These are condensations of endopelvic fascia and contain fibrous tissue and muscle fibres. There are three pairs of true ligaments namely:

1. **Mackenrodt's ligaments:** They are also known as **transverse ligaments.** Each ligament forms a fan shaped, fibromuscular band and extends laterally from the supravaginal part of cervix and upper part of lateral vaginal wall to the fascia covering the levator ani. These ligaments keeps the cervix in position and prevent downward displacement of uterus.

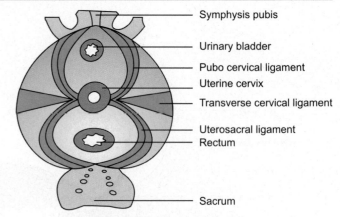

Fig. 19.4: Ligaments of uterus

2. **Utero-sacral ligaments:** Each utero-sacral ligament extends from posterior surface of cervix to 3rd sacral vertebra. These ligaments pull the cervix backwards and help in maintenance of anteversion and anteflexion.
3. **Pubo-cervical ligaments:** A pair of thin fibrous bands extend from anterior aspect of cervix to pubic bone. These ligaments help pull the cervix forwards and counter act the excessive traction of utero-sacral ligaments.

False Ligaments

These are primarily folds of peritoneum which do not provide any support to the uterus. They are
1. **Utero-vesical fold:** Also known as anterior ligament.
2. **Recto-vaginal fold:** Also known as posterior ligament.
3. **A pair of broad ligaments**
4. **A pair of round ligaments**

Broad Ligament

Developmentally, they are the mesentery of para mesonephric ducts. Each ligament is a broad fold of peritoneum consisting of two layers which extend from the lateral border of uterus to the lateral pelvic wall. It is quadrilateral in shape and has two surfaces and four borders as follows (Fig. 19.2).
1. **Anteroinferior surface:** It is related to urinary bladder.
2. **Posterosuperior surface:** It continues over the ovary in its upper part and is attached to the hilum of the ovary. This part is named **mesovarium.**
3. **Upper border:** It is free and encloses the uterine tube in medial 3/4th. This part is named **mesosalpinx.** Laterally, it extends over suspensory ligament of ovary.
4. **Lower border or base:** It is attached to the pelvic floor. Uterine artery passes just below the lower

border to reach isthmus from where it ascends up along the lateral wall of uterus.

5. **Medial border:** It is attached to the lateral border of uterus and contains the tortuous uterine blood vessels.
6. **Lateral border:** It is attached to the lateral pelvic wall.

Contents of Broad Ligament
1. Uterine tube
2. Round ligament
3. Ligament of ovary
4. Ovarian vessels
5. Uterine vessels
6. Tubules and ducts of epoophoron (remnants of mesonephric duct)
7. Tubules of paroophoron
8. Lymphatics nerves and unstriped muscles
9. Accessory supra-renal tissue - occasionally

Round Ligaments

Each ligament is 10 to 12 cm long. It is a fibromuscular band attached proximally to the lateral angle of uterus, below and in front of the uterine tube. It passes on each side through the broad ligament and enters the deep inguinal ring. It runs in the inguinal canal and comes out of the superficial inguinal ring to the perineum. It ultimately attaches to subcutaneous tissue of labium majus.

Functions: It maintains anteversion and anteflexion of the uterus.

Arterial Supply of Uterus
1. Uterine artery, branch of internal iliac artery.
2. Ovarian artery, branch of abdominal aorta.

Venous Drainage of Uterus
1. Uterine veins, drain into internal iliac vein.
2. Ovarian vein, drains into inferior vena cava on right side and left renal vein on left side.

Lymphatic Drainage of Uterus

From fundus and upper part of body: Lymphatics drain into pre aortic and lateral aortic group of lymph nodes. Few vessels from lateral angle (cornu) drain into superficial inguinal group of lymph nodes.
From lower part of body: Lymphatics drain into external iliac group of lymph nodes.
From the cervix: Lymph reaches external iliac, internal iliac and sacral lymph nodes.

Nerve Supply of Uterus
1. **Sympathetic supply:** Preganglionic fibres are derived from T_{12} to L_1 spinal segments.
2. **Parasympathetic supply:** Preganglionic fibres are derived from S_2, S_3, S_4 spinal segments.

Structure of Uterus

The uterine wall is thick and muscular and can be divided into three layers namely endometrium, myometrium and perimetrium.
1. **Endometrium:** It is the inner most mucus membrane of uterus and consists of epithelium made up of single layer of columnar cells lying over lamina propria. The lamina propria consists of connective tissue with numerous fibroblasts and has a rich vascular supply. It also has endometrial glands which are invaginations from the surface epithelium. They are of simple tubular variety lined by columnar epithelium of secretory type. The endometrium undergoes cyclical changes during the menstrual cycle and can be divided into two zones:
   a. **Pars basalis:** It is the deep zone inner to myometrium. It consists of stroma and proximal part of endometrial glands.
   b. **Pars functionalis:** It is the superficial zone made up of endometrial epithelium with subjacent lamina propria containing superficial or distal part of uterine glands. The pars functionalis increases in thickness due to increase in stroma and gland size during menstrual cycle and is shed during menstruation.
2. **Myometrium:** It is the thickest layer as the uterus is mainly made up of bundles of smooth muscle fibres with interspersed connective tissue. It has a rich network of blood vessels nerves and lymphatics.
3. **Serosa:** It is the outermost peritoneal covering of uterus and is made up of thin connective tissue layer with mesothelium.

Structure of Cervix

The epithelial lining of cervix is mostly ciliated columnar epithelium. The lower 1/3rd of cervix is lined by simple columnar epithelium while the mucosa over vaginal part of cervix is made up of stratified squamous epithelium. This epithelium is not shed during menstruation. The lamina propria is thin. Middle layer is thick and fibro muscular. The outer most layer consists of serosa.

UTERINE (FALLOPIAN) TUBES

They are two in number, one originating on each side of fundus of uterus. Each tube is situated in the medial 3/4th of the upper free margin of broad ligament of uterus. Uterine tube extends first laterally then upwards, backwards and then downwards (Fig. 19.2).
Length: 10 cm

Presenting Parts

Each tube presents from medial to lateral the following:

1. **Uterine opening:** It is 1 mm in diameter. It communicates the intramural part of uterine tube to lateral angle of uterine cavity.
2. **Intra mural part:** It is 1 cm long and lies with in the uterine wall.
3. **Isthmus:** It is 3 cm long, cord like, extending from intramural part to ampullary part. It has a thick wall.
4. **Ampulla:** It is 5 cm in length. It is the longest part and is thin walled, tortuous and dilated.
5. **Infundibulum:** It is 1 cm long. It is wide and trumpet like.
6. **Abdominal opening:** It is situated at the bottom of infundibulum. It is 2 to 3 mm in diameter. This end is known as fimbriated end due to presence of fimbriae. It lies in relation to ovary.

Arterial Supply of Fallopian Tube

1. Ovarian artery.
2. Uterine artery.

Venous Drainage of Fallopian Tube

Ovarian and uterine veins.

Lymphatic Drainage of Fallopian Tube

1. The lymphatics primarily drain into preaortic and lateral aortic group of lymph nodes.
2. Intramural part drains into superficial group of inguinal lymph nodes.

Nerve Supply of Fallopian Tube

1. **Sympathetic supply:** Preganglionic fibres are derived from T_{10} to L_2 spinal segments.
2. **Parasympathetic supply:** Lateral part is supplied via vagus nerve while medial part is supplied via pelvic splanchnic nerve.

Structure of Uterine Tubes

Each tube is made up of three layers:

1. **Mucosa:** It is the inner most layer made up of single layer of columnar epithelium lying over a thin layer of lamina propria. The epithelium is mostly ciliated columnar epithelium interspersed with secretory cells. The mucosa is thrown into numerous longitudinal folds (most pronounced in the infundibulum) with a central core of lamina propria lined by columnar epithelium.
2. **Muscular layer:** It is a relatively thick, intermediate layer consisting of inner circular and outer longitudinal layer of smooth muscles.
3. **Serosa:** It is derived from visceral peritoneum.

VAGINA

Vagina is a fibromuscular canal extending from the vulva to uterus. It is the female copulatory organ. Vagina lies between the urethra and bladder, in front and the rectum and anal canal, behind. The vagina is directed upwards and backwards from the vulva making an angle of 45° with the uterus (Fig. 19.2).

Measurements

Length	:	Anterior wall is 8 cm while posterior wall is 10 cm long.
Diameter	:	Upper end is wider, 5 cm and lower end is narrower 2.5 cm.

Shape of lumen: The lumen of vagina is circular at the upper end and H-shaped in the rest of the length. This is because the anterior and posterior walls are normally in apposition.

Relations of Vagina

Anterior: Bladder and urethra.
Posterior:
1. Rectouterine pouch in upper 1/4th.
2. Rectum in middle 1/4th.
3. Perineal body and anal canal in lower 1/4th.

Lateral
1. Transverse cervical ligament
2. Pubococcygeus
3. Bulb of vestibule, bulbospongiosus and greater vestibular gland.

Hymen: It is a thin annular fold of mucus membrane present just above the vaginal opening in vestibule. In sexually active women, especially after child birth the hymen is torn and only tags of membrane are seen known as carunculae myritiformis.

Fornices of Vagina

The cervix protrudes into the upper part of vagina and this results in formation of a circular groove at the upper part of vagina or vault of vagina. This is divided into four parts and is named as follows:

1. Anterior fornix: It is shallowest
2. Posterior fornix: It is deepest
3. Two lateral fornices

Blood Supply of Vagina

It is derived from vaginal branches of
1. Internal iliac artery
2. Uterine artery

3. Middle rectal artery
4. Internal pudendal artery

Veins accompany arteries and drain into internal pudendal veins.

Lymphatic Drainage of Vagina

1. From upper 1/3rd lymphatics drain into external iliac nodes.
2. From middle 1/3rd lymphatics drain into internal iliac nodes.
3. From lower 1/3rd lymphatics drain into superficial inguinal nodes.

Nerve Supply of Vagina

1. **Pudendal nerve:** It supplies lower 1/3rd of vagina.
2. **Sympathetic (L_1, L_2) and parasympathetic (S_2, S_3) supply:** Upper 2/3rd receives autonomic nerve supply.

OVARIES

Ovaries are a pair of female reproductive glands situated in the lesser pelvis, one on each side of the uterus. They are almond in shape (Fig. 19.2).

Dimensions

Vertical	:	3 cm
Anteroposteriorly	:	1.5 cm
Transversely	:	1 cm

Positions of Ovary

1. In early fetal life, ovaries lie in lumbar region near kidneys.
2. In new born, ovaries are situated above the pelvic brim.
3. In nulliparous women, ovaries lie in **ovarian fossa** below the pelvic brim.
4. During pregnancy, ovaries become abdominal structures after 14 weeks of gestation along with the uterus.

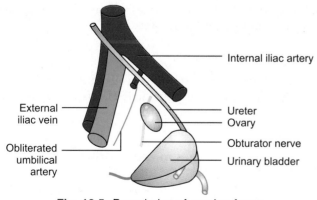

Fig. 19.5: Boundaries of ovarian fossa

5. After childbirth (in multiparous women), ovaries get displaced from ovarian fossa and usually lie in rectouterine pouch.

Boundaries of Ovarian Fossa (Fig. 19.5)

Superoanteriorly	:	Obliterated umbilical artery.
Superiorly	:	External iliac vein.
Posteriorly	:	Ureter and internal iliac vessels.
Lateral wall or floor	:	Parietal peritoneum, obturator nerve.

Presenting Parts

Each ovary has two ends, two borders and two surfaces.
1. **Tubal end:** It is directed upwards and related to uterine tube, fimbria and suspensory ligament of ovary
2. **Uterine end:** It is directed downward and connected to the lateral angle of uterus.
3. **Mesovarian border:** It is also known as anterior border. A fold of posterior layer of broad ligament is attached to the border which serves as passage for vessels and nerves. A white line known as **line of Furre** is present along this border.
4. **Free border:** It is also known as posterior border. It is convex in shape and is related with the uterine tube in upper part and ureter posteriorly.
5. **Medial surface:** It is related to the posterior part of uterine tube, separated by the bursa ovarica.
6. **Lateral surface:** It is convex and lies in ovarian fossa.

Arterial Supply of Ovary

1. Ovarian artery.
2. Uterine artery.

Venous Drainage of Ovary

A plexus of veins drains each ovary. It is known as pampiniform plexus. This plexus forms the ovarian vein. Right ovarian vein drains into the inferior vena cava while the left ovarian vein drains into left renal vein.

Lymphatic Drainage of Ovary

Lymphatics from ovary drain into pre-aortic and lateral aortic group of lymph nodes.

Nerve Supply of Ovary

It is derived from **sympathetic supply.** Preganglionic fibres come from T_{10} and T_{11} spinal segments.

Structure of Ovary (Fig. 19.6)

Each ovary is oval in shape. Its outer surface is covered by a single layer of cuboidal cells known as germinal

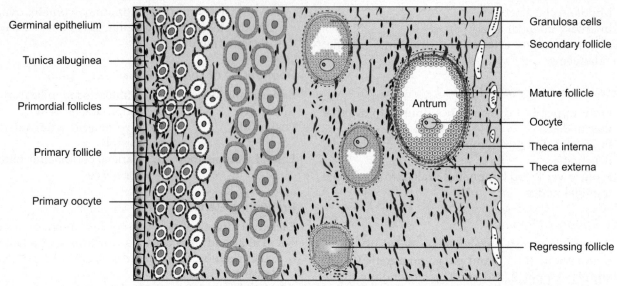

Germinal epithelium

Tunica albuginea

Primordial follicles

Primary follicle

Primary oocyte

Granulosa cells

Secondary follicle

Mature follicle

Antrum

Oocyte

Theca interna

Theca externa

Regressing follicle

Fig. 19.6: Histological section of ovary-showing different stages of development of oocyte

epithelium. A layer of dense connective tissue named tunica albuginea lines the inner aspect of germinal epithelium. The ovary can be further divided into an outer cortex and an inner medulla.

Cortex

Cortex is covered by tunica albuginea. It is made up of stroma and ovarian follicles. Stroma consists of reticular fibres and numerous fusiform shaped fibroblasts. Ovarian follicles with the developing oocyte at various stages of development are scattered throughout in this stroma.

Medulla

It is made up of connective tissue and has a rich network of blood vessels lying in loose connective tissue made up of elastic fibres. Few smooth muscle fibres are also present.

PHYSIOLOGY OF FEMALE REPRODUCTIVE SYSTEM

Functions of Female Reproductive Tract

External Genitalia
1. The external structures provide protection to the vaginal canal from invasion by infections and from foreign bodies, specially in young girls.
2. The secretions of bulbourethral and paraurethral glands help to lubricate the vulva.
3. Erectile tissue of clitoris and labia minora help in sexual arousal.

Vagina: It forms an important passage from uterus to exterior that helps in:

1. Birth of baby.
2. Flow of menstrual blood to exterior.
3. It acts as receptacle for the male copulatory organ, penis, for deposition of sperm.

Uterus: After puberty uterus undergoes cyclical changes known as menstrual cycle. These changes prepare uterus to receive fertilized ovum and nourish the embryo and maintain pregnancy till birth of baby (Fig. 19.8).

Uterine (fallopian) tubes: They are the site for receiving the ovum from ovary. Fertilization of ovum occurs in the ampulla of the tubes. The secretions of fallopian tubes provide nutrition to the fertilized ovum and helps in its propulsion to the uterus.

Ovarian Function

Two ovaries contain ovarian follicles in various stages of development and are the store house of female gametes or ova. There are about 1 to 2 million primordial follicles at birth which develop into primary follicles at puberty. There are about 3 to 4 lakh primary follicles in ovary at puberty. Ovary secretes two steroid hormones, estrogen and progesterone (Fig. 19.7).

Estrogen

It is produced by the granulosa cells of the developing follicles (Fig. 19.6), in response to FSH. It is also produced by placenta, adrenal and testes.

Actions of Estrogen
1. Stimulates changes in endometrium in a cyclical manner.
2. Facilitates growth of ovarian follicles.
3. Increases motility of fallopian tubes.

4. Promotes and maintains growth of internal genitalia.
5. Increases secretion of thin cervical secretions favouring penetration by sperms.
6. Promotes mitotic activity in vagina, increases breakdown of glycogen and production of lactic acid. This maintains an acid medium (pH-4.5) and the integrity of epithelium, preventing invasion by external organisms.
7. Promotes growth of external genitalia.
8. Provides negative feedback to pituitary for secretion of FSH.
9. Provides positive feedback to pituitary for secretion of LH causing LH surge.
10. Has an important role in maintaining pregnancy, in growth of myometrium and also in labour.
11. Responsible for appearance and development of secondary sexual characteristics in females especially breast enlargement.

Effect on breast: It is responsible for growth of duct system in breast resulting in breast enlargement during puberty.
12. Miscellaneous actions:
    a. Causes salt and water retention.
    b. Increases thin secretions of sebaceous glands and keeps skin elastic.
    c. Has anti atherogenic action by maintaining low circulating cholesterol levels and promoting endothelial vasodilatation.

Progesterone

It is a steroid hormone secreted by the corpus luteum of ovary. It is also produced by adrenal cortex and testes in small amounts normally and by placenta in large quantities during pregnancy.

Actions of Progesterone

1. It produces secetory changes in uterine endometrium which is primed by estrogen, making it receptive for implantation of fertilized ovum.

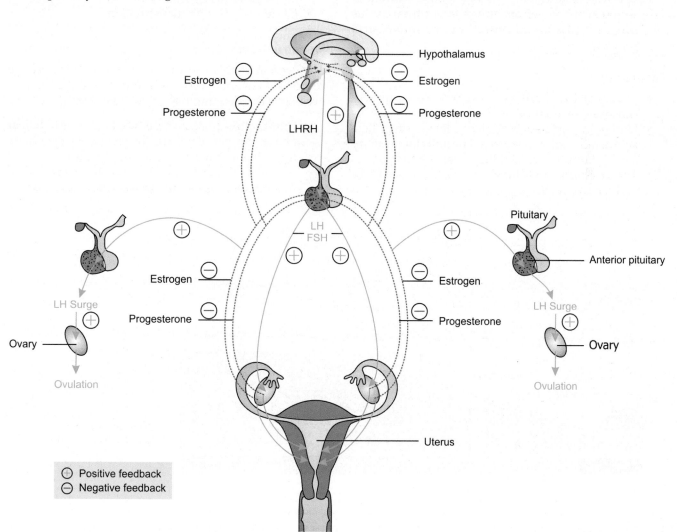

Fig. 19.7: Diagrammatic representation of hormonal control of ovarian and uterine function

2. It makes the cervical secretions thick and viscous. This creates a barrier for entry of further spermatozoa. It also protects against invasion by organisms.
3. It promotes development of glandular tissue of the breast increasing the alveolar mass.
4. It antagonizes the following effects of estrogen:
   a. Decreases myometrial contractility
   b. Decreases estrogen receptors on myometrium
5. Miscellaneous functions:
   a. Increases basal body temperature
   b. Stimulates respiration

Regulation of Ovarian Function

Synthesis and secretion of ovarian hormones is under control of pituitary gonadotropins, FSH and LH (Fig. 19.7).

1. **FSH:** It stimulates development of ovarian follicles and production of estrogen. It is inhibited by high estrogen levels. Inhibin B produced by granulosa cells of ovary inhibits FSH secretion.
2. **LH:** It is responsible for ovulation. It stimulates secretion of estrogen and progesterone from corpus luteum. LH is inhibited by estrogen and progesterone levels.

Ovarian Cycle

- The cyclical changes in ovary after puberty constitute ovarian cycle.
- Under the influence of rising levels of follicle stimulating hormone secreted by anterior pituitary a cohort of primordial follicles are stimulated.
- The primordial follicles grow and form secondary and tertiary follicles.

- The follicles secrete estrogen. Under the influence of hormones one follicle grows maximally to mature to Graffian follicle.
- When estrogen level attains a peak, it leads to stimulation of LH surge. There is a sudden increase in secretion of leutenizing hormone from pituitary due to positive feedback from estrogen.
- Ovulation occurs in response to LH surge. It is characterized by rupture of follicle and release of secondary oocyte from the ovary.
- After ovulation the walls of ovarian follicle collapse and fold. The granulosa cells increase in size and acquire a cytoplasmic carotenoid pigment, leutin, which is responsible for their yellow color. It is called corpus luteum. The cells now produce progesterone hormone.
- The lutein cells undergo fatty degeneration and autolysis in the absence of fertilization and atrophy by 12 to 14 days post ovulation.
- The atretic corpus is seen as a white scar called corpus albicans.
- Cycle restarts with menstruation.

Menstrual Cycle

The cyclical changes in the endometrium of uterus in response to ovarian hormones constitute the menstrual cycle. It is divided into the following phases (Fig. 19.8).

1. **Proliferative phase:** This is also known as follicular phase. This phase follows the last menstrual phase. It has the following characteristic features:
   — There is generalized active proliferation of endometrium which grows from 1 to 3 mm.

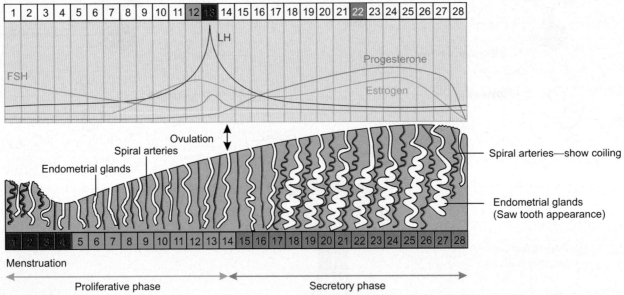

Fig. 19.8: Diagrammatic representation of changes in hormonal levels and corresponding changes in endometrium during menstrual cycle

— Uterine glands increase in length and remain straight
— Cells of endometrial stroma are arranged in following three layers, from superficial to deep
  a. **Stratum compactum:** Superficial compact layer
  b. **Stratum spongiosum:** Intermediate spongy layer
  c. **Stratum basale:** Deep basal layer
— Changes in this phase occurs under the influence of estrogen derived from maturing ovarian follicles.
— This phase generally lasts for 14 days in a 28 days menstrual cycle.

2. **Secretory phase:** This is also known as progestational phase. It is characterized by the following features:
— There is futher growth of endometrium.
— Endometrium grows upto 5 to 7 mm in thickness.
— Endometrial glands become dilated and convolute.
— There is increased amount of tissue fluid in the stroma.
— Increase in size of stromal cells occurs due to accumulation of glycogen and lipid droplets in their cytoplasm. This change in stromal cells is known as the **decidual reaction.**
— This phase is influenced by progestrone hormone, secreted by corpus luteum of ovary.
— This phase lasts for 14 days in a 28 days cycle.
— By the end of progesterone phase regression of endometrium starts due to decreasing concentration of progesterone hormone.

3. **Menstrual phase**
— This phase follows the secretory phase and lasts for 3 to 5 days.
— It is characterised by the shedding of stratum compactum and stratum spongiosum of endometrium along with some amount of blood.

— The average amount of blood loss during menstruation is about 50 to 60 ml.
— The onset of menstrual phase occurs due to decreasing concentration of progestrone because of degeneration of corpus luteum.

The duration of mestrual cycle on an average is 28 days. The duration of cycle is estimated from the first day of the menstrual bleeding to the onset of menstrual bleeding in the next cycle.

Duration of secretory phase remains constant (14 days) whereas the duration of proliferative phase is variable according to hormonal levels and is responsible for alterations in total duration of the cycle.

Menopause

There is a constant decline in the number of primordial follicles in ovaries with increasing age. Usually, at 45-50 years of age there are no ovarian follicles left. Hence, the ovaries become unresponsive to FSH. Decline in ovarian function and fall in inhibin B levels result in increase FSH levels in blood. The ovaries stop production of estrogen and progesterone resulting in atrophic changes in uterus and vagina. This results in irregular menstrual cycles and finally cessation of menstruation which is known as menopause.

MAMMARY GLAND

In males and immature females mammary gland is rudimentary. Nipple is small but areola is fully formed in both males and prepubertal females.

Female Mammary Gland

It is a modified sweat gland which lies in the superficial fascia in pectoral region.

Extent (Fig. 19.9)
Vertical: 2nd to 6th rib in mid clavicular line.

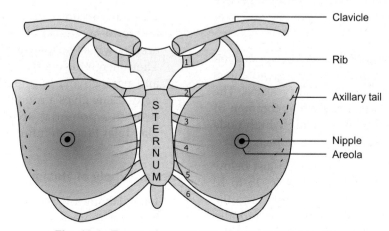

Clavicle

Rib

Axillary tail

Nipple
Areola

Fig. 19.9: Extent of mammary gland in relation to ribs

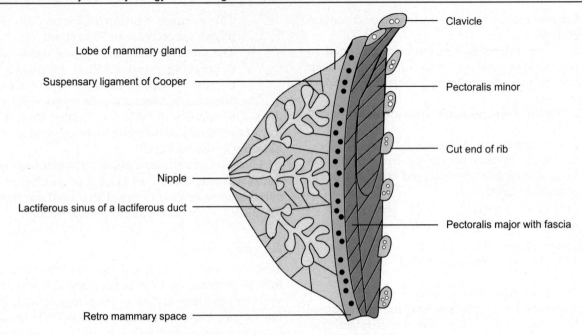

Clavicle

Lobe of mammary gland

Suspensary ligament of Cooper

Pectoralis minor

Cut end of rib

Nipple

Lactiferous sinus of a lactiferous duct

Pectoralis major with fascia

Retro mammary space

Fig. 19.10: Sagittal section of an adult female mammary gland

Horizontal: Lateral border of sternum to the mid axillary line along the 4th rib.

Mammary Bed

Three muscles form the mammary bed on which mammary gland lies (Fig. 19.10)
1. Pectoralis major covered by pectoralis fascia lies in relation to medial 2/3rd of the gland
2. Serratus anterior muscle is present in relation to the lateral 1/3rd of the gland
3. External oblique muscle lies in relation to the inferomedial part of the gland

Retromammary space (Fig. 19.10): This space lies between the deep aspect of the breast and fascia covering the mammary bed. It primarily contains loose connective tissue. This allows for the free movement of gland over the fascia.

Axillary tail of Spence (Fig. 19.9): A tail like projection from the upper and outer quadrant of the gland enters the axilla through an opening in axillary fascia. The opening in the axillary fascia is known as **foramen of Langer.** It can be confused with a axillary lymph node specially when it is swollen in lactating women.

Nipple (Fig. 19.10): The erectile projection just below the centre of the breast is known as nipple. 15 to 20 lactiferous ducts pierce the nipple and open onto the surface. Nipple is made up of circular and radially arranged smooth muscle fibres covered by the skin.

Circular muscle fibres erect the nipple and radial muscle fibres retract the nipple.

Areola (Fig. 19.9): It is the pigmented circular area around the nipple. It contains modified sebaceous glands at its outer margin.

Structure of the Mammary Gland

It is made up of glandular and fibrofatty tissue (Fig 19.10).
1. **Glandular tissue:** It is a tubo-alveolar type of gland and arranged in 15 to 20 pyramidal lobes. Each lobe is drained by a separate lactiferous duct. Each duct dilates towards areola and forms a lactiferous sinus which opens into the nipple. Large ducts are lined by stratified columnar epithelium

2. **Fibrofatty tissue:** Fibrous tissue supports the lobes and forms a number of septa. These fibrous bands are known as **suspensory ligaments of Cooper.** They anchor the overlying skin to the parenchyma and parenchyma to underlying pectoralis fascia. Fatty tissue gives a rounded shape to the organ. It provides potential space for proliferation of glandular tissue in future pregnancy.

Arterial Supply of Mammary Gland (Fig 19.11)

1. Lateral thoracic branch of 2nd part of axillary artery.
2. Superior thoracic artery from 1st part of axillary artery.

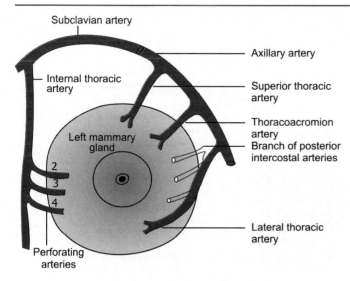

Fig. 19.11: Arterial supply of mammary gland

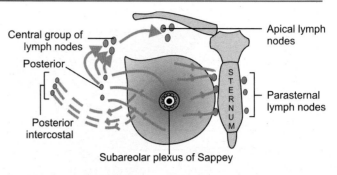

Fig. 19.13: Deep lymphatic drainage of mammary gland (parenchyma, nipple and areola)

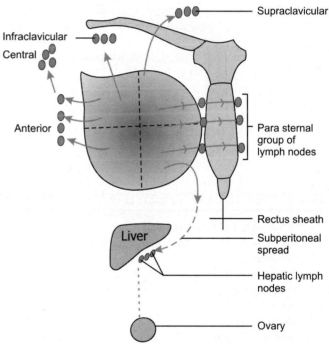

Fig. 19.12: Superficial lymphatic drainage of mammary gland

3. Perforating branches of internal thoracic artery to 2nd, 3rd and 4th intercostal spaces.
4. Lateral branches of 2nd, 3rd and 4th posterior intercostal arteries.
5. Thoraco-acromion artery.

Venous Drainage of Mammary Gland

Circulus venosus is formed beneath the areola which drains into axillary vein, internal thoracic vein and intercostal veins.

Nerve Supply of Mammary Gland

4th, 5th, 6th intercostal nerves: They supply the overlying skin and convey sympathetic fibres also. Sympathetic supply is primarily vasomotor.

Lymphatic Drainage of Mammary Gland (Figs 19.12, 19.13)

Lymphatic drainage can be divided into a deep and a superficial part.

1. **Deep part:** This drains the parenchyma, nipple and areola. Lymphatics from areola and nipple form a **subareolar plexus of Sappey.** Parenchyma is drained by vessels present in the interlobular connective tissue and walls of lactiferous ducts.
   — 75% of deep lymphatics drain into the axillary lymph nodes.
   — 20% of deep lymphatics drain into parasternal lymph nodes.
   — 5% of deep lymphatics drain into the posterior intercostal nodes.
2. **Superficial part:** Drainage from overlying skin except areola and nipple is divided into four quadrants as shown in figure. Outer part drains into axillary nodes. Upper part drains into supraclavicular group of lymph nodes. Inner part is drained by parasternal group of lymph nodes. This communicates with the opposite parasternal group of lymph nodes. Lower part communicates with sub peritoneal plexus of lymphatics and drains into sub-diaphragmatic nodes. Some pass through the falciform ligament to reach the hepatic nodes.

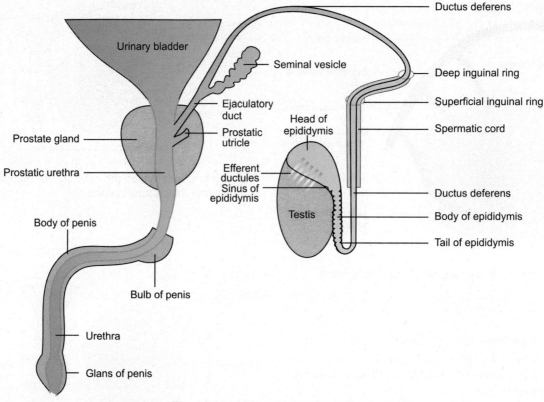

Fig. 19.14: Male reproductive organs

MALE REPRODUCTIVE SYSTEM (FIG. 19.14)

It consists of the following parts:
1. Penis
2. Scrotum
3. Testes
4. Epididymis
5. Spermatic cord
6. Ductus deferens
7. Seminal vesicles
8. Ejaculatory duct
9. Prostate gland
   First five form external genitalia of male.

PENIS (FIGs 19.14 to 19.16)

It is the male organ to excrete urine out side the body and to release the sperms in female genital tract. It is made up of two parts namely,
   a. Root of penis
   b. Body of penis

Root of Penis

It is situated in superficial perineal pouch and consists of two crura and one bulb of penis (Fig. 19.15).
   1. **Two crura:** Each crus is attached to the inner aspect of everted ischio-pubic ramus. It is covered superficially by ischiocavernosus muscle. The two crura are approximated in mid line and continue as corpora cavernosa. Deep artery of penis traverses forward within the crus.
   2. **Bulb of penis:** It is the expanded part and is attached to the perineal membrane. Superficially, it is covered by bulbo-spongiosus muscle. Bulb of penis continues as the corpus spongiosum of penis. Urethra enters through the upper surface of the bulb after piercing the perineal membrane.

Body of Penis

It is made up of a pair of corpora cavernosa and a single corpus spongiosum (Figs 19.15, 19.16). Corpora cavernosa lie on the dorsal surface and the corpus spongiosu, lies on the ventral surface. Each corpus cavernosus is divided into a number of intercommunicating cavernous spaces which are lined by endothelium. Cavernous spaces receive blood from capillaries of **helicine arteries** and are drained by deep dorsal vein of penis. Corpus spongiosus is traversed by the spongy urethra. Traced in front and behind it is expanded to form **glans penis** and the **bulb** respectively. When prepuce is retracted from the base of glans penis, it presents a raised margin known as **corona glandis.**

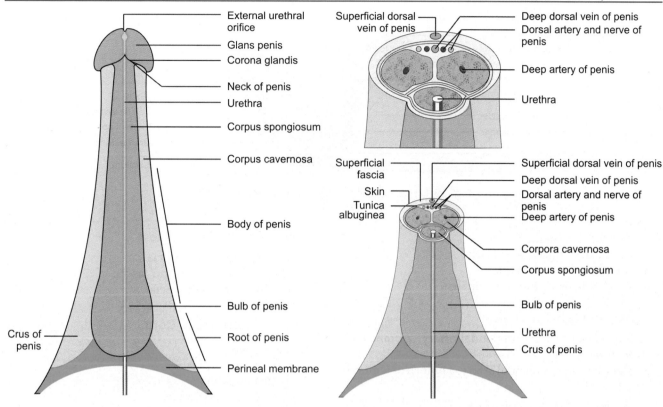

Fig. 19.15: Ventral surface of penis showing different parts

Fig. 19.16: Transverse section of penis

Body of the penis is covered by: outside inward
1. **Skin**
2. **Superficial fascia**
3. **Fibrous envelope**

Ligaments of Penis
1. Fundiform ligament of penis
2. Suspensory ligament of penis

Arterial Supply of Penis

It is derived from three paired arteries
1. **Arteries of bulb:** They supply the corpus spongiosus and spongy urethra.
2. **Deep arteries of penis:** They supply the corpora cavernosa as helicine arteries.
3. **Dorsal artery of penis:** They supply the skin, prepuce, glans penis.

Venous Drainage of Penis
1. Superficial dorsal vein
2. Deep dorsal vein

Lymphatic Drainage of Penis
1. **Glans penis:** Drains into deep inguinal group of lymph nodes.
2. **Rest of the penis including skin:** Drains into superficial inguinal group of lymph nodes.

Nerve Supply of Penis
1. **Dorsal nerve of penis:** Branch from pundendal nerve. It is the somatic nerve and supplies the skin, prepuce, glans.
2. Urethral branches of perineal nerve supply urethra and bulb of the penis.
3. **Parasymphathetic supply:** Preganglionic fibres are derived from S_2 S_3 S_4 spinal cord segments. Parasympathetic supply is vasodilator.
4. **Sympathetic supply:** Preganglionic fibres are derived from L_1 spinal cord segment. It is vaso-constrictor.

Functions of Penis
1. It is a passage for urine to exterior.
2. It is responsible for ejaculation of semen deposition in vagina.

SCROTUM

It is a cutaneous pouch that contains testes, epididymis and lower part of spermatic cords (Fig. 19.17).

Layers of Scrotum (From Outside Inward)
1. Skin
2. Dartos muscle

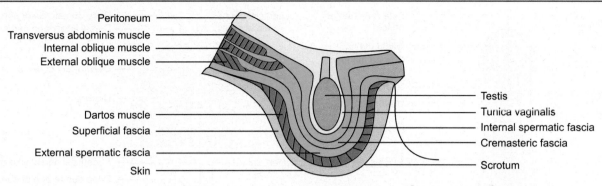

Fig. 19.17: Layers of scrotum and covering of testis

3. External spermatic fascia
4. Cremastric muscle and fascia
5. Internal spermatic fascia
6. Parietal layer of tunica vaginalis

Arterial Supply of Scrotum

1. Superficial external pudendal artery, a branch of femoral artery.
2. Deep external pudendal artery, a branch of femoral artery.
3. Posterior scrotal branch, a branch of Internal pudendal artery.

Venous Drainage of Scrotum

The corresponding veins drain into:
1. Great saphenous vein
2. Internal iliac vein

Lymphatic Drainage of Scrotum

Superficial inguinal group of lymph nodes

Nerve Supply of Scrotum

1. Anterior 1/3rd of scrotum is supplied by ilioinguinal nerve (L_1) and genito femoral nerve (L_1).
2. Posterior 2/3rd of scrotum is supplied by scrotal branch of pudendal nerve (S_2) and perineal branch of posterior femoral cutaneous nerve of thigh (S_3, S_4).

Functions of Scrotum

1. Protect testes from external voilence
2. Helps in temperature regulation of testes

SPERMATIC CORD

It is a tubular sheath, 7.5 cm in length and extends from the deep inguinal ring, inguinal canal and external inguinal ring to the upper posterior part of testis (Fig. 19.14).

Coverings of Spermatic Cord

1. External spermatic fascia.
2. Cremasteric muscle and fascia.
3. Internal spermatic fascia.

Contents of Spermatic Cord

1. Vas deferens
2. Pampiniform plexus
3. Testicular artery
4. Artery to vas deferens
5. Cremasteric artery
6. Lymphatics of testes and epididymis
7. Genital branch of genitofemoral nerve
8. Loose connective tissue
9. Processus vaginalis some times
10. Accessory suprarenal cortical tissues may be present

EPIDIDYMIS

It is a comma shaped body made up of highly coiled tubes, situated along the lateral part of the posterior border of testis (Fig. 19.14, 19.18).

Parts of Epididymis

It has following parts:
1. **Head** is formed by coiling of efferent ductules from testis.
2. **Body** is also called middle part.
3. **Tail:** It is the lower part which continues with vas deferens that ascends up on the medial aspect of epididymis.

Body and tail are made up of a single coiled epididymal duct. The canal of epididymis is 20 feet long when uncoiled. Sometimes head gives attachment to a sessile mass known as **appendix of epididymis**, a remnant of paramesonephros.

Functions of Epididymis

Maturation of sperms takes place in the epididymis.

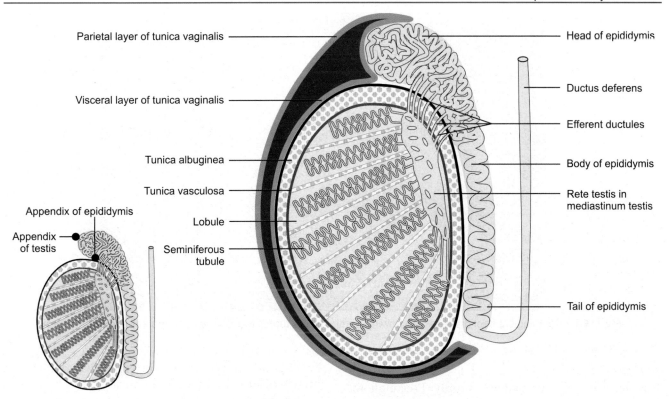

Fig. 19.18: Longitudinal section of testis and epididymis

TESTES

Testes are the male reproductive glands. They lie in the scrotum suspended by spermatic cords. Left testis is slightly lower than the right. They lie obliquely such that the upper pole is situated slightly laterally and forwards (Figs 19.14, 19.18).

Dimensions (in adult)

Length	:	5 cm
Breadth	:	2.5 cm
Anteroposteriorly	:	3 cm
Weight	:	10 to 14 gm

Coverings of Testis

Testis covered by three layers from outside inward (Fig. 19.18).

1. **Tunica vaginalis:** It is made up of two layers, parietal and visceral with a cavity in between. It is the persistent lower part of processus vaginalis which is invaginated by testis from behind. Therefore it covers the testis from all sides except at posterior border

2. **Tunica albuginea:** It is a thick fibrous membrane which invests the entire testis and projects into the organ from its posterior border forming the mediastinum testis. Numerous fibrous septae divide the testis into lobules. These septae arise from tunica albuginea from its anterior convex surface.

3. **Tunica vasculosa:** It is a vascular and areolar membrane which lines the individual lobules of testis.

Arterial Supply of Testis

1. Testicular artery, branch of abdominal aorta
2. Artery to vas deferens, branch from superior or inferior vesical artery
3. Sometimes cremasteric artery, branch from inferior epigastric artery.

Venous Drainage of Testis

Testis is drained by a plexus of 15 to 20 veins known as the pampiniform plexus. At the level of superficial inguinal ring they join to form four veins and at the deep inguinal ring they form two veins. A single testicular vein is formed in the posterior abdominal wall.

1. Right testicular vein drains into inferior vena cava
2. Left testicular vein drains into left renal vein at right angle.

Lymphatic Drainage of Testis

Lymphatics from each testis drain into the pre-aortic and para-aortic lymph nodes.

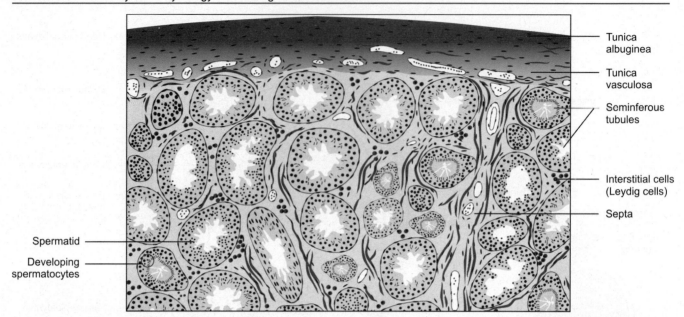

Fig. 19.19: Histological section of testis showing seminiferous tubules and various stages of spermatogenesis

Nerve Supply of Testis

It is derived from **sympathetic supply.** Preganglionic fibres come from T_{10} and T_{11} spinal segments.

Structure of Testis (Fig. 19.19)

The tunica albuginea divides the testis to 200 to 300 lobules. Each lobule contain 2 to 3 seminiferous tubules. Each tubule measures about 2 feet in length. Each seminiferous tubule is a highly convoluted structure surrounded by an outer connective tissue layer. Between connective tissue layer and lumen of the tubule there are several layers of the cells. Most cells represent stages in the formation of spermatozoa. Specialized cells which lie on the basement membrane are known as sustentacular cells or **cells of Sertoli.** Between the lobules there is connective tissue containing blood vessels and lymphatics. There are scattered group of cells lying in the connective tissue known as **interstitial cells of Leydig.** The straight part of tubules ascend in mediastinum, join with adjacent tubules and form a plexiform network of tubules known as **rete testis** 12-20 efferent ductules arise from the upper end of rete testis and enter the head of epididymis. The efferent ductules unite to form a single duct, the canal of epididymis.

VAS DEFERENS

It is also known as ductus deferens. It is a thick cord like tubular structure, 45 cm long. It begins from the tail of epididymis and ends at the base of prostate by joining with duct of seminal vesicle to form the ejaculatory duct (Figs 19.14, 19.18).

Arterial supply is from artery to vas deferens, a branch of superior or inferior vesical artery.

Venous drainage is via pelvic plexus of veins.

Nerve supply is derived from sympathetic via pelvic plexus.

SEMINAL VESICLES

These are a pair of pyramidal shaped organs which lie in relation to base of the urinary bladder and ampulla of rectum (Fig. 19.14). It presents the following parts:
1. Base is directed upwards
2. Apex points downward, towards the base of prostate, joins with ductus deferens and forms ejaculatory duct

Measurement
Length : 5 cm, When uncoiled its length is 10 to 15 cm
Breadth : 2 to 3 cm

Arterial Supply of Seminal Vesicles

1. Inferior vesical artery
2. Middle rectal artery

Nerve Supply of Seminal Vesicles

1. Sympathetic supply is derived from superior hypogastric plexus.
2. Parasympathetic supply is derived from pelvic splanchnic nerve.

EJACULATORY DUCTS (FIG. 19.14)

It is formed by union of vas deferens and duct of seminal vesicles on each side. Both the ducts open at colliculus

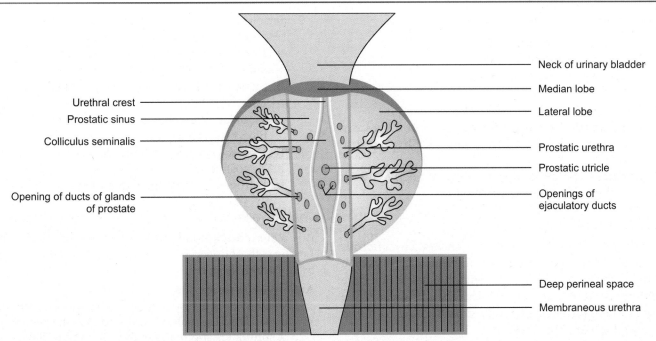

Fig. 19.20: Lobes of prostate and prostatic urethra

seminalis on each side of prostatic utricle. Each duct is 2 cm long and is lined by columnar epithelium (Fig. 19.14).

PROSTATE

It is a fibro-musculo-glandular organ and corresponds in development with the paraurethral glands of female. It is the accessory gland of male reproductive system (Figs 19.14, 19.20). It lies in lesser pelvis, below the neck of bladder, behind the lower part of symphysis pubis and in front of rectal ampulla.

Shape: Resembles an inverted cone. It has an apex, a base and anterior and posterior surfaces and two infero lateral surfaces.

Dimensions

Anterio-posterior	:	2 cm
Vertical	:	3 cm
Transverse	:	4 cm
Weight	:	8 gm

Lobes of Prostate

Anatomically prostate has three lobes, one median lobe and two lateral lobes.

Surgically, it is divided into five lobes namely:

1. **Median lobe:** It is wedge shaped with apex downwards and base upwards which forms uvula vesiace.
2. **2 lateral lobes:** These cover the side of the urethra.
3. Anterior lobe
4. Posterior lobe

Coverings of Prostate

1. **True capsule:** It is formed by the condensation of fibrous stroma of the gland. It intimately invests the entire gland.
2. **False capsule:** It is derived from the visceral layer of pelvic fascia. False capsule is connected to pubic bone by pubo prostatic ligaments.

Space between the true and false capsule is occupied by prostatic venous plexus.

Structures Passing Through Prostate

1. Prostatic urethra
2. Prostatic utricle
3. Ejaculatory duct

Arterial Supply of Prostate

1. Inferior vesical artery
2. Middle rectal artery
3. Internal pudendal artery

Venous Drainage of Prostate

The prostate is drained by prostatic venous plexuses. They have the following characteristics features:

- They receive the deep dorsal vein of penis.
- They communicate with vesical venous plexus.
- The plexus drains into internal iliac vein.
- Few veins pass backwards and communicate with the internal vertebral venous plexus via **para-vertebral veins of Batson.**

CHAPTER-19

Lymphatic Drainage of Prostate

1. Internal iliac lymph nodes
2. External iliac lymph nodes
3. Sacral group of lymph nodes

Nerve Supply of Prostate

1. **Sympathetic supply:** Preganglionic fibres are derived from L_1, L_2 from superior hypogastric plexus.
2. **Parasympathetic supply:** Fibres are derived from S_2, S_3, S_4. They are secretomotor.

Structure of Prostate

On histological section prostate is enclosed by a fibrous capsule. The capsule forms numerous septae which divide the gland into lobules. Smooth muscle fibres are interspersed between the lobules. Tha glandular tissue of prostate is arranged in three concentric layers or zones around the urethra. These are:

1. **Inner mucosal layer of glands:** It consists of simple tubular follicles.
2. **Intermediate submucosal layer of glands:** It consists of few follicles with small ducts.
3. **Outer main glands:** It is the largest zone which has numerous follicles and large ducts.

Changes in Prostate with Age

New born: The prostate primarily has ductal system in a fibromuscular stroma.

After birth: Rudimentory follicle buds apppear in the ducts which lie in the stroma.

At puberty: There is growth of follicles with increase in size of ducts and the glandular tissue is arranged in the adult pattern.

> 45 yrs.: There is involution of the glandular tissue with appearance of protein bodies known as corpora amylacea.

In old age: Prostate usually regresses but may also increase in size (known as benign hypertrophy of prostate).

PHYSIOLOGY OF MALE REPRODUCTIVE TRACT

The male reproductive tract is primarily concerned with production of mature sperms, their transport and ejaculation into the female copulating organ, that is vagina. The site of formation of sperms is testes. The sperms are then transferred successively to epididymus, vas deferens, ejaculatory duct and penile urethra.

Functions of Testes (Fig. 19.19)

1. Testes produce sperms or spermatozoa.

2. Sertoli cells in the seminiferous tubules of testes are responsible for following functions:
   a. Provide nourishment (are rich in glycogen) and support to the germ cells.
   b. Synthesize androgen binding protein that maintains high testosterone levels in testes.
   c. Tight junctions between sertoli cells provide the blood testes barrier.
3. Testes also produce two hormones:
   a. Testosterone
   b. Estrogen: In very small quantities.

Testosterone

It is a steroid hormone produced by the interstitial or Leydig cells of testes. To some extent it is also produced by the adrenal cortex.

Actions of Testosterone

1. In fetal life: It is responsible for the development of gonads and the male internal and external genitalia.
2. It stimulates spermatogenesis along with FSH.
3. It promotes and maintains growth of internal genitalia at puberty.
4. It is responsible for development of secondary sexual characteristics at puberty.
5. It exerts anabolic effects in the form of :
   a. Increases synthesis and decreases breakdown of proteins.
   b. It causes mild retension of Na^+, K^+ and water.
   c. Facilitates growth spurt at puberty.

Estrogen

Most of the circulating estrogen in males is obtained by the peripheral conversion of testosterone. Little estrogen is produced by Sertoli and Leydig cells.

Regulation of Testicular Function

Testicular function is controlled by pituitary gonadotrophins, FSH and LH.

1. **FSH:** FSH helps in the growth and maintainance of testes and Sertoli cells. It promotes spermatogenesis with testosterone.
2. **LH:** It stimulates growth and secretion of Leydig cells. Inhibin produced by Sertoli cells inhibits FSH secretion while testosterone inhibits LH secretion.

Spermatogenesis

It is an orderly sequential process which gives rise to spermatozoa from primordial germ cells. The entire process is divided into the following three phases:

1. **Spermatocytosis (Figs 19.21, 19.22):** Primodial germ cells divide mitotically in seminiferous tubules of testis during embryonic, fetal and early postnatal life to maintain their population and form sperma-

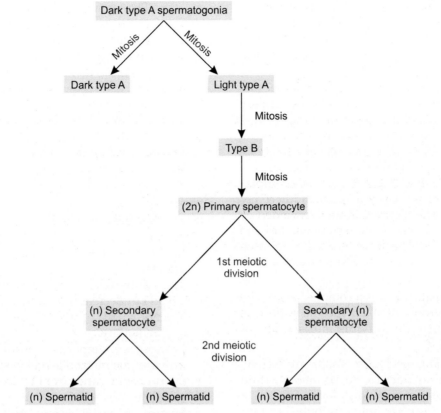

Fig. 19.21: Schematic diagram showing formation of spermatid from spermatogonia

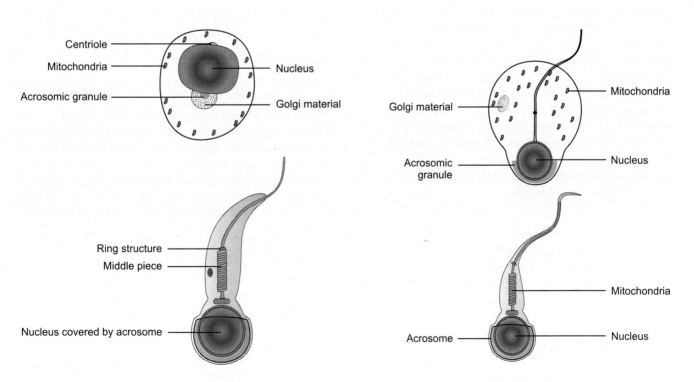

Fig. 19.22: Schematic diagram showing spermiogenesis

togonia. Spermatogonia are precursors of spermatozoa. At puberty their population increases dramatically under the influence of testosterone. The supermatogonia give rise to primary spermatocytes.
2. **Meiosis:** The primary spermatocyte undergoes 1st meiotic division and gives rise to two secondary spermatocytes with (n) number of chromosomes. The secondary spermatocytes then undergo a second meiotic division to give rise to a total of 4 spermatids with (n) number of chromosomes.
3. **Spermiogenesis (Fig. 19.22):** It involves a complex series of changes by which a spermatid becomes spermatozoon. The spermatids are surrounded by Sertoli cells which engulf the residual bodies and degenerating cells. The spermatozoa are released from Sertoli cells. The release is known as spermiation.

Maturation of spermatozoa: It is a complex process by which the spermatozoon attains a specific pattern of independent motility. Epididymis is essential for spermatozoon motility.

Motility of spermatozoa: Spermatozoa are largely transported in genital tract by ciliary action, fluid currents and muscular contractions. Rate of travel of human spermatozoa is 1.5 to 3mm/ minute and they reach the tubal ostia of uterus in 70 minutes following ejaculation.

Capacitation: It is the terminal event in the maturation of spermatozoa by which it attains the capacity to fertilize ova. The exact mechanism of capacitation is still uncertain.

Effect of temperature: The testes are present in scrotal sacs which have a counter current mechanism of heat exchange from arteries to veins. The interior of scrotum is thus kept at 4 to 5°C below the body temperature, i.e., around 32°C. This temperature favours development of sperms. The spermatogenesis is usually hampered in cases of abnormal position of testes, e.g., if it is lying in abdomen or in males exposed to high temperatures due to tight clothes or hot baths.

Functions of Accessory Male Glands

These are exocrine glands and consists of:
1. **Seminal vesicles:** They contribute about 60% of total semen volume. They secrete thick, sticky fluid which is rich in:
   a. Potassium, fructose, phosphorylcholine, citric acid and ascorbic acid which are energy sources to spermatozoa.
   b. Hyaluronidase that lyses mucopolysaccharides and help in penetration of cervical mucus.

c. Prostaglandins: These produce contractions in the uterine musculature leading to movement of sperm inside.
2. **Prostate gland:** It contributes to 20% of total semen volume. It secretes a thin, opalescent fluid which is acidic and gives semen its characteristic fishy order. The fluid contains calcium, ions like Na^+, zinc, citric acid, fibrinolysin and acid phosphatase.
3. **Bulbourethral (Cowper's) glands:** They produce a mucoid alkaline secretion which helps in lubrication during coitus.

Semen

- It is the fluid ejaculated from penile urethra during coitus.
- It contains sperms and secretions from the accessory glands.
- The volume of an ejaculate usually varies form 2.0-3.5 ml but decreases with frequent ejaculations.
- The normal pH of semen is alkaline which favours sperm motility.
- Fructose is an important constituent of semen and provides the metabolic fuel to sperms.
- Sperm count varies from 60 to 120 million/ml of ejaculate.
- Sperms remain viable for upto 24 to 48 hours in the female genital tract.

Functions of Seminal Tract

This is formed by epididymis, vasdeferens, and ejaculating duct. It stores the mature sperms before ejaculation.

PHYSIOLOGY OF PUBERTY

After birth the gonads in both sexes remain in a quiescent stage till they are activated again by the release of gonadotropins from the hypothalamus-pituitary axis. Puberty is the period of final maturation of endocrine and reproductive systems that ultimately makes the individuals capable of reproduction. The age of puberty is around 9 to 14 years in males and 8 to 13 years in females. Onset of puberty is characterised by a growth spurt, seen as increase in height and weight of an individual.

Changes in Males at Puberty

1. Male secondary sexual characters develop:
   a. Hair distribution: Hair appears on pubic and axillary areas. It also appears over lips, chin, chest and anal area.
   b. There is deeping of voice.
   c. There is enlargement of penis. The skin of scrotum thickens with increase in pigmentation there is appearance of rugae on the skin.

d. Body contours become manly with broad shoulder and increase in muscle mass.

2. Changes in internal genitalia.
   a. There is increase in size of testes.
   b. Seminal vesicles, prostate gland and bulbo-urethral glands increase in size and start producing secretions.

Changes in Females at Puberty

The following changes are seen in the external and internal genitalia.

1. Thelarche: There is appearance and development of breasts.
2. Pubic and axillary hair appear (adrenarche).
3. There is enlargement of external genitalia, labia majora and minora.
4. The uterus and ovaries increase in size. There is maturation of uterus and functioning of pituitary – ovarian–endometrial axis with cyclic changes that bring about menarche. Menarche is the appearance of first menstrual cycle.
5. Female body habitus is acquired with wider pelvic area and fat distribution over abdomen and hips.

DEVELOPMENT OF GONADS

The differentiation of primitive gonads to testes in male and ovaries in females is determined by sex chromosomes X and Y. The Y-chromosome bears the testes determining gene sequence called sex determining region of Y-chromosome or SRY.

Development of gametes involves meiosis, meiotic division results in reduction of chromosome number. In females, each ovum contains 23 chromosomes with 22 autosomes and one X-chromosome. In males, each sperm contains 23 chromosomes with 22 + X-chromososme in one and 22 + Y-chromosome in other. When Y-containing sperm fertilizes ovum the resultant zygote has 46 chromosomes with XY giving rise to genetic male sex while fertilization of ovum with X-containing sperm results in 46, XX-genetic female. Hence, genetic sex is determined at fertilization. However, the external appearance,that is phenotypical sex is determined by the production and action of sex hormones.

Embryology of Gonads

The genetic sex as explained is determined at fertilization. Primordial germ cells migrate from Epiblast to urogenital ridge via yolk sac in developing embryo. This leads to formation of primitive gonads which appear at 6 weeks. Presence of Y-chromosome initiates development of testes and appearance of Leydig cells and Sertoli cells in the gonad. Leydig cells produce testosterone that stimulates development of male genitalia while sertoli cells secrete MIS (Mullerian inhibiting substance) that inhibit Mullerian duct

development. In females, presence of XX chromosome results in differentiation of gonad to ovary.

Embryology of Genitalia

By 7th week of intrauterine life two sets of primordial duct systems are seen in fetus, the Wolffian duct and the Mullerian duct. Wolffian duct gives rise to the male genital tract structures (epididymus, vas deferens) while Mullerian duct gives rise to female genital tract structures (uterus, fallopian tubes and vagina). The secretion of MIS by Sertoli cells in males results in regression of Mullerian duct and development of Wolffian ducts. In females Mullerian ducts differentiate while Wolffian duct disappears. Development of external genitalia depends on secretion of testosterone that differentiates it to male pattern while absence of testosterone in females leads to formation of female external genitalia.

MALE GAMETE AND SPERMATOGENESIS

Male Gamete (Fig. 19.23)

It is also known as sperm, spermatozoon, spermatoid, spermium. A single ejaculate contains about 300 million spermatozoa (60 to 120 million/ml). It consists of the following parts:

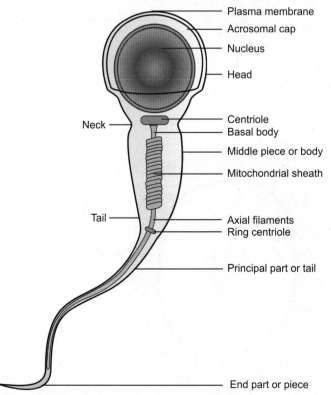

Fig. 19.23: Schematic diagram showing parts of spermatozoon

a. **Head or caput:** It is ovoid or piriform in shape. It has an elongated, flattened nucleus covered by a bilaminar acrosomal cap with minimal cytoplasm. The acrosomal cap contains acid phosphatase, hyalunronidase and protease enzymes.
b. **Neck:** It is a small constriction, 0.3 m, present between the head and middle piece of spermatozoon. It has little cytoplasm and is covered with plasma membrane continuous with head and tail.
c. **Tail or cauda:** It is 45 to 50 m in length. It is divided into three parts, middle piece, tail and end part.

Spermatogenesis

It has been described above.

FEMALE GAMETE AND OOGENESIS

Female Gamete

It is known as ovum.

Oogenesis

After migration of germ cells from yolk sac to the gonadal ridges at 6th week post conception they proliferate and by 8 to 10 weeks about 6,00,000 oogonia are present in the ovary. At 12 weeks of gestation the oogonia start differentiating to primary oocytes. By 5th month of gestation, continuous proliferation leads to presence of 70,00,000 primary oocytes in ovary. At birth, only 1,000,000 remain and by puberty there are about 40,000 primary oocytes in ovary.

The primary oocytes, seen as early as 12 weeks of gestation, undergo DNA replication and enter 1st phase of meiotic division. The primary oocyte gets arrested in the diplotene stage of meiotic prophase from 20 weeks of gestation till further stimulation. Thus a fully grown primary oocyte contains double stranded diploid number of chromosomes at birth. The further stimulus to resume meiosis occurs after puberty in the developing

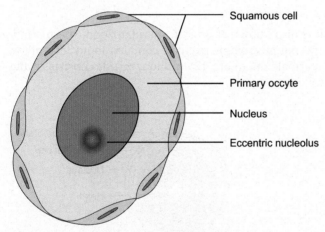

Squamous cell

Primary occyte

Nucleus

Eccentric nucleolus

Fig. 19.24: Primordial follicle

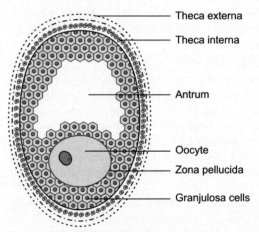

Theca externa

Theca interna

Antrum

Oocyte

Zona pellucida

Granjulosa cells

Fig. 19.25: Secondary or antral follicle

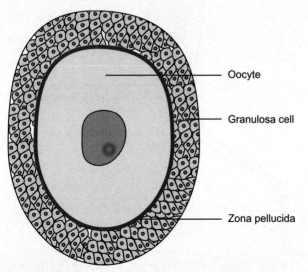

Oocyte

Granulosa cell

Zona pellucida

Fig. 19.26: Primary follicle

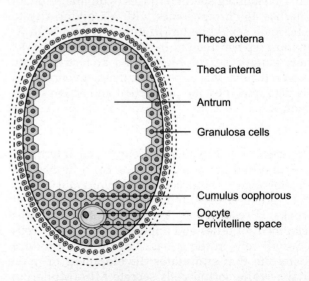

Theca externa

Theca interna

Antrum

Granulosa cells

Cumulus oophorous

Oocyte
Perivitelline space

Fig. 19.27: Tertiary or Graffian follicle

follicle at the time of LH surge. The primary oocyte completes the first meiotic division and gives rise to a large secondary oocyte and a smaller polar body. Secondary oocyte now has double stranded n haploid number of chromosomes It straight away enters the 2nd meiotic division. It gets arrested in the metaphase of 2nd meiotic division prior to ovulation. The secondary oocyte completes its second meiotic division only when it is fertilized and give rise to second polar body and ovum.

Development of Ovarian Follicle (Figs 19.24 to 19.27)

1. **Primordial follicle (Fig. 19.24):** Primary oocyte in fetal stage is enveloped by single layer of squamous cells and this unit is primordial follicle
2. **Primary follicle (Fig. 19.25):** After puberty, as the oocyte grows, the enveloping cells called granulosa cells become cuboidal and also proliferate. It is now called primary follicle
3. **Secondary (antral or vesicular follicle) (Fig. 19.26):** A cohort of about 15 to 20 primary oocytes start growing under influence of gonadotrophic hormones in each menstrual cycle. The granulosa cells proliferate, cavities form in between them which coalesce to form a single fluid filled space called antrum. They are surrounded by spindle shaped cells from ovarian stroma, called theca cells. At this stage the follicle is about 200 microns and oocyte is 80 microns.
d. **Tertiary follicle (also called Graffian follicle) (Fig. 19.27):** Only one follicle out of the many secondary follicles matures to tertiary stage. The antrum enlarges, oocyte is surrounded by clusters of cells known as cumulus oophorous and outer cells are called granulosa cells. Cell immediately surrounding the oocyte are called corona radiata. A perivetalline space is created beneath the zona pellucida after extrusion of 1st polar body. The mature fully grown oocyte breaks away and floats in follicular fluid. It completes its 1st meiotic division.

FERTILIZATION

It is the fusion of mature spermatozoon and mature ovum to form zygote (Fig. 19.28).

Mechanism of Fertilization

It is divided into following stages:
1. **Approximation of spermatozoon and ovum (secondary oocyte):** It includes transport of sperms and secondary oocyte to uterine tube. The commonest site of fertilization is ampullary region of uterine tube.

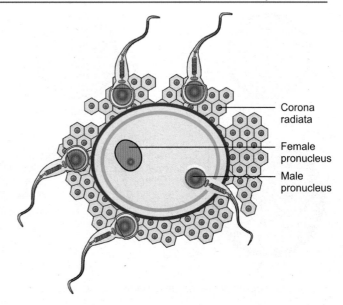

Corona radiata

Female pronucleus

Male pronucleus

Fig. 19.28: Fertilization

2. **Fusion of spermatozoon and ovum:** Secondary oocyte is surrounded by zona pellucida, corona radiata and cummulus oophorus. Spermatozoa undergo capacitation before traversing through above three barriers.
   The sperm now fuses with oocyte microvilli. The second meiotic division of oocyte is completed and polar body is extruted.
3. **Effects of fertilization:**
   a. Completion of second meiotic division of secondary oocyte.
   b. Restoration of diploid number of chromosomes.
   c. Determination of chromosomal sex.
   d. Initiation of cleavage division of zygote.

Preimplantation Development

It includes following stages:
   a. **Cleavage divisions (Fig. 19.29):** A process of repeated mitotic divisions of zygote within the zona pellucida which results in increase in number of cells.
   b. **Morula stage (19.29):** At about 12 to 16 cell stage, the mass is called as morula.
   c. **Blastocyst (19.29):** Cells in morula continue to divide and intercellular spaces appear between the inner cell mass and outer cell mass. Fluid from uterine cavity reaches intercellular spaces and give rise to a fluid filled cavity which is known as blastocele. This stage is known as blastocyst. It occurs at the 32 to 64 cell stage.

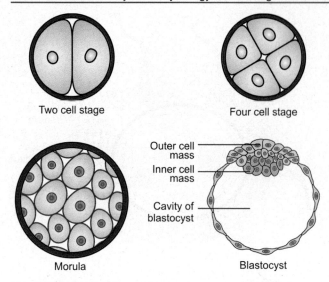

Two cell stage

Four cell stage

Outer cell mass
Inner cell mass
Cavity of blastocyst

Morula

Blastocyst

Fig. 19.29: Pre-implantation development of fertilised ovum

IMPLANTATION

Zygote enters uterine cavity on 3rd to 4th day of fertilization. It is in the stage of morula. At blastocyst stage zona pellucida disappears and implantation occurs on 6th to 7th day. On the 6th post ovulatory day, the blastocyst adheres to the uterine mucosa, zona pellucida undergoes dissolution and the trophoblast cells help in penetration of blastocyst into the endometrium. Blastocyst migrates into endometrium.

PHYSIOLOGY OF PREGNANCY

Pregnancy is associated with a number of anatomical, physiological and endocrinological changes in the body of mother in order to provide nutrition and sustenance to the growing fetus and also to prepare the body for delivery and lactation. Fertilization and implantation have been already discussed. The following text deals with maternal adaptations to pregnancy. The normal duration of pregnancy is 40 weeks or 280 days from the start of last menstrual period. Following changes are seen:

Reproductive Tract

1. Uterus enlarges in size which is brought about by hypertrophy and stretching of muscle cells and increase in connective tissue of myometrium. The weight increases from 70 gm in non pregnant to about 1000 gm at 40 weeks in pregnancy.
2. Cervix shows increase vascularity and edema with hypertrophy and hyperplasia of the glands.
3. Vulva and vagina: There is increase vascularity and congestion of vulva and vagina.
4. Ovaries: Ovulation stops during pregnancy.

Skin

1. There is increase pigmentation specially seen over cheeks (chloasma) and midline of abdomen (linea nigra).
2. With increasing size of fetus, the skin of abdomen, breast and thighs shows reddish-brownish streaks known as stria gravidarum (stretch marks).

Breast

1. The breast increase in size due to growth of glandular and connective tissue.
2. They start secreting watery, milky secretion called colostrum, in some as early as 20 weeks.
3. Nipples and areola show increase pigmentation.

Metabolic Changes

1. Weight gain: Average weight gain in pregnancy is 10 to 12 kgs.
2. Water metabolism: There is water retention in pregnancy leading to increase in total body water.
3. Protein metabolism: There is positive nitrogen balance with increase protein synthesis.
4. Carbohydrate metabolism: There is mild fasting hypoglycemia (due to glucose being taken up by fetus at night. After meals there is hyperglycemia and hyperinsulinemia. As pregnancy advances, there is insulin resistance brought about by increasing levels of hormones like progesterone, estrogen, cortisol, human placental lactogen. This allows for increase circulating glucose levels that can be transported to fetus. Hence, pregnancy is mildly diabetogenic.
5. Fat metabolism: There is an increase in circulating cholesterol, phospholipids and lipoprotein levels.
6. Electrolyte and mineral metabolism :
   a. There is increase filtration and reabsorption of Na^+ and K^+ with retention of these ions.
   b. Though uptake of calcium, magnesium and iron is increased, plasma levels show decline due to total volume expansion.

Hematological Changes

1. Blood volume: Increases during pregnancy, starts as early as 8 weeks and peaks at 32 weeks. About 40% increase is seen at term (40 weeks). This is achieved by increase in both plasma volume and red cell mass.
2. Iron requirements are increased in pregnancy total requirement being 900-1000mg.
3. Though total plasma protein and hemoglobin content of blood increases there is a fall in their concentration due to expansion of blood volume.
4. Coagulation factors, all clotting factors (except factors XI, XIII) are increased in pregnancy.

Cardiovascular Changes
1. Heart rate is increased by 10 beats per minutes.
2. Cardiac output increases by 25 to 30%.
3. Apex beat gets shifted laterally to left due to pushing up by diaphragm.
4. Blood pressure: There is a net fall in both systolic and diastolic blood pressures by 10 mm Hg.

Respiratory Functions
1. There is no change in respiratory rate or vital capacity in pregnancy.
2. There is an increase in minute ventilatory volume leading to increase O_2 uptake brought about by increase tidal volume.
3. O_2 carriage is increased due to increased red cell mass.

Urinary System
1. Renal plasma flow and GFR increases during pregnancy.
2. Mild hydroureter, dilatation of ureters may be seen in USG during pregnancy normally.
3. There is increase urinary frequency and occasionally incontinence during pregnancy.
4. Renal threshold for glucose is reduced, leading to glycosuria.

Gastrointestinal Functions
1. Gastroesophageal reflux due to loss of lower esophageal sphincter tone is common in pregnancy.
2. Haemmorrhoids due to increase venous pressure are common in pregnancy.
3. There is cholestasis, that is stasis of bile in bile canaliculi of liver resulting in slight elevation of liver enzymes and bile salts in blood circulation.

Endocrine Functions
1. There is slight increase in size of major endocrine glands, e.g., thyroid, pituitary during pregnancy with increase in their functions.
2. Hormones produced by placenta are:
   a. Human chorionic gonadotrophin (HCG): It helps to maintain corpus luteum of pregnancy which secretes progesterone to sustain pregnancy.
   b. Human chorionic somatomammotrophin on human placental lactogen.
   c. Human chorionic thyrotrophin.
   d. Estrogen.
   e. Progesterone.

PHYSIOLOGY OF PARTURITION

Parturition means the process of birth of baby.
- Duration of normal pregnancy is 280 days or 40 weeks.
- The uterus is quiescent almost till end of pregnancy that is there are not myometrial contractions and cervix is firm and closed.

- In the last 6 to 8 weeks of pregnancy there are changes in myometrium and cervix of uterus. There is a gradual increase in myometrial contractions which are of short duration and are usually painless. The cervix becomes soft and there is thinning and relaxation of its tissues.
- The exact physiological process that initiates changes of parturition resulting in onset of labour is not very clear.
- Active labour is defined as progressively increasing uterine contractions (labour pains) that result in dilatation of cervix and descent and expulsion of the fetus to exterior.
- The various probable contributes to initiation of labour are:
   a. Gradual increase in stretching of uterine muscle fibers which increases the intercellular gap junctions.
   b. Increase oxytocin receptors in myometrium. The high levels of estrogens in pregnancy result in increase synthesis and expression of oxytocin receptors in the myometrium. This makes the musculature increasingly sensitive to the circulating oxytocin levels. Oxytocin is a uterotonic and leads to increase myometrial contractions. Oxytocin stimulates production of myometrial contractile proteins. It also stimulates production of prostaglandins from decidua.
   c. Prostaglandins help to increase uterine contractions and soften the cervix allowing easy dilatation.
   d. Role of fetal hypothalamic-pituitary-adrenal axis and placental CRH (corticotrophin hormone). CRH is produced by placenta. It acts on fetal adrenals that stimulates ACTH secretion by fetal pituitary resulting increase production of cortisol by fetal adrenals at term. Cortisol helps in maturation of lungs of the fetus. Another hormone DHEAS (dihydroepiandrostenedione) is also produced in significant amounts by fetal adrenals at term. This increases maternal estriol levels further.
   e. Positive feed back mechanism: Uterine contraction result in stretching of cervix which further enhances uterine activity. This could be via stimulation of pelvic nerves and production of prostaglandins which further increase secretion of oxytocin.

Labour pains: These are painful uterine contractions that help in delivering of baby. Normally, labour pains begin at term which is defined as 37 to 40 weeks.

Preterm labour is when labour pains start before 37 weeks of pregnancy.

PHYSIOLOGY OF LACTATION

After delivery the breasts begin to secrete milk for nutrition of baby. The establishment of lactation or breast feeding involves the following changes:

1. Mammogenesis: This is the increase in the glandular tissue of breast during pregnancy preparing it for milk production.
2. Lactogenesis: It is the synthesis of milk.
3. Galactokinesis: It is the expulsion of milk from breast which is established by the sucking of new born.
4. Galactopoesis: It is the maintenance of synthesis and secretion of milk.

Lactation is controlled by the various hormones like progesterone, estrogen, placental lactogen, prolactin, cortisol and insulin.

PHYSIOLOGY OF CONTRACEPTION

Contraception is prevention of occurrence of pregnancy. The various contraceptive methods available are:

1. **Natural family planning method:** This method is useful when the woman has regular menstrual cycles. Ovulation usually occurs 14 days prior to menstruation and the ova is viable only for 24 to 48 hours. The couple should avoid intercourse for 1 week around the day of ovulation. Ovulation and menstrual cycle may not follow the same pattern every month and hence this method has high failure rates.
2. **Barrier methods:** These are mechanical or chemical substances that are used to prevent contact of sperm and ova.
   a. **Methods used by male:**
   - **Condoms:** They are made up of latex and are applied over erected penis before intercourse.
   b. **Methods used by female:**
   - **Diaphragms or cervical caps:** They are made up of rubber and are cup like in shape to fit into the vagina or over cervix. They have to be inserted by female before coitus.
   - **Spermicides:** These are chemical compounds mostly made up of nonoxynol-9 available as jellys, creams or vaginal tablets (today) that are applied locally or placed high in vagina before coitus. Reapplication is required if the act is repeated.

   Advantages: They are easy to use and have no systemic side effects. Condoms also help to prevent spread of HIV and other sexually transmitted diseases.

   Disadvantages: They have to be used with every coital act and hence compliance may be poor leading to relatively high failure rates.

They may also cause local allergies or infections.

3. **Hormonal contraception:** These are methods used by females. Male pills are still in experimental phases. The various mode of hormonal contraception are:
   a. **Oral contraceptive pills:** These are pills containing a combination of estrogen and progesterone.
   b. **Injectables:** These are depot preparations of medroxy progesterone acetate 150 mg. It is given as intramuscular injection at 3 monthly interval.
   c. **Implants:** These are elastic implants placed subdermally containing synthetic progesterone, levonorgestrol and last for 5 years.

Mode of action: The synthetic hormone preparations help contraception by:
- Inhibiting ovulation
- Thickening cervical mucus: Making it hostile to sperm and preventing its entry into uterine cavity.
- Rendering the endometrium unfavorable for implantation.

Advantages: They are highly effective.

Disadvantages: They may lead to side effects like migraine, nausea and vomiting, irregular bleeding, rarely jaundice and increase clotting in veins (thrombosis).

4. **Intrauterine contraceptive devices (IUD) (Fig. 19.30):** Most common example is copper-T (CuT). It is a T-shaped device made up of chemically inert polyethylene wrapped with thin copper wire. The device is inserted into uterine cavity just after bleeding of normal menses has stopped.

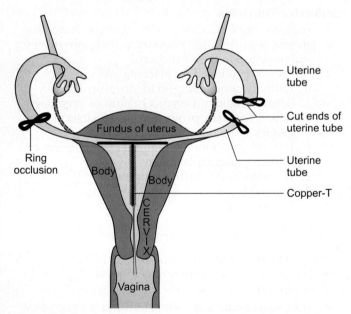

Fig. 19.30: Copper-T in uterine cavity, tubectomy and ring occlusion

Mode of action: The copper initiates an intense inflammatory response in the endometrium which helps to destroy the sperms or fertilized ova in uterine cavity preventing pregnancy.

Advantages: CuT is highly effective method and provides long term contraception.

Disadvantages: It can cause irregular and heavy bleeding, pain during periods, expulsion and infection.

5. **Sterilization:** This is a surgical method that is a permanent, method of contraception, usually irreversible.

   a. **In females,** methods are:
      • **Tubectomy (Fig. 19.31):** The fallopian tubes a cut, about 1cm length removed and the two ends are ligated.
      • **Tubal occlusion (19.31):** This is occlusion by a fallopian ring place in the tube via laparoscopy.

   b. **In males,** methods are:
      • **Vasectomy:** It involves cutting and ligating ends of vas deference
      • **Nonscalpel vasectomy:** It involves occlusion of vas without cutting it.

CLINICAL AND APPLIED ASPECT

VULVA AND VAGINA

• **Episiotomy (Fig. 19.31)** It is a planned surgical incision on the posterior vaginal wall and perineum.

  Structures cut: (From without inward)
  1. Skin
  2. Subcutaneous fat
  3. Superficial perineal muscles
  4. Bulbospongiosus muscle
  5. Deep perineal muscles, in deep episiotomy
  6. Fibres of levator ani, in deep episiotomy
  7. Transverse perineal branches of pudendal vessels and nerves.
  8. Vaginal mucosa

  Aim of episiotomy: To enlarge the introitus in order to prevent stretching and rupture of perineal muscles and vagina during delivery.

  Indications
  1. Tight introitus, e.g., in primigravida.
  2. Difficult delivery, e.g., forceps application, breech delivery.

• **Bartholin cyst:** It is the enlargement of Bartholin's gland due to retention of its secretions. This occurs after repeated infections which leads to blockage of the duct of the gland. It is treated by excision.

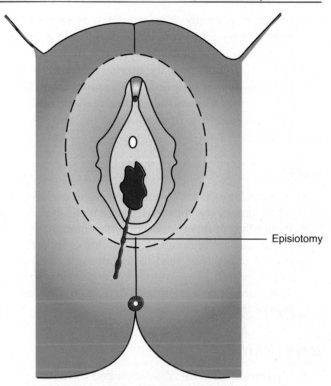

Fig. 19.31: Episiotomy

• **pH of vagina:** It varies with age
  — In reproductive age group, it is 4.5 to 5.
  — In pre pubertal and post menopausal women it is as high as 5 to 6.

  Normal vaginal flora consists of Doderlin's bacillus which utilise glycogen in vaginal epithelium to produce lactic acid. Thus, the pH of vagina is normally acidic which helps to prevent invasion by exogenous microorganisms.

UTERUS AND FALLOPIAN TUBES

• Round ligaments and uterosacral ligaments are responsible for anteflexion and anteversion of uterus.

• **Prolapse of uterus:** It is the clinical condition characterised by descent of uterus and cevix with or without the vaginal walls towards the vulva and the exterior. The most common cause of prolapse is weakness of Mackenrodt's and utero-sacral ligaments due to repeated deliveries or due to old age.

• **Endometriosis:** It is the presence of endometrial tissue outside the endometrial lining of uterus. The most common site of endometriosis is pelvic peritoneum and ovaries. This condition is associated with pelvic pain, painful menses and heavy bleeding during periods.

- Infection of uterine tube is known as **salpingitis.** Pain is referred to umbilicus due to same spinal segment involvement. Sympathetic preganglionic fibres T_{10} to L_2 supply the uterine tube and skin of the umbilicus is supplied by T_{10} spinal segment.
- Ligation of fallopian tubes during sterilization is done at junction of medial 1/3rd and lateral 2/3rd.

OVARY

- At birth 200,000 follicles are present in each ovary while at puberty, they to decrease to 40,000.
- **Anovulation:** It is the absence of ovulation.
- Ovary lies in the floor of ovarian fossa. Inflammation of ovary may lead to irritation of obturator nerve which is present in the ovarian fossa. Therefore, patient complains of pain on the medial side of the thigh and knee joint.

MALE GENITALIA

- **Varicocele:** It is the dilatation and tortuousity of pampiniform plexus of veins of testis. It is more common on the left side because the left testicular vein drains into the left renal vein at a right angle. Also, loaded sigmoid colon may compresses the left testicular vein.
- **Descent of testes:** Testes develop in the lumbar region, they lie in the iliac fossa at 4th month of intrauterine life. At 7 month they reach the deep inguinal ring. In the 8th month of intrauterine life testes traverse inguinal canal and superficial inguinal ring and reach scrotum at birth or just after birth. Factors responsible for descent of testis are
  a. Contractions from below, produced by gubernaculum of testis which is a musculo-fibrous cord, attached inferiorly to scrotum and superiorly to testis and adjacent peritoneum.
  b. Differential growth of body wall.
  c. Intra-abdominal pressure.
  d. Male sex-hormones.
  e. Maternal gonadotrophins.
  f. Increased intra-abdominal temperature.
  g. Normally developed testis.
- **Cryptorchidism:** It is the arrest or incomplete decent of testis.
- Temperature of each testis is 2 to 3°C lower than the body temperature. This is important to facilitate spermatogenesis. Following factors are responsible for temperature regulation.

a. Pampiniform plexus of veins helps in temperature regulation by counter current principle. This is the most important factor.
b. Scrotal skin contains numerous sweat glands
c. Superficial fascia of scrotum is replaced by dartos muscle. Contraction of dartos muscle helps in regulation of temperature in cold weather.
d. Absence of deep fascia in scrotum.
- **Azospermia:** It is absence of sperms in the semen.
- Prostate undergoes a benign hypertrophy of its tissue in old age which can compress the prostatic urethra. It leads to urinary symptoms mainly, difficulty in urination, frequency of urination, recurrent infections and occasionally acute retention of urine. It is treated by surgically enucleating the gland.
- Carcinoma prostate spread to vertebral column due to retrograde venous drainage of prostate into internal vertebral venous plexus through para vertebral vein of Batson.

PHYSIOLOGY OF REPRODUCTION

- Chromosomal anomalies are described on page no. 611.
- **Testicular feminization:** It is a clinical condition in which the genetic sex is male (46 XY) but the external genitalia are similar to females. This occurs due to an enzyme deficiency that prevents the action of testosterone on the external genitalia.
- **Precocious puberty:** It is the appearance of mature secondary sexual characteristics before the age of 8 years. It can occur due to presence of various tumors and infections of hypothalamus resulting in premature activation of hormonal changes. It can also be caused by presence of gonadal or adrenal tumors secreting excess hormones.
- **Delayed puberty:** It is defined in females, as lack of development of secondary sexual characters by the age of 16 years or absence of menstruation by 18 years of age if external characters have developed. In male it is defined as lack of testicular development by 20 years of age.
- **Infertility or subfertility:** It is the inability to consive a child after twelve months of unprotected coitus. It can occur due to male factor deficiency, e.g., low sperm count or azoospermia or due to female factor deficiency, e.g., anovulation, blocked uterine tubes.

Chapter 20

Skin

INTRODUCTION

Skin is also known as integument or cutis. It is the outer covering of the body. It also covers the external auditory meatus and lateral aspect of tympanic membrane. It continues with the mucus membranes of the oral, nasal and urogenital orifices.

Skin acts as an interface between the body and environment. Epidermis of skin has a property of self repair and renewing.

Types of Skin

Skin is classified as thin or hairy skin and thick or hairless skin based on its structural and functional properties.

1. **Thin or hairy skin:** It covers the greater part of the body.
2. **Thick or hairless skin:** It forms the surface of palms of hands, soles of feet and flexor surfaces of digits.

This type of skin is necessary for manipulation of frictional surface and aids in locomotion.

STRUCTURE OF SKIN (FIG. 20.1)

Skin consists of two layers namely,
1. Epidermis: It is the superficial avascular layer of skin.
2. Dermis: It is the deep layer of skin.

Epidermis

Epidermis is made up of keratinized stratified squamous epithelium. The principal cells of this epithelium are called keratinocytes. It also has cells known as non keratinocytes which are usually derived from sites outside the skin and have migrated into it. They are:
1. Melanocytes.

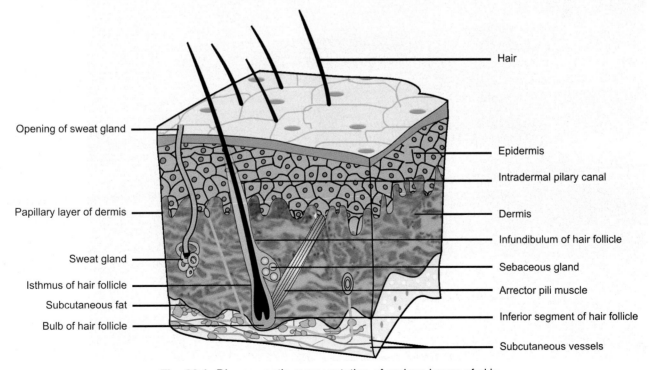

Opening of sweat gland

Papillary layer of dermis

Sweat gland

Isthmus of hair follicle

Subcutaneous fat

Bulb of hair follicle

Hair

Epidermis

Intradermal pilary canal

Dermis

Infundibulum of hair follicle

Sebaceous gland

Arrector pili muscle

Inferior segment of hair follicle

Subcutaneous vessels

Fig. 20.1: Diagrammatic representation of various layers of skin

2. Langherhans cells, derived from bone marrow.
3. Lymphocytes, derived from circulation.
4. Merkel cells or clear cells, are the sensory receptors.

Epidermis is made up of cells arranged into five strata (layers). From deep to superficial ,these layers are: **(Fig. 20.2)**

1. **Stratum basale:** It consists of a single layer of columnar to cuboidal shaped cells lying on a basement membrane. These cells are continuously dividing and provide for the cell population that differentiates to form the successive layers of epidermis. This layer also contains Langerhans cells, melanocytes, merkel cells and stem cells.

2. **Stratum spinosum (prickle cell layer):** It contains more mature keratinocytes. This layer is made up of several layers of cells that contain prominent bundles of keratin filaments in their cytoplasm. The cells are closely packed and connected to each other with the help of desmosomes. On routine histological staining these cells appear shrunk and give rise to a characteristic spinous appearance. Other cells present in this layer are Langerhans cells and lymphocytes.

3. **Stratum granulosum:** This layer consists of 3 to 4 layers of cells. The keratinocytes of this layer show disintegration of their nuclei and degeneration of mitochondria and ribosomes. Keratin filaments are compact and are associated with densely staining keratohyalin granules.

4. **Stratum lucidum:** It is present only in thick skin, e.g, over palms and soles. This layer often contains nuclear debris. It is a poorly understood stage in keratinocyte differentiation. On staining it appears as an ill defined zone below the densely staining cornified layer.

5. **Stratum corneum:** It is the most superficial layer and consists of closely packed layers of flattened, polyhedral corneocytes known as squames. The cells do not contain nucleus or any membranous organelles. They contain dense arrays of kerato-hyalin filaments embedded in the cytoplasm. This layer can vary from few cell thickness to more than 50 cell thick layer in the thin and in thick skins respectively.

Stratum basal, spinosum and granulosum are together known as stratum malpighii. The basal cells committed to differentiation pass successively through the various layers and finally form the cornified layer. The superficial cells are continuously shed and replaced with the full cycle taking about 28 days.

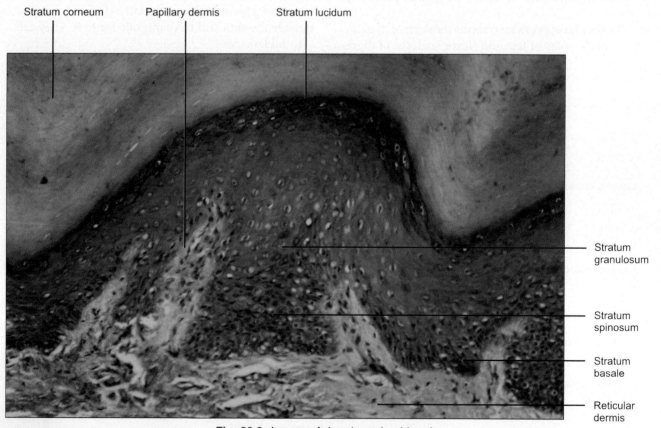

Stratum corneum   Papillary dermis   Stratum lucidum

Stratum granulosum

Stratum spinosum

Stratum basale

Reticular dermis

Fig. 20.2: Layers of dermis and epidermis

Melanocytes: These cells are derived from the neural crest and produce the pigment melanin. Melanocytes are present in the following sites:

1. Epidermis
2. Appendages of skin
3. Oral epithelium
4. Choroid of eyeball
5. Middle and inner ear lining
6. Arachnoid and pia maters

Melanin is produced by:

1. Melanocytes
2. Pigment layer of retina
3. Neuromelanin is produced by the substantia nigra of brain stem and basal ganglia

Dermis

Dermis lies deep to the epidermis (Figs 20.1 and 20.2). It is made up of irregular, dense connective tissue composed of collagen fibers, elastic fibers and ground substance. Ground substance consists of glycosaminoglycans, glycoprotein and water and has blood vessels, lymphatics, nerves and the skin appendages. Dermis gives passage to the neurovascular bundle. It is made up of the following two layers:

a. **Papillary layer:** It is the superficial layer, lying immediately deep to epidermis. In its superficial part it forms numerous papillae which interdigitate with recesses of the epidermis. This inter-digitation is known as the dermo-epidermal junction. It provides the nutritional support to the overlying epidermis which is avascular and provides passage for the free nerve endings.

b. **Reticular layer:** It lies deep to the papillary layer. The bundles of collagen fibres in this layer are thicker than those in the papillary layer and form a lattice. The deep reticular plexuses of nerves and blood vessels are present in this layer.

APPENDAGES OF SKIN

Appendages of skin consist of pilosebaceous unit, nails and sweat glands (Figs 20.1 and 20.3).

Pilosebaceous Unit

It consists of hair and its follicle with the associated sebaceous gland, arrector pili muscle and sometimes apocrine glands.

Hairs

They are keratinized filamentous structures. Hairs are present all over the body except palms, soles, flexor surfaces of digits, umbilicus, nipples, glans penis, clitoris, labia minora, inner aspect of labia majora and prepuce. Hairs vary in length from 1 mm to 1 meter. Hairs can be curly or straight.

Hair Follicle

It is an invagination of the epidermis into the dermis which contains hair. Hair follicles provide for the outer root sheath of hair. Structure of hair follicle varies with the stage of hair growth.

Phases of hair growth: It is cyclical and consists of three phases:

  i. **Anagen phase:** In this phase, hair is actively growing and follicle is at its maximum development.
 ii. **Catagen phase:** Hair growth ceases and follicle shrinks.
iii. **Telogen phase:** This is the resting stage during which inferior segment of the follicle is absent.

Structure of anagen follicle: Anagen follicle has the following regions (Fig. 20.1):

a. **Inferior segment:** It is the deepest part of the follicular epithelium that forms the hair bulb. It receives attachment of the arrector pili muscle.

b. **Isthmus:** It is the part of follicle that extends from the attachment of arrector pili muslce to the opening of the sebaceous duct. The shaft of hair is in close apposition to the follicular epithelium upto the isthmus. Above isthmus the hair shaft is surrounded by a pilary canal.

c. **Infundibulum:** Region above the opening of sebaceous duct is known as infundibulum. This region is also known as **dermal pilary canal.**

d. **Intra-epidermal pilary canal:** It is the upper most part which lies in the epidermis.

Hair Bulb

It is the lowermost expanded part of the hair follicle. The lower most end of follicular epithelium of the bulb encloses another structure known as the dermal papilla. Dermal papilla is an invagination of a layer of mesenchymal cells of dermis with a central core of capillaries. These cells are responsible for the growth of hair follicle growth and generate the hair shaft and its inner root sheath The hair bulb can be divided into two parts:

a. **Lower germinal matrix:** Consists of actively dividing pleuripotent keratinocytes.

b. **Upper bulb:** Consists of cells derived from the matrix. These cells migrate up and differentiate to form the medulla, cortex, cuticle and the inner root sheath of hair.

Structure of Hair

Hair is made up of hair shaft with the inner and outer root sheaths.

1. **Hair shaft:** Mature hair shaft is made up of three concentric zones. From within outwards these are, medulla, cortex and cuticle. In thinner hairs the medulla is usually absent. Cuticle and cortex are

made up of keratinized cells whereas medulla consists of discontinuous columns of partially disintegrated cells containing vacuoles.

2. **Inner root sheath:** It consists of three layers namely cuticle of inner root sheath, Huxley's layer and Henle's layer. It is made up of layers of cells with irregular demarcation. Above the level of isthmus the inner root sheath is fragmented.

3. **Outer root sheath:** It consists of undifferentiated cells containing glycogen. It is a single or double layer of cells at level of hair bulb and higher up it becomes multilayered showing stratification just like the epidermis with which it is continuous.

Sebaceous Glands

These are saccular structures present in the dermis, related to the hair follicle and arrector pili muscles. The gland is made up of clusters of acini(alveoli) which are enclosed in a basal lamina and a thin dermal capsule having a rich capillary network. Each acinus is made up of small flat to polygonal cells. The secretions of the acini are conduted by a thin duct which opens at the infundibulum of the hair follicle. In areas devoid of hair, the ducts of sebaceous glands directly open onto the surface of skin. These areas are lips, corner of mouth, buccal mucosa, nipples, areola of female breast, glans penis, glans clitoridis and labia minora.

These glands secrete sebum which forms the major part of skin surface lipid. The sebum provides a protective covering over the epidermis and prevents water loss from skin. It may also be inhibitory to invasion by fungal and ectoparasites present on surface of skin. Secretion of sebum is under the control of androgens produced by testes and adrenals.

Meibomian glands of eyelids are similar type of sebaceous glands.
Sebaceous glands are absent in palms, soles and flexor aspect of the digits.

Apocrine Glands

These are large glands of dermis and hypodermis. They develop as outgrowths of hair follicle and discharge the secretion into the hair canal. They are a subset of the sweat glands. Apocrine glands are present in axilla, perianal region, periumbilical region, prepuce and scrotum(in male), mons pubis and labia minora (in female).

The gland consists of an secretory part, made up of cuboidal cells, which are arranged as coiled structures and a conducting part, which consists of a thin straight duct that opens into the hair follicle above the opening of sebaceous gland duct. The secretions of apocrine glands are mainly produced after puberty and are controlled by local androgen and adrenaline levels. These secretions are responsible for the peculiar body odour.

Specialized subtypes of these glands are:
— Ceruminous glands of external auditory meatus
— Glands of Moll of eyelids.

Arrector Pili Muscle

It is made up of smooth muscle cells forming small fasciculi. It is diagonally placed between the papillary layer of dermis and dermal sheath of hair follicle. Arrector pili is attached to the bulge region of hair follicle and directed obliquely and superficially towards the side to which the hair sloped. Sebaceous gland lies in the angle between the muscle and hair follicle. Contraction of muscle leads to erection of hair and elevation of the surface where the superficial attachment of muscle is present. This muscle may be involved in the expression of secretions from sebaceous glands. The muscle is absent in areas of face, axilla, pubis, eyelashes, eyebrows, nostrils and external auditory meatus.

Nails (Figs 20.3 and 20.4)

Nails are homologous to the stratum corneum of general epidermis. They consist of anucleated keratin filled squames. Nails have following five components:

1. **Nail plate:** It is a rectangular shaped plate bounded by nail folds. It is composed of matrix protein with a high content of sulphur with lipids and mineral elements. Calcium is one of the main minerals in the plate.
   Nail plate is convex longitudinally and transversely. Its thickness increases from the proximal part to distal. The colour of nail plate is generally

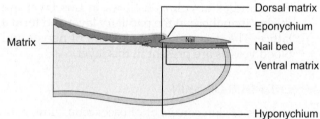

Fig. 20.3: Nail and its related structures

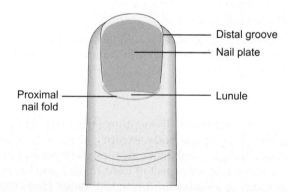

Fig. 20.4: Nail and its related structures

translucent pink. A cresentic white area is seen emerging from under the proximal nail fold. This is known as lunule.

2. **Nail folds:** The lateral margin on each side of the nail plate is bounded by a lateral fold of skin called lateral nail folds. The proximal margin is covered by the proximal nail fold which is formed by two epidermal layers with a core of dermis in between. Nail plate extends under this proximal nail fold. The superficial layer of epidermis forms the eponychium and deep layer merges with matrix of the nail.

3. **Matrix:** Matrix is seen a wedge of cells in which the deeper part of nail plate is embedded. Matrix lying dorsal to nail plate is known as dorsal matrix. The ventral epitheium of proximal nail fold is continuous with the dorsal matrix. Ventral matrix is continuous with the nail bed.

   The ventral and dorsal matrix give rise to the nail plate.

4. **Nail bed:** It extends from lunule to hyponychium underneath the nail plate. Nail bed cells differentiate and contribute to the nail plate. Nail bed consists of two to three layers of nucleated cells, which lack keratohyalin granules. Beneath the epithelium of nail bed is dermis, which is anchored to the periosteum of phalanyx. The dermis is richly vascularized and numerous sensory nerve endings are present in it.

5. **Hyponychium:** It is an area of epidermis, which extends from the nail bed to the distal groove. It underlies the edges of nail plate. It provides defence against microorganisms.

Sweat Glands

- They are a type of unbranched tuboalveolar glands and are situated deep in dermis or hypodermis. The secretory part is arranged in a convoluted or coiled form. It is drained by a thin, straight or slightly helical duct which passes through the dermis and epidermis and opens via a rounded aperture on the surface of skin.

- Sweat glands are numerous all over the body except over lip margins, nail bed, nipples, glans penis or clitorodis, labia minora ,and over the tympanic membrane.

- These glands secrete a clear, odourless hypotonic fluid known as sweat which contains Na^+, Cl^-, with small amounts of K^+, HCO_3^-, urea, lactate, amino acids, immunoglobulins etc. Sweat has a role in thermoregulation of body. Secretion of sweat is increased by action of aldosterone and sympathetic stmulation. The post ganglionic sympathetic secretomotor fibers to sweat glands are cholinergic that is they secrete acetycholine.

- In palms and soles sweat increases the sensitivity of skin and helps in proper grip.

Arterial Supply of Skin

Blood flow to skin is 10 times its nutritional requirements. Vascular supply of skin is derived from cutaneous branches of vascular trunks, from perforating branches of intramuscular vasculature and vessels of deep fascia of the corresponding area. The vessels come together and form three arteriolar plexuses within the dermis. From deep to superficial aspect they are, **deep dermal plexus, reticular dermal plexus and subpapillary plexus.** They supply the dermis, pilosebaceous unit and sweat glands.

Lymphatic Supply of Skin

It is drawn from the superficial and deep lymphatic plexuses of the corresponding area.

Nerve Supply of Skin

Skin is supplied by cutaneous branches of nerves of corresponding dermatomes. On reaching the dermis, these divide and branch extensively to form a deep reticular plexus and a superficial papillary plexus. Reticular plexus supplies sweat glands, hair follicles and large arterioles. Nerve fibres from papillary plexus pass horizontally and vertically and terminate either in relation to encapsulated receptors or as free nerve terminals reaching the basal lamina of epidermis.

Functions of the Skin

1. It protects the underlying structures from mechanical, chemical, osmotic, thermal and photopic injury, within limits.
2. It acts as an effective barrier against invasion of microbial organisms.
3. It is a major sense organ. It is richly supplied by sensory receptors and nerve endings for pain, touch, temperature, pressure and pleasurable stimuli.
4. It helps in regulation of body temperature by vascular mechanism and sweating.
5. It acts as an endocrine organ as it helps in the formation of vitamin D and also secretes certain cytokines and growth factors.
6. It helps in mounting a primary immune response.
7. It helps in excretion of substances like ions of Na^+, Cl^-, H^+, water and even urea in sweat.
8. It is not an actual absorptive surface but it can absorb certain drugs when administered as transdermal patches, e.g., hormonal patches, diclofenac patches.
9. It is involved in socio-sexual communication especially, facial skin helps in emotional signals.

10. Melanin present in skin helps protect against ultra-violet rays and also damage by free radicals.
11. The texture, elasticity and structure of skin is an important indicator of status of health of an individual. Change in color or appearance of the skin, loss of sensations can help in identifying certain clinical conditions. Skin biopsy helps in clinching the clinical diagnosis in certain disease conditions.
12. Skin is important in preventing water loss from body.

CLINICAL AND APPLIED ASPECT

- Dermatome is the part of skin supplied by a nerve from single spinal segment. Knowledge of the dermatomal supply of various parts provides clues in clinical conditions to determine origin of referred pain
- Following surfaces in the body do not bear any hair:
  — Palms, soles and dorsal surfaces of distal phalanges.
  — Umbilicus
  — Glans penis, inner surface of the prepuce, inner surfaces of the labia majora and labia minora
  — Surfaces of the eye-lids
  — Exposed margins of the lips
- Excessive shedding of superficial layers of epidermis is seen in **seborrhic dermatitis.** It usually occurs in areas bearing hair and is also known as dandruff. It is usually caused by fungal infection of superior layer of skin.
- **Stria:** The excess strain on elastic fibers due to over stretching of dermis leads to their rupture and formation of whitish lines on skin. These are known as stria. This is seen in obesity and pregnancy (on abdomen and breasts mainly).
- **Wrinkles:** These are fine folds of skin that appear during aging due to gradual loss of collagen fibers in the matrix of dermis. These are mostly seen over the areas of thin skin, e.g., around eyes and dorsum of hand.
- **Comedone/Acne:** This occurs due to blockage of the ducts of sebaceous of glands due to hyperkeratinization (usually due to hormonal or external environment changes). There is retention of sebum which results in formation of small papules known as comedone. Infection of these leads to acne.
- **Wound healing:** Destruction of an area of skin due to injury brings about complex and orderly processes that result in repair and regeneration of the area. This known as healing. The various stages of healing are described as:
  — **Stage of inflammation:** The wound is filled with blood clot. Within 24 hours of injury, neutrophils appear in the margins of wound that are responsible for phagcytosis of clot and debris in the wound. There is thickening of cut edges of epidermis due to increase mitotic activity. By day three neutrophils are replaced by macrophages which further the process of phagocytosis. Fibroblasts appear in the margins and start laying down collagen fibers.
  — **Stage of proliferation:** Granulation tissue fills up the wound. It is a specialized tissue consisting of proliferating new small blood vessels and proliferating fibroblasts. It provides the area with new vascular supply. The epidermal cells proliferate and regain normal thickness and differentiation and they cover the wound. The collagen fibers form bridges across the wound, under the epithelium.
  — **Stage of maturation:** There is continued accumulation of collagen and proliferation of fibroblasts during 2nd neck and it gradually replaces the granulation tissue. The inflammation settles down by end of one month. The bridging of wound is complete with scar formation and gets covered by the intact epidermis. The dermal appendages that are destroyed are lost permanently.

Factors affecting wound healing are:
Local factors:
— Presence of infection or foreign bodies delays healing.
— Type of wound: Clean incision heals by primary intention while large wound with separated margin heal by secondary intention. The basic process is same but the magnitude of inflammation and repair is more in healing by secondary intention.
— Local blood supply: Wound in areas with good vascular supply like face heal faster that areas with poor blood supply like foot.

Systemic factors:
— Nutritional status of individual.
— Metabolic status, e.g., Diabetes mellitus results in delayed healing.
— Immunity of individual: Anaemias and chronic debilitating diseases result in poor immunological response and poor healing.
— Circulatory status: Inadequate blood supply due to narrowing of blood vessels (atherosclerosis) as in old age leads to poor healing.
- **Fingerprinting:** It is the science of studying papillary ridges. PR are surface projections of epidermis that occur secondary to underlying dermal papillae and are seen in areas of palms, soles and flexion surfaces of digits. Each individual has a specific pattern of this papillary ridges which are arranged in arches, loops and whorls. These are not affected by aging and are unique to an individual. Study of patterns of papillary ridges in the form of their prints is dermatoglyphics. This is of considerable use in forensic medicine.

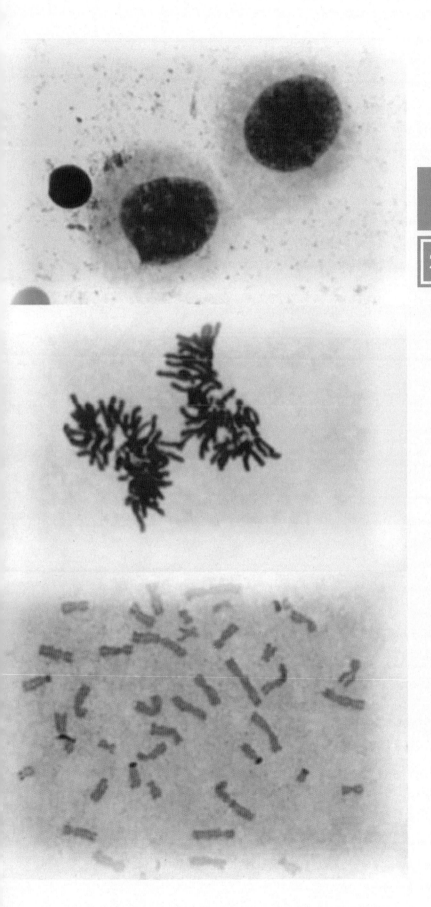

Chapter 21

Genetics

CHROMOSOME

The word chromosome is derived from the Greek words 'chroma' meaning colour and 'soma' meaning body. Chromosomes are vehicles of inheritance which facilitate reproduction and maintenance of species. They are thread like structures located in the cell nucleus and are made up of genes. Normal human cells contain 23 pairs of chromosomes, a total of 46, one member of each pair is inherited from each parent. Body characters and functions are regulated by genes on 22 pairs of chromosomes known as autosomes. The 23rd pair consists of sex chromosomes. These are of two types, namely X and Y, based on their role in sex determination. Females consist of 22 pairs of autosomes plus XX chromosomes while in males there are 22 pairs of autosomes plus XY chromosomes.

Cytogenetics

The study of chromosomes and cell division is known as cytogenetics.

Karyotyping

It is the characterization of chromosomes according to their size, shape and the distribution of stain taken up by them. Each pair of homologous chromosomes are arranged in a sequence and the chromosomal constitution of a cell is studied.

Structure of Chromosome

Each chromosome is made up of a double helix of DNA molecule wrapped around on a framework of histone proteins along with non histone proteins. In fact, chromosome is a complex structure which consists of coiled and supercoiled double stranded DNA along with its packaging protein. Two types of nuclear protein material are seen

1. **Non-histone proteins:** These are highly mobile group of proteins (HMG). Gene regulatory proteins, DNA and RNA polymerases form the non histone proteins.

2. **Histone proteins:** There are five histone proteins namely H, H_2A, H_2B, H_3 and H_4. They are basic in nature and are aggregated along with the DNA. These packaging proteins along with the DNA coil to form the following structures.
   a. **Nucleosomes:** two molecules, each of H_2A, H_2B, H_3 and H_4 histone proteins form an octomer. This octomer forms a core around which 146 base pairs of helical DNA are wrapped forming a nucleosome. Nucleosomes forms the structural framework of a chromatin fibre of 10 nm diameter.
   b. **Solenoid:** six nucleosomes radially arranged form a solenoid. This is 30 nm thick.
   c. **Chromatin fibre:** A series of solenoids form chromatin fibre of 30 nm diameter. It is composed of nucleosomes, histone H and DNA.
   d. **Chromatin loop** The 30 nm chromatin fibres are further packed into a system of supercoiled domains known as loops. Each loop contains 20,000 to 1,00,000 base pairs of DNA and are formed at the non-histone protein binding sites along the 30 nm fibre.
   e. **Chromosome:** The highly condensed form of chromatin loop is the chromosome.

Levels of Coiling of DNA in the formation of a Chromosome

1. **Primary coiling:** The double helical structure of DNA molecule is primary coiling.
2. **Secondary coiling:** Coiling of DNA around histone proteins to form nucleosomes is secondary coiling.
3. **Tertiary coiling:** It is the coiling of nucleosomes forming solenoids and thence chromatin fibres.
4. **Quaternery coiling:** Is seen in chromatin loops.

Euchromatin

Chromatin is combination of DNA and histone proteins. The uncoiled portion of a chromosome consisting of 10 nm chromatin fibre made up of nucleosomes forms the euchromatin. It is so named because it stains lightly on routine staining. It is the genetically active site (site of transcription) of a chromosome.

Heterochromatin

It is the coiled chromatin that is either devoid of genes or has inactive genes. It is characteristically located around the periphery of nucleus and nucleolus. Heterochromatin remains condensed in the interphase and replicates very late in the S-phase of the cycle. It stains darkly.

Types of Heterochromatin

There are two types of permanent hetero-chromatin observed in human chromosomes.
1. **Constitutive heterochromatin:** These are located around the centromere of all chromosomes, in the long arm of the chromosomes and in the satellites of acrocentric chromosomes. These heterochro-matin areas contain repetitive sequences of DNA bases. These repetitive DNA sequences code for ribosomal and transfer RNA.
2. **Facultative heterochromatin:** It is the euchromatin which is temporarily in a transcriptionally inactive state. In humans, the inactive X-chromosome in females is the best example of facultative hetro-chromatin. In early embryogenesis both X-chromosomes are actively involved in development of ovaries. At around 15 to 16 days of gestation inactivation of one X chromosome is initiated. Then it becomes permanently inactive and forms a heterochromatin known as the Barr body.

Appearance of Chromosomes in the Metaphase

Each pair of chromosome forms a condensed body with a common basic structure during cell division. The following parts are identified in each chromosome:

1. **Chromatids:** Each chromosome consists of two parallel and identical filaments known as chromatids. These two chromatids are also known as sister chromatids.
2. **Primary constriction:** Both chromatids are held together at a narrow region called as the primary constriction.
3. **Centromere:** A pale staining area seen in the centre of the primary constriction is known as the centromere. The centromeric proteins form the kinetochore which provides attachment to the mitotic spindle in metaphase.
4. **Telomere:** The extremity of a chromosome is referred to as telomere. Telomere helps to maintain the stability of the chromosomes. It has a polarity that prevents other segments of the chromosome from joining with each other. Telomere also provides the template for priming the replication of the lagging strand during DNA synthesis.
5. **Secondary constriction:** Some chromosomes show another constriction known as the secondary constriction. This is related to the site of formation of nucleoli. This region of chromosome is known as the nucleolar organising region. It is present in chromosome numbers 13, 14, 15, 21 and 22.

CLASSIFICATION OF CHROMOSOMES (FIG 21.1)

Chromosomes are variously classified according to variation in length and structure.

Classification According to the Position of Centromere

1. **Acrocentric:** In acrocentric chromosomes the centromere is present near one end. Therefore one arm is very short and other is very long.
2. **Metacentric:** Centromere is situated near the centre.
3. **Submetacentric:** Centromere is situated between the midpoint and one end of the chromosome.

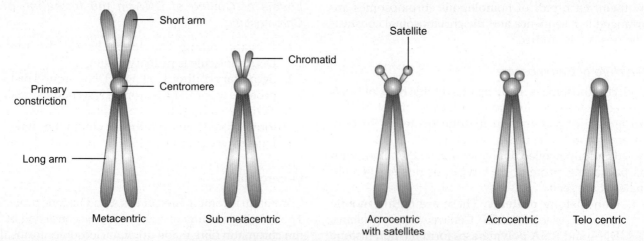

Fig. 21.1: Types of chromosomes according to the position of centromere

4. **Telocentric:** Centromere is situated at the end. The chromosome appears to have only one arm. This type is not present in human beings.

Denner-London System Classification

- It is the most common classification used in karyotyping. According to this system of classification chromosomes are classified in different groups according to their length. The chromosomes are placed in 7 groups described below.

Denner-London System Classification

Group	Number of chromosome	Character
A	1, 2, 3	Long, metacentric
B	4, 5	Long, sub-metacentric
C	6, 7, 8, 9, 10, 11, 12 and X	Medium size submetacentric
D	13, 14, 15	Medium size, acrocentric satellite present
E	16, 17, 18	Short, submetacentric
F	19, 20	Short and metacentric
G	21, 22 and Y	Very short acrocentric with satellite body except in Y

Symbols and abbreviations used in karyotyping. This is in accordance with the ISCN (International system for human cytogenetic nomenclature).

Symbol	Abbreviation
A-G	Chromosome groups
1-22	Autosome number
X, Y	Sex chromosome
46, XX	Normal female karyotype
46, XY	Normal male karyotype
46 / 47	Mosaic with 46 and 47 chromosomes cell line
del	Deletion
dup	Duplication
fra	Fragile site
i	Isochromosome
ins	Insertion
inv	Inversion
nar	Marker chromosome
mat	Maternal origin
mos	Mosaic
p	Short arm of chromosome
pat	Paternal origin
q	Long arm of chromosome
r	Ring chromosome
rep	Reciprocal
rec	Recombinant chromosome
rob	Robertsonian translocation
t	translocation

- Chromosome pair number 13, 14, 15, 21 and 22 possess satellite bodies which are responsible for nucleoli formations. These chromosomes are known as sat-chromosomes. X chromosome is classified in group C and Y chromosome in group G.
- Paris conference (1972) classification: This classification is based on the banding pattern of each chromosome. It provides more accuracy to the identification of parts of the each chromosome.

CHROMOSOMAL ABNORMALITIES

Chromosomal abnormalities are classified as
  a. Numerical abnormalities
  b. Structural abnormalities

Numerical Abnormalities

Alterations in the chromosomal number constitute numerical abnormalities. These are of two types:

1. **Aneuploidy:** It is a condition in which there is an addition or a loss of one or more chromosomes. Most of the aberrations of chromosomal number take place due to non-disjunction.

   Non-disjunction: It is the failure of separation of a pair of bivalent chromosomes during meiosis I or a pair of chromatids during mitosis. It may involve either the sex chromosomes or the autosomes. The daughter cell which receives the pair of bivalent chromosome will have extra-chromosome while the other daughter cell will lack the same.

   Examples: Trisomy, monosomy.

2. **Polyploidy:** It is the addition of one or more complete haploid set of chromosomes to the normal diploid number of chromosomes.

Clinical Conditions with Numerical Abnormalities

1. **Trisomy:** Presence of 3 copies of a chromosome instead of the normal 2 in a cell is called trisomy. Trisomy of all the autosomes has been recorded except in chromosome 1.

   Cause and Risk Factors of Trisomy
   a. Trisomy occurs due to the non-disjunction of a chromosome or a chromatid in one of the fertilizing gametes. The frequency of non-disjunction is more in oogenesis than in spermatogenesis.

b. Occurrence of trisomy increases with the age of the mother.

The common conditions are described below:

Trisomy 21: This is also known as Down's syndrome or Mongolism.

Cytogenetics: It usually follows fertilization of two gametes out of which one has two chromosome 21 (usually a result of non disjunction during its meiosis I). Rarely, it can occur due to the translocation of long arm of chromosome 21 to a D and G group of chromosome.

Clinical features of a child with Down's syndrome

a. Mental retardation (moderate)
b. Short stature
c. Brachycephaly
d. Presence of epicanthal folds
e. Protuding tongue, small ears and flat occiput
f. Flat nasal bridge
g. Brushfield spots in the eye (in the iris)
h. All males are infertile while females have reduced fertility

Risk Factors

a. Higher incidence with advancing maternal age (aging effect on oocyte)
b. Family history of Down's syndrome (usually a translocation abnormality)
c. Radiation injuries

Trisomy 13: Also called Patau's syndrome. It is less commonly seen. The newborn has central nervous system malformations, cleft palate, hairlip and lethal cardiac anomalies. There is profound mental retardation in survivors.

Trisomy 18: This condition is also known as Edward syndrome. Most trisomy 18 pregnancies result in spontaneous abortions or still births. The newborn has a small face with prominent occiput, flat nose, low set ears, micrognathia, overlapping of fingers and rocker bottom heels.

Klinefelter's syndrome: This is trisomy of sex chromosomes. The karyotype is 47, XXY. A young boy with Klinefelter syndrome presents with a mild developmental delay and behavioral immaturity. The adult male presents with small testes, dysgenesis of seminiferous tubules, gynecomastia and poor musculature. Most males are infertile.

47, XYY syndrome: This condition occurs with the same frequency as 47, XXY. Male presents with tall stature and mild social problems.

47, XXX female: Majority of 47, XXX females have no clinical manifestations. They have normal fertility and normal off springs.

2. **Monosomy:** It is characterized by the presence of only one member of the homologous pair of chromosomes in the karyotype.

— Autosomal monosomies are not seen in live births or in early spontaneous abortions because they are fatal to the conceptus.

— **Turner's syndrome:** Monosomy of the X-chromosome (karyotype 45, XO)is the most common form of monosomy seen. The patient is a female (as there is no Y chromosome) and presents with the following features

a. Short stature
b. Webbing of neck
c. Low hair line at the nape of neck
d. Primary or secondary amenorrhea
e. Streak ovaries
f. Majority are infertile

Causes and risk factor: Turner's syndrome results from the fertilization of two gametes out of which one lacks it's X-chromosome. This occurs due to non-disjunction or anaphase lag during cell division in which the X-chromosome is lost to the non fertilizing daughter cell of the original germ cell.

3. **Mosaicism:** It is the presence of two or more cell lines with different karyotypes in a single individual. It is usually in cases of trisomy of 13, 18 and 21 chromosomes. Mosaic Turner female has also been described. Cause and risk factors of mosaicism—It arises from the non-disjunction or chromosome lag in the early cleavage stages of zygote or during embryogenesis.

4. **Polyploidy:** Two clinical conditions that occur in humans:

i. **Triploidy:** There are 69 chromosomes with XXX, XXY or XYY sex chromosome complements. A triploid conceptus generally aborts early in pregnancy and very rarely does it lead to a live birth. The fetuses have a relatively large head, syndactyly and congenital heart defects and all die soon after birth.

Cause of triploidy: Triploidy results from failure of meiosis in a germ cell or from a fertilization defect such as diaspermy (two sperms fertilizing one ovum).

ii. **Tetraploidy:** There are 92 chromosomes with XXXX or XXYY sex chromosome complements. Most tetraploid fetuses are lost in the first trimester of pregnancy.

Cause of tetraploidy: It results from the failure of completion of usually the first cleavage division of zygote.

Structural Abnormalities

These abnormalities result from the breakage and abnormal fusion of chromosome segments. Various structural abnormalities are described below:

1. **Deletion:** It results from the loss of a segment of chromosome. Deletion may be of the following two types
   i. **Terminal deletion:** It is the loss of a terminal segment of a chromosome. It results from a single break in the chromosome. The acentric segments are later lost in the subsequent cell divisions.
   ii. **Interstitial deletion:** It occurs due to two breaks in the chromosome followed by the subsequent fusion at the break site with loss of the interstitial acentric fragment. Deletion can occur at two levels
      — **Microscopic deletions:** These are visualized on microscopy, e.g., Cri-du-chat syndrome (loss of short arm of chromosme).
      — **Microdeletion:** These are small deletions which require high resolution banding for cytogenetic diagnosis. These can also be detected by fluorescent in situ hybridization studies, e.g., Prader-Willi syndrome.
   iii. **Ring chromosome:** A ring chromosome is a type of deletion abnormality. It arises from breaks on either side of the centromere of chromosome and the subsequent fusion of the break points on the centric segment. The distal acentric segments are lost.
2. **Isochromosomes:** When the centromere divides perpendicular to the long axis of a chromosome instead of parallel to it, two chromosomes of unequal length are obtained. The resultant chromosomes, derived from the transverse splitting of centromere, are known as isochromosomes. This abnormality is usually encountered in X-chromosomes.
3. **Duplication:** It is the presence of a portion of a chromosome more than once. This results in trisomy of segments of chromosomes. This duplication results from gametogenesis in a carrier of translocation or inversion abnormality (occurs due to abnormal crossing over).
4. **Inversions:** Inversion is a reversal of the order of chromatin between two breaks in the chromosome. A part of the chromosome gets detached breaking at two points and later reunites with the same chromosome in an inverted position. They can occur as a new mutation or may be present in multiple generations of a family. Inversions are of two types:
   a. **Pericentric inversion:** When the breaks and rearrangement occurs on both sides of the centromere.
   b. **Paracentric inversion:** When the breaks and rearrangement occurs on the same side of the centromere. Inversions rarely cause problems in carriers unless one of the break points affects an important functional gene. However, they can cause significant chromosomal imbalance during gametogenesis leading to duplications or deletions after crossing over during meiosis. It is significant in pericentric inversions and mostly results is miscarrage of the conceptus.
5. **Translocation:** It is the exchange of segments between two non homologous chromosomes.

Reciprocal Translocation

It results from breakage and exchange of segments between chromosomes. There is no loss of genetice material. The points of exchange can be at any location along the chromosomes. This may be heterozygous or homozygous. Balanced reciprocal translocations involving the long arms chromosomes 11 and 22 are the commonest encountered abnormality

Robertsonian Translocation

It results from breakage in two acrocenteric chromosomes at or close to their centromeres and the subsequent fusion of their long arms. The short arms are usually lost. It usually involves 13–15, 13–14, 21–22 chromosomes.

Translocations may not affect the carrier however, the variable segregation pattern during meiosis results in various forms of unbalanced chromosome complements, e.g., monosomy, trisomy or translocation abnormalities.

Various clinical conditions and their structural defects in chromosomes

Structural chromosomal anomaly	Clinical condition	Genetic constitution and clinical features
1. **Deletion**	Cri-du-chat or cat cry syndrome of short arm of chromosome 5 (5p-)	It is due to deletion of the terminal portion The new born presents with — Round face — A cry that resembles the of a cat — Hypertelorism — Micrognathia — Severe mental retardation — Cardiac defects
	Wolf-Hirschhorn syndrome	There is deletion of the short arm of chromosome 4 (4p-) Infant has the following features — Prominent forehead and broad nasal root — Short philtrum — Mouth is downturned — Severe mental retardation — Cardiac defects — Growth failure
2. **Microdeletion**	Prader-Willi syndrome	This syndrome involves microdeletions of the proximal part of long arm of chromosome 15 (15q). The infant presents with: — Profound hypotonia — Mental retardation — Trunkal obesity
3. **Interstitial deletion**	WAGR syndrome	Chromosomal analysis shows an interstitial deletion of a particular region of the short arm of one of the chromosomes no. 11. The child usually develops — Wilm's tumour — Aniridia — Genital abnormalities — Growth retardation

MOLECULAR BASIS OF GENETICS

Genetic information is stored in the DNA (deoxyribose nucleic acid) helix which form chromosomes. Molecular genetics deals with the study of this genetic material, its structure, replication and the process of dissemination of the genetic information by formation of RNA (ribonucleic acid) and ultimately proteins.

STRUCTURE OF DNA (FIG. 21.2)

The DNA molecule consists of two long, parallel, complimentary polynucleiotide chains twisted about each other in the form of a double helix (twisted ladder model).

Each chain is composed of nucleotides, each of which contains a deoxyribose residue, a phosphate and a pyrimidine or a purine base. The sides of the twisted ladder consist of a backbone of deoxyribose residues linked by phosphate bands while the rungs of ladder are the bonds between the bases. The pyramidine bases are thymine (T) and cytosine (C) and the purine bases are adenine (A) and guanine (G). The two strands of DNA run in opposite directions and are held together by hydrogen bonds between the nitrogenous bases. (Adenine forms two hydrogen bonds with thymine while cytosine forms three hydrogen bonds with guanine). There are 10 nucleiotide pairs in a single complete turn of the double chain. The ends of the DNA strands are designated 5' and 3' depending on the depending on the number of the free carbon in the deoxyribose sugar residue at the terminal end. By convention the 5' end is written on the left and it indicates the sequence closer to the beginning of a gene. The 3' is written to the right and it indicates the sequence closer to the end of the gene. New DNA is synthesized in the 5' to 3' direction during replication.

Mitochondrial DNA: Nuclear DNA forms the bulk of DNA present in a cell. In addition to nuclear DNA, the mitochondria also contain a ring shaped DNA molecule. Mitochondrial DNA is entirely derived from the ovum. Therefore, it has maternal inheritance.

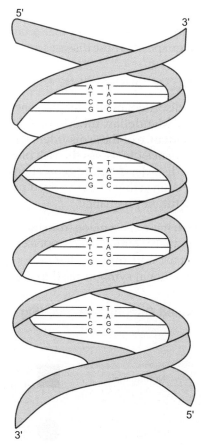

Fig. 21.2: Structure of DNA

Classes of DNA: DNA is classified into two types of sequences:
1. **Repetitive DNA:** It does not contain genes but is present as either short or long interspersed, repeated DNA sequences. These are of two types
   a. Short interspersed repeated sequences or SINEs
   b. Long interspersed repeated sequences or LINEs
      Their function is largely unknown.
2. **Non-repetitive DNA or unique DNA sequences:** It constitutes only 5% of the total human genome and consists of genes which code for mRNA and the specific proteins.

GENES

Genes are the units of hereditary. A gene consists of a specific sequence of DNA which codes for a specific sequence of amino acids forming a particular protein. The various genes are arranged in a linear series within the chromosomes.

Locus: The position of a gene in the chromosome is called locus. It is described in reference to the centromere.

Alleles: Genes occupying identical loci in a pair of homologous chromosomes are called as alleles or allelomorphs. One pair of allelic genes regulate the synthesis of a particular polypeptide chain and hence are responsible for a particular character of an individual.

Homozygous Alleles: When both allelic genes regulating a particular character or trait are similar, they are called homozygous alleles, e.g., presence of two genes representing tall height in an individual.

Heterozygous Alleles: When both allelic genes regulating a particular character are dissimilar, they are called heterozygous alleles, e.g., presence of two genes with one representing tall and other representing short height in an individual.

Multiple alleles: When in a population, more than two different alleles exist at a given locus of a chromosome. Such alleles are said to be multiple. In a given individual only two of these alleles are present. For example, the blood groups are coded by four alleles A1, A2, B and O out of which only two, e.g., AO, AB, OO etc. are present in a individual.

Organization of Genes

Genes are made up of exons and introns with following characteristic features.

Exons: Exons are the functional portions of a gene sequence that code for the protein.

Introns: Introns are the non-coding DNA sequences of unknown function. The number and size of introns vary in different genes.

Types of Genes According to the Mendelian Pattern of Inheritance

1. **Dominant gene:** An allele which is always expressed both in the homozygous and the heterozygous combination.
2. **Recessive gene:** When an allele is expressed only in the homozygous state it is known as recessive gene.
3. **Carrier gene:** In the heterozygous state, the recessive gene acts as a carrier gene which is not expressed in the individual but may be expressed in subsequent generations.
4. **Co-dominant genes:** When both the allelic genes are dominant but of two different types, both traits may have concurrent expression, e.g., blood group AB.
5. **Sex-linked genes:** The genes located on the X or Y-chromosomes are known as sex-linked genes.

6. **Sex-limited genes:** These genes are borne by the autosomes, but the trait is expressed preferentially in one sex only, e.g., baldness found predominantly in males.

MODES OF INHERITANCE

Mendel's laws of inheritance: Three principal laws of inheritance were established on the basis of Mendel's plant experiments.

1. **The law of uniformity:** The crossing over between two homozygotes of differing types results in offsprings that are identical and heterozygotic. The inherited characters do not blend.

2. **The law of segregation:** During formation of gametes the two members of a gene pair separate into different gametes. Therefore, in an individual each of the allelic pair in originally derived from separate parents.

3. **Law of independent assortment:** This law states that different traits conveyed by members of different gene pairs segregate to the offspring independent of one another.

   Lyon's hypothesis: This hypothesis was given by Mary F. Lyon. It proposed that in the somatic cells of female mammals, only one X chromosome is active. The other X chromosome is condensed and inactive. It is seen in the interphase cells as the sex chromatin or Barr body. The inactivation of chromosome occurs early in the development during embryonic life at around 15th -16th day of gestation. Normally either of the two X chromosomes can be inactivated. The process of X inactivation is often referred to as lyonization.

Classification of Genetic Diseases

1. **Chromosomal abnormalities** (See page no. 611)
2. **Single gene disorders:** This is usually a consequence of a point mutation in the base pair of a gene which may result in following changes in gene expression.
   a. No alteration in gene expression.
   b. Altered protein synthesis with reduced or complete loss of biological activity
   c. Termination of protein synthesis
   d. Increase or decrease in synthesis of particular enzymes with subsequent effects.
3. **Multifactorial disorders:** Some diseases, e.g., diabetes mellitus and schizophrenia and some conditions, e.g., cleft lip have a multifactorial inheritance with interaction of many genes.
4. **Acquired somatic genetic disease:** Recent research has identified the occurrence of various point mutations occuring in the somatic cells during life

with no involvement of the germ cells. These account for various diseases that occur in old age. e.g., malignancies. These diseases are not inherited.

INHERITANCE OF SINGLE GENE DISORDERS

Most human disorders exhibit single gene unifactorial inheritance or Mendelian inheritance. Studying the pattern of inheritance of these disorders within families enables the geneticist to assess the risk of transmission of a particular disorder in future generations. This helps in the genetic counselling of the affected parents before they plan any future pregnancy.

Pedigree chart: It is a chart made from the data collected from an individual or family which represents successive generations, past and future. There are certain international conventional symbols used to draw the chart.

Commonly used Genetic Symbols (Fig. 21.3)

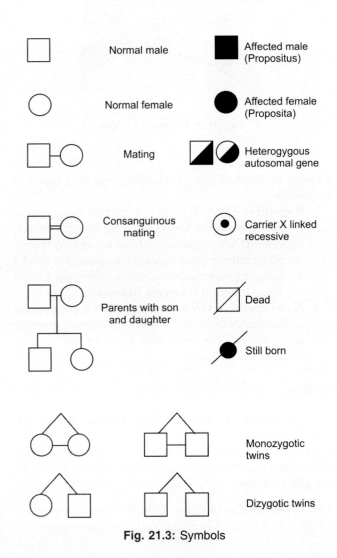

Fig. 21.3: Symbols

1. Autosomal dominant inheritance (Fig. 21.4)
— This occurs due to mutation in a dominant gene on an autosome leading to a particular trait.
— This trait is transmitted from one generation to the other equally to male and female offsprings (vertical transmission).
— The risk of transmission of the disorder is 50% if one of the parents has the dominant trait.
— The unaffected family members do not transmit the disorder.

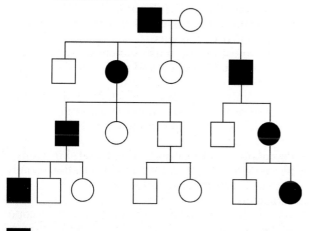

■ Affected male

● Affected female

Fig. 21.4 : Family tree of autosomal dominant trait

2. Autosomal recessive inheritance (Fig. 21.5)
— The mutated gene is expressed only in a homozygous state.
— The affected individuals are usually siblings (horizontal transmission) with equal distribution in males and females.

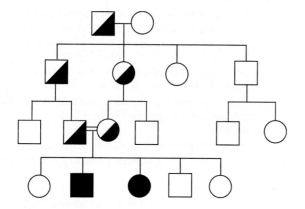

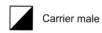 Carrier male

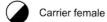 Carrier female

Fig. 21.5 : Family tree of autosomal recessive trait

— Successive generations may skip having the disorder till two carrier partners meet.
— The parents of an affected individual are apparently healthy as they are heterozygotes.
— The risk of transmission of the trait by 2 carrier parents to their offspring is 25%. There is 50% risk of offsprings being carriers and 25% offsprings are normal.
— It is often associated with consanguinous marriages.

3. Sex-linked inheritance: X-linked recessive disorders are the most common form of sex linked abnormalities. X-linked dominant and Y-linked traits are rarely encountered.

X-linked Recessive Inheritance (Fig. 21.6)
— The disorder affects only males while females are unaffected in families.
— The disorder is transmitted by carrier females to their sons.
— The affected males, on survival, can transmit the disorder to their male grandchildren via obligate carrier daughters.

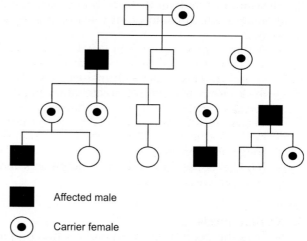

■ Affected male

⊙ Carrier female

Fig. 21.6: Family tree of X-linked recessive trait

PRENATAL DIAGNOSIS
Genetic abnormalities in a conceptus can result in the following:
1. **Spontaneous miscarriages:** First trimester losses are mostly associated with chromosomal abnormalities.
2. **Gross congenital abnormalities in newborn:** 2 to 3% of newborns have at least one major congenital anomaly. This leads to high perinatal morbidity and mortality.
3. Abnormalities in childhood and adult life, e.g., blindness, deafness, malignancies.

Congenital and genetic disorders are a great social and economic burden to the society. Prenatal diagnosis allows doctors to detect abnormalities in an unborn child in high risk cases. This helps in early detection and appropriate management. In developed countries pre-natal diagnosis offered to each couple planning a pregnancy.

Indications of pre-natal diagnosis
1. Advanced maternal age at conception. It is already known that Down's syndrome is characteristically associated with maternal age more than 35 years.
2. Previous history of a genetically abnormal child or child with gross congenital anomaly.
3. Multiple miscarriages.
4. Family history of genetic disorder.
5. Consanguinous couples.
6. Pre-implantation diagnosis in cases of in-vitro fertilisation.

PRENATAL DIAGNOSTIC PROCEDURES: THEY CAN BE NON-INVASIVE AND INVASIVE TESTS
Non-invasive Tests
1. **History:** A careful history can point to the pattern of inheritance of a genetic disorder and the risk associated. A pedigree chart helps in accurate prepregnancy evaluation which further helps in the proper counselling of the couples.
2. **Ultrasound:** It aids in the detection of structural anomalies which could point towards a genetic anomaly.
   — A transvaginal scan (TVS) usually performed at 11 to 14 weeks, can detect early skull and spinal defects. Nuchal transluscency (NT), thickness of skin and soft tissues at the nape of neck, is a marker for Down's syndrome.
   — Trans abdominal scan (TAS) is usually performed at 16 to 22 weeks for detection of congenital defects.
   — It however requires expensive equipments and an experienced operator.

Invasive Tests
1. **Amniocentesis**
   — It is the aspiration of amniotic fluid under ultrasound guidance.
   — It is generally performed at 16 to 18 weeks of gestation. About 10 to 20 ml of fluid is aspirated.
   — Amniotic fluid contains desquamated fetal cells from skin, respiratory and gastrointestinal tract besides water (98%) and electrolytes.
   — It is the most commonly performed procedure because it is an easy technique with a risk of fetal loss of only 0.5 to 1%.
   — The main disadvantage of this method is that the cells thus obtained need to be cultured for genetic analysis and results take 2 to 3 weeks.
   — Amniocentesis is now also performed at 10 to 14 weeks for earlier diagnosis.
2. **Chorionic villus biopsy or sampling (CVS)**
   — This enables prenatal diagnosis to be under-taken during the first trimester.

   — It is carried out at 10 to 14 weeks of gestation.
   — CVS involves aspiration of trophoblastic material from the placental site under ultra-sound guidance.
   — Detection of disorder in early pregnancy avoids need for second trimester abortions.
   — The risk of fetal loss is however higher, upto 1 to 2%. This method also requires an experienced operator.
   — The chorionic villus sample can be obtained via the transcervical or the transabdominal route.
3. **Percutaneous ultrasound guided fetal blood sampling/cordocentesis**
   — It is most useful in assessment of fetal haemo-gram, fetal infection and provides high quality karyotype in 48 to 72 hours.
   — It involves aspiration of fetal blood from the cord near its insertion in the placenta.
   — Cordocentesis is performed at 18 to 20 weeks of gestation.
4. **Percutaneous ultrasound guided fetal skin biopsy:** It is performed at 18 to 20 weeks of gestation usually to detect skin abnormalities.
5. **Fetoscopy**
   — It is the visualization of fetus by an endoscope.
   — Fetoscope is very rarely in use these days as ultrasound has superseded its relevance.

METHODS OF DETECTION OF GENETIC ABNORMALITY
The cultured cells obtained by various prenatal diagnostic procedures are evaluated by one of the following methods.
1. Karyotyping
2. Fluorescent in situ hybridization
3. Flow cytometry
4. Methods to detect DNA and RNA: These utilize recombinant DNA Technology. They are briefly described below:
   a. **Southern blot technique: It detects DNA.** The sample to be tested is treated with special restriction endonucleases which break the DNA into specific fragments. They are then exposed to an alkali and single stranded fragments are obtained. These are transferred onto a nitro-cellulose paper by blotting. A specific labelled DNA sequence (probe) is incubated with the sample.
   The probe gets hybridized with its comple-mentary fragment whose presence can now be identified.
   b. **Northern blot technique:** This is similar to southern blotting but helps in identifying RNA in the samples.
   c. **Western blot technique:** This technique is used to identify the size and amount of abnormal proteins that are present in a sample. It makes use of antisera specific for the proteins.

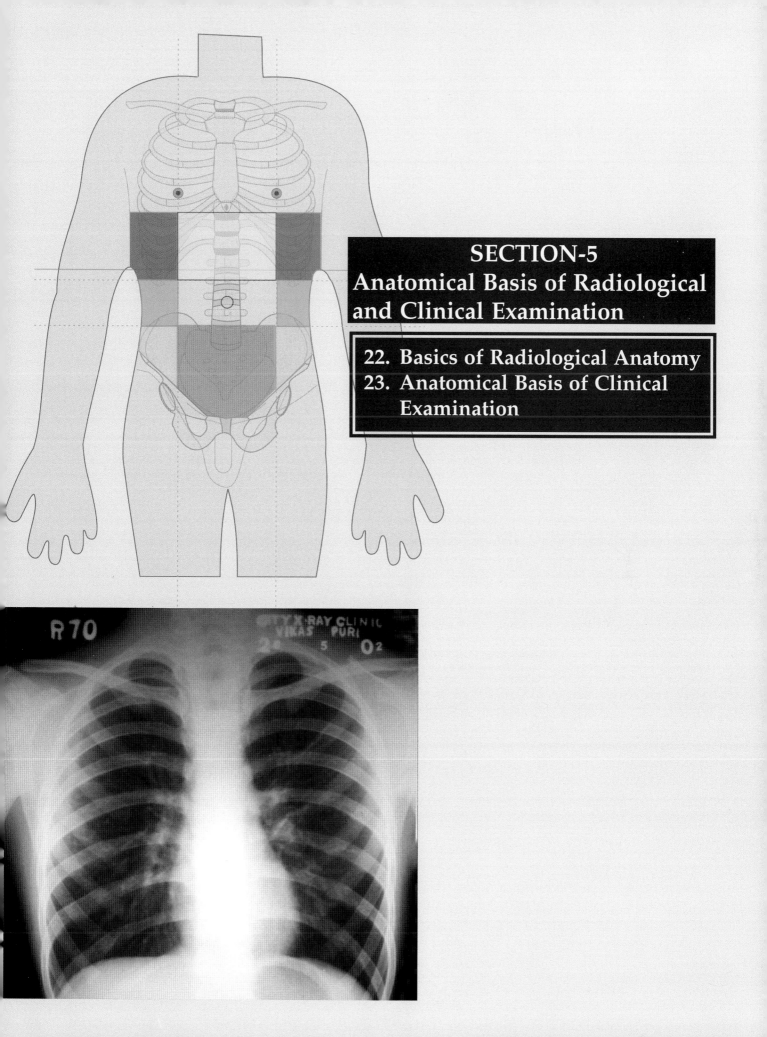

SECTION-5
Anatomical Basis of Radiological and Clinical Examination

22. Basics of Radiological Anatomy
23. Anatomical Basis of Clinical Examination

Basics of Radiological Anatomy

RADIOLOGICAL ANATOMY

Human anatomy can be studied by using various imaging techniques like X-rays, ultrasound and magnetic resonance imaging. Radiological anatomy deals with the study of human anatomy using X-ray imaging.

Techniques of imaging human body can be classified into the following categories:
1. **Techniques using ionizing radiations:**
   a. Simple X-ray.
   b. Computed X-ray tomography (CT).
   c. Radioisotope or radionuclide scanning.
2. **Ultrasound:** It utilizes the principle of high frequency or ultra-sonic sound waves.
3. **Magnetic resonance imaging:** It is based on the principle of variations in radiofrequencies of protons (hydrogen atoms, H) in an electromagnetic field.

X-ray Techniques

- X-rays were discovered in 1895 by a German physicist named Conrad Roentgen.
- X-rays are a part of the electromagnetic spectrum. The wireless radiofrequency waves are at one end of spectrum having long wavelengths while X-rays and cosmic rays are at the other end of the spectrum having very short wavelengths.
- X-rays have a very short wavelength of 1/10,000 of visible light. This characteristic permits X-rays to penetrate materials which otherwise do not transmit visible light.

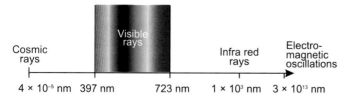

Fig. 22.1: Different rays of electromagnetic spectrum

Wavelength of different rays of electromagnetic spectrum (Fig. 22.1):

Type of rays	Wavelength
1. Cosmic rays	4×10^{-5} nm
2. Electronic rays	2.7×10^{-4} nm
3. Gamma rays	6×10^{-3} nm to 0.14 nm
4. X-rays	0.14 to 13.6 nm
5. Ultraviolet rays	13.6 to 379 nm
6. Visible rays	397 to 723 nm
a. Violet	397 to 424 nm
b. Indigo	424 to 455 nm
c. Blue	455 to 492 nm
d. Green	492 to 575 nm
e. Yellow	575 to 585 nm
f. Orange	585 to 647 nm
g. Red	647 to 723 nm
7. Infrared rays	723 to 1×10^3 nm
8. Wireless rays (Hertzian rays)	1×10^5 to 3×10^{13} nm
a. Short	1×10^5 to 1×10^{10} nm
b. Long	1×10^{10} to 3×10^{13} nm
9. Electromagnetic oscillations	Over 3×10^{13} nm

Features of X-ray Examination

- X-rays can easily pass through various substances due their short wavelength. The image of a substance fundamentally depends on two factors namely,
  1. Penetrating power of X-rays.
  2. Atomic weight of the substance. Higher the atomic weight of a substance, greater is the absorption of X-rays.
- When an X-ray beam is passed through the body, the beam gets partly scattered and partly absorbed. The amount of energy absorbed depends on the atomic weight of the structure.
- Higher the atomic weight, greater will be the absorption of the rays which cannot pass through the structure. As little or no rays will pass through, the structure is projected as a white or radio-opaque area on the developed film. Example, bone and teeth.

- Also in our body, calcium absorbs X-rays and since the concentration of calcium in bones is highest it absorbs more X-rays than skin, muscle, fascia.
- Structure with lower atomic weights allow passage of X-rays and appear as radiolucent or black to grey on the film. The rest of structures will appear in various shades of grey on the image. Examples of radiolucent structures which are readily penetrated by X-rays are cartilage, muscle and fascia (Figs 22.2, 22.3).
- The X-rays image is obtained on a silver impregnated plastic film known as the photographic plate. Hence, this type of image is actually a negative imprint of the X-rays. Thus a radiograph is also known as skiagram (skia – shadow, gram – a writing).

DIFFERENT METHODS OF X-RAY EXAMINATION

Simple Radiography

The X-ray beam is passed through the patient on to the photography plate (Fig. 22.2).
1. **Different views of radiography**
   a. **Anteroposterior view:** X-rays are projected from anteriort aspect of the subject and photographic plate is placed posteriorly to the subject. Posterior structures are better visualized in this view. Examples, Xrays of limbs, spine.
   b. **Posteroanterior view:** X-rays are projected from behind and photography plate is placed anterior to the subject. Anterior structures are better visualized in this view. The most common example is **chest X-ray** (Fig. 22.4) in which this view best delineates the lungs.

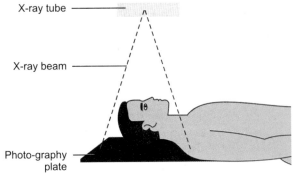

Fig. 22.2: Simple radiography

   c. **Lateral view:** It is done to assess depth of the structure. It is of two types:
      — Right lateral view: Photographic plate is place to the right side of the subject.

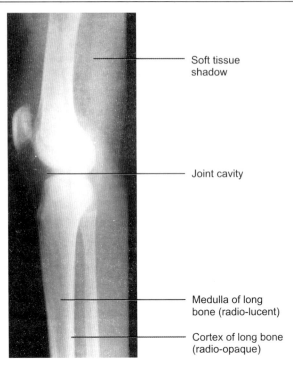

Fig. 22.3: X-ray of knee joint

      — Left lateral view: Photographic plate is placed to the left side of the subject.
   d. **Oblique view:** It is done to asses a particular structure, e.g., minimal fluid in pleural cavity.
2. **Screening and image intensifier:** In this method the beam of X rays is made to pass across the part of body on to a fluorescent screen to allow for instant view of the image. This image is captured via an electronic image intensifier on a closed circuit television monitor and can be seen simultaneously by the operator at a different place than the X ray dark room.
3. **Video-radiography:** As described above the same fluorescent image produced by an image intensifier can be utilized for video recording of multiple images. This is video-radiography.
4. **Xeroradiography:** The X-ray beam is passed through the subject onto an aluminum plate coated with a thin layer of selenium which is charged electrically. The X-ray beam causes an alteration of the electrostatic charges in correspondence with the structure being evaluated and an image is produced. The image is obtained by blowing a thin powder on to the plate receiving the rays. The powder adheres in proportion to local charge on the plate. This method is especially useful to delineate anatomy of soft tissues.

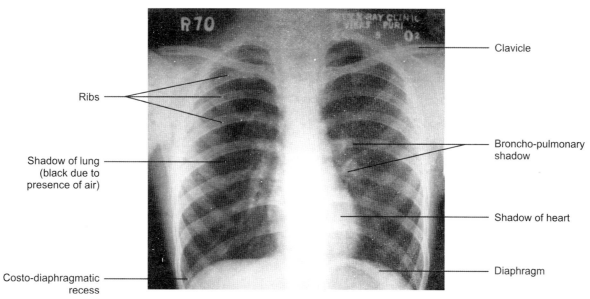

Fig. 22.4: X-ray of chest—PA view

5. **Digital vascular imaging (digital subtraction angiography):** This method is useful in the imaging of blood vessels. The area to be studied is imaged by an image intensifier screening and the picture stored in the computer. A second film is taken after injecting a bolus of contrast medium into the vessel. The first image is then electronically subtracted from the second and a clearer picture of the vessel minus soft tissue shadow, especially of the surrounding bones is obtained.

6. **Special radiography procedures using X-rays:** These include barium meal, contrast angiography, intravenous pyelography.

7. **Tomography:** This is the variation of simple X-ray radiography. In this method during X-ray exposure, X-ray tube and X-ray film are moved in opposite direction and image of a section of tissue is obtained.

Computed Tomography (CT) (Fig. 22.5)

This method was introduced by Godfrey Hounsfield in 1972 and is also known as computerized axial tomography. Computed tomography involves multi-directional X-ray scanning of the body. Multiple X-ray beams are received on special detectors which produce scintillations. These scintillations are quantified digitally and this digital data is passed to the computer. The computer analyzes the data and gives output in the form of two dimensional image display of the scanned area.

Spiral computed topography: In this method patient is moved longitudinally and X-ray tube moves circumferentially. Net result are according to the data from spiral path of X-ray beams which are studied.

Radioisotope Scanning

Radioisotopes are radioactive labeled isotopes of various substances. When injected they are taken up by specific areas of the body. The intensity of radio-activity after injection of these substances is evaluated by gamma cameras. Few examples where they are used are:

a. In detecting tumors example thyroid tumors which take up radioactive iodine in large amounts during study.

b. Study of myocardial perfusion which is performed using thallium isotope scan.

Ultrasound

Ultrasonic waves are sounds waves of very high frequency which is inaudible to human ear. They have a frequency of over 20,000 Hz. They are produced from a piezoelectric transducer which is capable of changing electrical signals to mechanical energy of sound waves and changing sound waves back to mechanical and electrical energy. The sound waves travel through human tissue at a velocity of 1500 meters / second. These waves are reflected back from various interfaces of body tissues depending on their density and are received by the same transducer and changed into electric currents. This is amplified and displayed on the cathode ray tube or screen of computer monitor as two dimensional

CHAPTER-22

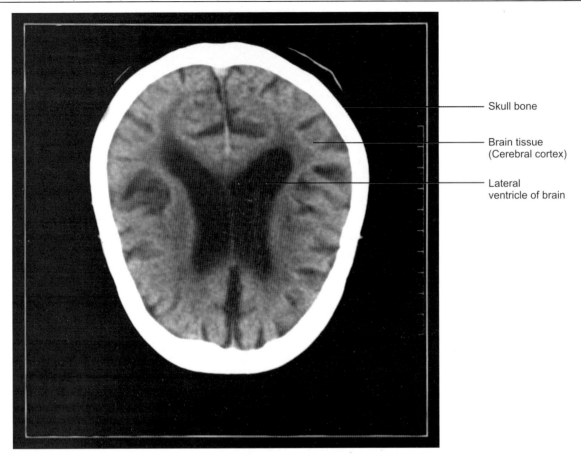

Skull bone

Brain tissue
(Cerebral cortex)

Lateral
ventricle of brain

Fig. 22.5: CT scan of head

images. The images are also in varying shade of grey. Several forms of ultrasound display are available. These are:

a. A-scan
b. B-scan
c. M-mode
d. Real time two dimensional scanning
e. Doppler
f. Duplex scanner
g. Continous wave doppler
h. Three dimensional ultrasound

MRI or Magnetic Resonance Imaging

Nuclei with unpaired electrons behave as magnets. Hydrogen atom nuclei are present in abundance in the body, mostly as water (H_2O) in extracellular and intracellular compartments. On application of an intense magnetic field these protons get excited and alter their alignment. This alteration is reversed with the cessation of the magnetic pulse and realignment results in the release of energy as radiofrequency waves. The energy changes per unit substance vary according to the proton content of the tissue which are quantified and converted to electrical wave forms. These are analyzed by a computer which then displays a two dimensional image of the scanned area in varying shades of grey and white. Magnetic field used in MRI is usually of the strength of 0.15 to 1.5 Tesla.

PACS

It stands for picture archiving and communications system. The X-ray images are computed digitally and stored as images on the hard disk of computer. This enables the storage of large number of images which can be easily retrieved when required at a later date without the dependency on paper or films. However this needs a high cost input and maintainance.

Use of Contrast Media in Radiology

Contrast media are substances that are injected into the lumen of various hollow organs, veins and arteries in order to facilitate better X-ray visualization of various structures like the interior of an organ (e.g., GIT, urinary tract) or blood vessels (e.g., Angiography).

Contrast media that are generally used are:
a. **Salts of heavy metals:** Barium as barium sulphate has long been used for barium enema, barium meal for evaluation of gastrointestinal tract.

b. **Organic iodide preparations:** These are used for urinary tract, gall bladder, angiocardiography, arteriography, phlebography, mylography.
c. **Gas:** Air and other gases are seen as black on X-ray exposure. Air is used identify lung, pharynx, paranasal sinuses.

Radiological Appearance of Normal Bones

- Bones are very well demarcated structures on X-rays because of their high calcium content which renders them highly radio-opaque.
- The long and short bones are made up of an outer cortex of compact bone which appears as a dense white homogenous image and an inner medulla made up of cancellous bone which appears as a transluscent area with fine white lines of trabecular bone scattered in between. (Figs 22.3, 22.6)
- Flat bones are seen as two white lines representing the outer and inner tables of compact bone separated by a translucent area of trabecular bone.

Radiographic anatomy of immature bone: Immature bones are made up of bone as well as cartilage. Cartilage is translucent. Therefore, the part of immature bone formed by cartilage is seen as translucent. It is thus important to know the timing of ossification of various long bones in order to evaluate the X-ray correctly otherwise a wrong diagnosis of fracture may be given to the translucent area which actually is the epiphyseal cartilage.

Radiographic appearance of joint: Joint is formed by articulation of two or more bones and has synovial membrane, articular cartilage, synovial fluid, ligaments and muscles. Ligaments and muscles are seen as soft tissue shadows. Articular cartilage is translucent and this gives an appearance of a radiolucent space between the two articulating ends of the bones. The width of joint space is an index of thickness of articular cartilage. Synovial membrane is not normally seen on skiagram unless thickened or inflamed by a disease process (Figs 22.3 and 22.6).

Radiological Anatomy of Head and Neck

- The anatomy of head and neck is best evaluated by CT scans or MRI. However, a plain radiograph of the area is still used as a preliminary tool of evaluation of a case and in the study of paranasal sinuses, pituitary fossa, skull fracture etc.
- Radiological anatomy of head and neck is studied with the help of anteroposterior and lateral views on plain radiograph.
- Paranasal sinuses are demarcated well in Caldwell position (posteroanterior view) of head and neck. (Fig. 22.7)

Anteriorposterior view of head and neck (Figs 22.7 and 22.8): Following features are identified for superior to inferior direction:
1. Outer and inner plates of skull vault bone.
2. Sagittal suture seen in the midline as a translucent line (till it ossifies).
3. Coronal suture meets the sagittal suture near the vertex.
4. Lambdoid suture is seen more anteriorly to the coronal suture.
5. Frontal air sinuses are seen on both sides above and between two orbits.
6. Orbits are distinctly visible on the face below and lateral to frontal air sinus.
7. Lesser wing of sphenoid, greater wing of sphenoid are seen within the orbital shadows as white lines.
8. Petrous temporal bone forms a white dense shadow running directly medially across the orbit and maxillary air sinus.
9. Nasal cavity is seen between two orbits separated by nasal septum, sphenoidal and ethmoidal air sinuses are seen superoinferioly.
10. Two maxillary air sinuses are seen as translucent areas, one on each side of nasal cavity below each orbit.
11. Two mandibular rami are seen extending upwards leading to mandibular condyles.
12. Mastoid process and air cells are visible laterally and inferiorly to mandibular condyle.
13. Anteriorly and inferiorly teeth of upper and lower jaw are visible. Body of mandible forms the lower most part of the face.

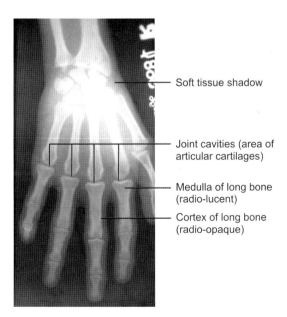
Fig. 22.6: X-ray of hand and wrist joint

- Soft tissue shadow
- Joint cavities (area of articular cartilages)
- Medulla of long bone (radio-lucent)
- Cortex of long bone (radio-opaque)

CHAPTER-22

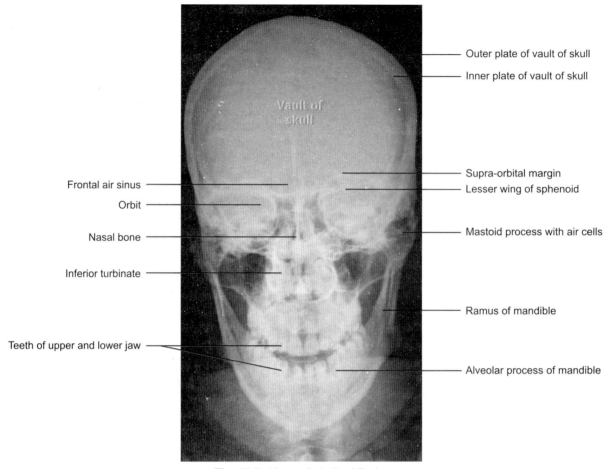

Outer plate of vault of skull
Inner plate of vault of skull

Frontal air sinus
Orbit
Nasal bone
Inferior turbinate

Teeth of upper and lower jaw

Supra-orbital margin
Lesser wing of sphenoid

Mastoid process with air cells

Ramus of mandible

Alveolar process of mandible

Fig. 22.7: X-ray of skull—AP view

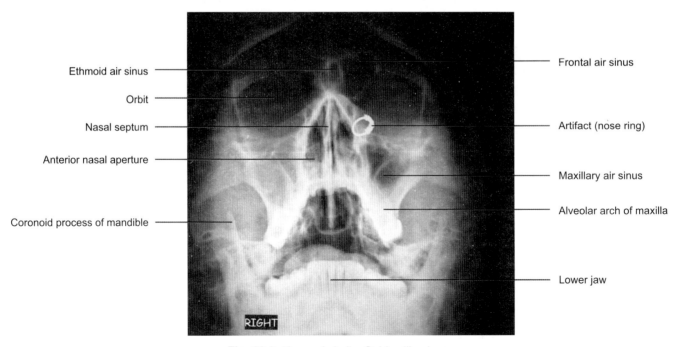

Ethmoid air sinus
Orbit
Nasal septum
Anterior nasal aperture

Coronoid process of mandible

Frontal air sinus

Artifact (nose ring)

Maxillary air sinus

Alveolar arch of maxilla

Lower jaw

RIGHT

Fig. 22.8: X-ray of skull—Caldwell's view

Lateral view of head and neck (Figs 22.8 and 22.9): In the lateral view following features are identified:

1. Outer and inner table of vault of skull are identified as two white lines.

2. Sutures are seen as translucent lines (till the time they do not ossify). The lambdoid suture extends downwards from the posterior part of vault of skull

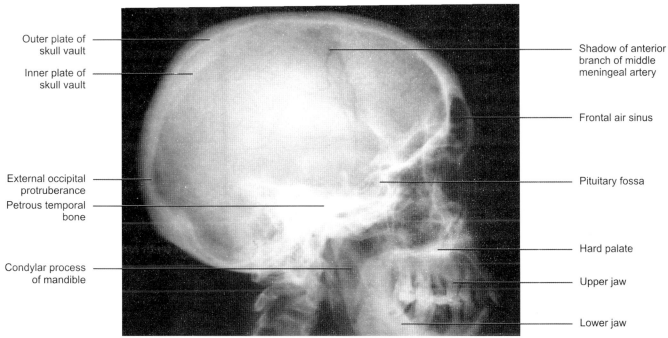

Outer plate of skull vault

Inner plate of skull vault

External occipital protruberance

Petrous temporal bone

Condylar process of mandible

Shadow of anterior branch of middle meningeal artery

Frontal air sinus

Pituitary fossa

Hard palate

Upper jaw

Lower jaw

Fig. 22.9: X-ray of skull—Lateral view

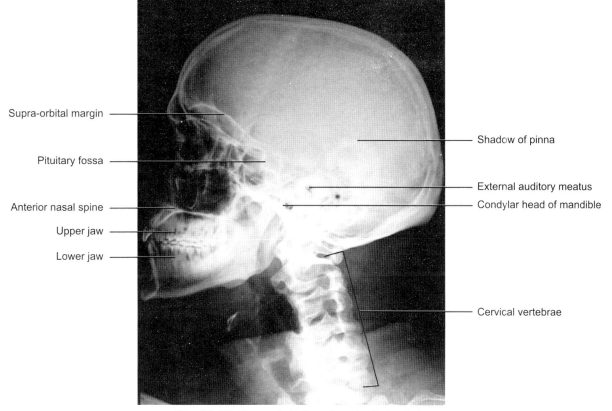

Supra-orbital margin

Pituitary fossa

Anterior nasal spine

Upper jaw

Lower jaw

Shadow of pinna

External auditory meatus

Condylar head of mandible

Cervical vertebrae

Fig. 22.10: X-ray of skull and neck—Lateral view

CHAPTER-22

to the base of skull, behind the shadow of petrous temporal bone.

3. In the anterior most part, near the base of the skull, a translucent triangle area is seen. This is the frontal air sinus. It lies in the frontal bone.

4. A white line extends from the frontal air sinus to the anterior clinoid process at the base of skull. This demarcates the anterior cranial fossa.

5. Anterior clinoid process forms the anterior boundary of pituitary fossa.

6. Pituitary fossa is seen as a round or oval depression which lies superior to the sphenoidal air sinus.

7. Posterior clinoid process is seen projecting from the posterior part of pituitary fossa. This forms the dorsum sella.

8. Sphenoidal air sinus are seen below the pituitary fossa.

9. A triangular, dense, white shadow seen behind posterior clinoid process is the petrous temporal bone.

10. At the center of petrous shadow, a circular translucent ring is present. This denotes the external acoustic meatus.

11. Behind and below the dense shadow of petrous temporal bone a honey comb translucent shadow of mastoid air cells is seen.

12. Coronal suture forms a zig-zag translucent line passing from vertex down to a variable distance.

13. Groove for middle meningeal vessels is seen as a dark line behind the coronal suture and extends to the vault of the skull.

14. Orbits casts shadow inferior to frontal air sinus and anterior to ethmoid air sinus.

15. Maxillary air sinuses are seen a translucent are below orbits.

16. Hard palate and teeth are seen below maxillary air sinuses.

17. Body and rami of mandible is seen.

18. Alveolar arches with teeth are clearly defined.

PALPATION OF ARTERIES IN BODY

Arteries of Head and Neck

Superficial Temporal Artery

- Pulsations of superficial temporal artery can be felt in front of the tragus of the ear. Here it crosses the root of zygoma. They can also be felt at the temple (Fig. 23.1).
- The course of anterior terminal branch of superficial temporal artery can clearly be seen on the forehead especially in bald men, during outbursts of anger.
- It also becomes noticeably more tortuous with increasing age.

Facial Artery

Pulsations of facial artery (Fig. 23.1) can be felt against the angle of mandible at the infero-medial border of masseter muscle. Ask the patient to clench his teeth and feel for the masseter muscle, follow it inferiorly and feel for the pulse at its anterior end, against the border of mandible.

Common Carotid Artery

Pulsations of common carotid artery (Fig. 23.1) can be felt at the level of superior border of thyroid cartilage, just in front of anterior border of sternocleidomastoid muscle.

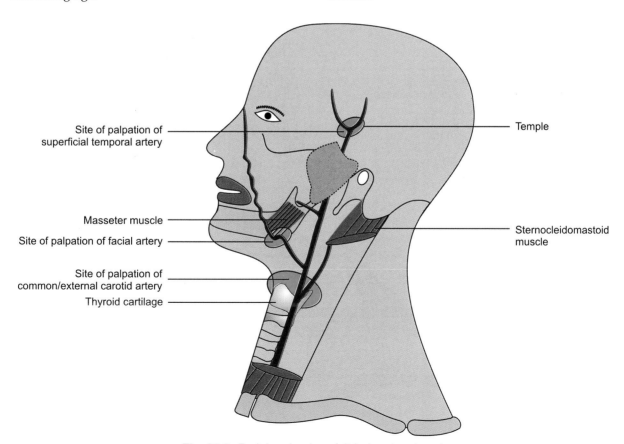

Fig. 23.1: Peripheral pulses felt in head and neck

Arteries of Upper Limb (Fig. 23.2 and 23.3)

Axillary Artery

Pulsations of axillary artery are felt in relation to lateral wall of axilla, at the junction of anterior 1/3rd and posterior 2/3rd.

Brachial Artery

Pulsations of brachial artery are felt in the cubital fossa, just medial to tendon of biceps brachii muscle. The biceps tendon can be easily felt in cubital fossa when the forearm is flexed against resistance (Fig. 23.2).

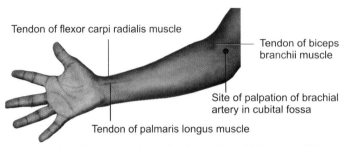

Fig. 23.2: Landmark tendons for palpation of brachial and radial arteries

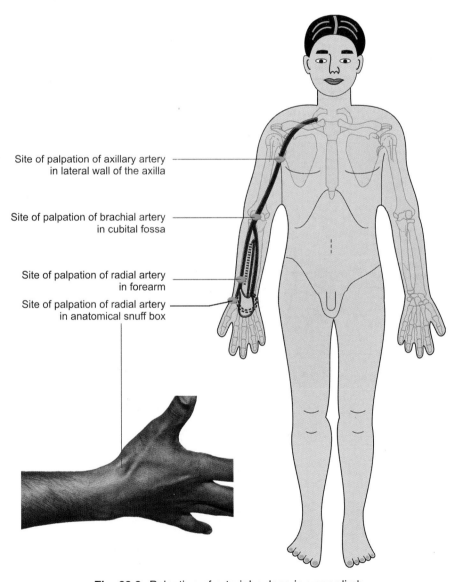

Fig. 23.3: Palpation of arterial pulses in upper limb

Radial Artery (Fig. 23.3)

Pulsations of radial artery are felt against the anterior surface of lower 1/3rd of shaft of radius in forearm, just lateral to tendon of flexor carpi radialis muscle.

Radial Artery in Anatomical Snuff Box (Fig. 23.3)

Pulsations of radial artery can be felt in the anatomical snuff box, on the lateral aspect dorsum of hand. Anatomical snuff box is a triangular depression present between tendon of extensor pollicis longus laterally and tendons of abductor pollicis and extensor pollicis brevis medially. It becomes visible when the thumb is extended.

Arteries of Abdomen (Fig. 23.4)

Abdominal Aorta

In a thin built person pulsations of abdominal aorta can be felt on deep palpation in the umbilical region.

Arteries of Lower Limb (Fig. 23.5)

Femoral Artery

Pulsations of femoral artery can be felt at the mid inguinal point, against the capsule of hip joint.

Popliteal Artery

- Pulsations of popliteal artery can be felt in the popliteal fossa in semiflexed position of knee joint.
- This artery is also used for measuring blood pressure in lower limb.

Dorsalis Pedis Artery

Pulsations of dorsalis pedis artery can be felt on the dorsum of the foot in front of ankle joint, between the tendon of extensor hallucis longus and first tendon of extensor digitorum longus. This point is about 5 cm distal to medial and lateral malleoli, over the intermediate cuneiform bone.

Posterior Tibial Artery

Pulsations of posterior tibial artery are felt behind the medial malleolus and in front of tendocalcaneus.

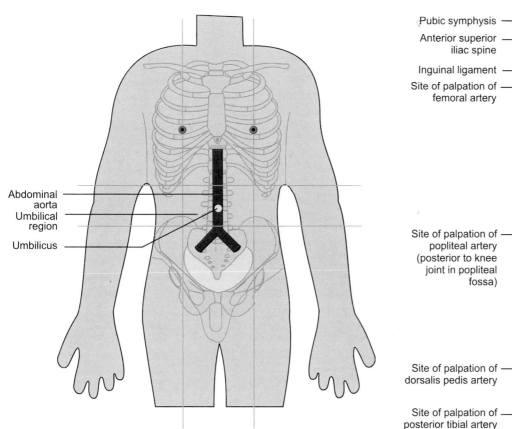

Fig. 23.4: Palpation of abdominal aorta

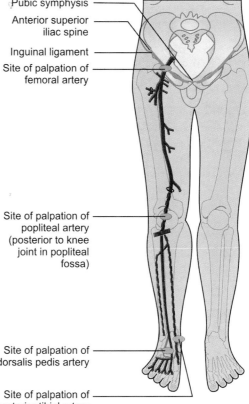

Fig. 23.5: Palpation of peripheral pulses in lower limb

Jugular Venous Pulse (JVP) (Fig. 23.6)

Atrial pressure rises during atrial systole. Further rise in pressure occurs during ventricular isovolumetric contraction, due to bulging of AV valves into the atria. Pressure falls rapidly in the atria during ventricular contraction as the AV valves are pulled down. Pressure again rises due to filling of atria till opening of AV valves. These pressure changes in the right atrium are transmitted in a retrograde manner into the superior vena cava and the internal jugular vein. The pulse of atrial pressure changes can be seen on the side of neck when an individual is placed in supine position with neck tilted up to an angle of 45°. This is known as jugular venous pulse and it has a three wave pattern as follows:

a. **a-wave:** due to atrial systole.
b. **c-wave:** due to rise in atrial pressure during isovolumetric ventricular systole.
c. **v-wave:** due to rise in atrial pressure while filling before the opening of tricuspid valve.

The usual height of JVP above sternum angle is 11 cm. It is increased and is more visible in conditions like mitral valve stenosis which results in dilatation of right atrium.

SURFACE ANATOMY OF HEART (FIG. 23.7)

It is the surface projection of the sternocostal surface of the heart.

Right Border

- Put a point 1.2 cm. lateral to the margin of sternum on the upper border of the right 3rd costal cartilage.
- Put a point in the right fourth intercostal space 3.7 cm. lateral to the median plane.
- Mark the sternal end of the right sixth costal cartilage.
  Draw a line joining these points with a gentle convexity to the right.

Lower Border

- Put a point on the sternal end of the right sixth costal cartilage.
- Mark the xiphisternal junction.
- Locate the apex beat.
  Draw a line joining these points.

Left Border

- Mark the apex beat.
- Put a point 1.2 cm. lateral to the sternal margin on the lower border of the left second costal cartilage. Join these points by a line with a gentle upward convexity.

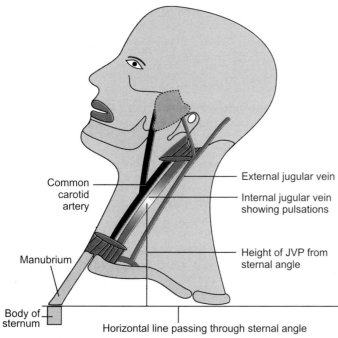

Common carotid artery

External jugular vein

Internal jugular vein showing pulsations

Height of JVP from sternal angle

Manubrium

Body of sternum

Horizontal line passing through sternal angle

Fig. 23.6: Measurement of JVP

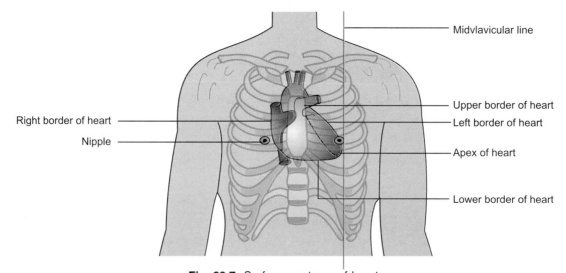

Midvlavicular line

Right border of heart

Nipple

Upper border of heart

Left border of heart

Apex of heart

Lower border of heart

Fig. 23.7: Surface anatomy of heart

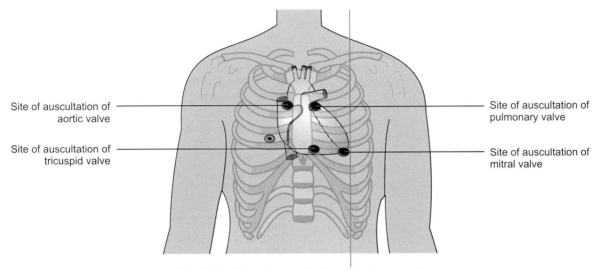

Fig. 23.8: Sites of auscultation of valve sounds

Upper Border

Join the upper ends of the right and left borders.

SITES OF AUSCULTATION OF HEART SOUNDS (FIG. 23.8)

The heart sounds are produced by closure of the various valves of the heart.

1. **Aortic valve sound:** It is heard in the right 2nd intercostal space, just next to the lateral margin of sternum.
2. **Pulmonary valve sound:** It is heard in the left 2nd intercostal space, just next to the lateral margin of sternum.
3. **Tricuspid valve sound:** It is heard in the left 5th intercostal space, just next to the lateral margin of sternum.
4. **Mitral valve sound:** It is heard at the apex of heart in the left 5th intercostal space, in midclavicular line.

On auscultation of heart, primarily two heart sound are heard namely, LUB (S1) followed by DUB (S2). First heart sound (S1) occurs due to simultaneous closure of atrioventricular valves and second heart sound (S2) occurs due to simultaneous closure of aortic and pulmonary valves.

SURFACE LANDMARKS OF ANTERIOR CHEST WALL AND ABDOMINAL WALL

Bony Landmarks of Anterior Chest Wall

Suprasternal notch: As a finger is slipped down along midline of neck, a depression is felt over superior aspect of manubrium. This is the suprasternal notch.

Sternal angle: As a finger is slipped down from suprasternal notch over manubrium sterni, a bony prominence is felt about 2.5 cm below it which is the sternal angle. This corresponds to lower border of T4 vertebra posteriorly.

The second costal cartilage is at level of sternal angle and lower ribs can be counted from this point.

Xiphisternum: As a finger is slipped downwards along the midline of sternum, the lowest bony point beyond which there is a depression is xiphisternum.

Costal margin: The costal margin can be traced as a bony margin from each side of xiphisternum passing the finger downwards and laterally.

Bony Landmarks of Abdomen and Pelvis

The upper limit of abdomen anteriorly is costal margin. The lower limit of abdomen presents the following bony landmarks:

1. **Pubic symphysis:** As a finger is passed downwards along the midline of anterior abdominal wall, the first bony prominence felt is the pubic symphysis.
2. **Pubic crest:** It may be felt as a small bony margin just lateral to pubic symphysis on each side.
3. **Pubic tubercle:** As the finger is passed laterally from pubic symphysis, a bony projection is felt about 2.5 cm lateral to it which is pubic tubercle. This rounded projection at the lateral end of pubic crest can be felt in obese individuals also.
4. **Anterior superior iliac spine:** Place your hand on the waist and slide the finger down, the bony prominence felt in front above the groin, is anterior superior iliac spine.
5. **Iliac crest:** It is a curved bony margin felt passing backwards from anterior superior iliac spine when the hand is kept on the waist.
6. **Posterior superior iliac spine:** A dimple is seen on back, on each side of vertebral spine, just above the buttocks. The posterior superior iliac spine lies underneath this dimple.

7. **Spine of S$_2$ vertebrae:** The line joining the two dimples passes through the spine of S$_2$ vertebra.

Soft Tissue Landmarks on Anterior Abdominal Wall

1. **Umbilicus:** It is the midline depression or defect in anterior abdominal wall, usually at the midpoint of a line joining xiphisternum and pubic symphysis. This corresponds to level of intervertebral disc of L$_3$ and L$_4$ vertebrae. It is lower in children and in obese individuals.
2. **Linea alba:** It is a midline raphe passing from xiphisternum to pubic symphysis which may be felt as a slight depression, more prominent above the level of umbilicus. The linea alba is seen better in muscular individuals.
3. **Linea semilunaris:** It corresponds to the lateral border of rectus abdominis muscle. It is marked as a line joining the tip of ninth costal cartilage to the pubic tubercle with a gentle convexity facing laterally. It is also better visible in muscular individuals.
4. **Midpoint of inguinal ligament:** It is the midpoint of a line joining the anterior superior iliac spine and the pubic tubercle. It corresponds to the deep inguinal ring.
5. **Mid inguinal point:** It is the midpoint of a line joining anterior superior iliac spine and the pubic symphysis. It corresponds to the site of origin of femoral artery.
6. **Mc Burney's Point (Fig. 23.9):** This point correspond to the junction of upper 2/3rd and lower 1/3rd of a line drawn from the right anterior superior iliac spine to the umbilicus. It is the usual site of referred pain of appendicitis.

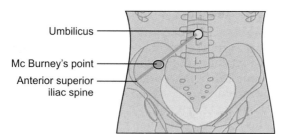

Fig. 23.9: Mc Burney's point

QUADRANTS AND PLANES OF ABDOMEN

For descriptive purposes the anterior abdominal wall is divided into four quadrants by a vertical midline and a horizontal line perpendicular to midline which passes through the umbilicus. The four quadrants are:
1. Upper right quadrant
2. Upper left quadrant
3. Lower right quadrant
4. Lower left quadrant

The anterior abdominal wall is also divided into nine regions for purpose of clinical description by two horizontal lines and two verticals lines.

Horizontal lines are:
1. Line joining the lowest point on costal margin on each side: corresponds to 10th costal cartilages.
2. Line joining the tubercles of iliac crest on each side, intertubercular line. Each tubercle of iliac crest may be felt or marked, as a bony point on iliac crest, 5 cm posterior to anterior superior iliac spine.

Vertical lines are lines passing vertically down from midpoint of clavicle on each side.

The nine regions of abdomen are:
1. Right hypochondrium
2. Epigastric region
3. Left hypochondrium
4. Right lumbar region
5. Umbilical region
6. Left lumbar region
7. Right iliac fossa
8. Hypogastric region
9. Left iliac fossa

Planes of Abdomen (Fig. 23.10)

The abdomen can be studied by the following horizontal and vertical planes.

Horizontal Planes

1. **Subcostal plane:** It is a horizontal plane passing anteroposteriorly from a line joining the lowest points of costal margins of each side. This corresponds to the 10th costal cartilage. The plane passes posteriorly through the lower border of L$_2$ vertebra.
   Clinical significance: It passes through the origin of inferior mesenteric artery and third part of duodenum.
2. **Trans-tubercular plane:** It is a horizontal plane passing antero-posteriorly from a line joining the two tubercles of iliac crest. Posteriorly, the plane passes through upper border of L$_5$ vertebra.
   Clinical significance: It passes the origin of inferior vena cava, joining of common iliac crest.
3. **Transpyloric plane:** It is a horizontal plane passing antero-posteriorly midway between suprasternal notch of manubrium and upper border of pubic symphysis. Anteriorly it passes through the tips of 9th costal cartilages while posteriorly, it passes at the lower border of L$_1$ vertebra.
   Clinical significance: This plane passes through:
   a. Pylorus of stomach

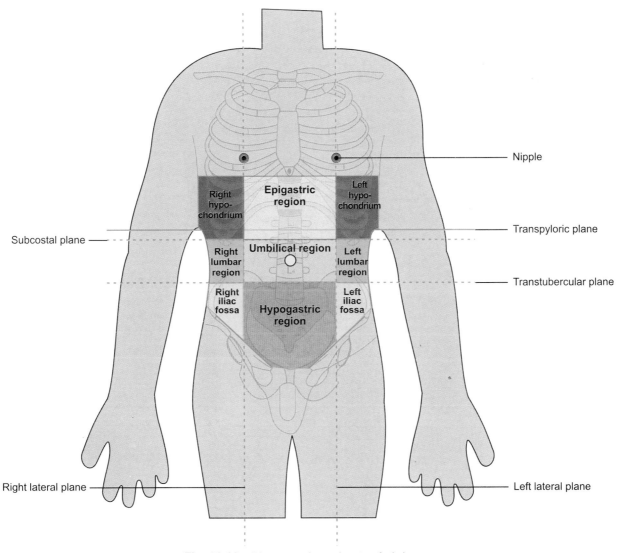

Fig. 23.10: Planes and quadrants of abdomen

b. Origin of superior mesenterior artery
c. Formation of portal vein
d. Hilum of kidneys
e. Head and neck of pancreas
f. Termination of spinal cord

Vertical Planes

1. Midsagittal plane: It is a midline vertical plane passing through a line joining midpoint of sternal notch of manubrium sterni and pubic symphysis.
2. Paramedian or right and left lateral vertical plane – These are vertical planes on either side, passing anteroposteriorly from a line joining midpoint of clavicle, and midinguinal point (midpoint of a line joining anterior superior iliac spine and pubic symphysis). It passes just lateral to tip of 9th costal cartilage.

DISPOSITION OF INTRA-ABDOMINAL VISCERA (FIGs 23.11 to 23.16)

Stomach (Fig. 23.11)

- It is placed on left upper quadrant of abdomen. It extends between epigastrium, left hypochondrium and umbilical regions.
- The upper or cardiac and is located 2.5 cm to left of median plane, at the level of 7th costal cartilage.
- The lower or pyloric is located 1.2 cm to right of median plane, on the transpyloric plane.

Duodenum (Fig. 23.12)

- It lies in the upper half of umbilical region.
- 1st part starts from pyloric end of stomach and extends along the tranpyloric plane for 2.5 cm to right.

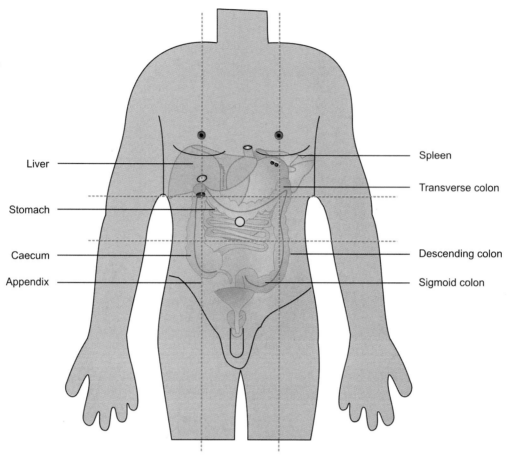

Fig. 23.11: Disposition of abdominal viscera

- 2nd part curves downwards, vertically to end 7.5 cm below the right end of the 1st part.
- 3rd part lies on the subcostal plane and extends from lower end of 2nd part crossing the midline to the left just above umblicus.
- 4th part curves upto 1 cm below the transpyloric plane from the 3rd part.

Liver (Figs 23.11, 23.12)

- It mostly lies in the right hypochondrium and is present behind the lower five ribs and the corresponding costal cartilages. The left lobe extends to the epigastrium and a little part lies in the left hypochondrium also.
- The lower edge may be just palpable below the left costal margin normally, especially in children.

Spleen (Figs 23.11, 23.12)

- It lies the left hypochondrium with the posterior end extending into the epigastric region.
- It lies horizontally at the level of spine of T_{10} vertebra, behind the 9th, 10th and 11th ribs on left side.

Caecum (Figs 23.11 and 23.12)

- It lies in the rigth iliac fossa.

Appendix (Fig. 23.12)

- It lies in the right iliac fossa.
- The base of appendix usually lies at the point of junction of upper 2/3rd and lower 1/3rd of a line joining umbilicus to right anterior superior iliac spine.

Ascending Colon (Fig. 23.15)

It extends up from the right iliac fossa at the level of transtubercular plane and passes vertically up in right lumbar region to right hypochondrium till the tip of 9th costal cartilage. The upper end correspondes to the hepatic flexure of colon.

Transverse Colon (Fig. 23.12)

It extends from the right hypochondrium to the left hypochondrium and hangs down as a loop. The lowest end of loop may reach upto the umbilicus.

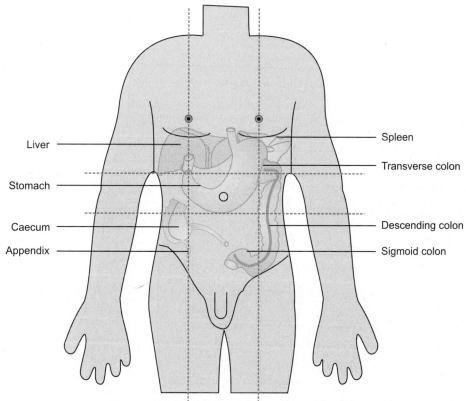

Fig. 23.12: Disposition of abdominal viscera

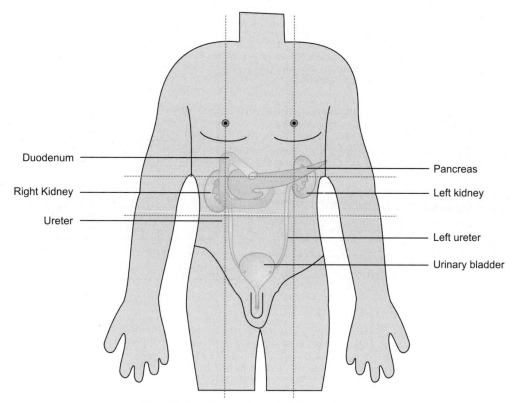

Fig. 23.13: Disposition of abdominal viscera

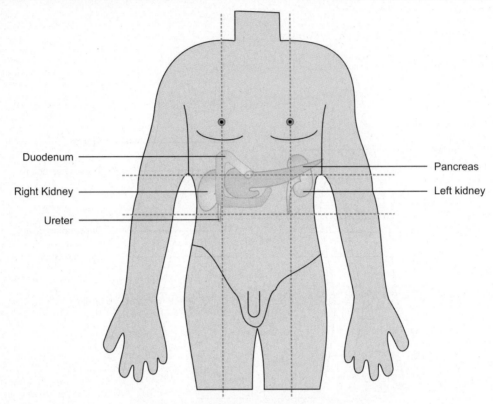

Fig. 23.14: Disposition of abdominal viscera

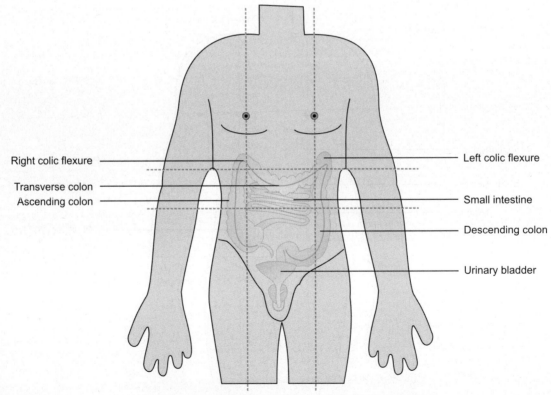

Fig. 23.15: Disposition of abdominal and pelvic viscera

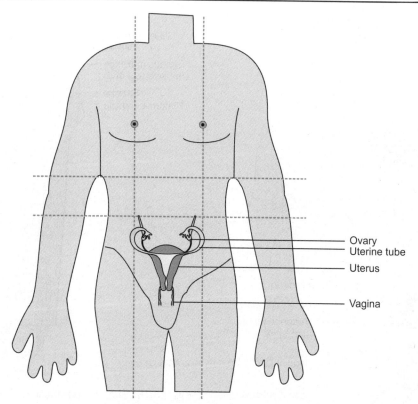

Fig. 23.16: Disposition of female reproductive organs

Descending Colon (Fig. 23.12)

It extends vertically down from the left end of transverse colon (splenic flexure) in left hypochondrium at level of 8th costal cartilage. It passes along left lumbar region till left iliac fossa.

Pancreas (Fig. 23.14)

It lies in the C-shaped curve of duodenum. It extends from the epigastrium to the left hypochondrium, at the level of transpyloric plane.

Kidneys (Figs 23.13, 23.14)

The right kidney lies slightly lower than the left due to presence of liver in the right hypochondrium.
  a. **Right kidney:** It lies in the right hypochondrium and right lumbar regions and extends medially into epigastric and umbilical regions. The transpyloric plane passes through upper end of its hilum.
  b. **Left kidney:** It lies in the left hypochondrium and left lumbar regions and extends medially into the epigastric and umbilical regions. The transpyloric plane passes through lower end of its hilum.

Urinary Bladder (Figs 23.13 and 23.15)

It lies in true pelvis behind pubic symphysis. When distended it extends into the hypogastric region of abdomen.

Uterus (Fig. 23.16)

It lies in the pelvic cavity between urinary bladder and rectum. During pregnancy it enlarges to become an abdominal organ.

Ovary (Fig. 23.16)

Ovaries lie in ovarian fossa one on each side of uterus in lesser pelvis.

SITES OF INTRAMUSCULAR INJECTION
Deltoid Muscle

Intramuscular injection is given in the lower half of deltoid muscle to prevent damage to axillary nerve (Fig. 23.17).

Gluteus Medius Muscle

Intramuscular injection is given in the outer and upper quadrant of gluteal region, in gluteus medius muscle. This minimizes any risk to sciatic nerve (Fig. 23.18).

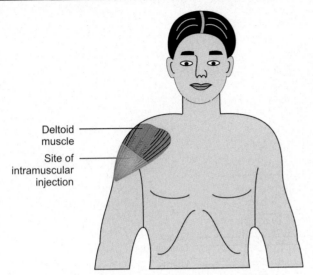

Fig. 23.17: Site of intramuscular injection

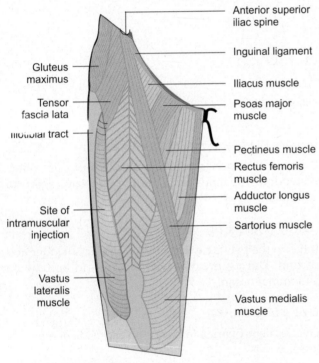

Fig. 23.19: Site of intramuscular injection in thigh

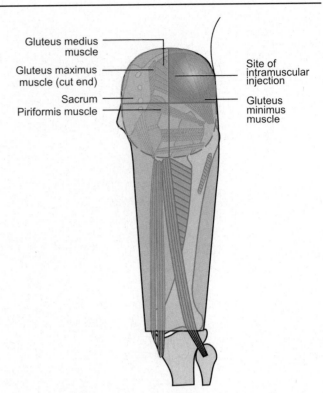

Fig. 23.18: Site of intramuscular injection in gluteal region

Hence, it does not slip away when intravenous injections are given. It acts as lifeline in emergency conditions to give intravenous injections and fluids. It is the most common site used for cardiac catheterization.

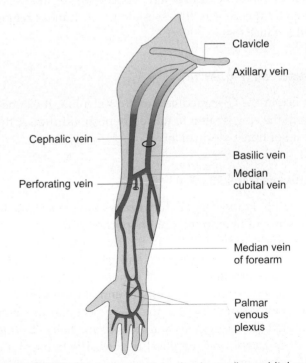

Fig. 23.20: Site of intravenous injection in median cubital vein

Vastus Lateralis Muscle

Intramuscular injection is given in vastus lateralis muscle in thigh. This is the preferred site in children (Fig. 23.19).

SITE OF INTRAVENOUS INJECTION (FIG. 23.20)

Median Cubital Vein

Median cubital vein is connected to the deep veins of the upper limb through a perforator which fixes it.

APPENDIX

BLOOD PRESSURE

Normal adult: 120 / 80 mmHg
Blood pressure above 140/90 is generally considered high, i.e., hypertension

HEART RATE

At rest	:	60 to 80 beats/min
Sinus bradycardia	:	< 60 beats/min
Sinus tachycardia	:	> 100 beats/min

RESPIRATION

Respiratory rate (at rest)	:	15 to 18 / min
Tidal volume	:	500 ml
Dead space	:	150 ml
Alveolar ventilation	:	5 to 6 l/min

pH (HYDROGEN ION CONCENTRATION)

Neutral	:	7
Acid	:	0 to 7
Alkaline	:	7 to 14

Normal pH of Various Body Fluids

Blood	:	7.35 to 7.45
Saliva	:	5.8 to 7.4
Gastric juice	:	1.5 to 3.5
Bile	:	6.0 to 8.5
Urine	:	4.5 to 8.0

BLOOD/SERUM LEVELS OF IMPORTANT MOLECULES AND IONS (IN ADULTS)

Fasting glucose	:	65 to 106 mg/100 ml
2 hr. PP glucose	:	106 to 140 mg/100 ml
Urea	:	15 to 45 mg/100 ml
Creatinine	:	0.5 to 1.2 mg/100 ml
Uric acid	:	2.5 to 6.5 mg/100 ml
Cholesterol	:	150 to 200 mg/100 ml
Calcium	:	8.5 to 10.5 mg/100 ml
Phosphorus	:	2.5 to 4.5 mg/100 ml
Sodium	:	135 to 143 mEq/l
Chloride	:	97 to 110 mEq/l
Potassium	:	3.5 to 4.5 mEq/l

ARTERIAL BLOOD GASES

PO_2	12 to 15 kPa	(90 to 110 mm Hg)
PCO_2	4.5 to 6 kPa	(40 to 46 mm Hg)
Bicarbonate	21 to 27.5 mmol/l	
H^+ ions	36 to 44 nmol/l	(pH = 7.35 to 7.45)

BLOOD COUNT
RBC Count

In female	:	3.8 to 5×10^{12} /l
In male	:	4.5 to 6.5×10^{12} /l

Platelet Count

Normal value	:	150 to 400×10^9 /l

WBC Count

Total WBC count	:	4 to 11×10^9/l
Neutrophils	:	2.5 to 7.5×10^9/l (40 to 75%)
Lymphocytes	:	1.5 to 3.5×10^9 /l (20 to 45%)
Eosinophils	:	0.04 to 0.44×10^9/l (0 to 6%)
Monocytes	:	0.2 to 0.8×10^9 /l (1 to 10%)
Basophils	:	0.015 to 0.1×10^9/l (0 to 1%)

ESR

In female	:	0 to 20 mm in first hr.
In male	:	0 to 10 mm in first hr.

DIET

1 kilocalorie (kcal) corresponds to 4.182 kilojoules (kJ)
1 kilojoule corresponds to 0.24 kilocalories

Energy source	Energy released	Recommended proportion in diet
Carbohydrate	1g = 17 kJ = 4 kcal	55 to 75%
Protein	1g = 17 kJ = 4 kcal	10 to 15%
Fat	1g = 38 kJ = 9 kcal	15 to 30%

URINE

Urine volume	:	1000 to 1500 ml / day
Specific gravity	:	1.020 to 1.030

Glucose, proteins, ketone bodies and blood are normally absent.

BODY TEMPERATURE

Normal	:	36.6 to 37.2°C (98.0 to 98.8°F)
Fever	:	> 37.2°C (99°F)
Hypothermia	:	Core temperature ≤ 35°C
Death	:	Core temperature ≤ 25°C

MISCELLANEOUS

Cerebrospinal fluid pressure	:	60 to 180 mm H_2O (when lying on the side)
Intraocular pressure	:	10 to 20 mmHg

INDEX

A

A-band 159
Abdomen 60
Abdominal aorta 410
Abdominal cavity 65
Abducent nerve 272
Abduction 15
Abductor digit minimia muscle 191, 202
Abductor hallucis muscle 202
Abductor pollicis brevis muscle 191
Abductor pollicis longus muscle 190
Aberrant obturator artery 98, 421
Absorption 482
Accessory azygos vein 435
Accessory lacrimal glands 322
Accessory nerve 280
Accessory obturator nerve 249
Accommodation 349
Acetabulum 130
Achalasia cardia 528
Acidophilic structures 43
Acquired immunity 475, 476
Acrocentric chromosome 610
Acromegaly 567
Acromioclavicular joint 141
Acromion process 127
ACTH 554
Action potential 206
Active transport 18
Addison's disease 570
Adductor brevis muscle 88, 196
Adductor canal 87
Adductor hallucis muscle 202
Adductor longus muscle 88, 196
Adductor magnus muscle 88, 196
Adductor pollicis muscle 191
Adenoids 389
ADH 555
Adipocytes 31
Adipose tissue 32
Adrenal androgens 563
Adrenal cortex 563
Adrenal medulla 563
Adventitious bursa 34
Ageusia 350
Aglossia 527
AIDS 480
Air embolism 451
Alleles 615
Amino acid derivatives 551
Amniocentesis 618
Amygdaloid body 220
Anabolism 523
Anal canal 505, 511
Anal triangle 71

Analgesia 317
Anaphase 24
Anatome 3
Anatomical planes 12
Anatomical position 11
Anatomical position of heart 395
Anatomical snuff box 81
Anconeus muscle 190
Android pelvis 137, 138
Anemia 460
Aneuploidy 611
Angiotensin II 443
Ankle joint 147, 150
Anosmia 350
Anteflexion 574
Antegrade degeneration 242
Anterior 13
Anterior abdominal wall 60
Anterior cervical nodes 471
Anterior commissure 219
Anterior corticospinal tract 309
Anterior cranial fossa 109
Anterior crural compartment 89
Anterior ethmoidal nerve 269
Anterior fontanelle 113
Anterior mediastinum 59
Anterior nasal spine 105
Anterior spinocerebellar tract or
     pathway 240, 296
Anterior spinothalamic tract 240, 293
Anterior superior alveolar nerve 269
Anterior tibial artery 90, 426
Anterior triangle of neck 55
Anteversion 574
Anthropoid pelvis 137, 138
Anticlotting mechanism in blood 459
Antidiuretic hormone 555
Antidromic conduction 206
Anuria 548
Aorta 408
Aortic body 386
Aortic vestibule 399
Ape-like hand 285
Aplastic anemia 460
Apnea 391
Apneustic centre 386
Apocrine gland 29, 604
Apoptosis 26
Appendicular skeleton 101
Appendix 503, 511
Aqueous humor 329
Arachnoid mater 209
Arachnoid villi and granulations 211
Arch of aorta 409
Arches of foot 94
Archicerebellum 234

Area for taste 217
Areola 582
Argentaffin cells 508
Arm 76, 79
Arrector pili muscle 604
Arterial pulse 406
Arteries 440
Arterioles 440
Arthritis 153
Arthrography 155
Articular genu 196
Arytenoid cartilages 363
Ascending aorta 409
Ascending colon 503
Ascites 97
ASD or atrial septal defect 449
Asphyxia 391
Association fibres 217, 218
Asterion 106
Asthma 392
Astigmatism 349
Astrocytes 209
Atavistic epiphysis 38
Athetosis 243
Atlanto-axial joint 152
Atlanto-occipital joint 152
Atrial arrythmias 450
Atrial systole 405
Atrio-ventricular block 449
Atrio-ventricular node 403
Atrium 396
Auditory pathway 317, 342
Auriculotemporal nerve 271, 299
Auscultation of heart 406, 632
Autoimmune diseases 479
Autonomic nervous system 204, 310
Autoregulation 443
Autosomal dominant inheritance 617
Autosomal recessive inheritance 617
Axial skeleton 101
Axilla 77
Axillary artery 417
Axillary group of lymph nodes 473
Axillary nerve 249, 251
Axillary tail of spence 582
Axillary vein 433
Axons 205
Azospermia 600
Azygos vein 435

B

Babinski's sign 319
Back of neck 57
Ball and socket joint 140
Baroreceptors 444

Barr bodies 22
Bartholin's glands 572
Basal ganglia 219, 306
Basal metabolic rate 523
Basilic vein 434
Basophilic structures 43
Basophils 457
Bell's palsy 288
Beri-beri 530
Biaxial joint 140
Biceps brachii muscle 187
Biceps femoris muscle 199
Bifid tongue 527
Bile canalculi 516
Bile duct 517
Bilroth's cords 468
Binocular vision 332
Bipennate muscle 158
Black eye 95
Blastocele 596
Blastocyst 595
Blood 453
Blood brain barrier 446
Blood flow dynamics 440
Blood groups 455
Blood pressure 441
Bohr's effect 385
Bones 36
Bony labyrinth 339
Bony orbit 323
Bony pelvis 135
Botulin toxin 242
Brachial artery 418
Brachial plexus 246, 247
Brachial veins 434
Brachialis muscle 187
Brachiocephalic vein 429
Brachioradialis muscle 189
Bradyapnea 391
Brain stem 307
Bregma 103
Bright-field microscope 44
Broad ligament 574
Broca's speech area 215
Brodmann's classification 242
Bronchial tree 369
Bronchoconstriction reflex 387
Brunner's glands 511
Buccal nerve 271
Buccal nodes 471
Buccinator muscle 168, 495
Bucket handle movement 380
Bulbo-spongiosus muscle 181
Bulbourethral or Cowper's glands 592
Bulbs of vestibule 572
Bursa 34

C

Caecum 502
Calcaneocuboid joint 147

Calcitonin 559, 566
Calcium metabolism 564
Caldwell position 625
Calf pump 439
Canines 484
Capacitation 592
Capillaries 440
Capillary circulation 442
Caput 95
Cardiac cycle 405
Cardiac failure 452
Cardiac muscle 161, 162, 165
Cardiac output 407
Cardiac plexus 403
Cardiovascular system 6, 393
Carotid body 386, 410
Carotid sheath 53
Carotid sinus 410
Carotid triangle 55
Carpal bones 129
Carpal tunnel syndrome 285
Carpometa carpal joint 141
Carrier gene 615
Carrier proteins 19
Carrying angle 97
Cartilage 34
Cartilaginous joints 139
Cartilaginous ossification 41
Catabolism 523
Cataract 349
Cauda equina 238
Caudate nucleus 219
Cavernous sinus 211, 432
Cell 17
Cell coat 18
Cell cycle 22, 23
Cell division 23
Cell membrane 17
Cellular or cell mediated
    immunity 476
Cementum 484
Central nervous system 203
Centriole 21
Centromere 610
Cephalhaematoma 95
Cephalic vein 434
Cerebellar nuclei 236
Cerebellum 234, 307
Cerebral circulation 445
Cerebral cortex 297
Cerebral hemispheres 213
Cerebrospinal fluid 211
Cerebrum 306
Ceruminosis 349
Cervical pleura 375
Cervical plexus 246
Cervical spinal nerves 246
Cervical vertebrae 119
Cervix 573
Chalazion 347

Cheeks 483
Chemoreceptor trigger zone 317
Chemoreceptors 291, 444
Chief cells or Zymogen cells 508
Cholecystectomy 529
Cholecystokinin (CCK) 522
Chondroblasts 34
Chondrocytes 34
Chorda tympani nerve 275, 487
Chordae tendinae 398
Chorea 243
Chorionic villus biopsy or
    sampling 618
Choroid 327
Choroid plexus 211
Chromatids 610
Chromatin fibre 609
Chromosomal abnormalities 611
Chromosomes 21, 609
Chvostek's sign 570
Chylothorax 391, 479
Chyluria 479
Cilia 21
Ciliary body 327
Ciliary ganglion 265
Circle of Willis 416
Circulation of CSF 212
Circumduction 16
Circumflex humeral artery 251
Cisterna chyli 464
Claustrum 220
Clavicle 125
Clavipectoral fascia 77
Claw hand 284
Cleavage divisions 595
Cleft lip 527, 528
Cleft palate 528
Clinical anatomy 10
Clitoris 572
Clivus 110
Cloquet's gland 475
Clotting of blood 459
Co-arctation of aorta 449
Coccygeal plexus 246, 251
Coccygeal spinal nerve 246
Coccygeus muscle 180
Coccyx 122
Cochlea 339
Cochlear duct 340
Co-dominant genes 615
Coeliac trunk 421
Collagen fibres 32
Collecting tubules 535
Colles fascia 73
Colles fracture 154
Colour vision 332
Columnar epithelium 27
Comedone (Acne) 606
Commissural fibres 217, 218
Common carotid artery 410

Common iliac artery 423
Common peroneal nerve 260
Compact bone 39, 36
Comparative anatomy 10
Compartments of eye ball 329
Complement system 478
Composition of body 49
Compound action potentials 206
Compound glands 30
Compound microscope 44
Compound tubular gland 31
Computed tomography 623
Concha 334
Conducting system of heart 403
Condylar joint 140
Cones 330
Congenital adrenal hyperplasia 570
Conjoint tendon 62
Conjunctiva 322
Connective tissue 31
Constipation 529
Constrictor muscles of the pharynx 360
Constrictor pupillae 328
Contralateral 14
Conus medullaris 238
Coraco-acrominal arch 142
Coracobrachialis muscle 187
Coracoid process 127
Cordocentesis 618
Cornea 327
Corneal reflex pathway 332
Corniculate cartilages 363
Corona radiata 218
Coronal 12
Coronal suture 103, 105
Coronary angiography 450
Coronary circulation 444
Coronary sinus 402
Coronoid process 129
Corpus callosum 219
Corpus striatum 219
Corticospinal tract 241, 309
Corticotropes 553
Costal cartilages 125
Costal pleura 375
Costocervical trunk 416
Coughing and sneezing reflexes 387
Counter irritants 317
Counter–current mechanism 545
Cranio-sacral outflow 314
Cremaster muscle 177
Crenitism 568
Cribriform fascia 85
Cricoid cartilage 363
Cricothyroid membrane 364
Crico-tracheal ligament 364
Cruciate muscle 158
Crus cerebri 227
Crux of the heart 400
Cryptorchidism 600

Crypts of Leiberkuhn 511
Cubital fossa 80
Cubital tunnel syndrome 284
Cuboid 135
Cuneiform bone 135
Cuneiform cartilages 363
Cushing's syndrome 570
Cutaneous nerve supply of body 292
Cutaneous receptors 292
Cyanosis 392
Cystic duct 517
Cystitis 548
Cystoscopy 547
Cytogenetics 609
Cytokines 478
Cytoplasm 17, 20
Cytoskeleton 21
Cytotoxic T-lymphocytes 478

D

Dacryocystitis 347
Dangerous layer of the scalp 51
Dark adaptation 331
Deep 14
Deep cervical fascia 51
Deep cervical lymph nodes 470
Deep fascia 42
Deep inguinal ring 61
Deep palmar arch 420
Deep perineal space 74
Deep peroneal nerve 261, 305
Deep transverse perinei muscle 181
Defecation reflex 513
Deglutition reflex or swallowing 389
Dehydration 43
Deltoid muscle 78, 185
Demilunes 493
Dendrites 205
Denner-London system 611
Dense irregular connective tissue 32
Dental caries 527
Dentine 484
Depression 16
Dermatomes 301
Dermis 603
Descendens cervicalis nerve 246
Descending aorta 410
Descending colon 503
Developmental anatomy 10
Diabetes mellitus 569
Diakinesis 26
Diaphragm 379
Diaphragma sellae 210
Diaphragmatic pleura 376
Diaphysis 38
Diarrhea 529
Diarthroses 138
Diastole 406
Diencephalon 220

Dietary fibre 527
Digastric muscle 171
Digastric triangle 55
Digestion 482
Digestive system 481
Digital synovial sheaths 83
Digital vascular imaging 623
Dilator pupillae 328
Diplotene 26
Direct inguinal hernia 96
Dislocation of joint 153
Distal 14
Distal convoluted tubule 534
DNA 614
Dominant gene 615
Dorsal 13
Dorsal digital expansion 192
Dorsal interossei 192, 202
Dorsal nerve of perineum 251
Dorsal nucleus of vagus 279
Dorsal ramus 246
Dorsal root of spinal nerve 245
Dorsal scapular artery 416
Dorsal scapular nerve 249
Dorsal subaponeurotic space 83
Dorsal subcutaneous space 83
Dorsal thalamus 220
Dorsal venous arch 434
Dorsalis pedis artery 426
Dorsum of foot 91
Dorsum of hand 81
Down's syndrome 612
Duct of Santorini 518
Duct of Wirsung 518
Duodenum 500, 501
Dupuytren's contracture 96
Duramater 209
Dysgeusia 350
Dysmetria 244
Dysosmia 350
Dyspnea 391

E

Ear 333
Ear ossicles 338
ECF volume 547
ECG 404
Ectopic excitation 450
Edema 452
Effector organ 309
Ejaculatory ducts 588
Elastic cartilage 36
Elastic fibres 32
Elbow 141
Elbow joint 144
Electrocardiogram 403
Electron microscope 46
Electrotonic potential 207
Elevation 16

Ellipsoid joint 140
Emboli 462
Enamel 484
Endochondral ossification 41
Endocrine glands 29, 551
Endocrine system 6, 551
Endocytosis 19
Endometriosis 599
Endomysium 159
Endoplasmic reticulum 20
Endothelins 443
Energy balance 523
Energy requirement 526
Energy transfer 523
Eosinophilia 457
Eosinophils 456, 457
Eosionopenia 457
Ependymal cells 209
Epidermis 601
Epididymis 586
Epigastric region 634
Epiglottis 362
Epimysium 159
Epiphyseal arteries 39
Epiphyseal cartilage 38
Epiphysis 38
Epiploic foramen 71
Episiotomy 599
Epithalamus 220
Epithelial tissue 27, 28
Erb's duchenne palsy 284
Erb's point 283
Erector spinae muscle 65, 175
Eruption of teeth 485
Erythroblastosis fetalis 462
Erythrocyte sedimentation rate 454
Erythropoesis 455
Erythropoietin 566
Esophagus 497, 508, 512
Essential amino acids 525
Estrogen 578
Ethmoid bone 117
Ethmoidal air sinuses 357
Euchromatin 21, 609
Eversion of foot 16
Exocrine glands 29
Exocytosis 19
Exons 615
Exophthalmos 568
Experimental anatomy 10
Expiration 381
Expiratory capacity 381
Expiratory reserve volume 381
Extension 15
Extensor carpi radialis brevis muscle 189
Extensor carpi radialis longus muscle 189
Extensor carpi ulnaris muscle 190
Extensor digiti minimi muscle 190
Extensor digitorum muscle 190
Extensor digitorum brevis muscle 199

Extensor digitorum longus
    muscle 89, 199
Extensor hallucis longus muscle 89, 199
Extensor indicis muscle 190
Extensor pollicis brevis muscle 190
Extensor pollicis longus muscle 190
Extensor retinaculum 80
External 13
External auditory/acoustic meatus 335
External carotid artery 410
External ear 333, 334
External iliac artery 424
External intercostal muscle 377
External jugular vein 429
External nasal nerve 299
External nose 352
External oblique muscle 61, 177
Exteroceptors 292
Extorsion 326
Extra hepatic biliary system 517
Extra pyramidal tract 307
Extracellular fluid 49
Eye ball 326
Eye movements 333
Eyelids 321

F

Face 51
Facial artery 411
Facial expression 170
Facial nerve 273
Facilitated diffusion 18
Fallopian tube 575
False or greater pelvis 135
False ribs 123
Falx cerebelli 210
Falx cerebri 209
Falx inguinalis 62
Fascia 42
Fascia adherens 22
Fascia lata 85
Fascia of Zuckerkendl 532
Fascia transversalis 61
Fasciculus cuneatus 241
Fasciculus gracilis 241
Female gamete 594
Female reproductive system 571
Female urethra 541
Femoral artery 424
Femoral canal 86
Femoral hernia 97
Femoral nerve 249, 256
Femoral sheath 86
Femoral triangle 87
Femoral vein 439
Femur 132
Fenestra vestibuli 338
Fertilization 595
Fetal circulation 448

Fetoplacental circulation 447
Fetoscopy 618
Fibroblasts 31
Fibrous flexor sheath of digits 82
Fibrous pericardium 393
Fibula 134
Fibular border 14
Filariasis 452, 479
Filtration 20
Fimbria 218
Fingerprinting 606
First cervical vertebra 119
Flagellum 21
Flat bones 37
Flat foot 154
Flexion 15
Flexor digitorum superficialis muscle 188
Fleexor carpi radialis muscle 188
Flexor carpi ulnaris muscle 188
Flexor digiti minimi muscle 191
Flexor digiti minimi brevis muscle 202
Flexor digitorum accessorius muscle 202
Flexor digitorum brevis muscle 202
Flexor digitorum longus
    muscle 90, 91, 201
Flexor digitorum profundus muscle 188
Flexor hallucis brevis muscle 202
Flexor hallucis longus muscle 90, 91, 201
Flexor pollicis brevis muscle 191
Flexor pollicis longus muscle 188
Flexor retinaculum 81, 92
Floating ribs 123
Fontanelles 112
Foot 91
Foot drop 286
Foramen of Magendie 213
Forced expiratory volume in one
    second (FEV$_1$) 382
Forearm 80
Foramen of Luschka 213
Fornices of vagina 576
Fornix 218
Fossa of Rosenmuller 359
Fourth ventricle 213
Fracture 153
Frank-Starling law of heart 166
Free nerve endings 292
Frenulum linguae 486
Front of thigh 86
Frontal air sinuses 357
Frontal bone 115, 214
Frozen shoulder 154
FSH (Follicle stimulating hormone) 553
Functional anatomy 10
Functional residual capacity 382

G

Galea aponeurotica 50
Gall bladder 517, 518

Ganglion nodosum 279
Gap junctions 22
Gas exchange 384
Gastric inhibitory polypeptide (GIP) 522
Gastrin 522
Gastrocnemius muscle 90, 200
Gastrointestinal or digestive
    system 8, 481
Gastrosplenic ligament 70, 467
Genes 615
Genioglossus muscle 486
Geniohyoid muscle 171
Genitofemoral nerve 249, 305
Gingiva 483
Glands 29
Glaucoma 349
Glenohumeral joint 141
Glenoid labrum 142
Glial cells 209
Gliding 141
Gliosis 242
Globus pallidus 219
Glomerular filtration rate 541
Glomerulus 534
Glossopharyngeal nerve 276
Glucocorticoids 563
Glucose reabsorption 542
Gluteal region 88
Gluteus maximus muscle 197
Gluteus medius muscle 197
Gluteus minimus muscle 197
Golfer's elbow 155
Golgi apparatus 20
Golgi tendon organ 310
Gomphosis 138
Gonadotropes 553
Gout 153
Gracilis muscle 196
Graffian follicle 595
Grave's disease 479, 568
Great auricular nerve 246, 299, 300
Great cerebral vein of galen 433
Great saphenous vein 438
Greater occipital nerve 299
Greater omentum 68
Greater petrosal nerve 275
Greater sac 66
Greater vestibular glands 572
Grey matter 209
Growth hormone 554
Gynaecoid pelvis 137, 138

H

Habenular commissure 219
Habenular nuclei 222
Haemoglobin 454, 461
Haemolysis 455
Haemolytic anemia 479
Haemothorax 391

Hairs 603
Hammer toe 154
Hamstring muscles 198
Hand 76, 81
Hard palate 489
H-band 159
Hearing and equilibrium 333
Heart 394
Heart sounds 406
Helix 334
Hematoxylin stain 43
Hemiazygos vein 435
Hemidesmosomes 22
Hemiplegia 318
Hemoglobinopathies 461
Hemophilia A 462
Hemopoesis 454
Heparin 462
Hepatic circulation 446
Hepatic lobule 516
Hepatorenal pouch or Morrison's
    pouch 67
Hering-Breuer reflexes 387
Hesselbach triangle 96
Heterochromatin 21
Hiatus rectalis 180
Hiatus urogenitalis 180
Hiccup 389
Hinge joint 140
Hip 88
Hip bone 130, 146, 147
Hippocampal commissure 219
Hippocampus formation 225
Histological techniques 43
Histology 10, 43
Histone proteins 609
HIV 480
Holocrine gland 29
Homeostasis 49
Hormones 551
Horner's syndrome 319
Humerus 126
Humoral immunity 476
Hunter's canal 87
Hyaline cartilage 34
Hyaline membrane disease 391
Hydrothorax 391
Hymen 572, 576
Hyoepiglottic ligament 364
Hyoglossus muscle 486
Hyoid bone 117
Hyperaldosteronism 570
Hypermetropia 348
Hyperparathyroidism 570
Hyperprolactinemia 567
Hypersensitivity reaction 479
Hypertension 452
Hyperthyroidism 568
Hypogastric region 634
Hypogeusia 350

Hypoglossal nerve 282, 487
Hypoglycemia 569
Hyponychium 605
Hypoparathyroidism 570
Hypophysis cerebri 552, 566
Hypoplastic anemia 460
Hyposmia 350
Hypotension 452
Hypothalamus 220, 222, 556
Hypothyroidism 568
Hypoxia 392

I

I-band 159
IgA 477
IgD 477
IgE 477
IgG 477
IgM 477
Ileum 500
Iliac crest 130
Iliacus muscle 179, 196
Ilio tibial tract 85
Ilioinguinal nerve 305
Ilium 130
Immunity 458, 475
Immunoglobulins (Ig) 477
Implanation 596
Incisors 484
Incus 338
Inferior 13
Inferior alveolar nerve 271
Inferior cerebral veins 433
Inferior epigastric artery 421
Inferior extensor retinaculum 91
Inferior gemellus muscle 198
Inferior gluteal nerve 251
Inferior meatus 355
Inferior mediastinum 59
Inferior mesenteric artery 422
Inferior mesenteric vein 437
Inferior nasal concha 355
Inferior nasal conchae 117
Inferior oblique muscle 325
Inferior oblique part 172
Inferior orbital fissure 325
Inferior peroneal retinaculum 92
Inferior petrosai sinus 211
Inferior radio-ulnar joint 141, 145
Inferior rectal nerve 251
Inferior rectus 325
Inferior sagittal sinus 209, 431
Inferior vena cava 427
Infertility or subfertility 600
Infraglottic compartment 366
Infrahyoid muscles 172
Infraorbital nerve 299
Infraspinatus muscle 78, 185
Infratemporal fossa 107

Infratrochlear nerve 269, 299
Ingestion 482
Inguinal canal 62
Inguinal ligament 61
Inguinal hernia   96
Inguinal lymph nodes 475
Innate immunity 475
Inspiratory capacity 381
Inspiratory reserve volume 381
Insular lobe 214
Insulin 560
Integumentary system 9
Interatrial septum 396
Intercalated disks 161
Intercostal arteries 378
Intercostal muscles 377
Intercostal nerves 255, 378
Intercostal spaces 377
Intercostal veins 378
Intercostobrachial nerve 300
Intermediate and medial femoral
    cutaneous nerves 304
Internal 13
Internal capsule 218, 219
Internal carotid artery 413
Internal ear 333, 339
Internal haemorrhoids 529
Internal iliac artery 424
Internal intercostal muscle 378
Internal jugular vein 430
Internal oblique muscle 61, 177
Internal thoracic artery 415
Interneurons 239
Interoceptors 292
Interosseous membrane 145
Interpeduncular fossa 228
Interphalangeal joint 146
Interstitial fluid 49
Interventricular septum 400
Intervertebral disc 139
Intestinal circulation 141, 446
Intorsion 326
Intracellular fluid 49
Intracranial dural venous
    sinuses 210, 431
Intramembranous or membranous
    ossification 40
Intramuscular injection 639
Intrauterine contraceptive devices 598
Intrinsic muscles of hand 83
Intrinsic muscles of the larynx 366
Introns 615
Inversion and eversion 151
Inversion of foot 16
Inversions 613
Investing layer of deep cervical fascia 51
Ionotropic drugs 407
Ipsilateral 14
Iris 328
Irregular bones 38

Irregular connective tissue 32
Irritant receptors in nose 343
Ischemic heart disease 452
Ischio femoral ligament 147
Ischio rectal fossa 72
Ischiocavernosus muscle 181
Ischium 130
Islets of Langerhans   519, 560
Isochromosomes 613
Isometric contraction 164
Isotonic contraction 164
Itching 298

J

Jacobson's cartilage 353
Jejunum 500, 501
Joints 138
Jugular pulse 406
Jugular venous pulse 632
Jugulo-digastric nodes 470
Jugulo-omohyoid node 470
Juxta glomerular apparatus 534
Juxta glomerular cells 534
Juxta-capillary receptor responses 387

K

Karyotyping 609
Kesselbach's plexus 389
Kidneys 531
Kinins (bradykinin) 443
Klinefelter's syndrome 612
Klumpke's paralysis 284
Knee joint 146, 148
Kocher's incision 529
Korotkoff sounds 441
Krause's end-bulbs 292
Kupffer's cells 516

L

Labia majora 572
Labia minora 572
Labour pains 597
Labrum 140
Lacrimal apparatus 322
Lacrimal bones 117
Lacrimal canaliculus 323
Lacrimal gland 322
Lacrimal nerve 267, 299
Lacrimal puncta 323
Lacrimal sac 323
Lacunar ligament 61
Lambda 104
Lambdoid suture 103
Large intestine 502, 511, 513
Laryngeal inlet 359, 365
Laryngopharynx 359, 496
Larynx 362

Lateral 13
Lateral atlanto-axial joints 153
Lateral corticospinal tract 309
Lateral crural compartment 90
Lateral cutaneous nerve of calf 305
Lateral cutaneous nerve of forearm 300
Lateral femoral cutaneous nerve 249, 304
Lateral geniculate body 222
Lateral longitudinal arch 94
Lateral medullary syndrome 244
Lateral pectoral nerve 249
Lateral pharyngeal space 54
Lateral plantar artery 426
Lateral plantar nerve 262, 306
Lateral pterygoid muscle 494
Lateral rectus muscle 325
Lateral root of median nerve 249
Lateral rotation 15
Lateral spinothalamic tract 240, 293
Lateral ventricles 213
Lateral wall of the nasal cavity 354
Latissimus dorsi muscle 78, 185
Law of independent assortment 616
Law of projection 292
Left atrium 398
Left coronary artery 400
Left hypochondrium 634
Left iliac fossa 634
Left lumbar region 634
Left ventricle 399
Leg 89
Lens 329
Lentiform nucleus 219
Leptotene 26
Lesser occipital nerve 246, 299
Lesser sac 66, 70
Lesser omentum 67
Leucocytes 456
Leucopoesis 457
Leuteinizing hormone (LH) 554
Levator anguli oris muscle 168
Levator ani muscle 179
Levator labii superioris alaeque
    nasi muscle 168
Levator labii superoris muscle 168
Levator palpebrae superioris
    muscle 168, 326
Levator scapulae muscle 78, 185
LH 554
Lienorenal ligament 70, 467
Ligamentum nuchae 57, 174
Light adaptation 331
Light microscope 44
Limbic lobe 214
Limbic system 224
Linea alba 64
Lingual nerve 271, 487
Lingual papillae 483
Lingual thyroid 527
Lingual tonsil 472

Lips 483
Lithotomy position 12
Littre's hernial 96
Liver 514
Locking of knee joint 149
Long bones 37
Long ciliary nerves 269
Long thoracic nerve 249
Longus capitis muscle 172
Longus colli muscle 172
Loop of henle 534
Loose areolar connective tissue 32
Lower subscapular nerve 249
Lower lateral cutaneous nerve of arm 300
Lower limb 84
Lower subscapular nerve 249
Lumbar plexus 246, 249
Lumbar spinal nerves 246
Lumbar vertebrae 120
Lumbo-sacral trunk 249
Lumbricals 192
Lung 370, 374
Lung compliance 382
Lung volume 381
Lymph 464
Lymph capillaries 464
Lymph node 466
Lymphatic blockade 452
Lymphatic circulation 442
Lymphatic system 463
Lymphocytes 457
Lymphocytosis 457
Lymphoid tissue 465
Lymphopenia 457
Lyon's hypothesis 616
Lysosomes 21

M

M phase 23
Mackenrodt's ligaments 574
Macrophages 32
Macula adherens 22
Macula densa cells 535
Macula lutea 347
Major duodenal papilla 501
Male gemete 593
Male reproductive system 583
Male urethra 540
Malleus 338
Mammary gland 77, 581
Mammotropes 553
Mandible 113
Mandibular nerve 270
Manubrium 122
Marginal artery of Drummond 423
Marginal mandibular branch 275
Masseter muscle 494
Masseteric nerve 271
Mast cells 32

Masticatory mucosa 483
Mastoid fontanelles 113
Mastoid nodes 471
Matrix 32, 605
Maxillary air sinuses 357
Maxillary artery 412
Maxillary nerve 269
Maxillary sinus 357
Mc Burney's point 529, 633
Mechanism of respiration 380
Mechanoreceptors 292
Medial 13
Medial cutaneous nerve of arm 249, 300
Medial cutaneous nerve of forearm 249, 300
Medial geniculate body 222
Medial longitudinal arch 94
Medial pectoral nerve 249
Medial plantar artery 426
Medial plantar nerve 262, 306
Medial pterygoid muscle 494
Medial rectus muscle 325
Medial root of median nerve 249
Medial rotation 15
Median antebrachial vein 434
Median cubital vein 434
Median nerve 253
Mediastinal pleura 375
Mediastinum 59
Medulla oblongata 230
Medullary respiratory centre 386
Megaloblastic anemia 530
Meibomian glands 322
Meiosis 24
Meissner's corpuscles 292
Meissner's plexus 512
Melanocytes 601
Membranous labyrinth 340
Membranous part of urethra 540
Meninges 209
Menopause 581
Menstrual cycle 580
Menstrual phase 581
Mental point 105
Mentalis muscle 168
Merkel's discs 292
Merocrine glands 29
Mesangial cells or Lacis cells 535
Mesencephalon 203
Mesenchymal stem cells 31
Mesentery 68
Metabolic acidosis 549
Metabolic alkalosis 550
Metabolism 523
Metacarpals 129
Metacarpo phalangeal joints 141, 146
Metacentric 610
Metaphase 24
Metaphyseal arteries 39
Metaphysis 38

Metatarsals 135
Metatarso-phalangeal joints 147
Metathalamus 220, 222
Methylene blue 43
Metopic suture 103
Microdeletion 613
Microglia 209
Microvilli 22
Micturition 546
Mid palmar space 83
Midbrain 226
Middle cervical ganglion 313
Middle concha 355
Middle cranial fossa 110
Middle ear 333, 337
Middle meatus 355
Middle mediastinum 60
Middle meningeal artery 413
Middle superior alveolar nerve 269
Middle tibiofibular joint 146
Midsagittal or median plane 12
Mineralocorticoids 563
Minerals 526
Mitochondria 20
Mitosis 23
M-line 160
Modes of inheritance 616
Molars 485
Molecular basis of genetics 614
Moll'glands 322
Monocular compound light microscope 44
Monocytes 457
Monoplegia 318
Monosomy 612
Monosynaptic reflexes 310
Mons pubis 571
Morula stage 595
Mosaicism 612
Motilin 522
Motion sickness 350
Motor cortex 306
Motor pathway 307
Motor unit 164
Motor-end plate 209
MRI or magnetic resonance imaging 624
Mucoid tissue 32
Mucosa 42
Mucus glands 31
Multicellular glands 30
Multifidus muscle 175
Multipennate muscle 158
Mumps 528
Murmurs 449
Muscles of facial expression 167
Muscles of hand 190
Muscles of larynx 366
Muscles of mastication 494
Muscles of the orbit 325
Muscles of the tongue 486

Muscular system 5
Muscular tissue 42, 157
Muscular triangle 56
Musculocutaneous nerve 249, 251
Myasthenia gravis 242
Myelin sheath 205
Myenteric plexus of Auerbach 508, 512
Mylohyoid muscle 171
Myocardial circulation 401
Myocardial infarction 450
Myopia 348
Myringotomy 349

N

Na⁺ reabsorption 542
Nails 604
Naked pleura 390
Nasal bones 117
Nasal cavity 353
Nasal septum 353
Nasalis muscle 168
Nasion 105
Nasociliary nerve 269
Nasolacrimal duct 323
Nasopharynx 359, 496
Navicular bone 135
Navicular fossa 540
Near vision reflex pathway 333
Neck 51
Neocerebellum 235
Nephron 534
Nerve 207
Nerve excitation 206
Nerve fiber 207
Nerve injury 242
Nerve supply of the heart 402
Nerve to obturator internus 251
Nerve to piriformis 251
Nerve to quadratus femoris 251
Nerve to subclavius 249
Nerve trunk 207
Nervi erigentes 314
Nervous spinosus 271
Nervous system 5, 203
Nervous tissue 42
Neuromuscular junction 208
Neuron 204
Neutropenia 456
Neutrophils 456
Newborn skull 112
Night blindness 348
Nipple 582
Nissl bodies 204
Nitrogen balance 525
Nociceptors 292
Non-striated or involuntary muscle 161
Norma basalis 107
Norma frontalis 104
Norma lateralis 105

Norma occipitalis 103
Norma verticalis 103
Northern blot technique 618
Nose 352
Nostrils 352
Nuclear bag fibers 310
Nuclear chain fibers 310
Nuclear envelope 21
Nuclear sap 22
Nucleolus 22
Nucleosomes 609
Nucleus 21
Nucleus ambiguus 279
Nucleus dentatus 236
Nucleus dorsalis 239
Nucleus emboliformis 236
Nucleus fastigii 236
Nucleus globosus 236
Nutrient artery 39
Nutrition 523, 526

O

O₂ debt 164
Obturator externus muscle 88
Obturator foramen 132
Obturator internus muscle 197, 179
Obturator nerve 249, 258, 305
Occipital artery 411
Occipital bone 116
Occipital lobe 214
Occipital nodes 471
Occipital sinus 210, 431
Occipital triangle 56
Occipitofrontalis muscle 50, 166
Oculomotor nerve 264
Odontoid process 119
Olecranon process 128
Olfactory bulb 225
Olfactory cortex 225
Olfactory epithelium 342
Olfactory nerves 225, 263
Olfactory pathway 224, 343
Oligodendrogliocytes 209
Oliguria 548
Olivo-spinal tract 242
Omental bursa 70
Omohyoid muscle 172
Oogenesis 594
Ophthalmic artery 414
Ophthalmic nerve 267
Opioid analgesia 318
Opponens digiti minimi muscle 191
Opponens pollicis muscle 191
Opposition 16
Optic nerve 263
Oral cavity 482, 512
Oral mucosa 483
Orbicularis oculi muscle 167
Orbicularis oris muscle 168

Oropharynx 359, 496
Orthodromic conduction 206
Orthostatic hypotension 452
Osmotic diuresis 543
Ossification of bone 40
Osteoblasts 36
Osteoids 41
Osteomalacia 570
Osteomyelitis 153
Otic ganglion 272
Otitis media 349
Oval window 338
Ovarian fossa 577
Ovaries 577
Oxidative phosphorylation 523
Oxyntic or parietal cells 508
Oxytocin 555

P

Pacemaker 165
Pachytene 26
Pacinian corpuscles 292
Packed cell volume 454
Pain sensation 298
Painful arch syndrome 154
Palate 489
Palatine bones 117
Palatine tonsils 472
Palato-glossal arch 359
Palatoglossal fold 490
Palatoglossus muscle 487
Palato-pharyngeal arch 359
Palatopharyngeal fold 490
Paleocerebellum 234
Palm of hand 81
Palmar 14
Palmar aponeurosis 82
Palmar cutaneous branch of median nerve 300
Palmar cutaneous branch of ulnar nerve 300
Palmar interossei 192
Palmar or volar aspect of hand 14
Palmaris brevis muscle 191
Palmaris longus muscle 188
Palpation of arteries in body 629
Pancreas 518, 519
Papillary muscles 397
Para-aortic lymph nodes 474
Paracrine glands 29
Paraffin 43
Paransal air sinuses 357
Paraplegia 318
Parasympathetic nervous system 204, 314
Parathormone 565
Parathyroid glands 565
Paravertebral muscles 172
Parietal bones 114

Parietal lobe 214
Parietal peritoneum 65
Parietal pleura 375
Parietomastoid suture 105
Parieto-squamosal suture 105
Parkinsonism 243
Parotid gland 490
Parotid/preauricular lymph nodes 471
Passavant's ridge 360
Passive diffusion 18, 543
Passive transport 18
Patella 133, 135
Payer's patches 469
Pectineus muscle 196
Pectoral region 77
Pectoralis major muscle 77, 183
Pectoralis minor muscle 77, 183
Pedigree chart 616
Pelvic cavity 135
Pelvic diaphragm 74, 179
Pelvic inlet 135
Pelvic outlet 136
Pelvic splanchic nerve 251
Pelvimetry 136
Penile part of urethra 540
Penis 584
Pennate muscles 157
Peptic ulcer 528
Percutaneous ultrasound guided fetal
    blood samplin 618
Percutaneous ultrasound guided fetal
    skin biopsy 618
Pericardial effusion 407
Pericardium 393
Perikaryon 204
Perimysium 159
Perineal body 71
Perineal branch of S$_4$ nerve 251
Perineal membrane 73
Perineal nerve 251
Perinephric fat 532
Perineum 71
Periodontal membrane 484
Periosteal arteries 39
Periosteal bud 41
Periosteum 40
Peripheral 13
Peripheral nerves 246
Peripheral nervous system 203
Peristalsis 512
Peritoneal cavity 66
Peritoneal folds 66
Peritoneum 65
Peroneal artery 426
Peroneus brevis muscle 90, 200
Peroneus longus muscle 90, 200
Peroneus tertius muscle 89, 199
Peroxisomes 21
Pes cavus 154
Peyer's patches 511

Phaeochromocytoma 569
Phagosomes 21
Phalanges 130
Pharyngeal tonsils 472
Pharyngotympanic tube 359, 362, 496, 497
Pharynx 358, 495
Phase contrast microscope 44
Photoreceptors 292
Phrenic nerve 246, 247
Phsyiology of exercise 448
Physical anthropology 10
Physiology of exercise 389
Physiology of eye 330
Physiology of growth 555
Physiology of muscle 163
Physiology of nerve cell 205
Pia mater 209
Piles 529
Pilosebaceous unit 603
Pineal body 222, 556
Pinna 334, 335
Pinocytosis 20
Piriform fossa 359, 496
Piriformis muscle 179, 197
Piston movement 381
Pituitary gland 552, 556
Pivot joint 140
Plane synovial joint 140
Plantar aspect 14
Plantar aponeurosis 92
Plantar arterial arch 427
Plantar aspect of foot 14
Plantar interossei 202
Plantaris muscle 90, 201
Plasma 49, 459
Plasma cells 32
Plasma proteins 459
Platelets 458
Pleura 375
Plica fimbriate 486
Pneumatic bones 38
Pneumotaxic centre 386
Pneumothorax 390
Polyaxial joints 140
Polycystic kidney 547
Polycythemia 462
Polyploidy 611, 612
Polysynaptic reflex 310
Polyuria 548
Pons 229
Popliteal artery 426
Popliteal fossa 88
Popliteus muscle 90, 201
Porta hepatis 514
Portal circulation 451
Portal triads 517
Portal vein 436
Portocaval anastomosis 437
Post auricular lymph nodes 470
Postaxial border 14

Posterior 13
Posterior abdominal wall 64
Posterior auricular artery 412
Posterior auricular nerve 275
Posterior commissure 219
Posterior cranial fossa 110
Posterior cutaneous nerve of arm 300
Posterior cutaneous nerve of forearm 300
Posterior cutaneous nerve of thigh 251
Posterior ethmoidal nerve 269
Posterior femoral cutaneous nerve 305
Posterior fontanelle 113
Posterior interosseous nerve 255
Posterior mediastinum 60
Posterior spinocerebellar
    pathway 241, 296
Posterior tibial artery 426
Posterior triangle of neck 56
Postsynaptic membrane 207
Pouch of Douglas 69
Prader-Willi syndrome 614
Preaortic group of lymph nodes 474
Preauricular lymph nodes 470
Preaxial border 14
Precocious puberty 600
Prefrontal cortex 216
Preimplantation development 595
Premolars 485
Premotor area 215
Premotor cortex 306
Prenatal diagnosis 617
Presbyopia 349
Pressure epiphysis 38
Presynaptic membrane 207
Pretracheal fascia 53
Prevertebral fascia 53
Prevertebral muscles 173
Primary auditory area 217
Primary cartilaginous joint 139
Primary immune response 477
Primary motor area 214
Primary somesthetic area 216
Primary visual area 217
Procerus muscle 168
Profunda femoris artery 426
Progesterone 579
Projection fibres 217, 218
Prolactin 554
Prolapse of uterus 599
Promontory 338
Pronation 16, 145
Pronator quadratus muscle 188
Pronator teres muscle 188
Prone position 12
Prophase 23
Proprioceptors 292
Prosencephalon 203
Prostate 589
Protein and polypeptide hormones 551
Protein energy malnutrition 529

Proteinuria 549
Protrusion 16
Proximal 13
Proximal convoluted tubule 534
Pseudostratified epithelium 28
Psoas major muscle 178, 179, 196
Psychical cortex 217
Pterion 106, 153
Pterygopalatine fossa 107
Pterygopalatine ganglion 270
Ptosis 347
Puberty 592
Pubis 130
Pubo femoral ligament 147
Pubo-analis 180
Pubo-cervical ligaments 574
Pubo-vesicalis or vaginalis 180
Pudendal canal 72
Pudendal nerve 251
Pulp cavity 484
Pulp spaces 83
Pump handle movement 380
Pupillary light reflex pathway 332
Putamen 219
Pyelonephritis 548
Pyothorax 391
Pyramidal tract 307, 309
Pyramidalis muscle 177
Pyriform lobe 224

Q

Quadrangular membrane 364
Quadrants of abdomen 634
Quadrate lobe 514
Quadratus femoris muscle 198
Quadratus lumborum muscle 179

R

Radial 14
Radial artery 418
Radial border 14
Radial bursa 83
Radial nerve 249, 255
Radial notch 129
Radical mastectomy 452
Radiological anatomy 10, 621
Radio-ulnar joints 144
Radius 128
Recessive gene 615
Reciprocal translocation 613
Recto-vaginal fold 574
Rectum 504, 511
Rectus abdominis muscle 177
Rectus capitis anterior muscle 172
Rectus capitis lateralis muscle 172
Rectus femoris muscle 196
Rectus sheath 63
Recurrent laryngeal nerve 280
Red blood corpuscles 453
Referred pain 317

Reflex arc 310
Reflexes 309
Refractive error 348
Refractory period 206
Regional anatomy 4, 10
Regular connective tissue 32
Regulation of cardiovascular function 443
Regulation of respiration 386
Renal angle 547
Renal clearance tests 549
Renal corpuscle 534
Renal fascia 532
Renal sinus 533
Renal tubule 534
Renin: Angiotensin system 566
Reproductive system 8
Residual volume 381
Respiration 380
Respiratory acidosis 549
Respiratory alkalosis 549
Respiratory minute volume 382
Respiratory system 6, 351
Resting membrane potential 163, 206
Reticular fibres 32
Reticular formation 225, 317
Reticulo-spinal tract 242
Retina 328
Retraction 16
Retroauricular/mastoid nodes 471
Retrograde degeneration 242
Retromammary space 582
Retropharyngeal space 54
Rheumatic heart disease 449
Rheumatoid arthiritis 479
Rhombencephalon 203
Rhomboideus major muscle 78, 185
Rhomboideus minor muscle 78, 185
Ribs 123
Rickets 570
Right atrium 396
Right coronary artery 400
Right hypochondrium 634
Right iliac fossa 634
Right lumbar region 634
Right lymph duct 465
Right ventricle 397
Rigor 164
Rima glottidis 365
Rima vestibuli 365
Ring chromosome 613
Risorius 168
Robertsonian translocation 613
Rods 330
Root of the penis 584
Rostral spinocerebellar tract 297
Rotator cuff 142
Rotatores 175
Round ligaments 575
Rubrospinal tract 241
Ruffini's endings 292

S

S phase 23
Saccule 340
Sacral canal 122
Sacral plexus 251
Sacral spinal nerves 246
Sacrum 121
Saddle joint 140
Sagittal plane 12
Sagittal suture 103
Salivary glands 490, 512
Salpingopalatine fold 359
Salpingopharyngeal fold 359
Saltatory conduction 206
Saphenous nerve 257, 304
Saphenous opening 85
Sarcomere 161
Sarcoplasmic reticulum 161
Sarcotubular system 161
Sartorius muscle 196
Saturday night palsy 285
Scalenus anterior muscle 172
Scalenus medius muscle 172
Scalenus posterior muscle 172
Scalp 50
Scapula 127
Scapular region 78
Sciatic nerve 251, 258
Sciatica 286
Sclera 327
Scrotum 585
Sebaceous glands 604
Secondary active transport 19
Secondary cartilaginous joint 139
Secondary immune response 477
Secondary somesthetic area 217
Secretin 522
Secretory phase 581
Sella turcica 110
Semimembranosus muscle 199
Seminal vesicles muscle 588
Semispinalis muscle 175
Semitendinosus muscle 199
Sense organs 291
Sensory area 216
Sensory pathway 293
Sensory system 291
Serosa 42
Serous glands 31
Serous pericardium 393
Serratus anterior muscle 77, 183
Sesamoid bones 38
Sex chromatin 22
Sex-linked genes 615
Sex-linked inheritance 617
Shock 452
Short bones 37
Short ciliary nerves 266
Short saphenous vein 438
Shoulder girdle 143

Shoulder joint 142
Shoulder region 78
Shunt muscles 158
Sialorrhea 528
Sigmoid colon 504
Sigmoid mesocolon 68
Sigmoid sinus 211
Simple radiography 622
Sino-atrial node 403
Sinus of larynx 366
Sinus venosus 396
Sinusoids 516
Skeletal muscle 157, 162, 163
Skeletal system 4, 101
Skeleton 101
Skin 601
Skull 102
Small intestine 500, 508, 513
Smell 342
Smooth muscle 161, 162
Soft palate 490
Sole of foot 92, 202
Solenoid 609
Soleus 90, 200
Somatic nervous system 204
Somato sensory system 291
Somato motor system 306
Somatostatin 522
Somatotropes 553
Southern blot technique 618
Space of Parona 83
Special Senses   321
Sperm 593
Spermatic cord 586
Spermatogenesis 590
Spheno-ethmoidal recess 355
Sphenoid bone 116
Sphenoidal air sinuses 357
Sphenoidal fontanelles 113
Spheno-parietal sinus 211
Sphincter urethrae muscle 181
Spinal cord 237
Spinal ganglion 245
Spinal nerves 245
Spinal shock 548
Spinocerebellar pathway 296
Spinothalamic pathway 293
Spiral computed topography 623
Spiral organ of Corti 340
Splanchnic circulation 446
Spleen 467
Splenic vein 437
Splenius capitis muscle 175
Splenius cervicis muscle 175
Squint 347
Stapedius muscle 338
Stapes 338
Stellate ganglion 311, 313
Stereognosis 298
Steroid hormones 551

Sternoclavicular joint 141
Sternocleidomastoid muscle 170
Sternohyoid muscle 172
Sternothyroid muscle 172
Sternum 122
Stomach 498, 508, 513
Straight sinus 209, 431
Stratum basale 602
Stratum corneum 602
Stratum granulosum 602
Stratum lucidum 602
Stratum spinosum 602
Stretch reflex 310
Striate cortex 217
Student's elbow 155
Stye 347
Styloglossus muscle 487
Stylohyoid muscle 171
Styloid process 106
Subarachnoid cisternae 211
Subarachnoid space 209
Subclavian artery 414
Subclavian vein 429
Subclavius muscle 77, 183
Subcostal nerve 304
Subcostal plane 634
Subdural space 209
Sublingual salivary gland 493
Submandibular ganglion 271
Submandibular nodes 471
Submandibular salivary gland 492
Submental nodes 471
Submental triangle 55
Submetacentric 610
Suboccipital triangles 57
Subscapularis muscle 78, 185
Subsidiary ganglia 311
Substantia gelatinosa 239
Substantia nigra 227
Subtalar joint 146
Subthalamus 220, 222
Sulcus tubae 108
Superficial 14
Superficial branch of radial nerve 300
Superficial cervical nodes 471
Superficial fascia 42
Superficial inguinal lymph nodes 475
Superficial inguinal ring 62
Superficial middle cerebral vein 433
Superficial pain 298
Superficial palmar arch 420
Superficial perineal pouch 74
Superficial peroneal nerve 90, 305
Superficial temporal artery 412
Superficial transverse perinei
    muscle 181
Superficial perineal nerve 261
Superior 13
Superior cerebral veins 433
Superior cervical ganglion 313

Superior concha 355
Superior epigastric artery 421
Superior extensor retinaculum 91
Superior gemellus muscle 197
Superior gluteal nerve 251
Superior meatus 355
Superior mediastinum 59
Superior mesenteric artery 422
Superior mesenteric vein 422, 437
Superior oblique muscle 325
Superior orbital fissure 324
Superior peroneal retinaculum 91
Superior petrosal sinus 210, 211
Superior radioulnar joint 141, 145
Superior rectus muscle 325
Superior sagittal sinus 209, 431
Superior vena cava 427
Supination 16, 145
Supinator muscle 190
Supine position 12
Supplementory motor cortex 306
Supraclavicular nerve 246, 300
Supraclavicular space 52
Supraclavicular triangle 56
Suprahyoid muscles 171
Suprameatal triangle 105
Supraorbital nerve 267, 299
Suprapleural membrane or Sibson's
    fascia 58
Suprarenal glands 561
Suprascapular nerve 249
Supraspinatus muscle 78, 185
Suprasternal space 52
Supratrochlear nerve 267
Supratrochlear nerve 299
Sural nerve 305, 306
Surface anatomy 10
Surface anatomy of heart 632
Surfactant 383
Suspensory ligament of Treitz 501
Suspensory ligaments of Cooper 582
Sutures 138
Swallowing 316
Sweat glands 605
Sympathetic nervous system 204, 311
Symphysis menti 105
Synapse 207
Synaptic cleft 207
Synaptic knobs 205
Synarthroses 138
Syndesmosis 138
Synovial joint 139
Synovial sheath of flexor tendons 83
Systemic anatomy 4

T

Tachypnea 391
Talipes equinovarus 154
Talocalcaneonavicular joint 146

Tarsometatarsal joints 146
Taste 344
Taste buds 486
Tectospinal tract 241
Tectum 227
Teeth 483
Tegmen tympani 108
Tegmentum 227
Tela choroidea 211
Telereceptors 292
Telophase 24
Temporal bones 114
Temporal fossa 106
Temporal lobe 214
Temporalis muscle 494
Temporomandibular joint 151
Tendocalcaneus 201
Tennis elbow 155
Tenon's capsule 327
Tensor fascia lata 196
Tensor tympani muscle 338
Tentorium cerebelli 210
Teres major muscle 78, 185
Teres minor muscle 78, 185
Terminal ventricle 213
Testes 586
Testicular feminization 600
Testosterone 590
Tetanus 164
Tetraploidy 613
Thalamus 220, 297
Thalassemias 461
Thenar space 83
Thermoreceptors 292
Thigh 85
Third ventricle 213
Thomson's ligament 61
Thoracic cage 58, 122, 376
Thoracic cavity 58
Thoracic duct 464
Thoracic inlet 58
Thoracic outlet 58
Thoracic spinal nerves 246, 304
Thoracic vertebrae 120
Thoraco-dorsal nerve 249
Thorax 58
Thoroughfare vessels 440
Threshold potential 206
Thrombocytopenia 462
Thrombosis 462
Thymus 468, 559
Thyrocervical trunk 415
Thyroepiglottic ligament 364
Thyrohyoid muscle 172
Thyrohyoid membrane 364
Thyroid cartilage 363
Thyroid gland 556
Thyrotoxicosis 568
Thyrotropes 553
Tibia 133

Tibial border 14
Tibial nerve 259, 306
Tibialis anterior muscle 89, 199
Tibialis posterior muscle 91, 201
Tibiofibular joints 147
Tidal volume 381
Toludine blue 43
Tomography 623
Tongue 485
Tongue tie 527
Tonsil 359, 496
Tonsillar fossa 359
Tonsillectomy 479
Tourniquet test 451
Trabecular bones 36
Trachea 368
Tract cells 239
Traction epiphysis 38
Tracts of spinal cord 239
Tragus 335
Transfusion reaction 456
Transitional epithelium 28
Translocation 613
Transport across cell membrane 18
Transpyloric plane 634
Transtubercular plane 634
Transverse cervical nerve 246
Transverse colon 503
Transverse cutaneous nerve of neck 300
Transverse mesocolon 68
Transverse planes 13
Transverse sinus 210
Transversus abdominis muscle 61, 177
Trapezius muscle 78, 185
Triceps brachii muscle 80, 187
Trigeminal nerve 267, 299
Trigone 539
Triploidy 612
Trisomy 13, 18, 21, 612
Trochlear nerve 266
Trochlear notch 129
Trousseau's sign 570
True pelvis 135
True ribs 123
True vocal cords 365
TSH 554
Tubal occlusion 599
Tubal tonsils 472
Tubectomy 599
Tunica albuginea 587
Tunica vaginalis 587
Tunica vasculosa 587
Two point discrimination 298
Tympanic cavity 337
Tympanic membrane 336

U

Ulna 128
Ulnar artery 418
Ulnar border 14
Ulnar bursa 83
Ulnar nerve 249, 252
Ulnar paradox 285
Ultrasound 618, 624
Umbilical region 634
Umblicius 64
Unicellular glands 29
Unipennate muscle 157
Unlocking 150
Upper back 78
Upper lateral cutaneous nerve of arm 300
Upper limb 76
Upper subscapular nerves 249
Urea 525
Uremia 549
Ureters 536
Urethra 540
Uric acid 526
Urinary bladder 537
Urinary system 8, 531
Urine 541
Urogenital diaphragm 74
Urogenital triangle 73
Uuterine tubes 575
Utero-sacral ligaments 574
Utero-vesical fold 574
Uterus 572
Utricle 340
Uveal tract 327

V

Vagina 576
Vaginal orifice 572
Vagus nerve 277
Varicocele 600
Varicose veins 451
Vas deferens 588
Vasectomy 599
Vasomotor centre 444
Vastus intermedius 196
Vastus lateralis muscle 196
Vastus medialis muscle 196
Venous circulation 442
Ventilation 383
Ventral 13
Ventral ramus 246
Ventral root 245
Ventricular arrythmias 450
Ventricular system 213
Ventricular systole 405
Venules 440
Vertebra 118
Vertebral artery 414

Vertebral column 101, 117
Vertebrochondral ribs 123
Vertex 103
Vertigo 350
Vestibular area 217
Vestibular folds 365
Vestibular ligaments 365
Vestibular pathway 342
Vestibule of ear 339
Vestibule of mouth 366
Vestibule 482
Vestibulo-cochlear nerve 275
Vestibulo-spinal tract 241
Video-radiography 623
Vincula longa and brevia 83
VIP (vaso-intestinal peptide) 522
Visceral peritoneum 65
Visceral pleura 375
Vision 321
Visual acuity 331
Visual fields 332
Visual pathway 264, 331
Visual receptors 330
Vital capacity 381
Vitamin D 565
Vitamins 526

Vocal folds (cords) 365
Vocal ligaments 364
Vomer 117
Vomiting 316
VSD or ventricular septal defect 449
Vulva 571

W

Waldeyer's lymphatic ring 472
Wallerian degeneration 242
Warfarin 462
Water diuresis 543
Watershed line 97
Western blot technique 618
Wharton's duct 492
White blood cells 456
White fibro-cartilage 36
White matter 209
White rami communicantes 246
Wilson's disease 243
Withdrawl reflex 310
Wrinkles 606
Wrist 141
Wrist drop 285
Wrist joint 145

X

Xeroradiography 623
Xerostomia 528
Xiphoid process 123
X-linked recessive inheritance 617
X-ray techniques 621

Y

Yawning 389

Z

Zies glands 322
Z-line 160
Zona fasciculata 562
Zona glomerulosa 562
Zona reticularis 562
Zonula adherens 22
Zonula occludens 22
Zygomatic bone 115
Zygomatic nerve 269
Zygomaticus major muscle 168
Zygomaticus minor muscle 168
Zygotene 26